MDR
MASSAGE DESK REFERENCE
your guide to complete knowledge

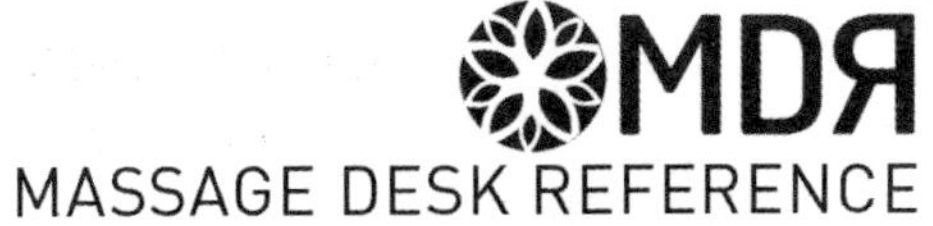

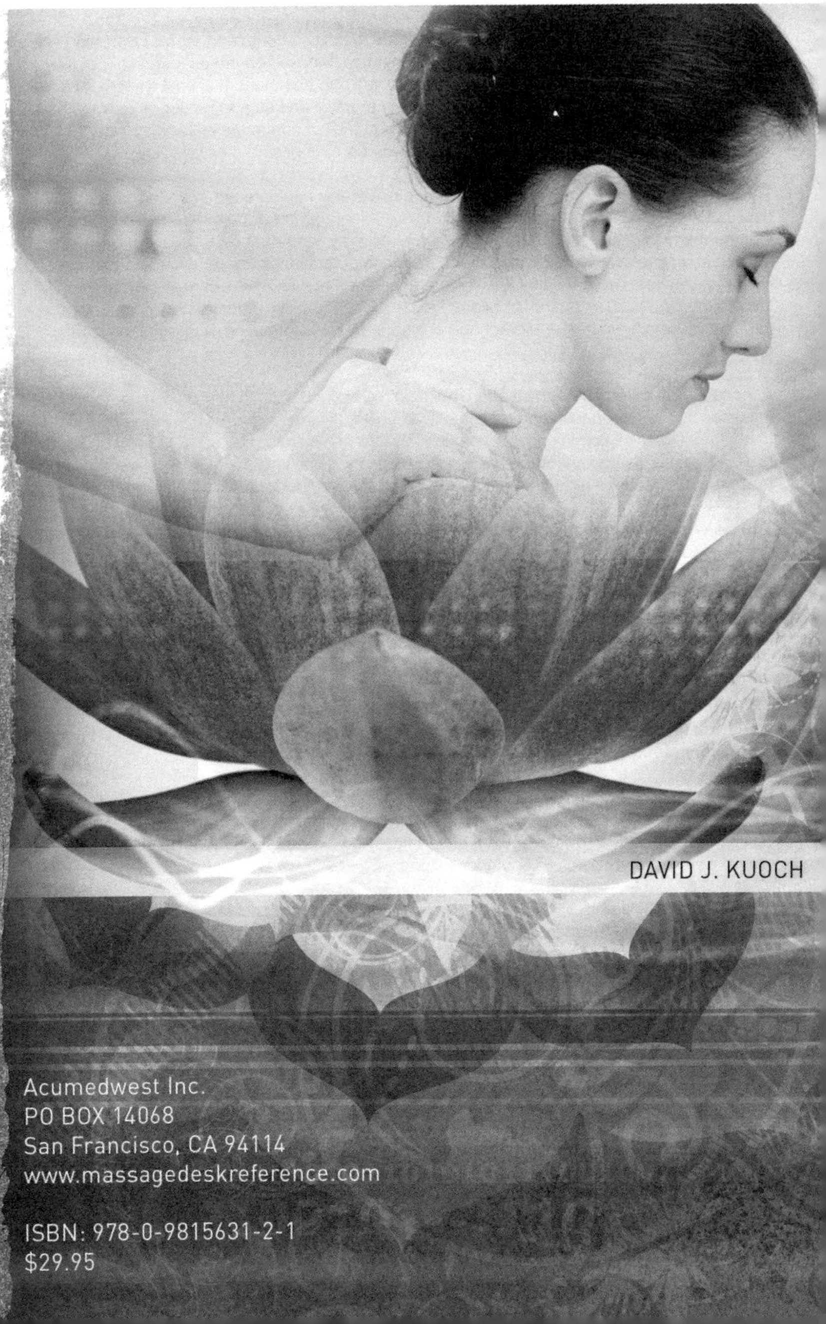

DAVID J. KUOCH

Acumedwest Inc.
PO BOX 14068
San Francisco, CA 94114
www.massagedeskreference.com

ISBN: 978-0-9815631-2-1
$29.95

Massage Desk Reference
by David J. Kuoch

Acumedwest Inc.

Disclaimer: This book is intended as a quick-reference volume for educational purposes only and not as medical information. It is designed to help students and professionals in the massage field make informed decisions about health based on the assumption that the reader has thorough training in massage procedures and treatment. It is best treated as a supplemental source for information used in daily practice and as a reminder of knowledge gained elsewhere. The information in this book is compiled from reliable sources, and exhaustive efforts have been put forth to make the book as accurate as possible.

The ideas, procedures, and suggestions contained in this book are not intended as a substitute for consulting with your physician. Health care professionals should use sound judgment and individualized therapy for each specific patient/client care situation. If you suspect that you have a medical problem, seek competent medical help. Neither the author nor the publisher shall have any liability to any person or entity with regard to claims, loss, injury, or damage caused, or alleged to be caused, directly or indirectly by the use of information contained herein, or damage arising from any information or suggestion in this book.

Although great care has been taken to maintain the accuracy of the information contained in this book, the information as presented in this book is for educational purposes only. We cannot anticipate all conditions under which this information might be used. In view of ongoing research, changes in governmental regulation, and the constant flow of information relating to massage, the reader is urged to check with other sources for all up-to-date information.

The staff and authors of Acumedwest Inc. recognize that practitioners accessing this content will have varying levels of training and expertise; therefore, we accept no responsibility for the results obtained by the application of the material within this book. Neither Acumedwest Inc. nor the authors of Massage Desk Reference can be held responsible for human, electronic or mechanical errors of fact or omission, nor for any consequences arising from the use or misuse of the information herein.

The statements in this book have not been evaluated by the Food and Drug Administration. These products are not intended to diagnose, treat, cure or prevent any disease and they are not intended to replace the diagnosis, treatments, prescriptions and services of a trained practitioner or physician.

Acumedwest Inc. is a division of Retired Hipster Inc.

Published by Acumedwest Inc.
PO Box 14068
San Francisco, CA 94114
Tel: 310-395-9573
www.massagedeskreference.com

Library of Congress Control Number: 2010900267
ISBN 978-0-9815631-2-1

Printed in China

"Live with intention. Walk to the edge. Listen hard. Practice wellness. Play with abandon. Laugh. Choose with no regret. Appreciate your friends. Continue to learn. Do what you love. Live as if this is all there is." ~ Mary Anne Radmacher

Purpose of the Book

Massage Desk Reference is a quick reference book for massage therapists and massage practitioners. This is not a medical book; rather, it is designed for educational purposes to help massage professionals make informed decisions on client care. This book is a collection of information assembled to help the practitioner become effective and successful in Massage practice. The authors assume the reader has familiarity with massage procedures and treatments, as well as cautions and contraindications of massage. This text is best used as a supplemental source for information used in daily practice and as a reminder of knowledge and information learned elsewhere. As a massage therapist, massage technician, and health care provider, I wrote this book primarily for the licensed practitioner.

To the practitioner who wants to discriminate between massage techniques and systems, clinical practice, Western medicine, office procedure, and alternative remedies, Massage Desk Reference is "user friendly." After years of compiling the information from multiple sources and organizing it in a database, I am able to offer a reference book with easily accessible tables that has integrated both the massage classics and Western methodology.

How the Book Came About

I started working on Massage Desk Reference after completing Acupuncture Desk Reference. I found it cumbersome to need different texts for the variety of different subjects that massage encompasses. It became an exhausting task seeking out information on a variety of massage modalities and organizing them into one place. As a student, I quickly became overwhelmed by the amount of information we needed to know in each area involved in becoming a good practitioner. I started compiling the information into a database to help organize what I thought would be pertinent in my practice at a later date.

As my computer database grew, so did the sources of information and volumes of books that I had begun to collect. By the time I graduated from massage school and acupuncture school, the volumes of information grew to nearly 100 massage and Western books. Some of these books represent the core of massage and Western medicine, while others are more obscure in content but still contain invaluable information. As you can imagine, in clinical practice, looking up the information while treating clients at the same time became a difficult task. I needed a way to refresh my memory on the options for treatment. Eventually, I created one cohesive resource from which I could access both massage and Western medical theory without pulling several books off the shelf every time.

My approach was integrative in theory, but in clinical practice the Western medicine was used sparingly and strictly adhered to massage principles. While it is outside our scope of practice to diagnose, the information in this book will be useful in daily practice. As health care providers, I felt that we have an obligation to educate our clients, whether massage, Western, or alternative, offering our clients healthcare options. If we needed to do orthopaedic tests, recall a cranial nerve test, look for signs of cancer, or identify a vitamin for a common ailment, this information could be integrated with the appropriate manual therapy, technique and treatment procedures for our clients/patients.

Format of Massage Desk Reference

In practice, a massage therapist already knows the information. He/she needs something to refresh his/her memory having gone through extensive training and practice with the hundreds and thousands of hours of massage. Many therapists, technicians, and practitioners have books and notes on the varying modalities but rarely open them unless they need to confirm what they have already read in their medical text in massage schools or in CEUs. We have many great massage reference books but need to condense the information and develop a practitioner's guide that can fit in the palm of the hand, which a practitioner can reference with ease: a comprehensive and usable handbook that includes massage techniques, clinical practice, useful reference and Western methodology. Thus began the development of Massage Desk Reference.

The comments I have received from my colleagues during the peer review are invaluable. I realize that this book could have been organized in a different manner: certain techniques, therapies, and massage basics were not included because of space limitations.

This is by no means a book lengthy in explanation, but instead, a handbook with material that can be easily referenced. Tables and brevity of content seem the most logical way of disseminating the information without overwhelming the reader. Some readers may enjoy the format and some may find the text too brief or requiring further explanation. It assumes that most of the information is common knowledge to the massage practitioner. For those who require more information, I have included a section towards the back of the book, "Resources," which will direct the reader to a detailed explanation of the subject at hand. I encourage you to build your library for those times when you need to reference what you already know and treat your patients/clients with confidence.

Please be advised: If you are an unlicensed practitioner or anyone without the proper training in massage therapy, the ideas, procedures, and suggestions contained in this book are not intended as a substitute for consulting with your healthcare professional.

Acknowledgement

I would like to express my gratitude to my friends and family, colleagues, and associates for the support and encouragement. A special thank you to Amy Gayheart Kuoch, for your love, light, patience and wisdom to guide me through the process. Without her encouragement, this book would not have been produced. Thank you to Rebecca Smith and Cory Bilicko, co-editors extraordinaire for the many generous hours, eagle eyes, and organization skills. Thank you to Chrissy Biro and Ariel F. Hubbard for their contributions with the peer reviews and tremendous input on the chapters. Thank you to Andrew Moulton for your enormous contribution to MDR and ADR. Thank you to David Pfister for his hard work in organizing the information and for the layout design. Thank you to Emily Burt, Gabe McIntosh, and Chris Tsuda for the incredible line drawings and concise illustrations. Thank you to my mom Lily for showing me how smart work pays off.

I would also like to thank all teachers, students, patients/clients, and associates for their valuable suggestions with this book. To everyone who continues to support and promote massage in this world, we are most grateful to all of you. Massage Desk Reference is dedicated to the promotion of professionalism and clinical excellence in massage therapy.

Thank you for your contribution

Amy Flanders, LMT
Amy D. Gayheart
Andrew Moulton, MD
Anthony O'Neill
Alejandro Morin, CMT
Ariel F. Hubbard, HHP
Brianna Noach, LAc, LMP
Carol Block, MD
Chris Tsuda
Claus Bigos, LMT
Conrad Santos
Cory Bilicko
Dane Sonnier
Daniel Herlihy, LMT, DO
Daniel Reid, MD
David Fedman
David Murray, MD
Deborah Weidhaas
Don Lee, LAc, QME
Douglas Andersen, DC
Elaine Pendergrast
Elizabeth Jacobs, LMT
Emily Burt
Erik Weissman, LMT
Fred Lerner, DC
Gabe McIntosh
Gustaf LaValle, MD
Heather Bree
Higgins Gayheart
Jean'e Freeman, LMT, RMT
Julie McGuiness
Kate McGregor, LMT
KC Chambers, LMT
Linda Morse, LAc
Linda Rikli
Manda Sherwood, LMT
Mark Durham
Martin Buitrago, MD
Michele Tilton, LMT
Michele T. Nowak-Sharkey
Mick Brackle, LAc
Mitchell D. Sonnier
Nick Scott
Patricia Saunders, LMT
Pete Whitridge, LMT
Rebecca Smith
Rene R. Bonetti
Rene Hicks, LMBT
Robert Amyes, LMT
Robert Berger, MD
Rory Aptekar
Ruth Black, PhD
Sandi Gayheart
Senika Hatfield, LAc
Stephanie Rush, LMT
Tanya Burke, LMT
Toni M. Milburn
Teri Polley-Michea MA, RN
Trina Cunningham, CMT
Vajra Matusow

Thank you for your contribution

Arizona School of Massage Therapy
ATI Career Training Center
Bastyr University
California Academy for the Healing Arts
Colorado Institute of Massage Therapy
Cortiva Institute
Center for Therapeutic Massage
Diamond Light School of Massage
Emperors College of Traditional Oriental Medicine
Esalen Institute
Everest College
Florida School of Massage
International Professional School of Bodywork
Lauterstein-Conway Massage School
Massage School of Santa Monica
Massage Connection - School of Natural Healing
Massage Therapy Institute of Colorado
Midline Massage and Bodywork
National Holistic Institute
National Massage Therapy Institute
Natural Touch School of Massage Therapy
Peninsula College
Ojai School of Massage
Swedish Institute
The Breema Center

This book belongs to: ....

If found please call: ....

TABLE OF CONTENTS

Table of Abbreviations

+ve	Positive
-ve	Negative
1/12	1 month. Similarly 2/12 means 2 months, 3/12 means 3 months, etc
1/24	1 hour. Similarly 2/24 means 2 hours, 3/24 means 3 hours, etc
1/52	1 week. Similarly 2/52 means 2 weeks, 3/52 means 3 weeks, etc
1/7	1 day. Similarly 2/7 means 2 days, 3/7 means 3 days, etc
a c	Before meals
A M A	Against medical advice
ad.	Freely as wanted
alt. die	Every other day
alt. h.	Every other hour
aq.	Water
aurist.	Ear drops
B M E	Bi-Manual Examination, i.e. A vaginal examination
B N O	Bowels not open - will be followed by a time span, e.g. B N O 4 days
B P	Blood pressure
b.d. or bd	Twice a day
b.i.d. or bid	Twice a day
c	A lower case c, especially with a line above it, in a medical text means "with" A lower case c, without a line above it, in a medical text means about or approximately An upper case C usually means century
C N S	Central nervous system
C O or C/O	Complains of
C V S	Cardio vascular system
Ca	Cancer
D R E	Digital rectal examination
Dx	Diagnosis
Dxx	Differential diagnosis
ext.	External
F H	Family history
G or gtt.	Drop or drops
G (number)	This is used in relation to childbirth and pregnancy. A woman described as G2 is in her second pregnancy. G stands for Gravida and is often used with P (see P below)
H O	History of
H P C	History of Presenting Complaint
h.	Hour
h.s.	At bedtime
Hx	History
i.d.	During the day or the same
I.D.	Infectious disease
i.d.	Intradermal, between layers of the skin
int.	Internal
Ix	Investigations
mg	Milligram or milligram - a measure of weight
mmHg	Millimeters of mercury, a measure of pressure, usually blood pressure
N A D	No Abnormality Detected (cynics version is Not Actually Done)
N B I	No bone injury
Nocte	At night
O E	On examination
o m	Every morning
o n	Every night
O T C	Over The Counter, i.e. A remedy available without prescription
o.c. or occ	Eye ointment
o.d. or od	Daily (or once a day)
O/E	On examination
P (number)	This is used in relation to childbirth and pregnancy. A woman described as P2 has given birth to two live children
P C	Presenting complaint
p c	After meals (on a prescription)
P H	Personal history
P M H	Past medical history
p.m.	Afternoon
p.o. or po	Orally
p.r. or pr	Rectally
p.r.n. or p r n	As required
p.v.	Vaginally
q.	Every
q.2.h.	Every two hours
q.4.h.	Every four hours
q.6.h.	Every six hours
q.8.h.	Every eight hours
q.d. or qd	Every day
q.d.s. or q d s	Four times a day
q.h.	Every hour, hourly
q.i.d. or qid	Four times a day
q.q.h.	Every four hours
q.s.	A sufficient quantity
R O S	Review of Systems or Removal of Sutures (stitches)
R S	Respiratory system
Rx	Prescription
S H	Social history
s.i.d. or sid	Once a day
Sig. or S.	Write on the label
SL.	Sublingual, under the tongue
spec	Short for speculum and will usually mean a visual examination of the vagina and cervix
Stat.	Immediately, with no delay
T	The capital letter T, when followed by an anatomical location, can occasionally stand for tuberculosis
T P R	Temperature, Pulse and Respiratory rate
t.d.s.	Three times a day
t.i.d. or tid	Three times a day
top.	Topically, applied to the skin
Ung.	Ointment
ut dict. or u.d.	As directed
V E	Vaginal examination

Active Release Therapy (ART)

Active Release Therapy is a movement-oriented, soft-tissue massage method used to treat issues with muscles, tendons, ligaments, fascia, and nerves. It is a mixture of observation, examination and myofascial technique. It is most often utilized by chiropractors and body workers who perform subtle, painless manipulation. ART addresses muscular and soft-tissue difficulties that are brought on by the development of adhesive tissues laid down from overuse or trauma. These techniques are similar to what massage therapists call "anchor and stretch," "pin and stretch," and other names. The ART practitioner uses hands to evaluate the texture, tightness, and movement of muscles, fascia, tendons, ligaments, and nerves by using palpation and subtle manipulation.

Acupressure

Acupressure is a healing approach that uses physical pressure points on the surface of the skin to stimulate the body's natural means of curing itself. Its principles are similar to those of acupuncture and Traditional Chinese Medicine, and it works without use of the acupuncture needles to stimulate specific reflex points located along 14 meridians, the lines of energy which run throughout the body. Each meridian line relates to a different organ of the body. When the vital energies can flow through the meridians in a balanced and steady manner, the outcome is good health. Pain and illness are considered indications that there is a block or leak in the energy flow within the body – so local symptoms are deemed an expression of the condition of the body as a whole.

Pressing points on the meridian lines relieves muscle tension and increases circulation. Stimulation of points along these pathways and meridians encourages the body to release endorphins. Other effects may include the release of anti-inflammatory and euphoric substances, increased circulation and decreased inflammation (sometimes referred to as the movement of qi). Release of neurotransmitters, serotonin and prostaglandins may also be influenced by the stimulation of acupressure points.

Acupressure's goal is to restore health and balance the energy flow. It is used to treat the body, mind, emotions, energy field, and spirit. Acupressure is said to help with many diseases or ailments, such as back or muscle aches, constipation, cramps, ulcer pain, and sinus problems. It can ease stress and promote overall wellness. Self-acupressure can be an effective way of addressing various injuries and ailments and may be performed by just about anyone, anywhere.

Aromatherapy Massage

Aromatherapy has historically been used outside of traditional massage and has recently become an accepted way to relax and rejuvenate, along with the benefit of massage. Aromatherapy massage incorporates essential oils from plants in order to provide a desired effect on the client. Essential oils are taken from flowers, seeds, herbs, woods, and roots, whose aroma is believed to encourage healing. During massage, essential oils are combined with carrier oils, such as almond or grapeseed oil, and selected based on the needs of the client and the therapeutic properties of the oils.

Despite aromatherapy being a form of alternative medicine, since many oils have antimicrobial characteristics, some clinicians in the Western medical community have started using some of them to treat infectious disease. When inhaled into the lungs these aromatherapeutic oils can provide physiological assistance (as when inhaling eucalyptus for easing congestion). Applied directly to the skin in diluted form, they are absorbed into the bloodstream. Aromatherapy can be used for a wide array of ailments because there are many different essential oils that can be mixed to aid with anything from headache relief to constipation to stress relief.

Aromatherapeutic treatments are selected based on their healing properties and to tap into the client's memory. These can be smells that remind the client of a time when he or she felt happy, safe, relaxed, peaceful or energized. The combination of the essential oils and the sensation of touch can make a client feel relaxed, stimulated, peaceful or euphoric, depending on their desired emotional response. This combination can also provide stress relief and pain relief, aid a sleeping disorder or physical condition, or energize the mind, body and spirit.

Ayurvedic Massage
Ayurvedic massage is based on Ayurveda ("life knowledge" or "right living"), a system of health and medicine developed in India. Ayurveda believes that problems occur in the body as a result of imbalances among the three toxins or doshas: Vata (wind), Pitta (bile), and Kapha (mucus). These three doshas combine into five different elements of ether, air, fire, water, and earth. Balance of the tridoshas creates a balance of these elements within the body, which creates health. Often one or two of the doshas dominate within an individual's body. The doshas constantly interact with each other and with the doshas in the outside environment, so this balance is constantly changing.

There are about 100 marmas, or points, which exist that connect different parts of the Ayurveda system. Some diseases can be controlled by treating marmas points that stimulate and treat the internal organs. Most marmas points are found along junctions of muscle, ligaments, bones, joints, and blood vessels – similar to trigger points. These points form the Prana, or seat of vital life force. Within the Prana are seven centers called chakras. The chakras are located along the spinal column and link the human body to the rest of the universe. They are centers of consciousness that preside over not just the physical body but also the emotional body. Chakras are believed to have a subtle energy called kundalini, which is focused along the backbone (though it may be expressed externally such as at the navel, heart, or throat). According to Ayurveda, digestion is a cornerstone of health – both what a person physically eats and what he consumes from the spiritual world. Ayurveda treatments include purging the body, such as through vomiting, enemas, or sweating, and then being aware of what is next put into the body. Ayurvedic massage focuses on these chakras through tapping, kneading, rubbing, and squeezing. The use of specific oils is important for the balance of the system.

Breema
Breema is a comprehensive bodywork system that was developed in California in 1980 by Jon Schreiber and a small group of colleagues. Breema is an acronym that stands for: Being Right now, Everywhere, Every moment, Myself Actually. The system has three components: Breema bodywork, Self-Breema exercises, and the Nine Principles of Harmony. These principles are Body Comfortable, Full Participation, No Extra, No Force, No Judgment, Mutual Support, Single Moment/Single Activity, Gentleness & Firmness, and No Hurry/No Pause. The focus is on encouraging and creating health, rather than curing or treating sickness or disease. Breema bodywork does not assume that a problem exists; instead, it attempts to help an individual focus on the unity of mind, body, and feelings and to elevate the level of consciousness.

The bodywork is done on the floor, with a range of techniques from simple holding of points on the body to techniques requiring flexibility and dexterity. Sessions are performed with the recipient fully clothed, either sitting or lying on a padded floor. Breema practitioners use their own relaxed body weight (rather than muscular strength) to work with the client while doing supported movements, gentle bending and stretching, holding postures, and rhythmic tapping. Sessions may last from 30 to 60 minutes. During these sessions, both the practitioner and the recipient wish to remain comfortable as well as engaged and aware of their bodies. The focus of the movements is to gently move and stretch the body, without causing any strain or discomfort.

Self-Breema exercises are based on the same Nine Principles as Breema bodywork, and are performed on one's own body, to experience not only being the recipient but also being the practitioner. The Self-Breema exercises are devised to: bring a person in touch with his or her own natural body postures; support and balance the flow of energy throughout the body; release tension; and increase dexterity. Combining Breema bodywork and Self-Breema allows a person to reach a higher level of health through awareness of body, mind, and feelings. Because of Breema's focus on wellness and not just on healing sickness, even those who consider themselves to be healthy can benefit from it.

Craniosacral (Cranial-Sacral) Therapy
Craniosacral therapy is a non-invasive manipulation technique for discovering and correcting cerebral and spinal imbalances. It was first developed by Dr. William Sutherland in the early 1900s. Dr. Sutherland was an osteopath who disputed the idea that cranial sutures were not intended to move. In fact, he argued, the subtle motion of the cranial bones is actually interconnected with the subtle movements of the fluids and tissues at the core of the body. He explored the cranial-sacral system that consists of the skull, vertebrae, meninges, cerebrospinal fluid, and all the structures related to cerebrospinal fluid; he concluded that the body has an inherent life force, which he termed the "Breath of Life," that fuels the rhythms of the body. At least three rhythms have been identified as part of the "Breath of Life": the cranial rhythmic impulse, the mid-die, and the long tide. Unimpeded flow of these tides is health; craniosacral therapy asserts that health is something active and not just an absence of disease.

Craniosacral practitioners work with the articulations of the skull sutures and the flow of cerebrospinal fluid. They try to liberate the imbalances that may cause sensory, motor, or intellectual dysfunction. Stresses or traumas that are overpowering can get locked into the body as a site of inertia, which blocks the free flow of Breath of Life impulses and affects the body at a physical level. Physical injuries, emotional and psychological stresses, birth trauma, and toxicity are some stresses that can become locked as sites of inertia. These experiences or stresses can get "stuck" in the tissues and be re-experienced each time the tissue is stimulated.

A craniosacral session involves the practitioner "listening through the hands" to the body's rhythms, trying to discover any areas of blockage or inertia. He seeks to find the restrictions in the cerebrospinal fluid flow. Treatment consists of gentle pressure on bones and soft tissues from the head to the base of the spine to aid cerebrospinal fluid circulation. Sessions usually last for up to one hour. Since craniosacral therapy is so mild, it can be used on children, babies, the elderly, and those individuals who are fragile or sick. Treatment can help many conditions and, in general, it improves the body's capacity for self-repair. It may help to treat head traumas, headaches, sinus congestion, TMJ, and behavioral or neurological issues. It has also been used to help treat infants with respiratory or digestive disorders.

Circulatory Massage
Circulatory Massage assists the body's natural blood flow in order to create more efficient and healthy circulation. One of the main ways the cells of the body get nutrients/oxygen and release waste products is through the blood. Circulatory massage facilitates this process to create a higher level of health for the client. Blood is pumped out by the heart through the arteries, where it distributes oxygen and nutrients to cells. On its return to the heart through the veins, the blood carries waste products to the liver and kidneys to be processed, and carbon dioxide to the lungs to be released. The blood pressure in the arteries is controlled mainly by the heart rate. However, the blood in the veins is controlled mainly by valve mechanisms and skeletal muscle constriction. Therefore, the techniques for affecting these two different types of vessels are different.

Compression is used to improve arterial blood flow. It is applied over the main arteries and moves from the heart distally to the tips of the fingers and toes. Gentle contraction compressions at the pace of the client's resting heart rate encourage arterial blood flow by changing the internal pressure in the arteries, stimulating them to contract. Short stripping and gliding strokes help the venous blood in its movement from valve to valve. Passive and active joint movements, along with lifting the limbs above the heart to utilize the effects of gravity, can be used to stimulate venous circulation. Circulatory massage is used by those who are bedridden or relatively inactive.

Chair Massage
For centuries, people have been receiving massages in seated positions or in chairs. Today's chair massage is a brief bodywork session, usually a shiatsu-based routine, in a seated position in which the client sits in a specially designed chair while the neck, back, shoulders, arms and hips are all accessible to the therapist. Sessions may last between five and 30 minutes to accommodate the client's schedule, without the hassle of getting undressed for massage that is done on a table. Originally pioneered as "on-site massage" for the workplace, it has grown into many other environments. Chair massage is now offered in storefronts, health-food stores, airports, airplanes and health fairs. It has come to be called "chair massage" or "seated massage" instead of "on-site." Because of the relatively low cost of a brief session, it is more affordable than the usual full-body massage. Since it is done in places where the client is already present, it is more convenient than table massage.

Deep Tissue Massage
Deep tissue massage is used to reach the connective tissue (the deeper layer of muscles) under the superficial layer of fascia on the body to release chronic tension. Deep tissue massage uses higher pressure, slower strokes and concentrates on specific areas of the body in comparison to relaxation or Swedish massage techniques. Pressure is applied using the hands, fingers, knuckles, elbow, or forearm, and movement is slow and deliberate. Sometimes tools such as ceramic, glass, or wooden props may be used. Just a small amount of oil or lotion is used to decrease the chance of the therapist slipping off of the muscle. Rather than moving along the length of the muscle, deep tissue massage necessitates that the therapist work across the muscle. The slow movement and the warmth created from the pressure allow the therapist to reach below the overlying fascia to the deeper muscle tissue. Since the work is unhurried and focused, a deep tissue massage will not necessarily address every area of the body as a relaxation massage would.

Deep tissue massage is used by athletes or individuals whose jobs require them to do a lot of physical activity. It also can be beneficial on injuries or emotional trauma that may be kept in the physical body. After a deep tissue massage, it is not uncommon for a client to be sore or even bruised, although the session itself should not cause any pain.

Esalen Massage
Also known as the art of "conscious touch massage," Esalen massage was first developed more than 40 years ago in California. Esalen massage is based on traditional massage, which works on the muscular and circulatory systems, and is enriched by emphasis on conscious, structured, and pleasant touch. Therapists are encouraged to quiet inner monologue and focus on awareness of the relaxation of the client. Esalen massage places value on the intuitive skills of the therapist, who may find it fitting to include other methods such as Feldenkrais, deep tissue, polarity, and acupressure, to create a holistic therapy for the client that includes physical relief as well as psychological wholeness. Traditionally, Esalen was received in the nude with no covering, to encourage acceptance of the whole body, as well as to allow the therapists to perform the long, gliding stroke that are part of the Esalen method.

Esalen massage is a combination that incorporates all of the massage methods found in Swedish massage and adds characteristics of energy work. The desired effect is a sense of harmony and balance for the client. Esalen massage may be used for relaxation massage and overall health and wellness. It is recommended for individuals who suffer from chronic pain, muscle and joint tension, or headache and migraine. Therapists also believe that Esalen strengthens the body to promote healing and psychological health. Through this conscious touching, stimulation occurs in the skin, blood, muscles, and nervous system. Stretch therapy positively affects the tendons, ligaments, and joints, leading to increased levels of relaxation. Esalen massage can be an intense experience as the body releases physical and psychological tension, and the therapist and client cooperate to make best use of the experience.

Feldenkrais

The Feldenkrais method was developed by Moshe Feldenkrais, a leading physicist of his time who began devising this system in mid-life. After a bus accident and careful exploration of his own body movement, his work highlighted the importance of a coherent body image and thinking a movement through. It also uses micro-movements for neuromuscular re-education. The method is most effective for pain relief, and it also promotes grace and ease of movement. The Feldenkrais method focuses attention on gentle movements to improve and enhance body functioning. Its effect is twofold: to improve coordination, flexibility, and posture; and to minimize physiological and psychological stress that stems from restricted functions. By creating awareness of restricted movement and carefully working the body into new postures, Feldenkrais offers a way to retrain the body to move in a less inhibited and healthier way.

The Feldenkrais method comprises two parts. First, the client attends Awareness Through Movement classes, in which students begin by lying on their backs on the floor, where they are guided through a full-body scan to draw awareness to their presence. They are then led through movement sequences that are devised to bring awareness to their normal movements and find restrictions in these movements. Movement through the postures is slow and gentle, and it includes rest when necessary. Students are taught to find alternative ways of moving that break their restrictive movements and allow them more freedom, flexibility, and health. The second part of the Feldenkrais method is Functional Integration, which involves a private session in which the practitioner gently manipulates the body to teach new postures and ways of moving. This supplements the re-education that is started in the Awareness Through Movement classes.

Practitioners of Feldenkrais usually do not diagnose clients, nor do they refer to the Feldenkrais method as therapy. Feldenkrais simply helps clients increase neuromuscular awareness and re-educate their bodies. The client is taught how to recognize and eliminate habitual patterns of movement. Users of the method include those who want to improve their movement capabilities, those who have pain or limitation in movement, and those who want to improve well-being and personal development. Clients have mentioned increased flexibility and energy, improved digestion and respiration, and decreased pain as results of the Feldenkrais method.

Hellerwork®

Hellerwork Structural Integration is a product of Rolfing, created by Joseph Heller. It incorporates movement and verbal communication with connective tissue work to restore the body's natural balance from the inside out. It is considered part of the field of Somatic Education, which addresses the whole person in relation to movement, as well as physical and psychological awareness of one's environment. Hellerwork is based on the notion that every person is innately healthy and emphasizes prevention and self-care through education. The power of the connection between body and mind is used to produce wellness, not just alleviation of symptoms.

Hellerwork practitioners are taught that, from the moment we are born, we begin to build up tension. This chronic tension (which differs from the acute tension we feel in an aching neck or a stiff back) pervades our beings without our awareness that it is there. It can be seen and felt by a trained eye or hand, and it affects the structural integration of our body and how our tissues are able to react to stimuli. Treatment merges three key elements: myofascial manipulation of the soft tissues; movement and awareness education; and client/practitioner dialogue that unites mind and body. Structure is viewed as relationship: the relationship of the whole to the gravitational field in which it exists; relationship between parts within the whole; and relationship of structure to function.

Hellerwork consists of eleven 90-minute sessions, during which the focus is on various parts of the body and their corresponding movements (breathing, standing, etc). The first sessions address the stages of development in early childhood and continue with systematic release and reorganization of muscle and connective tissue through deep-tissue bodywork techniques. Relieving unconscious chronic tension, reinforcing the structural integrity of the body, and creating awareness of the body are the objectives of the sessions. The goal of the session is not to address symptoms or acute pain, but, because of its healing of underlying tension issues, Hellerwork can relieve musculoskeletal and other acute pain. Each session begins with a discussion between client and therapist about how the sessions are progressing and how the body has been adapting between sessions. The client reclines on a massage table, or alternatively may be seated or standing during some exercises. The therapist will ask the client to make slow movements with the body, while guiding the client through stretches and holds. Hellerwork can supply relief from chronic pain and sports injuries since it lengthens core musculature, allows for postural improvements, and helps to free breathing.

Jin Shin Do
Jin Shin Do is an ancient method developed by psychotherapist Iona Marsaa Teeguarden which combines gentle but deep finger pressure on acu-points with simple body focusing techniques to release physical and emotional tension. Jin Shin Do encourages a pleasurable, deeply relaxed state during which the recipient can get in touch with the body and access emotions related to the physical condition. This body/mind approach, performed on the fully clothed client, is a combination of a traditional Japanese acupressure technique, classic Chinese acupuncture theory, Taoist yogic philosophy and breathing methods, and Reichian segmental theory. "The Way of the Compassionate Spirit" is based on the eight "Strange Flows," which regulate the entire body/mind energy. The "Strange Flows" teach the individual to harmonize the body energy. It is a simple, color-coded chart that lets anyone use Jin Shin Do to help themselves or others. Understanding of the "etheric" body as well as the physical body is vital, and recognition that our bodies are greater than just the physical part that we can see is crucial to benefiting from this practice.

The client lies fully clothed on his or her back on a massage table while the practitioner holds "local points" in tension areas together with related "distal points," which help the armored places to release easier and deeper. The client decides the depth of the pressure. A typical session is about 90 minutes. Jin Shin Do acupressure is effective in helping relieve tension and fatigue, stress-related headaches and gastro-intestinal problems, back and shoulder pain, eye strain, menstrual and menopausal imbalances, sinus pain and allergies. (If there are medical problems, the client is asked to consult a doctor.) Over a period of 10 or more sessions, armoring is progressively released in the head, neck, shoulders, chest, diaphragm, abdomen, pelvis and legs. After sessions, clients usually feel deeply relaxed and may even feel euphoric. If the client is receptive, there will be significantly less tension and pain together with an increased sense of well-being for hours or days. This response will likely extend after further sessions. In the case of chronic fatigue, originally the client may feel more tired after a session because the body is demanding rest. It is desirable to schedule sessions with time to rest and relax afterwards. Conversely, Jin Shin Do can be used before athletic events to enhance performance, for horses as well as for people.

Jin Shin Jyutsu
Jin Shin Jyutsu is a modern acupressure therapy based on ancient Japanese methods that unite the body, mind, and spirit on levels that many individuals are unaware exist within the body. Born of natural wisdom and passed down from generation to generation by word of mouth, Jin Shin Jyutsu had fallen into relative insignificance before being revived in the early 1900s by Master Jiro Murai in Japan. After clearing himself of life-threatening illness, Master Murai devoted the remainder of his life to the research and development of Jin Shin Jyutsu, gathering insight from a range of experiences and resources including the Kojiki (Record of Ancient Things).

Mary Burmeister, who studied the art with Murai, then brought the practice to the West in the 1950s. Burmeister began teaching the art of Jin Shin Jyutsu to others in the early 1960s and now there are thousands of students and practitioners throughout the United States and around the globe. Jin Shin Jyutsu is described as being an art rather than a technique, since it requires a more profound understanding and more creativity than application of a structured technique. It is often used with Qigong, an exercise of slow movement with focus on breathing, stretching, and posture.

Jin Shin Jyutsu brings balance to the body's energies, which promotes optimal health and well-being and facilitates a profound healing capacity. It is an important counterpart to conventional healing methods, inducing relaxation and stress relief. Jin Shin Jyutsu uses 26 "safety energy locks" along energy pathways that feed life into our bodies. When one or more of the paths become blocked, the consequential stagnation can disrupt the local area and eventually disharmonize the complete path of energy flow. Holding these energy locks in combination can bring stability to mind, body and spirit. Jin Shin Jyutsu can be applied as self-help and also by a trained practitioner. It is a very simple and gentle style of acupressure that works without needles, pressure, or rubbing.

A Jin Shin Jyutsu session normally lasts about an hour. Before the treatment begins, the practitioner takes the pulse of the client, who may enter into a meditative state. It does not involve massage, manipulation of muscles, or use of drugs or substances. It is a gentle art, practiced by placing the fingertips (over clothing) on selected safety energy locks, to harmonize and restore the energy flow. This makes possible the reduction of tension and stress that accumulate through daily life. The body's own healing mechanisms are able to come together and can positively affect the body in a more thorough manner. Because it is such a gentle treatment, Jin Shin Jyutsu can be used on the most fragile and sick individuals, as well as healthy individuals who seek to change the attitude that lies below their symptoms and not just heal the symptoms themselves.

Lomi Lomi and Hawaiian Massage

The goals of lomi lomi (which is the Polynesian word for "massage") are not just to heal the physical body, but also to create peace in the client's mind and spirit. Lomi lomi is influenced by the Hawaiian philosophy Huna, which is based on the primary belief that everything seeks harmony and love. It is believed that massage can unlock muscles to release thoughts that were hidden or stored in the muscle, thus giving physical relief and emotional peace. Practitioners of lomi lomi would say that what makes it unique is that much of the work is done by love (rather than a focus on technique), with the therapist concentrating on using loving hands and a loving heart while working with the client. Lomi lomi uses prayer, chanting, and the hula in conjunction with massage strokes.

The session begins with a prayer in which the practitioner calls upon the aid of a higher power to help to heal the client. The client may be asked to say her own prayer to specifically address the body parts that need healing. Lomi lomi massage makes use of aromatic oils, and the practitioner often will massage more than one area of the body simultaneously. Hands (often both at once), elbows, or forearms are used to create broad, long strokes. The therapist may chant or dance the hula during the massage, a technique used to help keep her body in sync with the client's body. Those who benefit from lomi lomi generally enjoy the process and are open to being healed both physically and emotionally.

Lymphatic Massage

Lymphatic massage, also known as Manual Lymphatic Drainage (MLD) or Lymph Drainage Therapy (LDT), is a gentle, relaxing form of massage that helps the body's lymphatic system get moving again while supporting immune function. The origins can be traced back to Dr. Frederic Millard and Dr. Emil Vodder. The lymphatic system is a system of vessels that circulate body fluids. Lymph is transported from in between the cells to the bloodstream and carries leftover fluid, bacteria, viruses, and waste products from body tissues. Lymph movement is vital for healthy immune system function, tissue repair, and maintenance of a proper fluid and chemical environment for the body's cells. Lymph movement is a gradual and mostly passive process since there is no central pump for the system; contraction of skeletal muscle (such as during exercise) and the action of the diaphragm in breathing both help the flow of lymph.

Lymphatic massage can be valuable in cases of edema, sports injury or for people experiencing poor immune system or those suffering from a lack of energy. Lymphatic massage helps to eliminate excess fluid in the tissues and to encourage healing by increasing the rate of waste disposal. Lymphatic massage is a slow, gentle process that aims to help move the lymph through the system of vessels and nodes. It is not simply a milder version of a relaxation massage; it is more precise (moving lymph towards the nodes) and uses very light pressure which directly affects the superficial vessels. It moves in a clockwise fashion to work with the natural flow of the lymph system. Lymphatic massage can be useful in clients with lymphedema, an abnormal accumulation of lymph fluid in tissues (which can be associated with treatment for diseases such as breast cancer). It can also help individuals with sports injuries, a sluggish immune system, or simply general fatigue.

Myofascial Massage

Also called myofascial release or myofascial unwinding, this modality is used to relax or loosen the fascia and connective tissue in the body. Fascia is the soft tissue component of connective tissue that protects and supports many structures within the body, in particular muscle. It is a thin layer that naturally can stretch and move without restriction, creating a constant pull that stabilizes the structures it surrounds. Because of disease, trauma, overuse, or inactivity, this tissue can become tense, tight, and misaligned, decreasing blood flow and causing the client pain. Local inflammation can become chronic and lead to fibrosis, or thickening of the connective tissue. This in turn causes more pain from decreased blood flow (ischemia) and continues a cycle of pain and tissue tightening, even if the original stimulus of muscle tension has gone

Myofascial massage stretches, releases, and realigns the fascia. The therapist starts by working on the most superficial layer of muscle, and slowly works down into the deeper layers. The fascia will feel as if it is "melting" and when ready can be realigned so it does not cut off circulation or cause tension in underlying muscle. Skin rolling and sustained stretch might be used to loosen the fascia from the underlying tissue. Normally, a small amount of oil or lubricant is used so the therapist can feel the "melting" of the fascia. The fascia also becomes more pliable because of the heat of the therapist's hand movements. As a result of these benefits, myofascial massage is often used on individuals who have restricted mobility or physical pain and dysfunction.

Neuromuscular Massage Therapy (NMT)

Neuromuscular massage therapy (NMT) is a series of treatment protocols that cooperate with the central nervous system to work on nerves in the body to achieve release. It specifically refers to the use of static pressure on specific myofascial points to relieve pain. Injury or stress to the body causes nerves to increase their impulses, making the body sensitive to pain and dysfunction. NMT emerged in both Europe and North America over the last half-century and combines holistic with traditional medicine to treat and prevent soft tissue injuries and chronic pain. There are five areas addressed under NMT: Ischemia, or lack of blood supply to soft tissue, leading to pain; trigger points, highly irritated points in muscle which refer pain to other parts of the body; nerve compression or entrapment, pressure on a nerve by soft tissue, cartilage or bone; postural distortion, or imbalance of the muscular system resulting from the movement of the body off the longitudinal and horizontal planes; and biomechanical dysfunction, or imbalance of the musculoskeletal system resulting in faulty movement patterns (such as poor ergonomic setup at a desk, or poor athletic mechanics).

NMT is a thorough program of recovery which uses massage therapy, flexibility stretching, and home care to ease or end pain. Manual therapy increases blood flow to decrease ischemic pain. Force must be applied perpendicular to the skin to stimulate the muscle. Identification of trigger points is followed by deep flushing work and stretching, to decrease the size of the trigger point and to elongate tissue that has been continually contracted. The practitioner checks for range of motion of joints to seek out any possible nerve entrapment or compression. NMT uses a resisted stretch called a muscle energy technique that improves range of motion through work with the neurons in the tendons. Postural distortion and biomechanical dysfunction are addressed through home care education, wherein the practitioner teaches the client the appropriate postures or mechanics necessary to keep the body healthy. Individuals with chronic pain and soft tissue injury have used NMT to prevent and treat their conditions. NMT is used in a broad range of places, including occupational and physical therapy, nursing, chiropractic, physical medicine clinics, and more.

Polarity Therapy

Polarity therapy acts on the assertion that the flow and balance of energy in the human body is the basis of good health. When energy is unbalanced, blockages occur and cause pain and disease. Polarity therapy is described as a “respectful, compassionate, and intentional laying of the hands on the body.” It encompasses some similar theory as Asian medicine and Ayurveda. In true health, the Human Energy Field (electromagnetic patterns of the body and mind) is balanced. The three types of energy are long lines (north-south on the body), transverse currents (east-west), and spiral currents (starting at the navel). Polarity therapy asserts that the body was designed to heal itself, so all treatment includes an underlying intention to support the client’s inherent self-healing intelligence as expressed in its energetic patterns.

Polarity therapy includes energy-based bodywork, diet, exercise and self-awareness. Manipulation, using light touch and medium and deep pressure, is used to release energy blockages and restore balance. Polarity has strong connections to many other healing and holistic health systems and is used by individuals who are looking for wellness in mind, body, and spirit. Because it is so gentle, polarity therapy can be used by most people, even those who are frail or elderly.

Pregnancy Massage

Pregnancy (or prenatal) massage commonly refers to Swedish or other relaxation massage done on a pregnant woman. Many of the stroke techniques are the same as in a normal relaxation massage. Positioning of the mother on the table will be different, as the ideal way to reach the back and hips is to have the client recline on her side. Certain areas of the body should not be massaged, and massage during the first trimester is generally not recommended.

Pregnancy massage has many benefits for the client. It can help relieve muscle cramps, spasm, and myofascial pain. The increase of blood and lymph circulation can reduce swelling and edema, and can reduce stress on weight-bearing joints. Pregnancy massage can induce relaxation and reduce stress on a mother-to-be, which can help improve the outcome of labor and delivery and provides the new mother with physical and emotional reprieve from the stress of mothering. Unless she has other diseases or conditions that counter-indicate massage, pregnancy massage can be very useful both physically and mentally for a mother-to-be.

Reflexology
Reflexology is based on the idea that specific spots (usually in the hands or feet) can be stimulated to activate corresponding areas of the body away from the stimulus site. In reflexology, the body is divided into 10 planes, or zones, which divide the body equally and which have endpoints at the hands, feet, and top of the head. By stimulating the endpoints on the hands and feet, the therapist can affect the rest of the plane on which that point lies, which is believed to help normalize function and increase circulation in the area of the body that is stimulated.

The scientific basis of reflexology is still somewhat unknown. Some believe the zones are more like energy meridians, while others believe that foot reflexology breaks up chemical or waste deposits that congest other parts of the body and hinder its function. The hands and feet have extensive nerve distribution comprised of 7200 nerve endings in each foot, 2500 in each hand and 435 in each ear that correspond to every part of the body, so stimulation of these areas of the body has a variety of functions, including activation of the parasympathetic nervous system and release of endorphins and other endogenous chemicals. It is the nerve endings in the hands, feet and ears that send the message to the brain about stress or pain found in the body during a reflexology session. These functions can lead to body-wide relaxation, healing, and positive mood.

After a point is identified, treatment is determined by the reaction of the point to pressure. A point that is hypersensitive or tender may be associated with a reflex structure that is hyper-reactive. This type of point requires relaxation and sedating methods. If the point feels numb, empty, or disconnected from the surrounding tissue, then stimulation methods should be used. Therapists respond to feedback from clients to decide appropriate techniques to use for each point.

Rolfing® Structural Integration
Dr. Ida P. Rolf, PhD, developed, practiced and taught a system of bodywork aimed toward achieving structural changes in the client by organizing and aligning the structure of the human being in the field of gravity. While Dr. Rolf originally called her system Structural Integration, it became more commonly called Rolfing®, and is more properly called Rolfing® Structural Integration. Rolfing Structural Integration, which includes movement work and education, works within the connective tissue matrix (including fascia, tendon, ligament, and cartilage) of the body to improve structure. Rolfing maintains that all aspects of the human being - physical; emotional; perceptual and cognitive; social and behavioral; energetic and spiritual - are interrelated, interdependent, and manifest in the physical body's structure, function, and its relationship with gravity.

Much of a Rolfer's repertoire consists of (1) hands-on interventions (applying direct pressure using fingers, knuckles, and elbows) to effect change in the connective tissue matrix; (2) qualities of touch and skills in observing and perceiving the structure, both in local tissues and through local tissues to the entire system, and (3) movement work directed toward shifting habitual patterns of function (which often originate in how we perceive and ascribe meanings to self, experience, and environment).

The purpose of Rolfing is to improve the organization of the person as a whole, rather than to alleviate symptoms. Rolfing is based on the fact that the body is not simply a collection of separate parts or anatomy, but rather a system of relationships that are all interconnected. Fascial layers that have been pulled out of balance due to habitual use, strain, scarring, or injury, result in effortful and inefficient motion, stress, tension, and a sense that something doesn't feel right or resolved. When the system is balanced, aligned, organized, and integrated within itself and with gravity, most symptoms no longer have an environment in which to persist. Rolfers work to access and improve the relationships and function among all the parts. This focus on overall structural and functional balance, as opposed to symptom relief, is a key distinguishing feature of Rolfing from medicine and from many other somatic approaches.

Structural integration can be done at any age and is good for all postural, limited mobility, chronic pain, and inflexibility issues. It is also used by many as fundamental to achieving overall well-being. Athletes, dancers, business professionals, and others who perform repetitive or continual actions are ideal candidates. This approach creates a more balanced structure which allows for the more efficient use of muscles and allows the body to cope better under stress, move more freely, and conserve energy.

Shiatsu
Shiatsu is a Japanese bodywork practice that uses principles of acupressure and TCM. Shiatsu means "finger pressure" and, as the name implies, it uses finger and palm pressure to energize pathways called meridians in order to enhance the flow of qi (vitality, stamina and energy). Traditionally, the sight-impaired were recruited as massage practitioners, as they were thought to have more sensitivity to the sense of touch. In the early 1940s, Shizuto Masunaga, trained as an Oriental medical practitioner, combined massage techniques with a knowledge of the meridian system and TCM, and called this Shiatsu. Since then, "Shiatsu" has been used as a general name for many different styles of massage that use the meridian system: Acupressure, Chi Nei Tsang, Five Element Shiatsu, Integrative Eclectic Shiatsu, Japanese Shiatsu, Jin Shin Do, Macrobiotic Shiatsu, Shiatsu Amma, and Zen Shiatsu.

In acupressure and Shiatsu, thumbs are most commonly used to apply pressure, although other fingers, knuckles, palms, elbows and even feet can be used in some of the therapies. The degree of pressure that is applied varies, as does the duration. Anything from moderate to penetrating pressure is utilized from several seconds to several minutes, and the treatment can be rhythmically performed once or repeatedly. Assisted self-stretching is also typically involved. Shiatsu can calm the sympathetic nervous system, improving circulation, relieving stiff muscles, and alleviating stress. Shiatsu can increase circulation of blood and lymph, reduce muscle stiffness, and release stress and fatigue (tsubo) that accumulate in the body. Shiatsu is conducted with the client fully clothed, usually in comfortable clothing that allows the client to stretch and move. It is performed on a mat on the floor or on a low table. No oil is used, and the shiatsu therapist applies pressure in a continuous rhythmic sequence. Shiatsu uses hand pressure and techniques to regulate the body's physical structure and its natural inner energies to maintain good health. By contrast to more traditional massage, Shiatsu uses fewer techniques and to an observer it would appear that little is happening – simply a still, relaxed pressure at various points on the body with the hand or thumb, an easy leaning of the elbows or a simple rotation of a limb. However, beneath the uncomplicated movements, much is happening internally to the body's energy on a subtle level to enhance physical vitality and emotional well-being.

Sports Massage
Sports massage is a type of Swedish massage that stimulates circulation of blood and lymph fluids. It can also include some deep tissue therapy or trigger point therapy to break down knots in muscle, and stretching to increase flexibility and range of motion. Sports massage stresses prevention and healing of injuries to the muscles and tendons. It also may decrease recovery time between workouts, maximize the supply of nutrients and oxygen through increased blood flow, and enhance elimination of metabolic by-products of exercise.

There are four main types of sports massage: pre-event, post-event, restorative (given during training), and rehabilitative. Generally, a sports massage therapist will focus on the area that is in pain or stiff/inflexible, rather than giving a full-body massage. It can be more vigorous than Swedish massage in the effort to increase circulation and healing. Although sports massage was designed with athletes in mind, it also can be very useful for individuals with many types of muscular injuries, chronic pain, or range-of-motion difficulties.

Thai Massage

Thai massage, one of the oldest massage techniques being used today, is one of four branches of traditional medicine in Thailand, along with herbs, nutrition, and spiritual practice. It evolved within the context of Buddhist monasteries and temples, with a goal of treating the body, mind, and spirit. The ultimate goal of Thai massage is for the receiver to attain spiritual enlightenment and harmony. On a base level, Thai massage is supposed to activate the capacity of the body to heal itself and to promote better health and well-being.

Electromagnetic or energetic fields are believed to surround and infuse the body, and Thai massage uses pressure and manipulative touch to affect these fields and bring health and peace to the body. Because of this focus on the energy fields, touching occurs less often (and in fact might be said to be "incidental") in Thai massage than in other traditional forms of massage; no oil is used and the client remains fully clothed. The massage combines assisted yoga postures, rocking, compressions, deep stretching, and mindfulness to create a physical and spiritual healing process. Typical sessions can run for at least two to three hours and occur with the client on a mat on the floor.

Structural Integration

Structural integration works with the fascia, the layer of tissue that surrounds and provides structure for the muscles, bones, and organs in the body. Gravity's effects, daily stress of activity and physical injury can pull the fascia out of alignment. These stressors cause the fascia to tighten and adjust to accommodate the misalignment, leading to stiffness, discomfort and loss of energy.

The practice of structural integration aligns and balances the body by lengthening and repositioning the fascia, which allows the muscles to move more effectively. Pressure is applied to the body, stretching the fascia and working the entire fascial system. As the fascia is released, it is able to lengthen and return to its appropriate positioning. Structural integration generally consists of 10 sessions, after which the body may continue to adjust for several months as fascia realigns. The goal is for the body itself to return to its structurally optimal position, leading to improved posture, easier breathing, better athletic performance, and higher levels of coordination. Individuals with poor posture or stiff joints, athletes, and those who repeatedly perform specific physical tasks can benefit from structural integration.

Swedish Massage

Swedish, or classical, massage is the style that comes to mind when most people think of massage. It was developed centuries ago by University of Stockholm physiologist Henri Peter Ling, who was in awe of Chinese massage techniques and benefits. Swedish massage is considered to be the basis for other types such as Western massage, aromatherapy, sports massage and deep tissue massage. It is used to reduce pain and joint stiffness, increase circulation and oxygen flow, and release toxins (especially lactic acid) from the muscles. It can aid in muscle recovery because it helps the body release lactic acid, uric acid, and other metabolic wastes more quickly. It also is used to relieve stress and improve mood, providing overall physical wellness and mental well-being.

Perhaps one of the most well-known modalities, Swedish massage incorporates five basic strokes: effleurage (sliding or gliding), petrissage (kneading), tapotement (rhythmic tapping), friction (cross fiber), and vibration/shaking. Oils or lotions are used, and the therapist may use hands, knuckles, elbows, or forearms with long, gliding strokes. Strokes go from distal (away from heart) to proximal (towards heart) to increase venous return and boost circulation. Pressure during Swedish massage can range from light to firm, and many practitioners will use deep tissue or trigger point therapy to add specific attention to certain areas of the body during a Swedish massage. This modality is beneficial for clients who are seeking to relieve stress, increase circulation, or recover from athletic workouts.

Trager Massage

Trager massage is a movement education developed in the 1920s by American medical practitioner Dr. Milton Trager. It makes wide use of touch-contact and encourages the client to experience the freeing-up of different parts of the body. The approach consists of simple exercises called Mentastics and deep, non-intrusive hands-on work that includes fluid, gentle, rocking movements. The idea is to use motion in the muscles and joints to produce positive sensory feelings that are then fed back into the central nervous system. The result is a feeling of lightness, freedom and flexibility. Trager work is movement re-education and is referred to as psychophysical integration therapy by its founder. When movement stops or is hindered because of injury or illness, the neural circuits that operate the body also slow down from lack of use. Unbalanced muscle tension can result. Through gentle, rhythmic, and supported movement, Trager massage allows the client's awareness of his own body to reawaken, helping to heal.

A Trager session generally lasts from 60 to 90 minutes. No oils or lotions are used. The client wears a swimsuit or underwear and lies on a well-padded table in a warm, comfortable environment. No long, broad strokes are used over the surface of the body and, unlike various techniques of deep tissue manipulation, it does not utilize extreme pressure or rapid thrusts to create structural change. It does not produce pain as a necessary adjunct to its effectiveness. During the session, the practitioner makes touch-contact with the client in such a gentle and rhythmic way that the person lying passively on the table in fact experiences the opportunity of being able to move each part of the body freely, easily and gracefully on their own. The practitioner moves the joints through a normal range of motion to find any areas that are stuck; the movements are passive, and the client does not assist the practitioner in any way. Gentle rocking, shaking, vibration, and traction are used. The practitioner works in a relaxed, meditative state of consciousness, which allows the practitioner to connect deeply with the recipient in an unforced way, to remain continually aware of the slightest responses, and to work efficiently without fatigue.

After getting up from the table, the client is given instruction in the use of Mentastics, a system of simple, effortless movement sequences to preserve and increase the sense of lightness, freedom and flexibility instilled by the table work. This is active work on the client's part, in contrast to the passive participation on the table. Mentastics is Dr. Trager's coinage for "mental gymnastics" a mindfulness in motion, designed to help clients re-create for themselves the sensory feelings produced by the motion of their tissue in the practitioner's hands. It is a powerful means of teaching the client to recall the pleasurable sensory state that produced positive tissue change. Since it is this feeling state that triggered positive tissue response to begin with, every time the feeling is clearly recalled, the changes deepen and become more permanent and more receptive to further positive change. Changes described have included the disappearance of specific symptoms, discomforts, or pains, heightened levels of energy and vitality, more effortless posture and carriage, greater joint mobility, deeper states of relaxation than were previously possible, and a new ease in daily activities.

Trigger Point Therapy

Trigger points are small spots in muscle that may be sore or radiate pain when they are pressed. The pain is due to excessive nerve stimulation of a muscle that is aggravated by stress of any sort. Pressure on the trigger point may cause pain in the immediate area or may cause referred pain if the areas are located near motor nerve points. Trigger point therapy is a type of neuromuscular therapy that is useful in the treatment of myofascial problems. The purpose of trigger point therapy is to get rid of pain and to re-educate the muscles into pain-free habits. The targeted muscle may be stiff, weak, have a restricted range of motion, or be resistant to stretch. Stimulation of trigger points might also cause spasm, vasoconstriction, coldness, sweating, hypersecretion, and other symptoms.

Trigger point therapy involves light and deep palpation, as well as gliding strokes. The trigger point is recognizable to the therapist as a tense band of tissue. Manipulation of trigger points is frequently used in conjunction with other therapies such as Swedish or deep tissue massage. After treatment, swelling and stiffness may be reduced, increasing range of motion, circulation, and flexibility. Individuals who may benefit from trigger point therapy include athletes or individuals who work in physically demanding jobs that overload certain muscle groups on a regular basis.

Tui na
Tui na uses Chinese taoist and martial arts principles to bring the body to balance. "Tui na" literally translates to "push pull" and is the name given to Chinese medical massage. Based on Traditional Chinese Medicine, (TCM) Tui na may actually predate the practice of acupuncture. It incorporates techniques that are similar to Western and Asian massage, chiropractic, osteopathic, and Western physical therapy. Tui na uses a variety of hand massage techniques and passive and active stretching to restore correct anatomical musculo-skeletal relationships and neuromuscular patterns, and to increase the circulation of qi and blood to remove biochemical irritants. It works not just on the muscles, bones, and joints, but also with the energy of the body at a deeper level. Its objective is to keep the body's energy in balance, preventing injury and maintaining good health. Tui na uses rhythmic compression along energy channels of the body and a variety of techniques that manipulate and lubricate the joints. The therapist directly affects the flow of energy by holding and pressing the body at acupressure points.

Tui na balances the eight principles of TCM where practitioners work on the areas between each of the joints, or "eight gates," to open the body's defensive qi, move the energy through the meridians, and get the muscles working. Brushing, kneading, rolling/pressing and rubbing are used to open the qi; then range of motion, traction, massage, and stimulation of acupressure points are used to treat the musculoskeletal physical conditions. In China, Tui na is used in hospital settings and is closer to the work of osteopaths, chiropractors and physical therapists. It may include some form of bone setting and manipulation. It is often used in conjunctive therapies in TCM with acupuncture, cupping, Chinese herbs, tai chi and qigong.

Zero Balancing
Zero balancing was developed by Fritz Smith, M.D. and has its roots in osteopathy, acupuncture, Rolfing and meditation. Relaxing, yet energizing, zero balancing integrates fundamental principles of Western medicine with Eastern concepts of energy. This technique provides clients the possibility of healing by addressing the energy flow of the skeletal system. While zero balancing does look at symptoms, it moves beyond them to address the body's more fundamental nature. By working with bone energy, zero balancing seeks to correct imbalances between energy and structure, providing relief from pain, anxiety, and stress. For the massage therapist or body worker, zero balancing may enhance other modalities and open new avenues of energetic and structural balancing through touch. Training takes one to two years and leads to certification as a zero balancer.

A zero balance (ZB) treatment generally takes between 30 and 40 minutes and is performed with the recipient fully clothed and lying on a massage table. The client begins in a seated position and then moves to a comfortable reclining position on his or her back. Through touch, the practitioner evaluates the energy fields and flows to find where they are disturbed or blocked the most, in order to find a focus for the session. The focus may be on the body, mind, spirit, or all three in any particular session. Touch during the ZB session is gentle and noninvasive and should feel enjoyable to both the therapist and the client. A session consists of gentle pressing, stretching and bending. Before or after the session, the client may want to enter into a state of meditation in order to receive the greatest benefits possible from the practice. The meditative state allows energy to flow freely and bring healing energies to body systems or organs that are not functioning at optimum. Zero balance is designed to complement primary health care, focusing on integrating the body, mind and spirit to promote unity and optimal functioning. ZB is described as ideal for helping to keep balance and wellness during stressful or difficult periods of life, as well as for those who simply want to continue along a path of self-realization. A minimum of three sessions is recommended, with maintenance sessions at intervals of every two to four weeks after the initial sessions.

MASSAGE STROKES

There is a variety of different massage strokes that can be used, ranging from light to deep with variations of speed and depth. The application of these strokes can be applied to soft tissues of the body, muscle, connective tissue, tendons, ligaments and joints. Not all terms for methods of strokes are consistent, nor the types of modalities ranging from Swedish, deep tissue, tuina, Thai, myofascial release to Structural Integration. The following section lists types of strokes, applications, physiologic effects, contraindications and indications associated with manual therapy and bodywork.

Effleurage is a slow, rhythmical gliding stroke, generally used in Swedish or classical massage

Application
- Finishing stroke is a smooth and gliding movement used with relaxed, flexible hands
- Provides integrative movements between different massage techniques
- Heavier pressure should be applied on upstroke with lighter pressure on downstroke
- Introduces the first touch by spreading oil or lotion

Indications	Contraindications
• Edema, muscle tension, pain control	• DVT/varicose veins
• Palpation assessment	• Unhealed wound
• Lethargic circulation	• All local and general CIs
• Inhibits adhesions and fibrosis	• High blood pressure

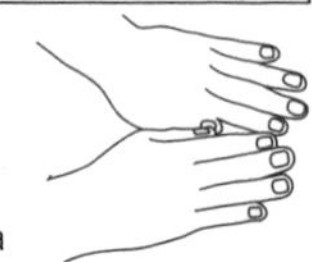

Physiologic Effects
- Stimulates the central nervous system
- Enhances superficial blood flow
- Raises then decreases blood pressure
- Increases the flow of lymph, removes waste products, decreases edema
- Motivates large mechanoreceptors, which temper pain

Petrissage is an alternating pressure and release technique similar to "kneading bread", applied with compression toward underlying structures or by raising soft tissues
- Kneading – compressive petrissage using palms, thumbs, fingertips or knuckles applied in rhythmic, rounded motions with alternating pressure and release
- Picking up – lifting petrissage using fingers, thumbs and palms away from underlying tissue
- Muscle compressions – pressing and releasing of soft tissues with fingers and palms
- Wringing - applying equal pressure on opposite sides of the tissue structure and lifting and pushing in contrary directions

Applications
Kneading
- May be done with one or two hands in circular movements, with alternate or reinforced contact
- Contact is constant
- Muscle compressions – pressing and releasing of soft tissues with fingers and palms

Picking up
- Squeezes the muscles and lifts it from underlying tissue
- Begins slowly and progresses to a deeper and firmer pick-up

Muscle compressions
- Pressure is downward towards belly of muscle
- No oil is required, full palmar contact, pressure is progressively amplified

Wringing
- Hand contact is unyielding but relaxed
- Hands lift tissue up and progressively release when tissues are raised to greatest height
- Hands glide past one another toward the opposite side of the part being treated
- Applied to the length of the muscle

Indications	Contraindications
Kneading • Hypertoned muscle, muscle contractures • Sluggish circulation, edema • Decreased active range of motion • Stimulated motor nerves • Digestive illnesses • Sleeping disorders • Spastic paralysis Picking up • Hypertoned muscle tissue • Intensify local circulation Muscle compressions • Lessen local edema and muscle spasm • Intensify local circulation • Decrease muscle guarding and hypertonicity • When applied vigorously, it can be used in pre-event sports massage Wringing • Poor or lethargic circulation • Hypertoned muscle tissue • Edema	Kneading • Severe varicosities • Avoid knuckle kneading over boney prominences or hypotonic tissue • Severely atrophied or flaccid tissue Picking up • All local and general CIs Muscle compressions • Avoid applying intense, unexpected pressure • All local and general CIs Wringing • All local and general CIs

Physiologic Effects

Kneading
- Stimulates lymphatic drainage
- Enhances and mobilizes muscle tone
- Less stiffness due to ischemia
- Relaxes adhesive muscle tissue, stretches muscle fibers
- Vasodilates arterial blood supply
- Decreases effects of fibrous thickenings and adhesions
- Soothing effect on the nervous system
- Improves circulation to nerves

Picking up
- Increases arterial flow
- Stimulates venous and lymphatic flow
- Loosens adhesive muscle tissue

Muscle compressions
- Increases interstitial flow
- Empties venous beds, lowering venous pressure and increasing capillary flow
- Relaxation of hypertoned issue
- Increases parasympathetic neural stimulation

Wringing
- Less stiffness due to ischemia
- Loosens adhesiveness in muscle tissue
- Extends muscle fibers
- Lessens effects of fibrous thickenings and adhesions
- Enhances muscle tone
- Soothing effect on the nervous system
- Increases circulation to nerves

MASSAGE STROKES

Tapotement is percussive tapping, cupping, flicking, slapping, pounding, pinching or beating. This procedure can be applied everywhere on the body to stimulate the nerves. It involves drumming hand movements on broad areas using fists, flat hands, fingertips, and edges of the hands over fleshy areas.

Application
- Pressure can differ, from light, moderate to heavy
- Releases congestion

Indications	Contraindications
• Decreased innervations of tissue • Dislodged mucus • Increased circulation • Decreased fatigue • Decreased hypertonicity • Maintains tone in hypotonic muscle • Atonic constipation	• Over boney prominences • Aggressive tapotement of flaccid tissue or decreased neurological sensation • Acute inflammatory areas • Cyst or tumors, severe varicose veins • Unstable cardiac condition • Kidney area and back of the knees • Lumbar during menstruation or pregnancy

Physiologic Effects
- Stimulates peripheral nerves
- Expectoration of mucous by shaking of lung walls
- Decrease in sinus congestion, increase in local circulation
- Increases peristalsis

Vibration is a quick, oscillating or trembling movement that is produced mechanically or manually. The objective of vibration is to loosen muscles and reduce pain. When performed manually, hands or fingers are placed against the specific area of the body, creating continuous shaking or trembling movements.

Application
- Degree of movement may be fine or course, in terms of vibration and pressure
- Movements consist of small quick flexions and extensions
- Surface may be static or running

Indications	Contraindications
• Course– flaccid or atrophied tissue, atonic constipation, chronic pulmonary disease • Fine– pain relief, acute muscle spasm, neuralgia, cutaneous inflammation, sinus congestion, nervous exhaustion, insomnia	• All local and general CIs • Course- acute muscle spasm, insomnia, lumbar or abdomen while pregnant

Physiologic Effects
Fine vibrations increase superficial lymphatic return, decrease lymph node congestion, have a soothing effect on cutaneous nerves, and sedative effect over nerve plexus
- Course vibrations provide stimulation to cutaneous nerves, stimulate peristalsis, decrease flatulence and increase expectoration
- Maintains muscular tone
- Loosens old scar tissues
- Increases peristalsis

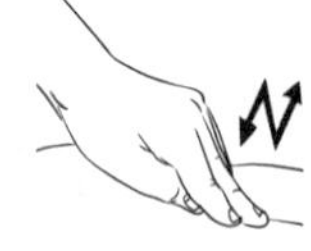

Shaking/Jostling refers to a back-and-forth type of vibration applied to muscle groups, limbs or torso with constant contact and physically shaking tissue. Jostling necessitates rapid shaking of a muscle back and forth, usually for a short period.

Application
- Grip limb securely and muscle group being shaken or jostled is held limply
- Movement is either steadily up and down or left to right
- Apply minor traction to limbs
- Shaking may be applied to abdomen

Indications	Contraindications
• Bronchitis and lung congestion • Muscle hypertonicity • Muscle guarding • Digestive disorders • Pre- and post-event athletic application	• Severe muscle spasm • Muscle atrophy accompanied by flaccid paralysis • Joint pathology • Maintain muscle or joint guarding

Physiologic Effects
- Helps to loosen mucus
- Encourages intestinal peristalsis
- Synovial fluid lubrication
- Reduces muscle guarding
- Motivates local circulation
- Brief duration stimulates nervous system and soft tissue
- Long duration has sedative effect

Skin Rolling is a type of petrissage motion in which cutaneous and subcutaneous tissues are held and lifted away from underlying tissues, then rolled between fingers with pressure towards the underlying structures

Application
- No oil
- Skin and underlying tissue is held between fingers of both hands and thumbs
- Fingers crawl down tissue and thumbs glide behind
- May be used in parallel, transversely, or indirectly with regard to tissue fiber direction

Indications		Contraindications
• Where cutaneous or subcutaneous adhesions have developed • Scar tissue formation • Overuse • Misuse • Prolonged absence of use	• Weak cutaneous circulation • Used to increase cutaneous and subcutaneous mobility • Improves range and fluidity of motion	• Hypersensitivity to pain • Increased histamine response • All local and general CIs

Physiologic Effects
- Releases adhered tissue in cutaneous and subcutaneous layers
- Stretching fascia lessens hypertonicity
- Decreases opposition to superficial lymph and venous flow
- Boosts lymphatic and venous return
- Enhances local skin temperature due to local hyperemia

MASSAGE STROKES

Compression refers to a form of downward pressure using therapist's thumbs, fingers, knuckles, forearms, hands, feet and elbows onto the subject's muscles. This is the primary method used in shiatsu, acupressure and pre- and post-sports massage treatments.

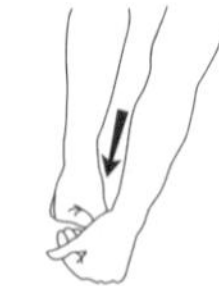

Application
- Lifting application stimulates muscle and nerve tissue
- Can be applied without lubricants or over clothing
- Broad and specific application can be controlled with varying pressures
- Excellent method for enhancing circulation

Indications	Contraindications
• Edema, muscle tension, pain control • Creates hyperemia for treating tenderness and trigger points • Palpation assessment • Lethargic circulation • Areas with body hair, without pulling the skin or the use of lubricants	• Over boney prominences • Unsupported tissues of the abdominal wall muscles • Quadratus lumborum which can injure the 12th rib • All local and general CIs

Physiologic Effects
- Stimulates muscle fibers and dilates capillaries
- Releases histamine and acetylcholine, both of which cause increased vasodilatation
- Accelerates healing and stimulates collagen production
- Bypasses tickle response and activates deep-touch receptors
- Increases the arterial blood flow and fluid exchange and decreases edema
- Rejuvenates fascia

Traction is a slow movement which involves drawing or pulling applied to a subject's body part. Traction can be applied to any part of the body or extremities.

Application
- Provides pulling force to cervical and lumbar spine
- Continuous traction is helpful for muscle relaxation
- Intermittent traction is used for the distraction of the spine

Indications	Contraindications
• Improves range of movement • Assists in relaxation of muscles	• Advanced age and severe osteoporosis • Disk herniation and spinal cord disease • Pregnancy • Active peptic ulcer • Untreated hypertension • All local and general CIs

Physiologic Effects
- Elongates muscles
- Stimulates proprioceptive receptors in ligaments and muscles

Musculotendinous Release is extending and softening muscles and their attachment sites.

Application
- Determine functional length
- Muscle in shortened position
- Administer to muscle belly before attachment, from origin to insertion or from most to least stable
- Apply frictions on short strokes at the attachment site
- Start frictions with longitudinal then progress to cross fiber, applying one direction at a time
- Work within client's tolerance for pain
- After treatment, reset neuromuscular feedback mechanisms with passive stretch and active range of motion

Indications	Contraindications
• Restriction of motion • Adhered, contracted muscles and attachment sites • Muscular hypertonicity • Previous injury • Overuse	• Edema • Tissue inflammation • Flaccid paralysis • Previous pathology sprain, strain, fractures • Onset of unusual symptoms, nausea, extreme pain

Physiologic Effects

- Reduces neuromuscular fixation from effect of muscular hypertonicity and irritability on attachment fiber

Myofascial Release is the stretching and releasing or unwinding of tight fascial layers that surround muscle and through a sustained pressure and gentle form of stretching that has a profound effect upon the body tissues. Myofascial release is a form of trigger point therapy consisting of strokes (rolling, shearing and stripping) which help the therapist find specific areas of trauma in connective tissues of muscle fibers. Most often feels like a smooth melting away of tightness or restriction in the muscles or "good hurt".

Application

- Muscle should be in neutral position
- Slower application is preferred
- No oil or lubrication is used
- Practictioners can use hands, knuckles, elbows, thumbs or other tools
- Use gradual application of technique, then stop and wait for release, holding from 90 seconds up to five minutes
- Basics steps include: feedback, stretch, hold, release, repeat and end-feel
- Pain should lessen with each application
- Stretching should be deep without force
- After treatment requires client to drink extra fluids

Indications	Contraindications
• Hardened scar tissue from trauma and tension • Adhesive fascia restriction due to postural abnormalities or immobilization • Joint restriction from immobilization • Areas can be contracted without putting strain to effected region • Painful complex postural asymmetries • Muscle weakness due to acute or chronic neuropathy	• Excessive hyperaemia or heat • Acute inflammation or inflammatory conditions • Patient that does not tolerate close contact or touch • Unhealed wounds, burns and acute skin conditions

Physiologic Effects

- Fascial tissue separated from adhered muscle fibers
- Restores tissue mobility
- Brings fresh fluids in and pushes toxic waste out
- Increases blood flow

MASSAGE STROKES

Types of myofascial release. Also referred to as unwinding, twist, or connective tissue massage.

	Rolling	Shearing	Stripping
Definition	• Skin rolling lifts deeper skin layers by physically picking tissue up and rolling it	• Sliding forces are applied to tissue and against the tissue that is causing restriction	• Deep thumb or fingers, palms, elbows, or forearms in stroking aimed at the deeper subdermal and muscle layers
Application	• Application to test fascia • Clasp tissue between index finger and thumbs to lift tissue off underlying tissue • Slowly roll through lifted tissue • Once fascia is flexible, move to other areas	• Contact is flat and broad in any direction • Once fascia is flexible, move to other areas	• Slow, moderate to deep, gliding stroke parallel to the fiber of the muscle, done passively or with movement of the muscle • Applied from origin to insertion to encourage elongation of the tissue • Once fascia is flexible, move to other areas
Effects	• Loosens fascia as it is picked up and rolled away from its surrounding tissue • Stabilizes and relaxes fascia	• Fascia tissue is separated from adhered muscle fibers • Stabilizes and relaxes fascia	• Fascial tissue is separated from adhered muscle fibers • Stretches little sections of myofascial tissue

Cross Fiber Friction is a method of massage used without oils or lubrication to evaluate and identify the specific tissue (muscle, tendon, ligament, etc.) causing an individual pain or dysfunctional movement.

Method
- Use reinforced thumb, index finger or knuckle, depending on client's tolerance for pain
- Taking the skin with it, allowing for the force to be transmitted directly to the deep tissue
- Use two to three cycles per second, for 5 to 10 minutes, in small movements
- Always stay within client's tolerance
- As client's tolerance increases, use increased pressure
- Can be followed up by some gentle stretching of the tissue and then icing

Frequency
- Two to three times a week for five to 10 treatments
- Treatment should not be performed on consecutive days to allow time for healing

Post-Treatment Considerations
- Ice Massage (up to 7 minutes)
- Inform clients of potential side-effects of soreness and mild bruising

Rationale
- This method promotes healing through proper remodeling by manually manipulating the tissues to both break down and form micro scar-tissue and promote circulation and decreasing collagen cross-linking, which will decrease adhesions and non-mobile scar formation. It separates ligament-to-bone adhesions and allows normal healing to occur and promotes the formation of properly aligned and mobile tissue.

Contraindications
- Don't use over acutely inflamed tissue due to trauma, open wounds or infection
- Deep friction should be avoided with clients on blood thiners or anticoagulants
- Avoid blood vessels that are large enough to feel a pulse on palpation
- Inflammatory arthritis, hematomas, calcification

Cautions and Contraindications for Massage

Always use good judgment in massage. If you are in any doubt, ask your client if he/she is under medical supervision or check with client's primary health care provider. Under certain medical conditions the therapist should request a written release from the health care provider prior to the treatment. Massage therapists often encounter situations when massage is inappropriate and should be avoided. While it is outside of your scope of practice to diagnose, you can still recognize the signs or symptoms. To this end, practitioners should always be wary of **contraindications:** specific situation in which a procedure should NOT be used, because it may cause harm. This stands in distinction from situations that merit **caution**: when a practitioner may proceed with the treatment but should modify techniques, pressure, and locations of treatment. Caution should be adjusted accordingly with the severity of open wound, fever, infection, inflammation, varicosity, nerve or tissue damage or clients under certain medical conditions.

Contraindications

Local contraindication – a situation in which a local area of the client's body should not be massaged under any circumstances to avoid spreading infection or to avoid further injury. *(acute inflammation, broken bone, recent surgery, inflammation of the skin, varicosities, local contagious conditions, open wound, local irritable skin conditions, undiagnosed lumps, acute lesions, malignancy over sites of active cancer, skin infection, tumor, rheumatoid arthritis, burns, and phlebitis)*

Total Contraindications – a situation in which no massage at all is appropriate. (*burns, infectious disease, anaphylaxis reaction, appendicitis CVAs, insulin shock, diabetic coma or complications, epileptic seizure, myocardial infarction, pneumothorax, severe asthmatic attack, syncope, acute pneumonia, kidney failure, respiratory failure, liver failure, eclampsia, hemophilia, hemorrhage, DVT, arthrosclerosis, hypertension, medical shock, high fever, certain cancers, and infectious conditions)*

- **High temperature & Fever:** High temperature and fever indicates a systemic infection introduced by an invading pathogen which the body is trying to isolate and eliminate. Therefore increasing overall circulation with massage would work against the body's immune defenses and exacerbate the condition.
- **Inflammation:** Avoid massaging over localized areas of inflammation, since irritation will further aggravate inflamed areas. As a general rule of thumb, you can recognize inflamed conditions as anything that ends in the suffix "–itis," such as dermatitis (inflammation of the skin), arthritis (inflammation of the joints), and so forth. It should be noted that in the case of localized inflammation massage can be given in surrounding areas but should not be administered directly.
- **Skin problems**: Skin infections such as rashes, fungal infections, wounds, bruises, burns, boils, and blisters should be avoided. These conditions are often localized, in which case the surrounding areas can be massaged.
- **Infectious diseases:** If clients are coming down with the cold or flu, massage can potentially exacerbate the spreading infection and expose the practitioner to the virus. It should thus be avoided in these situations.
- **Hernia:** Hernias (protrusion of an organ or any part of the organ through a muscular wall) present potentially harmful situations for massage. It is thus not advisable to try to push against the organs as it should be treated by surgery or inspected by a physician.
- **Osteoporosis:** Osteoporosis (when bones become porous, brittle, and fragile) presents a similar danger to recipients of massage. It should thus always be considered when administering, especially to elderly clients. Affected areas should be avoided.
- **Varicose veins:** Deep massage over varicose veins can be extremely painful and worsen the problem. Consult with a client if encountered. It should be noted, however, that applying light, directional massage toward the heart can be very beneficial.
- **Blood clot:** DVT is the formation of a blood clot in the deep vein usually found in the legs. Massaging over a thrombosis can potentially cause clots and displace the clot to other areas of the body which could induce a stroke or heart attack.
- **Broken bones:** Areas of mending bones should be avoided altogether. However, tender massage in surrounding areas is considered beneficial in some cases. Consult with the subject if such an area is encountered.
- **Other conditions and diseases**: Asthma, hemophilia, diabetes, and other serious conditions each entail its own series of precautionary steps and treatment. It is thus critical that you seek a health care provider's opinion before administering massage.
- **High blood pressure:** For treated, borderline or mild high blood pressure massage can be beneficial; however, untreated or severe high blood pressure places extra pressure against blood vessel walls and increase susceptibility to clotting. Massage affects the blood vessels, and so people with high blood pressure or a heart condition should receive light, sedating massages, if anything at all.

Massage Oils for Use

As you choose your massage oil, you need to be clear about what you need. Some massage oils may have unpleasant smells while others may cause irritation to your skin. Also, some massage oils are better for dehydrated skin, dry or mature skin or specific skin types and while some oils can be used on all skin types. Once you know the skin type that you are dealing with, it is possible to choose massage oil from the many that are available.

Massage oils that are thicker are good for use during cold weather while those that are light are good for use during warm weather. All these factors and many more go a long way in determining the massage oil that you choose. In addition, for people with oily skins, very thick massage oils may make them feel uncomfortable and it will be better for them to use the lighter massage oils.

On the other hand, almond massage oil is rather greasy and thus better used with a skin type that is dry or for purposes of moisturizing during dry weather. Always remember that your massage oil does not have to be expensive for it to produce the results that you need. Look at the ingredients of your massage oil to ensure that it does not have anything that you are sensitive to. If you notice anything that you are sensitive to, then that should tell that the given massage oil is not the best for you and you should seek other alternatives.

Oil	Use
Almond oil	Almond oil is the most popular massage oil due to its slightly oily but not greasy consistency. Although it spreads easily, it also has enough staying power so that reapplication is often not necessary. It is an effective moisturizer and softens, smoothes, and nourishes the skin. Almond oil is reasonably priced, readily available, and does not usually irritate the skin (should be avoided by those who are allergic to nuts). Its aroma is light, slightly sweet and nutty, and it can be used alone or as carrier oil.
Grape seed oil	Grape seed oil is rich in linoleic acid, an essential fatty acid that is vital to the skin and cell membranes. It is a non-greasy oil that can be used undiluted and is safe for use with all skin types. It can also be blended with other carriers like almond or wheat germ oil. Grapeseed oil has a nutty aroma and is rich in vitamins and minerals that help to restructure and moisturize the skin.
Apricot oil	Apricot oil is rich in both oleic and linoleic acid, essential fatty acids that are vital to the skin and cell membranes. It is especially helpful for very dry, dehydrated, or delicate skin. Apricot oil is a finely textured oil that spreads easily. It also has cooling properties that may be used to reduce inflammation.
Avocado oil	Avocado oil is a heavier oil that is usually mixed with other carrier oils such as almond or grape seed oil. It is usually used on individuals who have very dry or mature skin or who are suffering from eczema, psoriasis, or other skin-related problems. It can also be helpful in regenerating skin and softening the tissue after sun or climate damage. Avocado oil is more expensive than other lighter carrier oils and may irritate the skin of individuals who are sensitive to latex.
Jojoba oil	Jojoba oil is derived from the seeds of the jojoba plant. It is often used as carrier oil in aromatherapy treatments since it penetrates the skin easily. Its makeup resembles the skin and for this reason it can be used on almost all skin types. Because jojoba oil has some antibacterial properties, it is often used on individuals who have back acne or blemished skin. It has a silky texture and is rapidly absorbed, so it may need to be reapplied throughout a session; it also is more expensive than other nut oils. Thus it is often mixed with other carrier oils to make its use more effective and economical. Jojoba oil is an effective moisturizer and it has a long shelf life, so it is a good selection if it is not going to be used very often.
Wheat germ oil	Wheat germ oil is too sticky and thick to use on its own, but when blended with other carrier oils it is very effective. It is rich in vitamin E and other essential fatty acids and thus is used extensively in aromatherapy massage blends. It has been said to rejuvenate the skin, promote the formation of new cells, stimulate tissue regeneration, improve circulation, help repair sun damage, promote smoother and younger-looking skin, assist in healing scar tissue and stretch marks, and help relieve the symptoms of dermatitis. It is also said to have some antioxidant properties.
Hazelnut oil	Hazelnut oil is finely textured and has strong moisturizing qualities. It helps to tone and tighten the skin. It also helps to strengthen capillaries and assists in cell regeneration (should be avoided by those who are allergic to nuts).
Holy oil	Holy oil is an excellent carrier oil due to its unique molecular structure which allows it to carry essential oils deep into the skin. It is non-greasy, odorless and hypoallergenic. Holy oil spreads easily on any part of the body.

Oil	Use
Sunflower oil	Sunflower oil is a light, non-greasy oil that is rich in linoleic acid, palmitic acid, and stearic acids, important components of healthy skin. The amount of linoleic acid in skin declines with age, and can be stripped by commercial soaps, cosmetics, and cleansers; using sunflower oil helps to mitigate the effects of this decline. Adding vitamin E capsules to a bottle of sunflower oil and storing it in a cool, dark place can prolong its relatively short shelf life. Sunflower oil should be avoided by individuals who have allergies to the sunflower plant family.
Shea butter	Shea butter has a heavy, oily texture and is normally blended for massage or used on very small areas. It is extracted from a tree native to Africa and is a solid at room temperature. Shea contains a natural latex, so individuals who are allergic to latex may want to avoid its use.
Sesame oil	Sesame oil is a thick, strong-smelling oil that is often blended with lighter massage oils. It is prized in Ayurveda and is used in a daily Ayurvedic self-massage called abhyanga, as well as in shirodhara. It is used in to nourish and detoxify and for ailments associated with the Ayurvedic massage.

Massage Lotions, Creams and Gels for Use

As you choose your lotion, cream or gel, make sure your products are fresh. Massage oils, lotions, gels and creams do have a shelf life and will expire. Some products last longer than others and some are highly sensitive and should be stored in a dry and cool environment. There are a lot of different types of products on the market, hypo-allergenic to herbal blends. Some lotions will be better suited with a bottle pump or an applicator, others are better suited for mixture and blends. If you find that your lotion has a thick viscosity, add a little heat to thin it out. Some massage lotions are fragrant-free and some infused with essential oils, while other non-hypo-allergenic blends may cause irritation to your skin. Also, some massage lotions will be used with specific skin types, dehydrated, dry or mature skin types. Once you know the skin type that you are dealing with, it is possible to choose a massage lotion from the many that are available. Avoid products that contain high levels of parabens and synthetic ingredients which can be harmful to client's skin and can cause toxic exposure to the therapist after repeated use.

It is important to match the type of massage oil, cream, or lotion with the goals of the massage. Of the three types of lubricants, massage lotions provide the shortest glide and most absorption. These qualities make it ideal for deeper tissue work. The right type of lotion can minimize excessive drag on the skin, thus providing the greatest working grip and allowing the therapist to penetrate deeper into their client's muscles. Most lotions are blended with some forms of oils (sweet almond, sunflower, grapeseed) to develop a special texture without the feeling of being greasy.

Massage gels are a combination of an oil and a lotion and are ideal lubricants for light to semi-deep work. They tend to work well for clients with excessive body hair. Because of the viscosity of the gel, you are able to slide over hair and dry skin with less resistance, but it can be unsuitable for deeper work. One benefit of using gel is it offers the same workability as a high-quality massage oil in a similar light formula that moisturizes the skin at the same time. A small amount of massage gel will cover a larger surface area, plus it doesn't absorb into the skin quickly, which allows a prolonged massage. Massage gel nourishes the skin and refrains from leaving a greasy feeling after the massage. You can also blend your favorite lotion and oil together to create a gel that works best for you.

Massage creams are great to work with for all types of clients. Creams are thicker than lotions and cannot be used with a pump bottle. For sanitary purposes, you should always use a new cup or jar for each client. Since you use your fingers to scoop out the cream, any lotion remaining following that appointment should be discarded.

A listing of massage equipment suppliers and manufacturers/distributors who supply lotions, gels, creams and oils are available on page 394.

This table lists some of the more commonly used oils and their properties.

Oils	Properties
Basil	Aids concentration, clarity and helps fight colds, influenza and headaches.
Bergamot	A balancing and uplifting stress-relieving oil. Lifts depression and melancholy.
Cedarwood	An antiseptic, expectorant, astringent, and sedative. Normalizes sweat gland function. Good for bronchial problems and useful for controlling mildew and molds.
Chamomile	An analgesic, anti-inflammatory, and antispasmodic. Relieves muscular pain, as a sedative, which calms the mind and eases fear, eases anxiety, emotional stress, nervous tension, and insomnia. Excellent for headaches. A good remedy for gastrointestinal problems.
Cinnamon Bark	A useful scent enhancement in the home or office which makes a good air freshener and has antifungal properties.
Clary Sage	An aromatic oil that is used for healing eye problems. An antidepressant, anti-inflammatory, antispasmodic, and aphrodisiac. Helps relieve insomnia, menopause, PMS, and nervous exhaustion. Caution: Should not be used in the first months of pregnancy.
Cypress	An astringent, antiseptic, antispasmodic oil which is soothing and eases aches and pains and coughs. Used to increase circulation, relieve muscular cramps, bronchitis, whooping cough, painful periods, reduce nervous tension and other stress-related problems. Acts as an immune stimulant. Reduces coughing and excessive perspiration.
Eucalyptus	An antiseptic, antiviral chest rub, decongestant, and expectorant. Reduces fever, relieves congestion, muscle aches and asthma. Has a normalizing and balancing effect.
Frankincense	An anti-inflammatory, antiseptic, sedative and expectorant. Promotes cellular regeneration and elevates mind and spirit. Good to calm by slowing down breathing and controlling tension, it helps to focus the mind, enhance meditation, help breathing, and psychic cleansing. Also excellent for toning and caring for mature/aging skin.
Ginger	A fiery and fortifying oil used for massaging on the muscles and for nausea and sickness.
Geranium	An antidepressant, anti-diabetic, antiseptic, hormone balancer and insect repellant. A normalizing and balancing, flowery aroma which is both uplifting and calming oil good for PMS, hormone balancing, nervous tension, skin concerns, and neuralgia. Good as bath additive and in skin-care products for both its fragrance and cleansing properties.
Grapefruit	A citrus smell which is energizing and helps to elevate the spirits, reduces appetite and useful in treating obesity. Balances mood, relieves muscle fatigue, lifts depression, cleanses the body of toxins, reduces water retention, and detoxifies the skin.
Hyssop	An antiseptic, antidepressant, and sedative which promotes alertness and clarity of thought. Useful for anxiety, emotional imbalances, frigidity, and impotence. Benefits scalp and skin.
Jasmine	An antidepressant, aphrodisiac, antiseptic, and sedative which is emotionally warming, relaxing, soothing, uplifting and helps self confidence. Useful for anxiety, emotional imbalances, frigidity, and impotence. Benefits scalp and skin.
Juniper	An antiseptic, detoxifier, diuretic and internal cleanser which exerts a cleansing effect on the mental and spiritual planes as well as on the physical. Helps rid body of toxins and parasites, reduces spasms, improve arthritis and reduces cellulite. Caution: Do not use during pregnancies. Do not use if you have kidney problems.
Lavender	An overall first aid oil, antiviral and antibacterial, boosts immunity, antidepressant, anti-inflammatory, and antispasmodic which is relaxing and refreshing, uplifts the spirits, and helps to relieve the distress of muscle pain. Useful for improving immune system function, calming and normalizing the body fighting bacterial and fungal infect, easing depression and reducing inflammation. Good for acne, burns, eczema, skin healing, sleep disorders, and stress.
Lemon	An antiseptic, antibacterial, and astringent. Helps to increase the body's defenses against infections. Refreshing and uplifting for purification of the body. Good for varicose veins, stomach ulcers, anxiety depression and digestive disorders. Emulsifies and disperses grease and oil. Helpful in cleaning product and hair rinses and wound cleansing.
Lemongrass	An antiseptic and astringent oil which is refreshing, cleansing and stimulating body tonic. Serves as a good refreshing and deodorizing room fragrance.
Linden	A calming, sedating and soothing tonic. Moisturizes the skin.
Marjoram, sweet	A calming, soothing and warming effect on mind, body and spirit. It helps relieve common colds, including congestion and muscle aches and pains, and is also comforting in times of stress. Used to regulate the nervous system and treat insomnia.
Orange	Balances and uplifts emotions. Has an antispasmodic and regenerative property. Useful in skin-care products. Caution: This oil increases sensitivity to the sun. Do not use if you are spending considerable time outdoors.
Patchouli	An aphrodisiac used in personal fragrances to relieve stress and nervous exhaustion. Good for dry skin and athlete's foot. Has antidepressant, anti-inflammatory, antiseptic, aphrodisiac and anti-fungal properties.
Peppermint	An antiseptic, antispasmodic, mental stimulant and has regenerative properties which is energizing, penetrating, minty, and aromatic oil helpful for brightening moods, reduces pain, improves mental clarity, and memory. Good for headaches, congestion, fatigue, fever, indigestion, muscle soreness, sinus problems and stomach problems.
Pine	A refreshing and cleansing immune system stimulant which acts as an antiseptic, antiviral, expectorant, restorative, and stimulate. Helps to clear the mind. Repels lice and fleas.
Rose	An antidepressant, antiseptic, and tonic astringent which is soothing and cleansing oil which uplifts the spirit. Acts as a mild sedative. Good for female complaints, impotence, insomnia, and nervousness.
Rosemary	The ideal "pick you up" oil which is an antiseptic, antispasmodic, astringent, and mental stimulant. Enhances circulation. Energizing for muscle pains, cramps or sprains, brightens mood, for improving mental clarity and memory. Helpful for cellulite, dandruff, hair loss, memory problems, headache, and sore muscles. Caution: if irritation occurs, discontinue use. Do not use directly on the skin without diluting. Use caution if inhaling it if you have asthma or bronchitis. Do not use if you have epilepsy.
Rosewood	An antiseptic and regenerative. Helps relieve stress and balance the central nervous system. Calms and helps restore emotional balance. Good for jet lag, anxiety, cellular regeneration, depression headaches, nausea, PMS, and tension.
Sandalwood	An antidepressant, antiseptic, expectorant, aphrodisiac, and skin moisturizer. Lifts melancholy, enhances meditation, heals the skin, calms and reduces stress. Good for bronchitis and nervousness; it is soothing for both mind and body.
Tea Tree	A powerful, anti-infective, anti-inflammatory, antiseptic, antiviral, expectorant, antifungal, and anti-parasitic used as a cleansing agent. Powerful immuno-stimulant properties especially against bacteria and viruses. Good for athletes, foot, bronchial congestion, dandruff, ringworm, and yeast infection.
Thyme	An antiseptic, antispasmodic, and expectorant. Calming.
Yarrow	An anti-inflammatory and antispasmodic. Improves digestion and lowers blood pressure. Similar in function to chamomile
Ylang yiang	Antidepressant, antiseptic, aphrodisiac, and calming sedatives. Lifts mood, relieves anger, eases anxiety, relaxes muscles, reduces stress, normalizes the heartbeat, and lowers blood pressure. Good for frigidity, high blood pressure and impotence.

There are many different essential oils available, each with its own special properties. This table lists some of the more commonly used oils for common conditions.

Conditions	Oils
Allergies	Roman Chamomile, Lavender, Myrrh
Arthritis	Birch, Ginger, Juniper, Lavender, Marjoram
Asthma	Cypress, Frankincense, Lavender, Peppermint, Eucalyptus
Bacterial & Fungal Infections	Oregano, Tea Tree, Lemon, Eucalyptus, Niaouli, Lavender
Bone Breaks, Dislocation & Damage	Eucalyptus, Chamomile, Lavender
Bronchitis	Eucalyptus, Fir, Pine, Tea Tree, Niaouli, White Thyme, Myrtle
Burns & Sunburns	Lavender, Chamomile, Niaouli
Bruising	Lavender, Roman Chamomile, Myrtle
Candida	Tea Tree, Lemongrass, Marjoram, Myrrh, Niaouli
Cellulite	Fennel, Juniper, Lemon
Circulation (Poor)	Cypress, Lemongrass, Ginger
Colds, Flu	Eucalyptus, Lavender, Pine, Fir, Myrtle
Cold Sores	Lemon, Chamomile, Tea Tree, Lavender
Cystitis	Birch, Cedarwood, Juniper, Cypress, Lavender
Digestion (Poor)	Anise, Fennel, Ginger, Lemongrasss, Nutmeg, Pepper
Ear Problems	Chamomile, Lavender, Tea Tree, Niaouli, Marjoram, Juniper
Fatigue	Caraway Seed, Clove Bud, Cypress, Peppermint
Hair Loss	Cedarwood, Sage
Hair (Oily)	Sage, Lemon, Neroli, Cedarwood
Headaches	German Chamomile, Lavender, Peppermint, Cedarwood
Hemorrhoids	Cypress, Myrtle, Juniper, Myrrh
Immune System (Low)	Lemon, Tea Tree, Angelica, Niaouli
Inflammation	Blue and German Chamomile, Patchouli, Myrrh, Frankincense
Insomnia	Neroli, Marjoram, Tangerine, Lavender, Chamomile
Jet Lag	Melissa, Angelica, Peppermint, Ginger, Lemon
Laryngitis	Chamomile, Lavender, Lemon, Cypress, Lemongrass, Myrrh
Menopause	Clary, Chamomile, Fennel, Sage, Rose, Jasmine
Menstrual Pain (Light Periods)	Chamomile, Lavender, Marjoram, Clary Sage, Cypress
Menstrual Pain (Heavy Periods)	Chamomile, Lavender, Cypress, Marjoram
Migraine	Peppermint, Chamomile, Lavender, Marjoram, Angelica
Muscle & Tendon Damage	Eucalyptus, Peppermint, Ginger, Lavender, Chamomile
Nausea	Peppermint, Spearmint, Ginger
Obesity	Fennel, Lemon, Ginger, Peppermint, Cardamom
Pain (Muscular)	Birch, Chamomile, Clove, Ginger, Pepper, Lavender, Nutmeg
Post Operative Care	Chamomile, Lavender, Niaouli,
Rheumatism	Birch, Juniper, Chamomile, Lavender, Pine
Sinusitis	Lavender, Eucalyptus, Peppermint, Angelica, Myrtle, Tea Tree
Snoring	Myrtle, Marjoram, Lavender
Soft Tissue Damage	Chamomile, Lavender, Eucalyptus, Ginger
Sore Throat	Ginger, Myrrh, Pine, Eucalyptus, Tea Tree, Lemongrass
Sprains	Ginger, Nutmeg, Clove, Peppermint
Stretch Marks	Rose, Lavender, Tangerine, Neroli
Urinary Infections	Cedarwood, Juniper, Tea Tree, Myrtle
Varicose Veins	Cypress, Lemon, Peppermint, Lavender
Water Retention	Cypress, Orange, Juniper, Lemon
Wounds	Lavender, Fir, Tea Tree, Myrrh

TOPICAL APPLICATIONS

Massage products like topical analgesics, medicated oils, analgesic balms, and medicated plasters to support work on sore muscles, old injuries, as well as body aches and pains are commonly used by acupuncturist, herbalist, and alternative practitioner. Many of these products can be found online or through Chinese herbal pharmacies found in most Chinatowns in urban areas. The following list of products can be used with massage therapy for post and pre-treatment with great success.

Product	Indication	Notes
ABC Plaster	Injuries, aches and pains	Hot
Anti-Rheumatic Plaster (Tientsin Drug)	Re-injured joints or other tissues	Aromatic
Axe brand oil	Injuries, aches and pains	Warm
Bao Zhen Gao/ Shang Yao Plasters	Injuries, aches and pains	Warm
Chili Plasters	Injuries, aches and pains	Hot
Ching Wan Hung (Great Wall)	Abrasions, cuts, and open wounds	Best burn cream, heals tissue, can be applied to open wounds to reduce scarring, and heals bleeding hemorrhoids
Compound Prescribed Watermelon Frost (Guilin)	Abrasions, cuts, and open wounds	For non-healing or infected open wounds with redness and swelling
Dit Dat Jow	Tissue damage from trauma, strains, tears, contusions, and bruises	Good at tissue repair and healing burns, stopping bleeding, reducing pain and swelling as well as long term wound care. Based on formula Qi Li San, or Die Da Wan
Die Da Wan Hua (Jingxiutang Pharm.)	Tissue damage from trauma, strains, tears, contusions, and bruises	Good on burns
Die-Da Analgesic Essence (China National)	Tissue damage from trauma, strains, tears, contusions, and bruises	
Dr. Bob's Medicated oil (Blue Poppy)	Injuries, aches and pains	Warm to neutral
Dr. Shir's Liniment (Spring Wind brand)	Joint strain or sprain	
Dragon Fire Liniment (Oriental Herb Co.)	Injuries, aches and pains	Hot
Dragon's Blood Liniment (Blue Poppy)	Tissue damage from trauma, strains, tears, contusions, and bruises	For swelling and pain when there is no redness or heat
E Mei Shan Plasters	Injuries, aches and pains	Warm
Eagle oil	Over-worked, exhausted muscles, general after-workout soreness and pain	Strong pain reliever
Essential Balm	Over-worked, exhausted muscles, general after-workout soreness and pain	
Fast Patch (Wei Labs)	Tissue damage from trauma, strains, tears, contusions, and bruises	Long term use plaster for healing injuries
Felursa Plaster For Bruise (Zhanjiang)	Tissue damage from trauma, strains, tears, contusions, and bruises	
Feng Liu Sing Tincture	Tissue damage from trauma, strains, tears, contusions, and bruises	Warm
Flower oil (Shanghai medicines)	Injuries, aches and pains	Warm to neutral
Golden sunshine patches/ spray cream	Over-worked, exhausted muscles, general after-workout soreness and pain	Cool
Green Willow liniment (Blue Poppy)	Injuries, aches and pains	Hot
Hua To's Eight Immortal's Iron Palm (Oriental Herb Co.)	Tissue damage from trauma, strains, tears, contusions, and bruises	Designed for training as well as injury
Hua To's Eight Immortals Dit Da Jow (Oriental herb Co.)	Tissue damage from trauma, strains, tears, contusions, and bruises	For post trauma healing
Hua Tuo Plasters (Kwang Chow United)	Injuries, aches and pains	
Huo Lu Medicated Oil (East West USA)	Tissue damage from trauma, strains, tears, contusions, and bruises	
Huo Tuo Plasters (Jingxiutang Pharm.)	Injuries, aches and pains	Warm
Imperial Phoenix (Oriental Herb Co.)	Tissue damage from trauma, strains, tears, contusions, and bruises	Training formula, hot

Product	Indication	Notes
Iron Fist Liniment (Oriental Herb Co.)	Tissue damage from trauma, strains, tears, contusions, and bruises	Designed for training as well as injury
Iron Hand Liniment (East Earth)	Tissue damage from trauma, strains, tears, contusions, and bruises	Designed for training as well as injury
Jade Goddess (Oriental Herb Co.)	Tissue damage from trauma, strains, tears, contusions, and bruises	Training formula, tissue repair, cooling
Joseph's Si Chi Pain relieving oil	Over-worked, exhausted muscles, general after-workout soreness and pain	
King Care Arthritis Pain Formula	Injuries, aches and pains	Warm
King Care Original Formula	Over-worked, exhausted muscles, general after-workout soreness and pain	
King Care Sports Pain Formula	Over-worked, exhausted muscles, general after-workout soreness and pain	
Kou Pi Analgesic Plasters (Tientsin Drug)	Injuries, aches and pains	Warm
Kou Pi Analgesic Plasters (Beijing Tung Jen Tang)	Injuries, aches and pains	Warm
Kupico Plaster (Great Wall Brand)	Re-injured joints or other tissues	Aromatic
Kwan Loong	Injuries, aches and pains	Warm to neutral, also indicated for itching
Mao She Xiang San Xiong Dan Rheumatic oil (Kwangchow)	Injuries, aches and pains	Warm
Mopiko	Over-worked, exhausted muscles, general after-workout soreness and pain	Indicated for pain as well as itch from insect bites and eczema
Musk Anti-Contusion Plasters (Tianjin Drug)	Re-injured joints or other tissues	Aromatic
Musk plaster (Jingxiutang Pharm)	Re-injured joints or other tissues	Aromatic
Musk Rheumatic oil (Guangdong Medicines)	1. Re-injured joints or other tissues 2. Injuries, aches and pains	Aromatic and warm
Musk Rheumatism-Expelling Plasters (Guilin Fourth Pharm.)	Re-injured joints or other tissues	Aromatic
Ni Tian/Yee Tin Tong Oil	Joint strain or sprain	
Notoginseng Herbal Analgesic Liniment	Over-worked, exhausted muscles, general after-workout soreness and pain	Camphor free
Notoginseng Herbal Analgesic Liniment (Guangxi Med.)	Injuries, aches and pains	Warm to neutral
Po Sum On	Injuries, aches and pains	Warm to neutral, good massage oil for sore muscles
Porous Capsicum Plaster	Injuries, aches and pains	Hot
Red Dragon Balm	Injuries, aches and pains	Warm
Salonpas Plasters	Injuries, aches and pains	Warm to neutral, focused on pain
San qi powder	Bleeding, external and internal, severe bruising	
Shang Shi Bao Zhen Medicated Plaster (Shanghai Med. Works)	Re-injured joints or other tissues	Aromatic and warm
Shaolin Dee Dat Jow (Blue Poppy)	Tissue damage from trauma, strains, tears, contusions, and bruises	For acute injury with redness and swelling
Sprain Ointment (Blue Poppy)	Joint strain or sprain	
Spring Wind Herbal Muscle and Joint rub (Spring Wind)	Joint strain or sprain	
Stop Pain (Blue Poppy)	Over-worked, exhausted muscles, general after-workout soreness and pain	
Three Angels Liniment (Blue Poppy)	Red painful muscles and joints due to chronic injury, rheumatoid arthritis, gout	Cool - red painful muscles & joints due to chronic Injury, rheumatoid arthritis, gout

TOPICAL APPLICATIONS

Product	Indication	Notes
Tie Bi (Oriental Herb Co.)	Tissue damage from trauma, strains, tears, contusions, and bruises	Training formula, cooling
Tieh Ta Yao Gin (Chu Kiang Brand)	Tissue damage from trauma, strains, tears, contusions, and bruises	Great on severe bruises
Tieh Ta Yao Gin (United Pharm.)	Tissue damage from trauma, strains, tears, contusions, and bruises	
Tieh Ta Yao Jiu (Five Photos brand)	1. Abrasions, cuts, and open wounds 2. Tissue damage from trauma, strains, tears, contusions, and bruises	Great on "Qi burn" and abrasions
Tien chi powder	Bleeding, external and internal, severe bruising	
Tiger Balm Red	1. Injuries, aches and pains 2. Over-worked, exhausted muscles, general after-workout soreness and pain	Warm
Tiger balm white	Over-worked, exhausted muscles, general after-workout soreness and pain	
Tokhuon Plasters	Injuries, aches and pains	Warm
Wan Hua Oil (United Pharm)	1. Tissue damage from trauma, strains, tears, contusions, and bruises 2. Abrasions, cuts, and open wounds	Good for hard swellings, burns, necrotic wounds
White Dragon Balm	Over-worked, exhausted muscles, general after-workout soreness and pain	
White Flower oil	Over-worked, exhausted muscles, general after-workout soreness and pain	Cool
White Tiger Liniment (Oriental Herb Co.)	Red painful muscles and joints due to chronic injury, rheumatoid arthritis, gout	Cool - red painful muscles & joints due to chronic Injury, rheumatoid arthritis, gout
White Patch (Wei Labs)	Injuries, aches and pains	Warm
Wood lock oil	Over-worked, exhausted muscles, general after-workout soreness and pain	
Wu yang Plaster for bruise	Tissue damage from trauma, strains, tears, contusions, and bruises	Better than ice on acute injuries
Xi Shang Le Ding (Pham. Factory of TCM)	Joint strain or sprain	
Xin Fang Shang Shi Bao Zhen Gao Plasters (Shanghai Med. Works)	Injuries, aches and pains	Warm
Yang Cheng Medicated Herbal Plaster	Tissue damage from trauma, strains, tears, contusions, and bruises	Similar to Wu Yang brand
Yun Xiang Jin	Injuries, aches and pains	Warm
Yun Xiang Jing liniment (Yulin)	Injuries, aches and pains	Hot
Yunnan Baiyao liniment	Over-worked, exhausted muscles, general after-workout soreness and pain	
Yunnan Baiyao Plasters	Over-worked, exhausted muscles, general after-workout soreness and pain	
Yunnan Baiyao Powder,	1. Bleeding, external and internal, severe bruising 2. Abrasions, cuts, and open wounds	The stop-bleeding formula, open wounds
Zheng Gu Shui (Yulin Drug)	1. Joint strain or sprain 2. Re-injured joints or other tissues	Aromatic. "Heal bone water". Great on any joint pain including carpel tunnel, overuse soreness and tennis elbow. Apply to feet before standing for hours.
Zhitong Gao/ Shang Yao Plasters	Injuries, aches and pains	Warm

Effects and Benefits of Massage

There are many theories that have been proposed for how massage works its healing wonders. There's no denying the power of bodywork, as we journey down the path to see its effect on people that we touch. Regardless of the adjectives we assign to it (pampering, rejuvenating, therapeutic) or the reasons we seek it out (a luxurious treat, stress relief, pain management), massage therapy can be a powerful ally in health and well-being. It's important to understand the benefits of massage beyond relaxation and stress relief by educating clients on its physiological and psychological effects and benefits. There is clinical evidence that the effects and benefits enhance general health and well-being and its specific therapeutic effects should not be oversimplified. Not only affecting the obvious – the soft tissues (the muscles, tendons, and ligaments) and improved muscle tone. Although massage therapy affects those muscles just under the skin, its benefits may also reach the deeper layers of muscle and include physiological and psychological effects on the body. Consequently, the medical community is actively embracing bodywork, and massage is becoming an integral part of healthcare and well-being.

Research continues to show the enormous benefits of receiving massage, ranging from treating chronic diseases, neurological disorders and injuries, to alleviating the tensions of modern lifestyles. A massage increases metabolism, hastens healing, relaxes and refreshes the muscles, and improves the detoxifying function of the lymphatic system. Massage helps to prevent and relieve muscle cramps and spasms and improves circulation of blood and lymph. The delivery of oxygen and nutrients to the cells can increase and enhance the removal of metabolic waste.

One of the beneficial effects of pressure applied to the skin is the stimulation of the sensory receptors, which in turn provides general relaxation, body awareness, and pain reduction. Application of different massage strokes such as light rubbing, rolling and wringing movement during massage stimulates nerves. This, in turn, increases body heat, which promotes perspiration and increases sebaceous excretions. This suggests that there is an increase in metabolic rate. Tapotement applied to the body as light tapping, slapping, and beating movements increases nervous irritability. Strong tapotement for a short period of time excites nerve centers directly. Prolonged percussion tends to anesthetize the local nerves. Vibration by shaking, trembling, rocking or quivering movements stimulates peripheral nerves and all nerve centers with which a nerve trunk is connected. Furthermore, massage can assist the skin in the process of respiration, the exchanging of carbon dioxide and oxygen.

Massage can also provide physiological benefits to people with anxiety, emotional frustrations, and mental fatigue which exacerbate stress. Modern-day stress causes the release of hormones that create vasoconstriction and reduce circulation, making the heart work harder to facilitate optimal organ function. Manual therapy using a restorative and invigorating pace, varied rhythm in a shorter session assists in the release of endorphins, which will reduce stress to the central nervous system. Benefits such as mental alertness and clarity are related by increased sensory stimulation and circulation. The relaxation response is activated by the "fight or flight" parasympathetic nervous system, which brings balance to back into the body.

Specific health benefits of the relaxation response are as follows:

- Increased levels of serotonin which protects against depression
- Reduced stress and tension
- Increased endorphin levels
- Decreased oxygen consumption and metabolic rate, thus less strain on the body's energy resources
- Relieves chronic and temporary pain
- Eases medication dependency
- Increased intensity and frequency of alpha brain waves associated with deep relaxation
- Promotes tissue regeneration and reduces scar tissue and stretch marks
- Reduced blood lactates, blood substances associated with anxiety
- Significantly decreased blood pressure in hypertensive individuals
- Reduced heart rate and slower respiration
- Decreased muscle tension
- Increased blood circulation to arms and legs
- Enhanced immunity by stimulating lymphatic flow
- Decreased anxiety, fears, and phobias, and increased positive mental health
- Reduces post-surgery adhesions and swelling

Massage can provide benefits for everyone. The more frequent the visits, the more benefits received. This is the beauty of massage therapy. Just because massage feels like a pampering treat doesn't mean it is any less therapeutic. The focus of practitioners should include education on the benefits and provide managed health care utilizing techniques and principles learned in massage school and in our daily practice.

Acupressure and Shiatsu

Acupressure is a healing approach that uses physical pressure points on the surface of the skin to stimulate the body's natural means of curing itself. Its principles are similar to those of acupuncture and Traditional Chinese Medicine, (TCM) and it works without use of the acupuncture needles to stimulate specific reflex points located along 14 meridians, the lines of energy which run throughout the body. Shiatsu is a Japanese word made up of two written characters meaning finger (shi) and pressure (atsu) it uses finger and palm pressure to energize pathways called meridians in order to enhance the flow of qi (vitality, stamina and energy), sharing the principles of acupressure and TCM.

There are many legends about the origins of the meridian system and the acupressure points found along the meridians. One story is that the meridians were discovered by observing soldiers who were wounded by arrows and spears and recovered from ailments in other parts of their bodies. Trial and error over many centuries evolved into a refined and detailed clinical methodology based on this system of correspondences, traced to Chinese medicine, and *The Yellow Emperors' Classic of Internal Medicine*. Another tale holds that sages were able to map the pathways of energy transmission in the body while they were in heightened states of meditation.

Whatever the origins, the recording of these observations over the centuries led to a very sophisticated mapping which Chinese Taoist monks formalized into the meridian system. These systems and treatment was later introduced to Japan by Chinese monks and integrated into their existing massage techniques, known as anma massage. Thus the terms "acupressure and shiatsu" are often interchanged, whereas in shiatsu, the pressure is not limited to just acupressure points, but sometimes applied over a wider area, using palms, elbows, knees, and feet. In addition to the acupressure points, shiatsu involves gentle stretching and manipulation techniques used in Thai massage and Tui na.

Acupressure's goal is to restore health and balance the energy flow. The benefits of acupressure can calm the sympathetic nervous system, improving circulation, relieving stiff muscles, and alleviating stress. Each meridian line relates to a different organ of the body. When the vital energies can flow through the meridians in a balanced and steady manner, the outcome is good health. Pressing points on the meridian lines relieves muscle tension and increases circulation. Stimulation of points along these pathways and meridians stimulates the body to release endorphins. Other effects may include the release of anti-inflammatory and euphoric substances, increased circulation and decreased inflammation (sometimes referred to as the movement of qi / chi). Release of neurotransmitters, serotonin and prostaglandins may also be influenced by the stimulation of acupressure points.

Most Common Acupuressure/Shiatsu Points

There are a number of acupoints that are useful for acupressure/shiatsu that are easy to apply. The following section outlines the most commonly used acupoints and their usage. A complete listing of all acupoints with location, usage, illustratration, indication and function are on pages 47-109.

Points	Locations	Acupressure & Shiatsu Usage
Lu-5 **Chize** *Foot Marsh*	On the cubital crease, on the radial side of tendon of m. biceps brachii. This point is located with the elbow slightly flexed.	Elbow pain and swelling; tonsillitis; painful breathing; coughs; asthma; fever associated with lung problems; stiffness
Lu-7 **Lieque** *Broken Sequence* luo-connect	Superior to the styloid process of the radius, 1.5 cun above the transverse crease of the wrist, between brachioradialis and abductor pollicis longus.	Congestion; headaches; colds; coughing; Bell's palsy; stiff neck; sore throat; wind rash
Lu-9 **Taiyuan** *Greater Abyss* shu-stream, yuan	At the radial end of the transverse crease of the wrist, in the depression on the lateral side of the radial artery.	Reviving unconscious person; coughs; painful breathing; pharyngitis; pain and paralysis of wrist
Lu-11 **Shaoshang** *Lesser Metal*	On the radial side of the thumb, .1 cun posterior to the corner of the nail.	Sore throat; cough; painful breathing; fainting; loss of consciousness; nose bleeds; asthma; mania
LI-1 **Shangyang** *Metal Yang* jing-well	On the radial side of the index finger, about .1 cun posterior to the corner of the nail	High fever; diarrhea; toothache if infected only
LI-4 **Hegu** *Joining Valley* yuan	On the dorsum of the hand, between the 1st and 2nd metacarpal bones, approximately in the middle of the 2nd metacarpal bone on the radial side.	Normalizes intestines; major pain point and general well-being; facial problems; frontal headache; neuralgia; lower toothache; problems of back of hand.; diarrhea; rash; toothache; facial tension DON'T USE DURING PREGNANCY
LI-5 **Yangxi** *Yang Stream* jing-river	On the radial side of the wrist. When the thumb is tilted upward, it is in the depression between the tendons of muscle extensor pollicis longus and brevis.	Wrist point; good for smoking withdrawal; pain and swelling of the eye; sore throat
LI-10 **Shousanli** *Arm Three Miles*	On the line joining LI-5 and LI-11, 2 cun below LI-11.	Sore throat; general well-being; pain or fatigue in arms; sore legs
LI-15 **Jianyu** *Shoulder Transporting Point*	In the depression, anterior and inferior to the acromion, on the upper portion of the deltoid muscle when the arm is in full abduction.	Frozen shoulder; neuralgia of arm and shoulder; hemiplegia; shoulder joint pains
LI-20 **Yingxiang** *Welcome Fragrance*	In the nasolabial groove, at the level of the midpoint of the lateral border of the ala nasi.	Sinusitis; rhinitis; facial tension; neuralgia of face; paralysis of facial nerves; nasal obstruction
St-3 **Juliao** *Great Crevice*	Directly below St-2, at the level of the lower border of the ala nasi, on the lateral side of the nasolabial groove.	Sinus and nasal congestion; facial tension or paralysis; upper toothache; neuralgia of face; tension
St-25 **Tianshu** *Heavenly Pillar*	2 cun lateral to the center of the umbilicus.	All intestinal problems; constipation; gastritis; abdominal pain; menstrual pain; bowel irregularities; intestinal obstruction; diarrhea; vomiting; colitis; blood in stools; irregular menstruation; edema
St-34 **Liangqiu** *Beam Mound* xi-cleft	When the knee is flexed, point is 2 cun above the laterosuperior border of the patella.	Stomach pains; diarrhea; arthritis in the knee
St-35 **Dubi** *Calf Nose*	When the knee is flexed, the point is at the lower border of the patella, in the depression lateral to the patellar ligament.	Numbness and motor impairment of the knee

COMMON ACUPRESSURE / SHIATSU POINTS

Points	Locations	Acupressure & Shiatsu Usage
St-36 **Zusanli** *Three Miles of the Leg* he-sea	3 cun below St-35, one finger breadth from the anterior crest of the tibia, in tibialis anterior.	Well-being particularly for tonifying Stomach and Spleen; fatigue; tired legs; loss of appetite; nausea; vomiting; abscess; insufficient lactation
St-44 **Neiting** *Inner Courtyard* ying-spring	Proximal to the web margin between the 2nd and 3rd toes, in the depression distal and lateral to the 2nd metatarsodigital joint.	Stomach pain; toothache; frontal headache; sore throat; gum disorders
Sp-6 **Sanyinjiao** *Three Yin Meeting*	3 cun directly above the tip of the medial malleolus, on the posterior border of the medial aspect of the tibia.	Ankle pains; menstrual pain; digestive problems; female reproductive problems; insomnia; diseases of reproductive system; distension or pain in abdomen; diarrhea; hemiplegia; overweight. DON'T USE DURING PREGNANCY
Sp-9 **Yinlingquan** *Yin Mound Spring* he-sea	On the lower border of the medial condyle of the tibia, in the depression on the medial border of the tibia.	Pains in the knee; ascites; edema; retention of urine
Sp-10 **Xuehai** *Sea of Blood*	When the knee is flexed, the point is 2 cun above the mediosuperior border of the patella, on the bulge of the medial portion of the muscle quadriceps femoris.	All skin diseases (especially redness and itchiness); hives; menstrual pain; neurodermatitis
Ht-3 **Shaohai** *Lesser Sea* he-sea	When the elbow is flexed, the point is in the depression between the medial end of the transverse cubital crease of the elbow and the medial epicondyle of the humerus.	Heart palpitations; psychosis; intercostal neuralgia; ulnar neuralgia; important for hand tremors
Ht-7 **Shenmen** *Spirit Gate* shu-stream, yuan	At the ulnar end of the transverse crease of the wrist, in the depression on the radial side of the tendon of muscle flexor carpi ulnaris.	Reviving unconscious person; insomnia; hysteria; mania; high blood pressure; irritability; angina pectoris; constipation; palpitations; absent mindedness
SI-3 **Houxi** *Back Stream* shu-stream	When a loose fist is made, the point is on the ulnar side, proximal to the 5th MP joint, at the end of the transverse crease at the junction of the red and white and skin.	Paralysis of fingers; numbness; hardness of hearing; ringing in ears; low back pain; malaria; night sweats; tinnitus
SI-11 **Tianzong** *Heavenly Attribution*	In the infrascapular fossa, at the junction of the upper and middle third of the distance between the lower border of the scapular spine and the inferior angle of the scapula.	Shoulder pain; frozen shoulder; intercostals neuralgia; lung problems
SI-19 **Tinggong** *Listening Palace*	Anterior to the tragus and posterior to the condyloid process of the mandible, in the depression formed when the mouth is open.	Ringing in ears; difficulty in hearing; TMJ
Ub-1 **Jingming** *Eye Brightness*	0.1 cun superior to the inner canthus.	Any eye problems; poor or tired vision; swollen eyes
Ub-2 **Zanzhu** *Collecting Bamboo*	On the medial extremity of the eyebrow, or on the supraorbital notch.	Front or back headache; hay fever; eye strain; sinus allergies; hay fever; sinus headaches
Ub-10 **Tianzhu** *Heaven Pillar*	1.3 cun lateral to Du-15, in the depression on the lateral aspect of the trapezius muscle.	Common colds; headaches; insomnia; bronchitis; nasal congestion; neck ache; eye and nose problems
Ub-13 **Feishu** *Lung Back Shu*	1.5 cun lateral to Du-12, at the level of the lower border of the spinous process of T3.	Cough; asthma; breathlessness; bronchitis; pneumonia; Tonifies deficient Lungs; breathing problems
Ub-17 **Geshu** *Diaphragm Shu*	1.5 cun lateral to Du-9, at the level of the lower border of the spinous process of T7.	Irregular menstruation; measles; night sweats; hiccups

Points	Locations	Acupressure & Shiatsu Usage
Ub-23 Shenshu *Kidney Shu*	1.5 cun lateral to Du-4, at the level of the lower border of the spinous process of the L2.	Tonifies Kidneys; impotence; nocturnal emission; impotence; infertility; lack of sexual desire; physical weakness and exhaustion; depression; lack of will-power; chronic low back pain; weak legs; chronic ear problems; tinnitus; deafness; poor vision; vitalizing patient's energy
Ub-24 Qihaishu *Sea of Qi Shu*	1.5 cun lateral to the DU meridian, at the level of the lower border of the spinous process of L3.	Chronic or acute lower back pain; irregular menstruation; uterine bleeding; dysmenorrhea; asthma
Ub-25 Dachangshu *Large Intestine Shu*	1.5 cun lateral to Du-3, at the level of the lower border of the spinous process of L4.	Tonifies Large Intestine; constipation; diarrhea; abdominal distension; chronic or acute lower back pain; sciatica
Ub-27 Xiaochuangshu *Small Intestine Shu*	1.5 cun lateral to the DU meridian, at the level of the lower border of the 1st posterior sacral foramen.	Any small intestine problems; abdominal pain; low back pain over sacrum; urination and menstruation problems; nocturnal emission
Ub-40 Weizhong *Supporting Middle* he-sea	Midpoint of the transverse crease of the popliteal fossa, between the tendons of muscle biceps femoris and muscle semitendinosus.	Low back pain; calf spasms; sciatica
Ub-57 Chengshan *Supporting Mountain*	Directly below the belly of muscle gastrocnemius, on a line joining Ub-40 and Ub-60, about 8 cun below Ub-40.	Sciatica; tired legs; calf spasms; pain on sole of foot
Ub-60 Kunlun *Kunlun Mountains* jing-river	In the depression between the external malleolus and tendo calcaneus.	Sciatica; dizziness; backache; epilepsy; blurry vision; neck rigidity; difficult labor DON'T USE DURING PREGNANCY
Ub-67 Zhiyin *Reaching Yin* jing-well	On the lateral side of the small toe, 0.1 cun posterior to the corner of the nail	Malposition of fetus; headaches; blurred vision; pain in eyes and other eye problems; easy labor; nasal obstruction; epistaxis DON'T USE DURING PREGNANCY;
K-1 Yongquan *Bubbling Spring* jing-well	On the sole, between 2nd and 3rd toes, in the depression when the foot is in plantar flexion, approximately at the junction of the anterior third and posterior 2/3 of the sole.	General vitality; fear; dizziness; revival; epilepsy; menstrual pain
K-3 Taixi *Greater Stream* shu-stream, yuan	In the depression between he medial malleolus and tendo calcaneus, at the level of the tip of the medial malleolus.	General kidney function; pain in lower back; impotence; abnormal menstruation; nephritis; cystitis; irregular menstruation; spermatorrhea; enuresis; tinnitus; alopecia; impotence; constipation
K-27 Shufu *Transporting point Mansion*	In the depression on the lower border of the clavicle, 2 cun lateral to the Ren meridian.	Bronchitis; chest pain; asthma
Pc-3 Quze *Marsh on Bend* he-sea	On the transverse cubital crease, at the ulnar side of the tendon of muscle biceps brachii.	Acute gastritis and gastroenteritis; pain along the arm; cardiac pain; palpitation; febrile diseases; tremor of the hand and arm
Pc-6 Neiguan *Inner Gate* luo-connect	2 cun above the transverse crease of the wrist, between the tendons of palmaris longus and flexor carpi radialis	Nausea; vomiting; sea sickness; insomnia; chest pain; stuffiness in chest; pain in hypochondrium; asthma; nausea or vomiting; opens the chest; stomachache; hysteria; irritability; insomnia
Pc-8 Laogong *Palace of Toil* ying-spring	On the transverse crease and center of the palm, between the 2nd and 3rd metacarpal bones. When the fist is clenched, the point is just below the tip of the middle finger.	Heat exhaustion; shyness; high blood pressure; writer's cramp; excessive sweating of palms
Pc-9 Zhongchong *Center Rush* jing-well	In the center of the tip of the middle finger.	Shock; apoplectic coma
Sj-5 Waiguan *Outer Gate* luo-connect	2 cun above Sj-4, between the radius and the ulna.	Tinnitus; ear infection; migraine headaches; common colds; high fever (shao yang); tinnitus; temporal migraines; lateral stiff neck

ACUPRESSURE

COMMON ACUPRESSURE / SHIATSU POINTS

Points	Locations	Acupressure & Shiatsu Usage
Sj-14 **Jianliao** *Shoulder Crevice*	Posterior and inferior to the acromion, in the depression about 1 cun posterior to LI-15 when the arm is abducted.	Shoulder and upper arm pain and impairment
Gb-1 **Tongziliao** *Pupil Crevice*	0.5 cun lateral to the outer canthus, in the depression on the lateral side of the orbit.	Headache around temples; conjunctivitis; eye problems
Gb-2 **Tinghui** *Hearing Convergence*	Anterior to the intertragic notch, at the posterior border of the condyloid process of the mandible. The point is located with the mouth open.	Ringing in the ears; facial paralysis; mumps; dislocation or motor impairment of the jaw (TMJ)
Gb-12 **Wangu** *Mastoid Process*	In the depression posterior and inferior to the mastoid process.	Headache; toothache; ringing in ear; insomnia
Gb-14 **Yangbai** *Yang White*	On the forehead, directly above the pupil, 1 cun directly above the midpoint of the eyebrow.	Supraorbital neuralgia; headache; sinus headache; eye problems
Gb-20 **Fengchi** *Wind Pool*	In the depression between the upper portion of the SCM and muscle trapezius, on the same level with Du-16.	Eye disorders; common cold; front and side headaches; hypertension; tension in neck; dizziness; vertigo; swollen eyes; occipital headache; stiff neck; hypertension; seizures; hemiplegia
Gb-21 **Jianjing** *Shoulder Well*	Midway between Du-14 and the acromion, at the highest point of the shoulder.	Hemiplegia due to stroke; shoulder pain; frozen shoulder; mastitis; lack of milk; childbirth difficulties DON'T USE DURING PREGNANCY
Gb-30 **Huantiao** *Circling Jump*	At the junction of the lateral 1/3 and medial 2/3 of the distance between the greater trochanter and the hiatus of the sacrum (Du-2). When locating this point, put patient in lateral recumbent position with thigh flexed.	Sciatica; hip, lumbar, and thigh pain; diseases of the hip joint and surrounding tissue
Gb-31 **Fengshi** *Wind Market*	On the midline of the lateral aspect of the thigh, 7 cun above the transverse political crease. When the patient is standing erect with hands at sides, the point is where the tip of the middle finger touches.	Circulation in legs; tired legs; sciatica, especially with lateral leg pain
Gb-34 **Yanglingquan** *Outer Mound Spring* he-sea	In the depression anterior and in inferior to the head of the fibula.	Major point for musculoskeletal problems; ankle pains; headaches; knee problems; leg weakness
Gb-40 **Qiuxu** *Mounds of Ruins* yuan	Anterior and inferior to the lateral malleolus, in the depression on the lateral side of the tendon of m. extensor digitorum longus.	Pain in chest and ribs; tidal fevers; malaria; low back pain; aids function of liver and gall bladder; neck pain; calf pain
Liv-3 **Taichong** *Bigger Rushing* shu-stream, yuan	On the dorsum of the foot, in the depression distal to the junction of the 1st and 2nd metatarsal bones.	Headaches; dizziness; muscle cramps and muscle tension; insomnia; hepatitis; mastitis; major point for irregular menstruation due to stagnation
Liv-4 **Zhongfeng** *Middle Seal* jing-river	1 cun anterior to the medial malleolus, midway between Sp-5 and St-41, in the depression on the medial side of m. tibialis anterior.	Arthritis in the ankle; low back pain
Liv-8 **Ququan** *Spring and Bend* he-sea	When the knee is flexed, the point is located in the depression above the medial end of the transverse popliteal crease, posterior to the medial epicondyle of the tibia, on the anterior part of the insertion of m. semimembranosus and m. semitendinosus.	Inside knee problems; urine retention; burning urination; itchy genitals; genital herpes; vaginitis; local for medial knee pain
Liv-14 **Qimen** *Cyclic Gate*	Directly below the nipple, in the 6th intercostal space, 4 cun lateral to the midline.	Main point for intercostal neuralgia; hepatitis; rib pain; lactation problems; coughing; breathing difficulty; hypochondrium pain and distension; shingles

Points	Locations	Acupressure & Shiatsu Usage
Du-3 **Yaoyangguan** *Lumbar Yang Gate*	Below the spinous process of the 4th lumbar vertebrae, level with the iliac crest.	Low back pain; paralysis of lower limbs; muscular atrophy of the legs; impotence; nocturnal emission; epilepsy
Du-4 **Mingmen** *Gate of Life*	Below the spinous process of the 2nd lumbar vertebrae.	Strengthens Kidneys; lumbar weakness; lack of vitality; impotence; infertility; weak legs; headaches; ringing in the ears; low back pain or sprain; 5am diarrhea; enuresis; spermatorrhea; impotence; leukorrhea; irregular menstruation; endometriosis; peritonitis; sciatica; nephritis
Du-8 **Jinsuo** *Tendon Spasm*	Below the spinous process of the 9th thoracic vertebrae.	Epilepsy; gastric pain; back stiffness
Du-11 **Shendao** *Spirit Pathway*	Below the spinous process of the 5th thoracic vertebrae.	Stroke; anxiety; palpitation; pain and stiffness of the back
Du-14 **Dazhui** *Big Vertebra*	Below the spinous process of the 7th cervical vertebrae, approximately level with the shoulders.	Common cold; fever; asthma; headaches; clears mind and stimulates brain; allergies; pain in shoulder; neck pain and rigidity
Du-15 **Yamen** *Gate of Muteness*	0.5 cun directly above the midpoint of the posterior hairline, in the depression below the spinous process of the 1st cervical vertebrae.	Colds; headaches; nosebleeds; stimulates speech, so good for speech difficulties; mental disorders; epilepsy; deafness and muteness
Du-16 **Fengfu** *Wind Palace*	1 cun directly above the midpoint of the posterior hairline, directly below the external occipital protuberance, in the depression between m. trapezius.	Stimulates/calms brain; giddiness; tension in upper neck; common colds; strokes; headache; sore throat
Du-20 **Baihui** *Hundred Meetings*	On the midline of the head, 7 cun directly above the posterior hairline, approximately on the midpoint of the line connecting the apexes of the two auricles.	Vertex headache; frontal headache from sinus congestion; dizziness; hypertension; insomnia; giddiness; piles; prolapsed anus or vagina; heatstroke; hemorrhoids
Ren-4 **Guanyuan** *Gate to the Original Qi*	On the midline of the abdomen, 3 cun below the umbilicus.	For all Kidney problems; abdominal pain; pain from deficiency; fatigue; grounding; reproductive organ problems; menstrual cramps; frigidity; can use it to regulate almost any GYN problems
Ren-6 **Qihai** *Sea of Qi*	On the midline of the abdomen, 1.5 cun below the umbilicus.	Physical and mental exhaustion and depression; lower abdominal pain or distension; lack of willpower; impotence; irregular menstruation; intestinal paralysis; all urinary problems like incontinence; stomach pain; diarrhea; wet dreams; menstrual pain; constipation
Ren-14 **Juque** *Great Palace*	On the midline of the abdomen, 6 cun above the umbilicus.	Mental diseases; seizures; acts on stomach and heart; stomach spasm; stomach ulcers; emotional upset; calms mind
Ren-17 **Shanzhong** *Middle of Chest*	On the anterior midline, at level with the 4th intercostal space.	Asthma; bronchitis; intercostal neuralgia; wheezing; panting; spitting blood; difficulty or inability to swallow food; dilates bronchioles; insufficient lactation; hiccups; acts on Heart and Lungs; breathlessness; chronic cough or bronchitis; palpitations; high blood pressure; insufficient lactation
Ren-22 **Tiantu** *Heaven Projection*	In the center of the suprasternal fossa.	Acute and chronic cough and asthma; bronchitis; sore throat; goiter; hiccups; spasms of the esophagus; diseases of the vocal cords
E-Taiyang *Greater Yang*	In the depression about 1 cun posterior to the midpoint between the lateral end of the eyebrow and the outer canthus.	Headaches in the side of the head; over-active mind; deviation of eye & mouth
E-Xiyan/ Xiyuan *Eyes Of the Knee*	A pair of points in the two depressions, medial and lateral to the patellar ligament, locating the point with the knee flexed. Lateral xiyan overlaps with St-35.	Knee pain; weakness of the lower extremities; used for painful obstruction of the knee
E-Yintang *Seal Hall*	Midway between the medial ends of the two eyebrows.	Headache; epistaxis; insomnia; head heaviness; frontal headache; calms mind and tension in forehead; frontal headaches; blocked frontal sinuses

ACUPRESSURE

COMMON ACUPRESSURE / SHIATSU POINTS

Point Combinations / Conditions

Conditions	Points
Acne and other skin disorders	Ub-23, Ub-47, St-36, Ub-10
Allergies	LI-4, Liv-3, Sj-5, LI-11, Ub-10, K-27, Ren-6, St-36
Ankle problems	K-3, Ub-60, K-6, Ub-62, Gb-40
Anxiety and nervousness	Sj-15, Ub-10, Pc-3, Pc-6, Ht-7, E-Yintang, Ren-17
Arthritis	LI-4, Sj-5, St-36, LI-11, Gb-20
Asthma	K-27, Lu-1, Ub-13, Lu-9, Lu-10
Back pain	Ub-23, Ub-47, Ub-48, Ren-6, Ub-54, Gb-30
Chronic fatigue syndrome	Lu-1, Gb-21, Gb-20, Pc-6, Sj-5, Ub-23, Ub-47, St-36, Liv-3, Du-24.5, Ren-6
Colds and flu	Ub-2, St-3, LI-20, LI-11, LI-4, Gb-20, Du-16, Du-24.5, K-27
Constipation	Ren-6, St-36, LI-4, LI-11, St-25
Coughing	Ub-38, E-17, Ub-10, Ren-22, K-27
Cramps and spasms	Du-26, Ub-57, Liv-3
Depression	Ub-38, Ub-10, Gb-20, Du-19, Du-20, Du-21, K-27, Lu-1, Ub-23, Ub-47, E-Yintang, Ren-17, St-36
Dizziness	Gb-20, Gb-34, Liv-3
Diarrhea	Sp-16, Ren-6, St-36, Sp-4, Liv-2
Discomforts due to pregnancy	Ub-23, Ub-47, Ub-48, Ub-10, Ren-17, Pc-6, E-Yintang, Sp-12, Sp-13
Earaches	Sj-21, SI-19, Gb-2, Sj-17, K-3
Eyestrain	Ub-2, St-2, St-3, Ub-10, Du-16, E-Yintang, Liv-3
Fainting	Du-26, Ub-23, Ub-47, K-1, St-36, Liv-3
Fever	Du-14, LI-4, LI-11
Frustration and irritation	Gb-21, Ren-12, Ub-48, Gb-30, Lu-1, Gb-20, E-Yintang, Ren-17
Hangovers	LI-4, Ub-10, Gb-20, Sp-16, Liv-3, E-Yintang, Du-16, St-3, Ub-2
Headaches and migraines	Gb-20, Du-16, Ub-2, E-Yintang, St-3, LI-4, Gb-41
Hiccups	Sj-17, Sp-16, Ren-22, Ren-17, Ren-12, Lu-1, K-27
Hot flashes	K-1, K-27, LI-4, Gb-20, Ren-17, E-Yintang, Du-20
Hypertension	Pc-6, St-36, K-3
Immune system	K-27, Ub-23, Ub-47, Ren-6, St-36, K-3, Liv-3, LI-11, Sj-5, LI-4, Ren-17
Impotency	Ub-23, Ub-47, K-1, K-3, St-36, Ren-4, Ub-27 to Ub-34, Ren-6, Sp-12, Sp-13
Insomnia	Ub-38, Pc-6, Ht-7, Ub-10, Du-16, Gb-20, E-Yintang, Ren-17, K-6, Ub-62
Jaw problems	St-6, Sj-17, SI-19, Sj-21, Gb-2, Gb-20
Knee pain	Ub-54, Liv-8, K-10, Sp-9, Gb-34, Ub-53, St-35, St-36, E-Xiyan
Labor pain	Gb-21, Ub-27 to Ub-34, LI-4, K-3, Ub-67
Lower-body pain	Gb-20, St-36, K-3, Ub-60
Memory and concentration	Du-20, E-2, Du-26, Ub-10, Gb-20, E-Yintang, Ren-17, St-36, Liv-3
Motion sickness, morning sickness, and nausea	SI-17, Pc-5, Pc-6, Sp-16, St-36, Liv-3, St-45
Neck tension and pain	Gb-21, Ub-10, Gb-20, Sj-16, Du-16, Ub-2
Nosebleeds	Du-26, St-3, Ub-1, LI-4, Du-16
Nursing	Lu-1, St-16, Pc-1, E-Yintang, Ren-17
PMS	Sp-12, Sp-13, Ub-27 to Ub-34, Ren-6, Ren-4, Ub-48, Sp-6, Sp-4
Postpartum recovery	Ren-6, Pc-6, Ub-23, Ub-47, Ub-48, St-36, Liv-3
Sciatica	Ub-31, Ub-32, Ub-33, Ub-40, Gb-30
Shoulder pain	Sj-15, Gb-21, LI-14, LI-15, Gb-20, Gb-21
Sinus and hay fever	Ub-2, Ub-10, Ub-7, LI-20, St-3, Du-20, E-Yintang, Du-26, LI-4
Stomachaches, indigestion, and heartburn	Ren-12, Ren-6, Ub-23, Ub-47, St-36, Pc-6, Sp-4
Swelling and water retention	Ren-6, Sp-9, Sp-6, K-2, K-6
Tennis elbow	LI-10, LI-11, Gb-34
Tinnitus	K-3, SI-3, SI-19, Gb-20, Sj-17
Toothaches	St-6, St-3, LI-4, Sj-13
Upper-body pain	LI-4, E-Yintang, Gb-20, Du-16
Wrist pain	Pc-6, Pc-7, Sj-5, Sj-4, SI-5

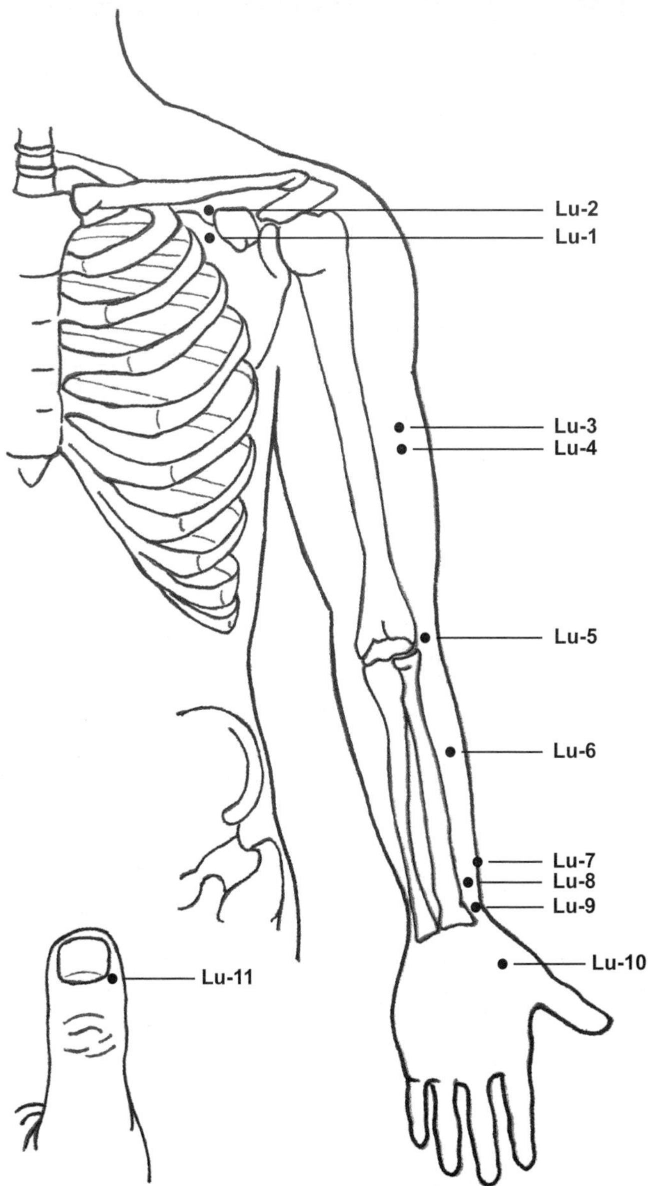

Jing Well	Ying Spring	Shu Stream	Jing River	He Sea
11	10	9	8	5
Yuan	**Luo-connect**	**Xi-Cleft**	**Front Mu**	**Back Shu**
9	7	6	Lu-1	Ub-13

Points	Location	Usage	Indications / Functions
Lu-1 Zhongfu *Central Residence*	6 cun lateral to the anterior midline, on the line lateral and superior to the sternum at the level of the 1st intercostal space.	Dry cough; cough with fullness in chest; asthma, lung heat; pulmonary TB (severe yin deficiency); coughing and wheezing with blood	• **Disperses fullness of the Lung**: used for late stage exterior patterns when the pathogen has penetrated into the interior such as retention of phlegm in the Lungs. • **Stops cough:** used for acute and chronic cough. • Treatment of chest pain due to stagnation of Heart blood or retention of phlegm in the chest. • Treats shoulder pain due to Lung channel dysfunction with lung-heat, damp-phlegm, or phlegm-heat obstructing the Lungs. • **Tonifies Lung and Spleen.**
Lu-2 Yunmen *Cloud Door*	In the depression below the acromial extremity of the clavicle, 6 cun lateral to the anterior midline.	Cough; asthma; pain in the chest; shoulder and arm; fullness in the chest	• **Clears Heat in the Lungs, Descends Lung Qi:** used to treat painful obstruction syndrome of the shoulder.
Lu-3 Tianfu *Heavenly Residence*	The point is on the medial aspect of the upper arm, 3 cun below the end of the axillary fold, on the radial side of the muscle biceps brachii.	Pain in the medial aspect of upper arm; asthma; epistaxis	• Clears Heat in the Lungs, Descends Lung Qi. • Cools the Blood, Stops bleeding.
Lu-4 Xiabai *Clasping the White*	On the medial aspect of the upper arm, 4 cun below the end of the axillary fold, on the radial side of the muscle biceps brachii.	Pain in the medial aspect of upper arm; cough; fullness in the chest	• Descends Lung Qi, Regulates Qi and Blood in the chest.
Lu-5 Chize *Foot Marsh*	On the cubital crease, on the radial side of tendon of m. biceps brachii. This point is located with the elbow slightly flexed.	Yellow phlegm maybe white and viscous; URI gone deeper; productive cough; asthma; bronchitis; pleurisy; pain in throat with cough; good for excess LU heat	• **Clears Heat in the Lungs**: for excess patterns characterized by heat in the Lungs with cough, fever, yellow sputum and thirst, and qi level patterns. It is also used in chronic conditions with phlegm and heat in the Lungs, bronchitis. • **Clears Lung and Nourishes Yin**: for injury to body fluids following febrile diseases. • **For excess-cold with retention of cold phlegm:** for Lung symptoms and cough with profuse white-sticky sputum and chilliness. • **Opens the water passages and facilitates urination**: for retention of urine caused by obstruction of the Lungs by descending and opening the water passages in the lower burner. • **Relaxes the tendons in the arm along the Lung channel**: used for painful obstruction syndrome.
Lu-6 Kongzui *Maximum Opening* xi-cleft	The point is on the palmar aspect of the forearm, on the line joining Lu-9 and Lu-5, 7 cun above the transverse crease of the wrist.	Dry cough; dryness in lungs; good elbow and biceps point	• For acute, excess patterns of the lung including asthma. • Stops bleeding due to its action as an accumulation point.

Points	Location	Usage	Indications / Functions
Lu-7 **Lieque** *Broken Sequence* luo-connect	Superior to the styloid process of the radius, 1.5 cun above the transverse crease of the wrist, between brachioradialis and abductor pollicis longus.	Wind cold; wind-heat; headache; coughing; asthma with little phlegm (allergic asthma); facial paralysis; stiff neck; taiyang s/sx; diseases of the wrist joint; sore throat; wind rash; empirical point for blood in urine	• **Releases the exterior in both Wind-heat and Wind-cold attacks**. For patterns including common cold and influenza, sneezing, stiff neck, headache, aversion to cold and a floating pulse, nasal obstruction, runny nose, headaches. • **Stimulates descending and dispersing of Lung Qi**: for all types of coughs and asthma. • Treats psychological and emotional disorders due to grief and sorrow, especially when there are repressed emotions. • Treats painful obstruction syndrome of the shoulder due to Large Intestine channel pathology. • **Opens the water passages:** for edema and water retention due to Kidney dysfunction (failing to grasp the qi).
Lu-8 **JingQu** *Channel canal* jing-river	1 cun above the transverse crease of the wrist in the depression on the lateral side of the radial artery.	Wrist pain; cough; asthma	• Treats cough, asthma, fever, pain in the chest, sore throat, pain in the wrist.
Lu-9 **Taiyuan** *Greater Abyss* shu-stream, yuan	At the radial end of the transverse crease of the wrist, in the depression on the lateral side of the radial artery.	Any LU problem due to deficiency; cold; weak deficient LU; cough; asthma; fever	• **Tonifies Lung Qi and yin.** • Resolves phlegm obstructing the Lungs with symptoms as chronic cough with yellow-sticky sputum. • **Tonifies Gathering Qi:** for deficiency with signs of weak voice and cold hands due to deficiency qi. • For weak and deep pulse.
Lu-10 **Yuji** *Fish Border* ying-spring	On the radial aspect of the midpoint of the 1st metacarpal bone, on the junction of the red and white skin.	Sore throat; loss of voice; fever	• **Clears Heat and fire in the Lungs:** cough, hemoptysis, sore throat, loss of voice, fever, feverish sensation in the palms.
Lu-11 **Shaoshang** *Lesser Metal*	On the radial side of the thumb, .1 cun posterior to the corner of the nail.	Fainting; loss of consciousness; nose bleeds; asthma; mania	• **Expels Exterior Wind-heat with sore throat.** • **For Interior Wind**: apoplexy and loss of consciousness from wind-stroke.

ACUPRESSURE

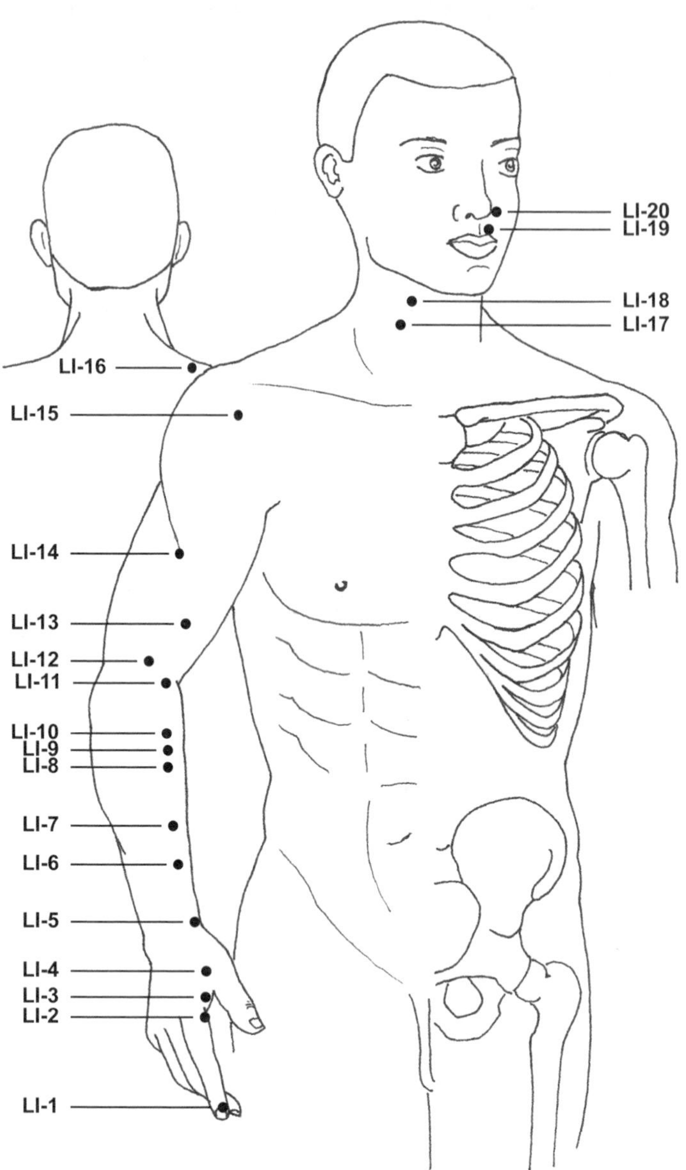

Jing Well	Ying Spring	Shu Stream	Jing River	He Sea
1	2	3	5	11
Yuan	**Luo-connect**	**Xi-Cleft**	**Front Mu**	**Back Shu**
4	6	7	St-25	Ub-25

Points	Location	Usage	Indications / Functions
LI-1 **Shangyang** *Metal Yang* jing-well	On the radial side of the index finger, about .1 cun posterior to the corner of the nail	Apoplectic or any coma; high fever (yang ming meridian) and often used for high fevers instead of others; toothache if infected only; bleed with LI-11 needled for tonsillitis (fire toxin situation)	• **Removes obstruction:** for acute stage of wind-stroke. • **Clears both interior and exterior heat:** sore throat, interior heat affecting the large intestine. • **Expels Wind and Cold from the channel:** painful obstruction syndrome of the shoulder.
LI-2 **Erjian** *Second Interval* ying-spring	In the depression of the radial side of the index finger, distal to the second metacarpal-phalangeal joint. The point is located with the finger slightly flexed.	Toothache; trigeminal neuralgia; febrile diseases; sore throat	• Clears heat from the Large Intestine: for constipation, dry stools, fever and abdominal pain.
LI-3 **Sanjian** *Third Interval* shu-stream	When a loose fist is made, the point is on the radial side of the index finger, in the depression proximal to the head of the second metacarpal bone.	Toothache; sore throat; redness and swelling of fingers and dorsum of the hand	• Toothache, opthalmalgia, sore throat, redness and swelling of fingers and dorsum of the hand [arthritis].
LI-4 **Hegu** *Joining Valley* yuan	On the dorsum of the hand, between the 1st and 2nd metacarpal bones, approximately in the middle of the 2nd metacarpal bone on the radial side.	Common cold; febrile disease with or without sweat; headache (used for non-OP frontal and vertex; and only otherwise if URI related); disease of the sensory organs; facial paralysis; any face related problem; hemiplegia; major pain point; pain in the neck or any part of the body	• **Expels Wind-heat and Releases the Exterior:** exterior patterns including nasal congestion, sneezing, burning eyes, allergic rhinitis, hay fever. • **Stimulates Dispersing and Descending:** for nasal congestion, sneezing, cough, stiff neck, aversion to cold and a floating pulse, common cold, influenza or other infectious diseases. • **Unblocks the channels**: stops pain due to spasm and relieves painful obstruction syndrome of the arm or shoulder. • **Treats facial problems:** rhinitis, conjunctivitis, mouth ulcers, sties, sinusitis, epistaxis, toothache, trigeminal neuralgia. • **Tonifies Qi and Consolidates the Exterior:** for chronic wind attacks. • **Harmonizes the ascending of Yang and Descending of Yin:** subdues ascending rebellious qi of the Stomach, Lung or Liver with symptoms of epigastric pain, Liver-yang rising in migraine headaches, and asthma. • Empirical point for promoting delivery during labor.
LI-5 **Yangxi** *Yang Stream* jing-river	On the radial side of the wrist. When the thumb is tilted upward, it is in the depression between the tendons of muscle extensor pollicis longus and brevis.	Diseases of the soft tissue of the wrist point; good for smoking withdrawal; pain and swelling of the eye; sore throat	• **Expels Wind and Releases the Exterior:** for headache, redness, pain and swelling of the eye, toothache, sore throat. • **Stops pain:** for painful obstruction syndrome of the wrist.
LI-6 **Pianli** *Slanting Passage* luo-connect	When the elbow is flexed with the radial side of the arm upward, the point is on the line joining LI-5 and LI-11, 3 cun above LI-5.	Facial edema; hand edema; tinnitus; deafness	• **Opens the water passages:** for edema of the face and hands due to impaired circulation of defensive qi in the skin. • Treats manic depression.
LI-7 **Wenliu** *Warm Flow* xi-cleft	When the elbow is flexed with radial side of the arm upward, the point is on the line joining LI-5 and LI-11, 5 cun above LI-5.	Headache; sore throat; swelling of the face; arm and shoulder pain	• **Stops pain and Removes obstructions from the channel:** painful obstruction syndrome of the channel and wind-heat causing painful and sore throat or swollen tonsils.

Points	Location	Usage	Indications / Functions
LI-8 **Xialian** *Lower Angular Ridge*	On the line joining LI-5 and LI-11, 4 cun below LI-11.	Elbow and arm pain; motor impairment of the upper limbs; abdominal pain	• Harmonizes Small Intestine, Expels Wind, Clears Heat
LI-9 **Shanglian** *Upper Angular Ridge*	On the line joining LI-5 and LI-11, 3 cun below LI-11.	Shoulder and arm pain; motor impairment of the upper limbs; abdominal pain	• Harmonizes Large Intestine, Unblocks the channels, Stops pain.
LI-10 **Shousanli** *Arm Three Miles*	On the line joining LI-5 and LI-11, 2 cun below LI-11.	Pain in the arm; neck pain; good for overuse injuries of the arm and forearm (often quite sore and is the bulky area of the muscle)	• **Removes obstructions from the channel:** for painful obstruction syndrome, atrophy syndrome and sequelae of wind-stroke affecting the arm. A major point for the treatment of any muscular problem affecting the forearm and hands.
LI-11 **Quchi** *Pool at Bend* he-sea	When the elbow is flexed, the point is in the depression at the lateral end of the transverse cubital crease, midway between Lu-5 and the lateral epicondyle of the humerus.	Paralysis; hemiplegia; arthritic pain in the upper limb; hypertension from excess yang (with St-36); high fever; any febrile disease; measles (heat toxin in TCM and showing up in the skin); main point for skin diseases involving redness; red eyes and pain	• **Expels exterior Wind-heat**: for exterior patterns with fever, chills, stiff neck, sweating, runny nose, body aches. • **Clears Internal Heat patterns**: including liver fire with hypertension. • **Cools the Blood:** for skin diseases due to heat in the blood such as urticaria, psoriasis and eczema. • **Resolves Dampness:** for patterns occurring in any part of the body including damp-heat causing skin eruptions or acne, damp-heat in the Spleen with digestive symptoms, or damp-heat in the urinary system causing cystitis or urethritis. Also for damp-heat causing fever, feeling of heaviness, loose stools, abdominal distention. • **Phlegm in the neck:** goiter. • **Benefits the sinews and joints:** for painful obstruction syndrome, atrophy syndrome and sequelae of wind-stroke paralysis, particularly of the arms and shoulders.
LI-12 **Zhouliao** *Elbow Seam*	When the elbow is flexed, the point is superior to the lateral epicondyle of the humerus, about 1 cun superolateral to LI-11, on the medial border of the humerus.	Numbness and contracture of the elbow and arm	• Unblocks the channels, Stops pain, Benefits elbow joint: for tennis elbow.
LI-13 **Shouwuli** *Arm Five Mile*	Superior to the lateral epicondyle of the humerus, on a line joining LI-11 and LI-15, 3 cun above LI-11.	Contracture and pain of the elbow and arm; scrofula	• Unblocks the channels, Stops pain, Stops coughing, Regulates Qi, Transforms Phlegm.
LI-14 **Binao** *Upper Arm*	On the line joining LI-11 and LI-15, 7 cun above LI-11, on the radial side of the humerus, superior to the lower end of the deltoid muscle, at the insertion.	Shoulder and arm pain; stiff neck; scrofula	• **Unblocks the channels:** for painful obstruction syndrome of the arm and shoulder. • Clears and enhances vision. • **Resolves Phlegm and disperses Phlegm masses:** for goiter.
LI-15 **Jianyu** *Shoulder Transporting Point*	In the depression, anterior and inferior to the acromion, on the upper portion of the deltoid muscle when the arm is in full abduction.	Hemiplegia; pain in shoulder; inflammation in shoulder; any shoulder problem	• **Benefits the sinews and joints, promotes Qi circulation, stops pain:** for painful obstruction syndrome of the shoulder.

Points	Location	Usage	Indications / Functions
LI-16 **Jugu** *Great Bone*	In the upper aspect of the shoulder, in the depression between the acromial extremity of the clavicle and scapular spine.	Disease of the shoulder and soft tissue of the shoulder; spitting blood	• Unblocks the channels: for painful obstruction syndrome of the shoulder. • Descends the Lung Qi: for breathlessness, cough or asthma caused by impairment of the Lung descending function.
LI-17 **Tianding** *Celestial Tripod*	On the lateral side of the neck, 1 cun below LI-18, on the posterior border of the SCM.	Sudden voice loss; sore throat; goiter; scrofula	• Benefits the throat and voice.
LI-18 **Futu** *Support the Prominence*	On the lateral side of the neck, level with the tip of the Adam's apple, between the sternal head and the clavicular head of the SCM muscle.	Cough; asthma; sore throat; goiter	• Benefits the throat, Stops coughing and wheezing: for tonsillitis, laryngitis, aphasia, hoarse voice and goiter.
LI-19 **Kouheliao** *Mouth Bone Hole*	Just below the lateral margin of the nostril, 0.5 cun lateral to Du-26.	Nasal obstruction; deviated mouth; epistaxis	• Expels Wind, Opens the nose.
LI-20 **Yingxiang** *Welcome Fragrance*	In the nasolabial groove, at the level of the midpoint of the lateral border of the ala nasi.	Rhinitis; sinusitis; can cause immediate clearing of the sinuses	• **Opens the nose:** for sneezing, loss of the sense of smell, epistaxis, sinusitis, runny nose, stuffed nose, allergic rhinitis and nasal polyps. • **Dispels Wind:** used for exterior patterns with nasal symptoms or trigeminal neuralgia and tics.

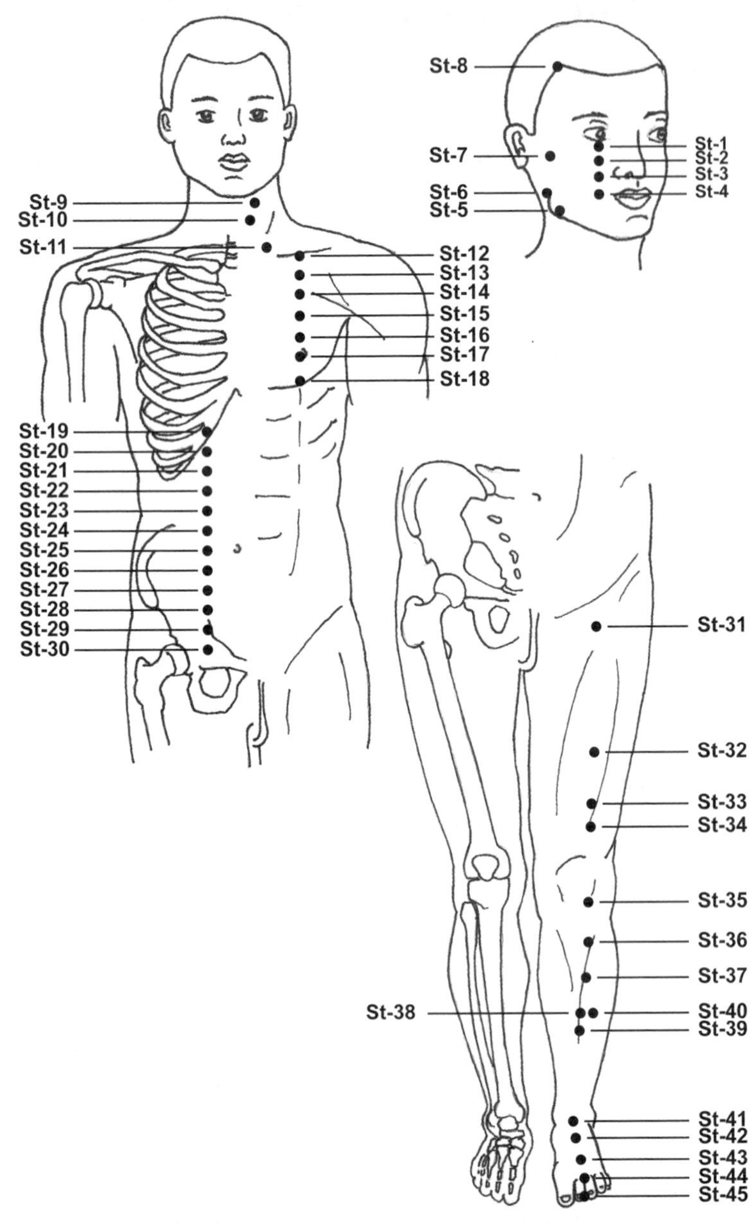

Jing Well	Ying Spring	Shu Stream	Jing River	He Sea
45	44	43	41	36
Yuan	**Luo-connect**	**Xi-Cleft**	**Front Mu**	**Back Shu**
42	40	34	Ren-12	Ub-21

Points	Location	Usage	Indications / Functions
St-1 Chengqi *Containing Tears*	With the eyes looking straight forward, the point is directly below the pupil, between the eyeball and the infraorbital ridge.	Conjunctivitis; sties; eyelid twitching; redness and swelling of eye; lacrimation; night blindness	• Treats problems of the eye including acute and chronic conjunctivitis, myopia, astigmatism, squint, color blindness, night blindness, glaucoma, atrophy of the optic nerve, cataract, keratitis and retinitis. • **Expels Wind:** both for exterior and interior wind-heat or wind-cold with symptoms of swelling, pain and lacrimation and paralysis of the eyelid.
St-2 Sibai *Four Whites*	Below St-1, in the depression at the infraorbital foramen.	Facial paralysis; spasms; trigeminal neuralgia; sinusitis (especially maxillary or ethmoid sinusitis)	• **Expels Wind:** for either external or internal wind with swelling of the eyes, allergic rhinitis or facial paralysis, twitching of the eyelids, facial paralysis and trigeminal neuralgia. • Also used for biliary ascariasis.
St-3 Juliao *Great Crevice*	Directly below St-2, at the level of the lower border of the ala nasi, on the lateral side of the nasolabial groove.	Rhinitis; facial paralysis; trigeminal neuralgia in this area; upper toothache	• Expels Exterior and Interior Wind: for facial paralysis and trigeminal neuralgia. Also for treatment of epistaxis and nasal obstruction.
St-4 Dicang *Earth Granary*	Lateral to the corner of the mouth, directly below St-3.	Facial paralysis; trigeminal neuralgia; excessive salivation; difficulty closing eyes; herpes; gum ulcers	• **Eliminates Exterior Wind:** facial paralysis with deviation of the mouth, or aphasia.
St-5 Daying *Great Reception*	Anterior to the angle of the mandible, on the anterior border of the attached portion of the masseter muscle, in the groove-like depression appearing when the cheek is bulged.	Local problems; parotitis; lock jaw	• Expels Wind, Reduces swelling.
St-6 Jiache *Jaw Chariot*	One finger breadth anterior and superior to the lower angle of the mandible where the masseter attaches, at the prominence of the muscle when the teeth are clenched.	Lower toothache; mumps; TMJ; grinding of teeth; facial paralysis	• Expels exterior wind affecting the face including mumps and spasm of the masseter muscle. • Toothache.
St-7 Xiaguan *Lower Gate*	At the lower border of the zygomatic arch, in the depression anterior to the condyloid process of the mandible, located with mouth closed.	Upper toothache; TMJ; TM arthritis; otitis media; tinnitus; earache; pus in ear	• **Removes obstruction:** for facial paralysis and trigeminal neuralgia, otitis, toothache, deafness and earache.
St-8 Touwei *Head Support*	.5 cun within the anterior hairline at the corner of the forehead, 4.5 cun lateral to Du-24.	Frontal and damp headache; psychosis if phlegm misting; facial paralysis; major headache point for frontal and vertex headache; other for dizziness especially with damp involvement; Meniere's disease (qi deficiency with damp)	• **Resolves Dampness and Phlegm:** for dizziness due to dampness and phlegm retained in the head and preventing the clear yang from rising to brighten the orifices, or causing frontal headaches.

Points	Location	Usage	Indications / Functions
St-9 **Renying** *Person's Welcome*	Level with the tip of the Adam's apple, on the anterior border of the SCM.	Blood pressure; sore throat; asthma; goiter; flushed face	• **Removes obstructions from the head to send Qi downwards:** stops hiccup, belching and nausea or asthma due to stomach channel obstruction. • **Removes Masses and resolves swellings:** heat and swelling affecting the stomach channel with tonsillitis, swollen and sore throat, adenitis, pharyngitis and swelling of the thyroid. • **Tonifies and Regulates Qi:** to regulate excess above and deficiency below.
St-10 **Shuitu** *Water Prominence*	At the midpoint of the line joining St-9 and St-11, on the anterior border of the SCM.	Sore throat; asthma; cough	• Descends Lung Qi, Benefits throat and neck.
St-11 **Qishe** *Qi Abode*	At the superior border of the sternal extremity of the clavicle, between the sternal head and the clavicular head of the SCM.	Sore throat; asthma; neck stiffness; cough; hiccups	• Descends Qi, Benefits throat and neck.
St-12 **Quepen** *Empty Basin*	In the midpoint of the supraclavicular fossa, 4 cun lateral to the Ren meridian.	Supraclavicular fossa pain; cough; asthma	• Descends Lung qi, Clears heat from the chest: used for excess patterns characterized by rebellious Stomach Qi going upwards causing breathlessness and asthma. • Used for anxiety, nervousness and insomnia due to a Stomach disharmony.
St-13 **Qihu** *Qi Door*	At the lower border of the middle of the clavicle, 4 cun lateral to the Ren meridian.	Chest and hypochondrium pain; chest fullness; hiccups	• Descends rebellious Qi, Unbinds the chest.
St-14 **Kufang** *Storeroom*	In the 1st intercostal space, 4 cun lateral to the Ren meridian.	Chest fullness and pain; cough	• Descends rebellious Qi, Unbinds the chest.
St-15 **Wuyi** *Room Scream*	In the 2nd intercostal space, 4 cun lateral to Ren meridian.	Chest and costal region fullness and pain; mastitis; asthma	• Descends rebellious Qi, Unbinds the chest. • Benefits the breast, Stops pain.
St-16 **Yingchuang** *Breast Window*	In the 3rd intercostal space, 4 cun lateral to the Ren meridian.	Mastitis; insufficient lactation	• Stops coughing and wheezing, Benefits the breast.
St-17 **Ruzhong** *Breast Center*	In the 4th intercostal space, 4 cun lateral to the Ren meridian.	Landmark for locating points; no moxa or acupressure	• Contraindicated for moxa or acupressure.
St-18 **Rugen** *Breast Root*	In the 5th intercostal space, directly below the nipple.	Breast problems; mastitis; insufficient lactation	• Stops coughing and wheezing, Benefits the breast, Reduces swelling: used mostly as a local point for breast problems, especially in relation to stomach qi with symptoms as mastitis, PMS swellings and lumps in the breasts. • Regulates lactation and can either promote or reduce it.
St-19 **Burong** *Not Contained*	6 cun above the umbilicus, 2 cun lateral to Ren-14.	Stomachache; vomiting; gastritis (stuck food); upper abdominal distension	• Harmonizes the middle jiao, Descends Qi, Stops cough and wheezing.
St-20 **Chengman** *Assuming Fullness*	5 cun above the umbilicus, 2 cun lateral to Ren-13.	Abdominal distension; gastric pain; vomiting	• Harmonizes the middle jiao, Descends rebellious Lung and Stomach Qi.

Points	Location	Usage	Indications / Functions
St-21 **Liangmen** *Beam Door*	4 cun above the umbilicus, 2 cun lateral to Ren-12.	Stomachache; stomach ulcers; gastritis; nervous stomach; nausea; vomiting; secondary back up support point used with Ren-12	• **Regulates Stomach Qi:** for excess patterns including nausea or vomiting, burning sensation in the epigastrium, epigastric pain.
St-22 **Guanmen** *Pass Gate*	3 cun above the umbilicus, 2 cun lateral to Ren-11.	Abdominal distension; lack of appetite	• Regulates Qi, Stops pain, Regulates the intestines, Benefits urination.
St-23 **Taiyi** *Supreme Unity*	2 cun above the umbilicus, 2 cun lateral to Ren-10.	Gastric pain; indigestion; irritability	• Harmonizes the middle jiao, Transforms Phlegm, Calms the Mind.
St-24 **Huaroumen** *Slippery Flesh Gate*	1 cun above the umbilicus, 2 cun lateral to Ren-9.	Gastric pain; vomiting; mania	• Harmonizes the Stomach, Transforms Phlegm, Calms the Mind, Stops vomiting.
St-25 **Tianshu** *Heavenly Pillar*	2 cun lateral to the center of the umbilicus.	All intestinal problems; constipation; gastritis; abdominal distension and stagnation; diarrhea; constipation; low back pain as related to constipation; vomiting; colitis; blood in stools; irregular menstruation; edema	• **Regulates Intestines:** for excess patterns of the stomach manifesting in abdominal problems such as diarrhea, abdominal pain, bloating, abdominal distention. • **Clears heat from the Stomach and Intestines:** for burning sensations in the epigastrium, thirst, constipation, or foul-smelling loose stools and a yellow tongue coating. • **Treats acute stomach patterns:** for yangming or Qi level patterns with high fever, thirst, profuse sweating and a full pulse. • When used with direct moxibustion, it tonifies and warms the Spleen and the Intestines, and is a special point for chronic diarrhea due to Spleen-yang deficiency.
St-26 **Wailing** *Outer Mound*	1 cun below the umbilicus, 2 cun lateral to Ren-7.	Abdominal pain; hernia; dysmenorrhea	• Regulates Qi, Stops pain.
St-27 **Daju** *Big Great*	2 cun below the umbilicus, 2 cun lateral to Ren-5.	Spermatorrhea; premature ejaculation; inguinal hernia	• Regulates Stomach Qi: for excess patterns of the stomach with lateral abdominal pain and genital or hernia pain.
St-28 **Shuidao** *Water Passage*	3 cun below the umbilicus, 2 cun lateral to Ren-4.	Opens water passages; edema; urine retention; UTIs; menstrual and fertility problems related to dampness	• **Opens the water passages of the lower burner:** stimulates excretion of fluids, for edema, difficult urination and retention or urine when caused by an excess pattern. • **Regulates Qi in the lower abdomen:** regulates menses due to stasis of qi or blood.
St-29 **Guilai** *Return back*	4 cun below the umbilicus, 2 cun lateral to Ren-3.	Irregular menstruation; dysmenorrhea; amenorrhea; orchitis from blood or cold stagnation; endometriosis; inguinal hernia	• **Relieves Blood Stasis:** for blood stasis in the uterus and irregular menses, dysmenorrhea with dark clotted blood, amenorrhea due to blood stasis. • **Tonifies and raises Qi:** prolapse of the uterus.
St-30 **Qichong** *Rushing Qi*	5 cun below the umbilicus, 2 cun lateral to Ren-2.	Diseases of the reproductive organs; essence point; impotence; external genitalia pain female or male; retained placenta	• **Regulates Qi and Blood in the lower abdomen and genitals:** for excess patterns with abdominal pain, abdominal masses, hernia, swelling of the penis, retention of placenta and swelling of the prostate. • **Promotes Kidney Essence:** for impotence. • Improves Stomach and Spleen Function

ACUPRESSURE

Points	Location	Usage	Indications / Functions
St-31 **Biguan** *Thigh Gate*	At the crossing point of the line drawn down from the ASIS and the line level with the lower border of the pubic symphisis, in the depression on the lateral side of sartorius, when the thigh is flexed.	Paralysis of the lower limb; atrophy and blockage of the muscles of the thigh and buttock if at least the thigh is involved	• **Removes obstruction from the channel:** for atrophy syndrome, painful obstruction syndrome, and sequelae of wind-stroke. • **Strengthens the Leg:** facilitates leg movement and raising of the leg.
St-32 **Futu** *Hidden Rabbit*	On the line connecting the anterior superior iliac spine (ASIS) and lateral border of the patella, 6 cun above the laterosuperior border of the patella, in muscle rectus femoris.	Lumbar and iliac region pain; knee coldness; beriberi; lower extremities motor impairment and pain	• Strengthens leg. • Expels Wind-heat: urticaria and heat in the blood.
St-33 **Yinshi** *Yin Market*	When the knee is flexed, the point is 3 cun above the latero superior border of the patella, on the line joining the laterosuperior border of the patella and ASIS.	Numbness; soreness; motor impairment of leg and knee	• Opens channels, Stops pain, Dispels Wind-Damp.
St-34 **Liangqiu** *Beam Mound* xi-cleft	When the knee is flexed, point is 2 cun above the laterosuperior border of the patella.	Gastritis (stomach); mastitis (meridian); diseases of the knee (meridian); excess and hot ST problems; stuck food (needle against the flow of the qi)	• **Subdues Rebellious Qi:** for acute patterns of the Stomach with pain, hiccup, nausea, vomiting and belching. • **Open Channels:** for painful obstruction syndrome of the knee due to exterior dampness, wind and cold from the knee joint.
St-35 **Dubi** *Calf Nose*	When the knee is flexed, the point is at the lower border of the patella, in the depression lateral to the patellar ligament.	Numbness and motor impairment of the knee	• **Invigorate the Channels:** for painful obstruction syndrome of the knee. Used to expel dampness and cold.
St-36 **Zusanli** *Three Miles of the Leg* he-sea	3 cun below St-35, one finger breadth from the anterior crest of the tibia, in tibialis anterior.	Gastritis; ulcers; enteritis; all digestive problems; shock; mania; hypertension (deficiency type); allergies; hay fever; asthma; cough (deficiency type); neurasthenia (nervous exhaustion); nausea; vomiting; abscess breasts (channel problem); insufficient lactation	• **Tonifies Qi and Blood:** for all cases of deficiency of Stomach and Spleen, and to strengthen the body in debilitated persons after chronic disease. • **Tonifies the Defensive Qi:** used for prevention of attacks from exterior factors when symptoms include sweating or edema. • **Brightens eyes:** blurred vision or declining vision in elderly. • **Regulates the Intestines:** for constipation due to deficiency. • **Raises the Yang:** for prolapse when used with direct moxibustion in combination with Ren-6 and Du-20. • **Expels Wind and Damp from the channels in painful obstruction syndrome.** Can be used either as a local point for the knee or a distal point for the wrist.
St-37 **Shangjuxu** *Upper Great Emptiness*	3 cun below St-36, one finger breadth from the anterior crest of the tibia, in the muscle tibialis anterior.	Colitis; and problem in the large intestine; abdominal pain or distension; diarrhea; appendicitis; dysentery like disorder (any damp-heat disorder); hemiplegia	• **Regulates the Stomach and Intestines:** for chronic diarrhea and damp-heat patterns of the Large Intestine with loose stools and mucus and blood. • Opens the chest to calm asthma and breathlessness.
St-38 **Tiaokou** *Narrow Opening*	2 cun below St-37, one finger breadth lateral to the crest of tibia, midway between St-35 and St-41.	Perifocal inflammation of the shoulder; frozen shoulder; limited ROM; good local point	• **Opens channels:** pain and stiffness of the shoulder joint.

Points	Location	Usage	Indications / Functions
St-39 **Xiajuxu** *Lower Great Emptiness*	3 cun below the St-37, one finger breadth from the anterior crest of the tibia, in muscle tibialis anterior.	Acute or chronic enteritis; paralysis of lower limb; mastitis in some books	• **Regulates Stomach and Intestines:** for all patterns of the Small Intestine including lower abdominal pain with borborygmi and flatulence, damp-heat in the Small Intestine with cloudy, dark urine.
St-40 **Fenglong** *Abundant Bulge* luo-connect	8 cun superior to the external malleolus, two finger breadth lateral to St-38.	All phlegm situations; coughing; asthma (excess or deficient; but with phlegm); abundant mucous; phlegm nodules; damp headache with tight band around head; vertigo; swelling of the limbs; any significant swelling	• **Resolves Phlegm and Dampness:** for profuse expectoration from the chest, lumps under the skin, thyroid lumps and uterus lumps, phlegm misting the mind causing mental disturbances or dizziness and muzziness of the head. • Opens the chest and relieves asthma in phlegm patterns. • **Calms the Mind:** for phlegm misting the mind causing anxiety, fears and phobias. • **Relaxes the chest:** for bruising of the chest and rib-cage injuries.
St-41 **Jiexi** *Dispersing Stream* jing-river	On the dorsum of the foot, at the midpoint of the transverse crease of the ankle, in the depression between the tendons of muscle extensor digitorum longus and hallucis longus, approximately at the level of the tip of the external malleolus.	Disease of foot and soft tissues; good distal point on the ST meridian; ankle joint pain; motor impairment; dizziness and vertigo	• **Opens channels:** for painful obstruction syndrome of the foot to remove cold-damp. Is frequently used for ankle problems. • **Clears Stomach-heat:** burning epigastric pain and thirst or headache or sore throats due to stomach heat.
St-42 **Chongyang** *Rushing Yang* yuan	Distal to St-41, at the highest point of the dorsum of the foot, in the depression between the 2nd and 3rd metatarsal bones and cuneiform bone.	Pain in upper teeth; facial paralysis; muscular atrophy and motor impairment of the foot	• **Tonifies the Stomach and Spleen.** • Powerfully tonifies the middle burner and dispels cold from the joints.
St-43 **Xiangu** *Sinking Valley* shu-stream	In the depression distal to the junction of the 2nd and 3rd metatarsal bones.	Facial edema; conjunctivitis with heat	• Expels Wind and Heat from the joints in painful obstruction syndrome.
St-44 **Neiting** *Inner Courtyard* ying-spring	Proximal to the web margin between the 2nd and 3rd toes, in the depression distal and lateral to the 2nd metatarsodigital joint.	Upper toothache; trigeminal neuralgia; gastric pain; stomach heat from overeating; acid reflux with heat involved; hot diarrhea and constipation; sore throat and tonsillitis combined with digestive symptoms; gum disorders	• **Clears heat from the Stomach:** for febrile diseases, epistaxis, gastric pain, acid regurgitation, abdominal distention. • **Expels Wind from the face:** toothache, pain in the face, trigeminal neuralgia, facial paralysis, deviation of the mouth, sore throat. • **Promotes Digestion:** diarrhea, dysentery.
St-45 **Lidui** *Strict Exchange* jing-well	On the lateral side of the 2nd toe, .1 cun posterior to the corner of the nail.	Tonsillitis; febrile disease with heat; toothache (bleed); facial inflammation; distal point for any yangming face problems; dream-disturbed sleep; sore throat and hoarse voice; mania; coldness in the leg and foot	• **Calms the Mind:** for excess patterns such as Stomach-fire resulting in Heart-fire, with insomnia, irritability. • Clears Heat and brightens the eyes.

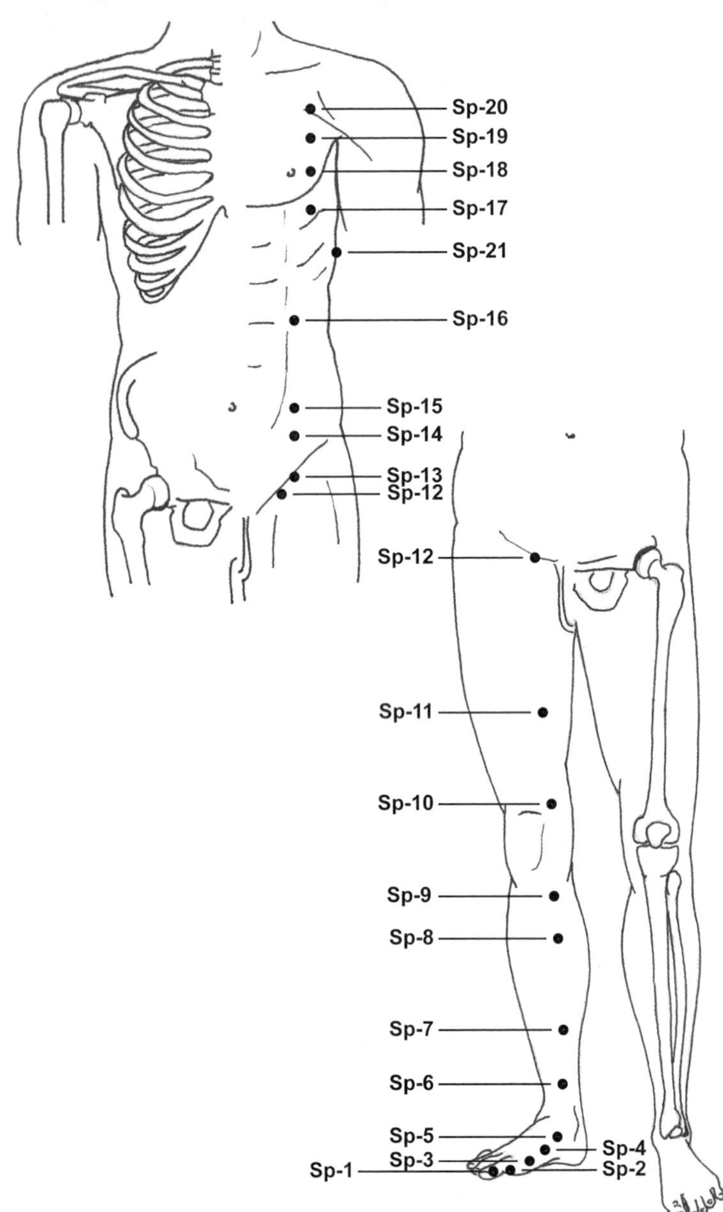

Jing Well	Ying Spring	Shu Stream	Jing River	He Sea
1	2	3	5	9
Yuan	**Luo-connect**	**Xi-Cleft**	**Front Mu**	**Back Shu**
3	4	8	Liv-13	Ub-20

Points	Location	Usage	Indications / Functions
Sp-1 **Yinbai** *Hidden White* jing-well	On the medial side of the great toe, .1 cun posterior to the corner of the nail.	Any kind of bleeding; especially uterine (mostly from deficiency); watery, thin, scanty menorrhagia; bleeding of GI tract (most common places for SP related bleeding); mental diseases (SP overthinking); continuous nose bleeds; blood in stool; dream-disturbed sleep; convulsions	• **Regulates Blood in cases of excess in the Spleen or Stomach**, especially in blood stasis in the uterus. • Used with direct moxa to stop bleeding from any part of the body. • Mental restlessness and depression due in excess patterns due to blood stasis.
Sp-2 **Dadu** *Great Metropolis* ying-spring	On the medial side of the great toe, distal and inferior to the first metatarso-digital joint, at the junction of the red and white skin.	Used for fever because the ying spring point; used locally for gout; foot pain; and cold feet	• Clears Heat in excess patterns to cause sweating in febrile diseases.
Sp-3 **Taibai** *Greater White* shu-stream, yuan	Proximal and inferior to the head of the first metatarsal bone, at the junction of the red and white skin.	Headache from damp; stomach or gastric pain; abdominal distension; usually due to damp; sluggishness damp feeling; mental obsessions (can't let it go); cloying kind of thing; like emotional dampness; deficient type constipation or diarrhea	• **Tonifies the Spleen in cases of deficiency:** includes stimulating mental faculties associated with Spleen function that is weakened by excess mental work. • **Resolves dampness in 3 jiaos:** for symptoms of confused thinking, muzziness of the head, stuffiness. • Treats chronic retention of phlegm in the Lungs. • **Strengthens and straightens the spine.**
Sp-4 **Gongsun** *Grandfather Grandson* luo-connect	In the depression distal and inferior to the base of the first metatarsal bone, at the junction of the red and white skin.	Fullness in chest and abdomen; great point for stomachache; acute and chronic enteritis; vomiting; endometriosis; amenorrhea (stuck type); intestines like a drum; abdominal pain and distension; Liv invading the SP; borborygmus; great point for gynecological problems	• **Tonifies Spleen and Stomach** • **For excess patterns of the Stomach and Spleen**: dampness in the epigastrium, stasis of blood in the Stomach, Stomach-heat and nausea or vomiting and stops abdominal pain. • **Opens the Chong:** regulates menstruation and stops excessive bleeding.
Sp-5 **Shangqiu** *Gold Mound* jing-river	In the depression distal and inferior to the medial malleolus, midway between the tuberosity of the navicular bone and the tip of the medial malleolus.	Edema; diseases of ankle and surrounding soft tissue	• **Painful obstruction syndrome:** for dampness, especially of the knee or ankle.
Sp-6 **Sanyinjiao** *Three Yin Meeting*	3 cun directly above the tip of the medial malleolus, on the posterior border of the medial aspect of the tibia.	Diseases of reproductive system; distension or pain in abdomen; diarrhea; hemiplegia; neurasthenia; eczema; urticaria; deficient and weak conditions of SP and ST; borborygmus; poor digestion; irregular menstruation; almost any reproductive system problem	• **Tonifies Spleen and Stomach, Resolves Dampness:** for diarrhea, distension, and weak stomach conditions. • **Harmonizes the Liver, Regulates menses, and harmonizes the lower jiao:** for irregular menstruation, and any reproductive problems. • **Calms the Mind, Moves the Blood.** • **Unblocks the Channels, Stops pain.**

Points	Location	Usage	Indications / Functions
Sp-7 **Lougu** *Leaking Valley*	3 cun above Sp-6, on the line joining the tip of the medial malleolus and Sp-9.	Abdominal distension; bloody stools; mental disorders; dream-disturbed sleep; convulsions	• Tonifies Spleen, Resolves Dampness. • Regulates menses, Harmonizes the Spleen, Moves the blood.
Sp-8 **Diji** *Earth Pivot* xi-cleft	3 cun below Sp-9, on the line joining the tip of the medial malleolus and Sp-9.	Irregular menstruation; dysmenorrhea; irregular menstruation; edema of the legs or abdomen; nocturnal emissions; stuck food; emotional stagnation	• **Removes obstructions and stops pain:** acute excess patterns including dysmenorrhea of either acute or chronic nature. • Regulates the uterus, stops pain by moving blood and reducing blood stasis.
Sp-9 **Yinlingquan** *Yin Mound Spring* he-sea	On the lower border of the medial condyle of the tibia, in the depression on the medial border of the tibia.	Distension and pain of the abdomen; ascites; edema; retention of urine; incontinence of urine; irregular menstruation due to damp; knee pain; diarrhea with undigested food; pain in the genitals; main diuretic point with Ren-9; main point for leukorrhea	• **Resolves Dampness in the lower burner:** damp-cold or damp-heat with symptoms of difficult urination, retention of urine, painful urination, cloudy urination, vaginal discharge, diarrhea, mucus in the stools and edema of the legs or abdomen. • Painful obstruction of the knee.
Sp-10 **Xuehai** *Sea of Blood*	When the knee is flexed, the point is 2 cun above the mediosuperior border of the patella, on the bulge of the medial portion of the muscle quadriceps femoris.	All skin diseases (especially redness and itchiness); irregular menstruation; dermatitis; menstrual and uterine bleeding disorders (from heat in blood)	• **Cools the Blood:** for blood heat patterns causing skin diseases such as eczema, urticaria and rashes. Also used for menorrhagia or metrorrhagia when due to heat in the blood. • **Removes Blood Stasis:** for stagnant blood especially in the uterus, including painful or irregular periods, chronic or acute dysmenorrhea.
Sp-11 **Jimen** *Winnower*	6 cun above Sp-10, on the line drawn from Sp-10 to Sp-12.	Dysuria; enuresis; lower extremities paralysis and pain; muscular atrophy	• Regulates urination, Drains Damp, Clears Heat.
Sp-12 **Chongmen** *Rushing Door*	Superior to the lateral end of the groove, on the lateral side of the femoral artery, at the level of the upper border of the symphisis pubis, 3.5 cun lateral to Ren-2.	Abdominal pain; hernia; dysuria	• Nourishes Yin: for Kidney deficiency. • Painful obstruction syndrome of the hip.
Sp-13 **Fushe** *Bowel Abode*	.7 cun laterosuperior to Sp-12, 4 cun lateral to the Ren meridian.	Lower abdominal pain; hernia	• Regulates Qi, Stops pain.
Sp-14 **Fujie** *Abdominal Bind*	1.3 cun below Sp-15, 4 cun lateral to the Ren meridian, on the lateral side of the muscle rectus abdominis.	Pain around umbilical region; hernia; diarrhea; constipation	• Regulates Qi, Subdues Rebellion, Warms and benefits lower jiao.
Sp-15 **Daheng** *Big Horizontal Stroke*	4 cun lateral to the center of the umbilicus, lateral to the muscle rectus abdominis.	Abdominal pain and distension; constipation; diarrhea; dysentery	• **Strengthens Spleen Function:** for chronic constipation due to deficiency. • **Strengthens Limbs:** for cold or weak limbs. • **Resolves Dampness:** for chronic diarrhea with mucus in the stools due to deficiency. • **Regulates Qi:** promotes the smooth flow of Liver qi manifesting in abdominal pain.
Sp-16 **Fuai** *Abdominal Lament*	3 cun above Sp-15, 4 cun lateral to Ren-11.	Abdominal pain; diarrhea; dysentery; constipation	• Regulates the Intestines.

Points	Location	Usage	Indications / Functions
Sp-17 **Shidou** *Food Hole*	In the 5th intercostal space, 6 cun lateral to the Ren meridian.	Chest and hypochondriac fullness and pain	• Reduces food stagnation, Promotes digestion.
Sp-18 **Tianxi** *Heavens Ravine*	In the 4th intercostal space, 6 cun lateral to the Ren meridian.	Insufficient lactation; chest and hypochondriac fullness and pain; hiccups; mastitis	• Regulates and Descends Qi, Benefits the breast, Promotes lactation.
Sp-19 **Xiongxiang** *Chest Village*	In the 3rd intercostal space, 6 cun lateral to the Ren meridian.	Chest and hypochondriac fullness and pain	• Regulates Qi, Subdues rebellion.
Sp-20 **Zhourong** *All Round Flourishing*	In the 2nd intercostal space, 6 cun lateral to the Ren meridian.	Chest and hypochondriac fullness and pain; cough; hiccups	• Regulates Qi, Descends Qi.
Sp-21 **Dabao** *Great Wrapping*	On the mid-axillary line, 6 cun below the axilla, in the 6th intercostal space, midway between the axilla and the free end of the 11th rib.	General body soreness; excess in the luo vessels	• **Moves Blood in the connecting channels:** for muscular pain moving throughout the body.

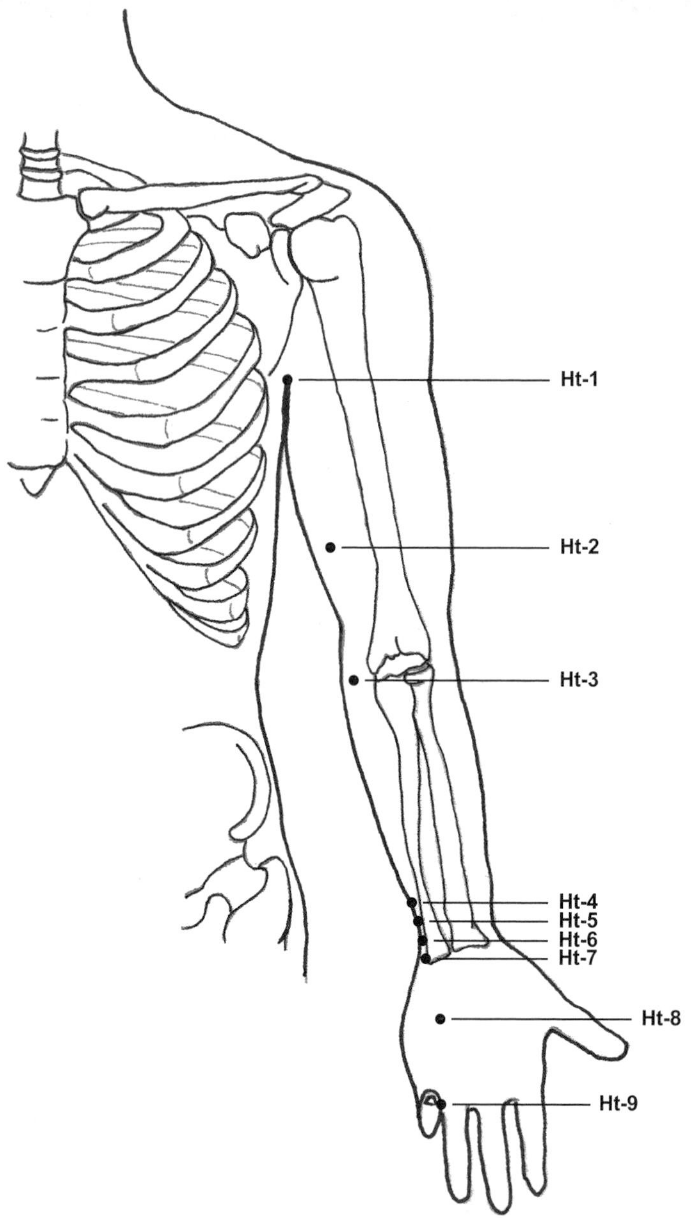

Jing Well	Ying Spring	Shu Stream	Jing River	He Sea
9	8	7	4	3
Yuan	**Luo-connect**	**Xi-Cleft**	**Front Mu**	**Back Shu**
7	5	6	Ren-14	Ub-15

Points	Location	Usage	Indications / Functions
Ht-1 Jiquan *Summit Spring*	When the upper arm is abducted, the point is in the center of the axilla, on the medial side of the axillary artery.	Arthritis; local shoulder joint problems; generally for armpit problems; not very common	• **Nourishes Heart Yin and Clears deficiency heat:** for dry mouth, night sweating, mental restlessness, and insomnia. • Also used in sequelae of wind-stroke for paralysis of the arm.
Ht-2 Qingling *Green Spirit*	When the elbow is flexed, the point is 3 cun above the medial end of the transverse cubital crease (Ht-3), in the groove medial to muscle biceps brachii.	Cardiac and hypochondriac pain; shoulder and arm pain	• Unblocks the Channels, Stops pain.
Ht-3 Shaohai *Lesser Sea* he-sea	When the elbow is flexed, the point is in the depression between the medial end of the transverse cubital crease of the elbow and the medial epicondyle of the humerus.	Neurasthenia; psychosis; intercostal neuralgia; ulnar neuralgia; important for hand tremors; good for trembling and shaking from Parkinson's; cardiac/chest pain; pain in axilla	• **Clears Heat:** for Heart-fire or Heart deficiency heat. • **Calms the Mind:** for epilepsy, depression, mental retardation or hypomania due to Heart fire.
Ht-4 Lingdao *Spirit Pathway* jing-river	When the palm faces upward, the point is on the radial side of the tendon of muscle flexor carpi ulnaris, 1.5 cun above the transverse crease of the wrist.	Aphasia; main point for speaking difficulties; bradycardia; hysterical aphasia; stuttering due to emotional issues; nervous anxiety; uptight nervousness	• Unblocks obstructions from the Heart channel: for spasm and neuralgia of the forearm and arthritis of the elbow and wrist.
Ht-5 Tongli *Penetrating the Interior* luo-connect	When the palm faces upward, the point is on the radial side of the tendon of m. flexor carpi ulnaris, 1 cun above the transverse crease of the wrist.	Palpitations; dizziness; blurry vision; sore throat; sudden voice loss; aphasia with stiff tongue; wrist and elbow pain	• **Main point to tonify Heart Qi:** for all symptoms of Heart-qi deficiency and especially aphasia due to its effect on the tongue. • **Benefits the Bladder:** for Heart fire causing heat in the Urinary Bladder via the Small Intestine channel with symptoms of thirst, bitter taste, insomnia, tongue ulcers, burning on urination and hematuria.
Ht-6 Yinxi *Yin's Crevice* xi-cleft	When the palm faces upward, the point is on the radial side of the tendon of m. flexor carpi ulnaris, 0.5 cun above the transverse crease of the wrist.	Night sweats; nosebleed; cardiac pain; hysteria	• **Nourishes Heart yin:** for Heart yin deficiency with symptoms including night sweating, dry mouth, insomnia. • **Clears Heart-fire and Heart yin deficiency heat:** for mental restlessness and feelings of heat from deficiency.
Ht-7 Shenmen *Spirit Gate* shu-stream, yuan	At the ulnar end of the transverse crease of the wrist, in the depression on the radial side of the tendon of muscle flexor carpi ulnaris.	Palpitations; absent mindedness; insomnia; excessive dreaming due to HT or Liv fire; angina and cardiac pain; mental illness of any kind; dementia; mania; irritability and insomnia; main point for insomnia; hysteria	• **Calms the Mind:** for any Heart pattern and nourishes Heart blood with symptoms of anxiety, insomnia, poor memory, palpitation, cardiac pain and hysteria and a pale tongue.
Ht-8 Shaofu *Lesser Palace* ying-spring	When the palm faces upward, the point is between the 4th and 5th metacarpal bones. When a fist is made, the point is where the tip of the little finger rests.	Tachycardia; dysuria; enuresis; itching of the groin; sweaty palms	• **Clears Heat in the Heart:** for both excess and deficiency heat patterns of the Heart with symptoms of insomnia, vivid dreams, thirst, bitter taste, mental restlessness or hypomania, dark urine, tongue ulcers, and a Red tongue with redder tip and yellow coating. • **Calms the Mind:** for more excess patterns including schizophrenia and psychosis.
Ht-9 Shaochong *Lesser Surge* jing-well	On the radial side of the little finger, .1 cun posterior to the corner of the nail.	Coma; apoplectic hysteria	• **For excess patterns of the Heart with Heat:** including wind-stroke due to internal wind.

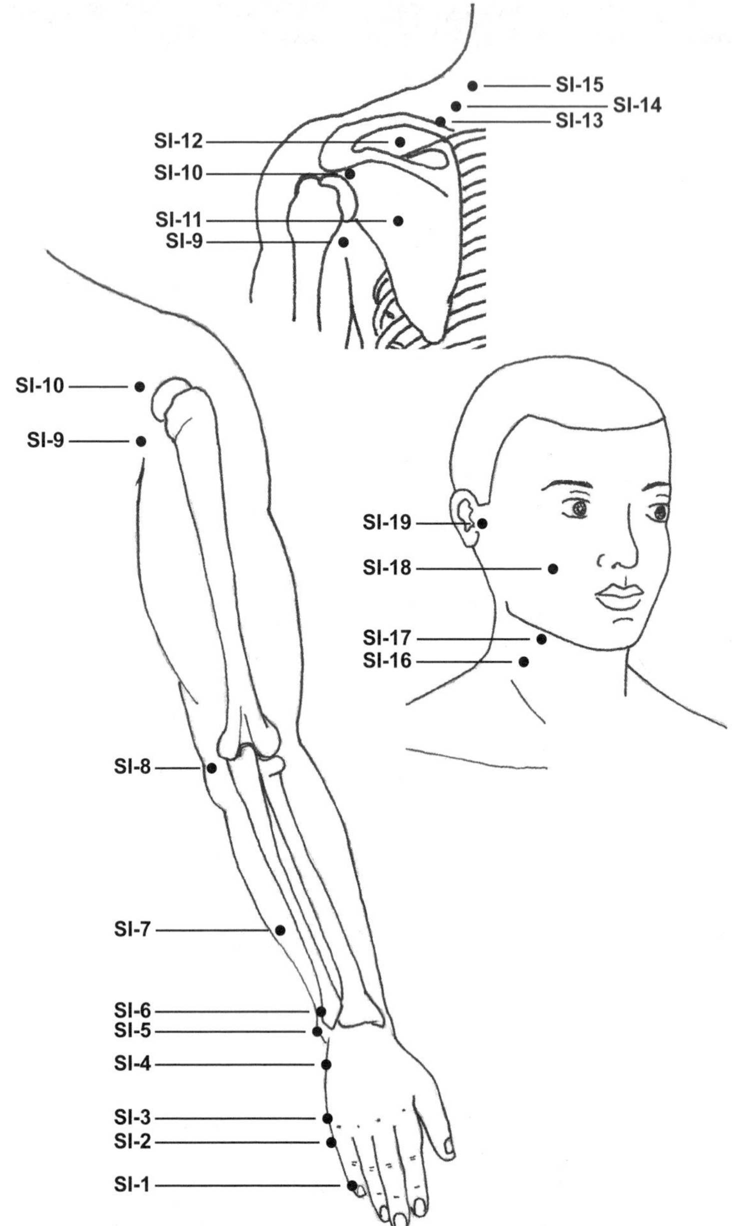

Jing Well	Ying Spring	Shu Stream	Jing River	He Sea
1	2	3	5	8
Yuan	**Luo-connect**	**Xi-Cleft**	**Front Mu**	**Back Shu**
4	7	6	Ren-4	Ub-27

Points	Location	Usage	Indications / Functions
SI-1 Shaoze *Lesser Marsh* jing-well	On the ulnar side of the little finger, about .1 cun posterior to the corner of the nail.	Mastitis; insufficient lactations; sometimes for PMS breast tenderness; swollen breasts including benign breast lumps and fibrocystic lumps; as jing well point can be used for loss of consciousness	• Expels Wind-heat: for exterior attacks, especially when the symptoms affect the head and neck, causing stiff neck and headache. Also used to treat tonsillitis from invasion of exterior wind-heat. • Opens the orifices and promote resuscitation: for internal wind and phlegm blocking the orifices and causing sudden unconsciousness, as in wind-stroke. • Used as a distal point for channel problems of the neck including chronic stiff neck or acute torticollis. • Promotes lactation: when lactation is inhibited by the presence of some pathogenic factor or stagnation.
SI-2 Qiangu *Front Valley* ying-spring	When a loose fist is made, the point is on the ulnar side, distal to the 5th MP joint, at the junction of the red and white skin.	Numb fingers; febrile diseases; tinnitus	• **Clears Heat:** for both interior and exterior heat patterns, especially when the neck and eyes are affected and also to clear interior heat from the Small Intestine, or acute febrile diseases. Also for clearing heat in the Urinary Bladder with burning on urination.
SI-3 Houxi *Back Stream* shu-stream	When a loose fist is made, the point is on the ulnar side, proximal to the 5th MP joint, at the end of the transverse crease at the junction of the red and white and skin.	Seizures; psychosis; mania; all kinds of sweating; stiff neck; low back pain (acute and chronic); mania; malaria; night sweats; tinnitus; deafness (meridian related); the strongest distal point on the SI meridian	• **Opens the Governing Vessel:** for all symptoms of the Du channel including eliminating interior wind from the channel with convulsions, tremors, epilepsy, stiff neck, and giddiness and headache. In combination with Ub-62 it can be used to affect the whole spine and back in both acute and chronic cases. • **Eliminates Exterior Wind:** for both wind-heat and wind-cold when there are symptoms affecting the neck and head such as stiff neck, occipital headache, aches down the spine and back, and chills and fever. • **Benefits the sinews and tendons:** especially along the Du, Small Intestine and Bladder channels. In particular, for the upper more than the lower back area along the Small Intestine and Bladder channels. More for acute than chronic conditions. • **Clears the Mind:** helps strengthen the mind to face up to choices and difficult decisions.
SI-4 Wangu *Wrist Bone* yuan	On the ulnar side of the palm, in the depression between the base of the fifth metacarpal bone and the triquetral bone.	Wrist pain; neck rigidity; finger contracture	• **Unblocks the Channels:** mostly used for channel problems of the Small Intestine including painful obstruction syndrome of the wrist or elbow. • **Clears Damp-heat:** for jaundice from damp-heat obstructing the Gallbladder, hypochondriac pain or cholecystitis.
SI-5 Yanggu *Yang Valley* jing-river	At the ulnar end of the transverse crease on the dorsal aspect of the wrist, in the depression between the styloid process of the ulna and the triquetral bone.	Hand and wrist pain; febrile diseases	• **Clears the Mind:** helpful in distinguishing correct action, direction, due to providing a sense of clarity. • Unblocks the channel. • **Expels Exterior Damp-heat:** eliminates dampness from the knees when they are swollen and hot.
SI-6 Yanglao *Nourishing the Old* xi-cleft	Dorsal to the head of the ulna. When the palm faces the chest, the point is in the bony cleft on the radial side of the styloid process of the ulna.	Pain in shoulder and back; arthritis; main point for acute low back sprains; used a lot for whiplash	• **Benefits the sinews and unblocks the channels:** used for any channel problems of the Small Intestine, particularly when there is tightness of the tendons and ligaments causing stiff neck and shoulders. • **Brightens eyes:** benefits the eyesight in patterns related to Heart or Small Intestine.
SI-7 Zhizheng *Branch to Heart Channel* luo-connect	On the line joining SI-5 and SI-8, 5 cun above SI-5.	Headache; spastic elbow and fingers	• Unblocks the channel: treats any channel problem, especially related to elbow problems. • Calms the Mind: for severe anxiety affecting the Heart. • Treats thyroid phlegm swellings.

Points	Location	Usage	Indications / Functions
SI-8 Xiaohai *Small Intestine Sea* he-sea	When the elbow is flexed, the point is located in the depression between the olecranon of the ulna and the medial epicondyle of the humerus.	Headache; nape pain; shoulder arm and neck pain; epilepsy	• **Clears Damp-heat:** effective in treating acute swelling of the glands of the neck and parotitis. • Removes obstruction from the channel: painful obstruction syndrome of the elbow and neck. • Calms the Mind: heart patterns with anxiety.
SI-9 Jianzhen *Upright Shoulder*	Posterior and inferior to the shoulder joint. When the arm is adducted, the point is 1 cun above the posterior end of the axillary fold.	Scapula pain	• Benefits the shoulder, Unblocks the channels, Stops pain: local point for painful obstruction syndrome of the shoulder.
SI-10 Naoshu *Upper Arm Hollow*	When the arm is adducted, the point is directly above SI-9, in the depression inferior to the scapular spine.	Swelling shoulders; shoulder and arm pain	• Benefits the shoulder, Unblocks the channels, Stops pain: local point for painful obstruction syndrome of the shoulder.
SI-11 Tianzong *Heavenly Attribution*	In the infrascapular fossa, at the junction of the upper and middle third of the distance between the lower border of the scapular spine and the inferior angle of the scapula.	Pain in the shoulder; insufficient lactations	• Benefits the shoulder, Unblocks the channels, Stops pain, Benefits the breast: local point for painful obstruction syndrome of the shoulder.
SI-12 Bingfeng *Grasping the Wind*	In the center of the suprascapular fossa, directly above SI-11. When the arm is lifted, the point is at the site of the depression.	Scapula pain; shoulder and arm motor impairment	• Benefits the shoulder, Unblocks the channels, Expels the Wind: local point for painful obstruction syndrome of the shoulder.
SI-13 Quyuan *Crooked Wall*	On the medial extremity of the suprascapular fossa, about midway between SI-10 and the spinous process of the 2nd thoracic vertebra.	Scapula pain and stiffness	• Benefits the shoulder and scapula: local point for painful obstruction syndrome of the shoulder.
SI-14 Jianwaishu *Outer Shoulder Shu*	3 cun lateral to the lower border of the spinous process of the 1st thoracic vertebra where Du-13 is located.	Shoulder and back pain; neck stiffness and pain	• Benefits the shoulder and scapula, Stops pain, Expels Wind: local point for painful obstruction syndrome of the shoulder and trapezius.
SI-15 Jianzhongzhu *Middle Shoulder Shu*	2 cun lateral to the lower border of the spinous process of the 7th cervical vertebra.	Cough; asthma; pain in shoulder and arm; hemoptysis	• Unblocks the channels, Stops pain, Descends Lung Qi: local point for painful obstruction syndrome of the shoulder and neck.
SI-16 Tianchuang *Heaven Window*	In the lateral aspect of the neck, in the posterior border of the SCM, posterior and superior to LI-18.	Tinnitus; stiff neck; loss of voice	• Benefits the ear, throat, and voice, Unblocks the channels, Stops pain, Clears Heat.
SI-17 Tianrong *Heavenly Appearance*	Posterior to the angle of the mandible, in the depression on the anterior border of the SCM.	Difficulty hearing; difficulty swallowing; sometimes goiter; tonsillitis	• Resolves Damp-heat: for both interior and exterior damp-heat and is indicated in swelling of the cervical glands, parotitis and tonsillitis.
SI-18 Quanliao *Zygomatic Crevice*	Directly below the outer canthus, in the depression on the lower border of the zygomatic bone.	Trigeminal neuralgia; facial paralysis; toothache in upper jaw	• **Expels Wind, Relieves Pain:** local point for treating facial paralysis, tics or trigeminal neuralgia.
SI-19 Tinggong *Listening Palace*	Anterior to the tragus and posterior to the condyloid process of the mandible, in the depression formed when the mouth is open.	Tinnitus; difficulty hearing; jaw problems like TMJ; otitis media	• **Benefits the ear:** local point for tinnitus and deafness.

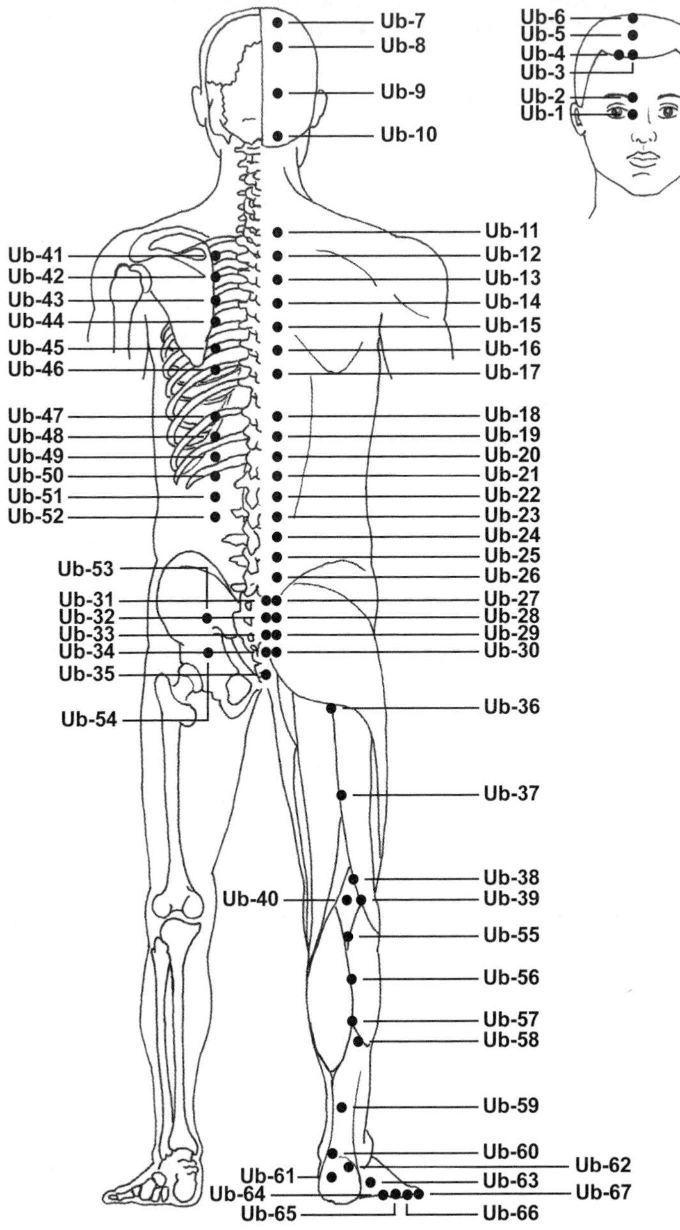

Jing Well	Ying Spring	Shu Stream	Jing River	He Sea
67	66	65	60	40
Yuan	**Luo-connect**	**Xi-Cleft**	**Front Mu**	**Back Shu**
64	58	63	Ren-3	Ub-28

Points	Location	Usage	Indications / Functions
Ub-1 **Jingming** *Eye Brightness*	0.1 cun superior to the inner canthus.	Any eye problems; blindness; blurring; itchy canthus	• **Expels Exterior Wind and Clears Heat:** for conjunctivitis and runny eyes due to exterior wind, red, painful, swollen and dry eyes due to Liver-fire, and stops pain and itching due to heat. • Treats insomnia and somnolence by opening the Yin and Yang Qiao vessels.
Ub-2 **Zanzhu** *Collecting Bamboo*	On the medial extremity of the eyebrow, or on the supraorbital notch.	Headache (local point); acute conjunctivitis; excessive tearing; excessive twitching; good point for sinus allergies; hay fever; sinus headaches	• Expels Wind from the face and removes obstructions from the channel: for facial paralysis, facial tics and trigeminal neuralgia. • Brightens the eyes and soothes the Liver: for any Liver pattern affecting the eyes such as floaters in the eyes, red eyes, blurred vision, and persistent headaches around or behind the eyes.
Ub-3 **Meichong** *Eyebrow Surging*	Directly above the medial end of the eyebrow, 0.5 cun within the anterior hairline between Du-24 and Ub-4.	Headache; giddiness; nasal obstruction	• Expels Wind, Clears the head, Stops pain, Benefits the eyes and nose.
Ub-4 **Quchai** *Deviating Turn*	1.5 cun lateral to Du-24 at the junction of the medial 1/3 and lateral 2/3 of the distance from Du-24 to St-8.	Headache; nasal obstruction; epistaxis; blurry and failed vision	• Expels Wind, Clears the head, Stops pain, Benefits the eyes and nose.
Ub-5 **Wuchu** *Five Places*	10.5 cun lateral to Du-23, or 0.5 cun directly above Ub-4.	Headache; blurry vision; epilepsy; convulsion	• Subdue Interior Wind: a local point to treat epilepsy, convulsions or rigidity of the spine in children during a febrile disease. • Restores Consciousness: for acute attacks of interior wind with unconsciousness.
Ub-6 **Chengguang** *Receiving Light*	1.5 cun posterior to Ub-5, 1.5 cun lateral to the DU meridian.	Rhinitis (nasal obstruction); any nose problem	• Expels Wind, Clears Heat, Benefits the eyes and nose.
Ub-7 **Tongtian** *Reaching Heaven*	1.5 cun posterior to Ub-6, 1.5 cun lateral to the DU meridian.	Headache; nasal obstruction; rhinorrhea	• Dispels Wind: for both exterior and interior wind patterns of the head causing severe headache or facial paralysis, dizziness, vertigo. A local point for vertex headaches due to liver yang rising or liver-wind or Liver-blood deficiency. • Subdues interior wind: local point for convulsions and unconsciousness. • For the eyes and nose, rhinitis.
Ub-8 **Luoque** *Declining Connection*	1.5 cun posterior to Ub-7, 1.5 cun lateral to the DU meridian.	Dizziness; blurry vision; mania; tinnitus	• Benefits sensory organs, Transforms Phlegm, Calms the Mind.
Ub-9 **Yuzhen** *Jade Pillow*	1.3 cun lateral to Du-17, on the lateral side of the superior border of the EOP.	Occipital headache; stiffness and soreness in back of neck; pharyngitis; URIs; common cold; seizures (wind)	• Expels Wind and Cold, Stops pain, Benefits the nose and eyes.
Ub-10 **Tianzhu** *Heaven Pillar*	1.3 cun lateral to Du-15, in the depression on the lateral aspect of the trapezius muscle.	With common cold; bronchitis; with pleurisy can be needled if tender; neck and back pain	• **Expels Wind:** for both exterior and interior wind in the head, for occipital or vertex headache from any origin. Also for wind causing stiff neck and headache due to wind-cold invasion. • **Subdues Interior Wind:** for occipital headaches deriving from Liver wind rising. • **Clears the brain:** stimulates memory and concentration. • Increases vision, especially due to Kidney deficiency. • **Invigorates the lower back:** for bilateral acute lower backache.

Points	Location	Usage	Indications / Functions
Ub-11 **Dazhu** *Great Shuttle*	1.5 cun lateral to Du-13, at the level of the lower border of the spinous process of T1.	Common cold; bronchitis; pleurisy; can use for taiyang stage disease (some say it is best used before the pathogen gets into the organ); URIs like wind-heat	• **Nourishes Blood:** for generalized muscular ache due to blood not nourishing the muscles. • **Releases the Exterior:** for wind-cold or wind-heat. • **Nourishes the Bones:** promotes bone formation and prevent bone degeneration in the elderly or in chronic arthritis. Also treats contractions of the tendons.
Ub-12 **Fengmen** *Wind Door*	1.5 cun lateral to the DU meridian, at the level of the lower border of the spinous process of T2.	Bronchitis; asthma; pleurisy; night sweats; pulmonary TB; steaming bone syndrome (severe kidney yin deficiency); spitting blood from lungs; any kind of cough; fullness in chest; throat blockage; anything that affects lungs	• For beginning stage of exterior invasion of wind-cold or wind-heat with symptoms of stuffy nose, sneezing, chills, aversion to cold and headache.
Ub-13 **Feishu** *Lung Back Shu*	1.5 cun lateral to Du-12, at the level of the lower border of the spinous process of T3.	Cough; asthma; chest pain; spitting blood	• For both exterior and interior patterns of the Lung, especially including cough, breathlessness or asthma. • **Clears Heat from the Lungs**: for acute bronchitis or pneumonia, high fever, thirst, a cough with sticky yellow sputum, breathlessness, restlessness, a rapid pulse and a red tongue body with a thick dry yellow coating. • **Tonifies Lung Qi:** for chronic deficiency of Lung qi or Lung yin.
Ub-14 **Jueyinshu** *Terminal Yin Shu*	1.5 cun lateral to the DU meridian, at level with the lower border of the spinous process of T4.	Neurasthenia (nervous system exhaustion); seizures; psychosis; hysteria; absent-mindedness; any mental problems; very good insomnia point; mania; memory loss; palpitations	• For Heart conditions, including arrhythmia, tachycardia, angina pectoris and coronary heart disease.
Ub-15 **Xinshu** *Heart Shu*	1.5 cun lateral to the Du-11, at the level of the lower border of the spinous process of T5.	Cardiac pain; loss of memory; palpitation; spitting blood; night sweat; epilepsy	• **Calms the Mind:** for nervous anxiety and insomnia due to excess conditions of the Heart such as Heart-fire, or Heart yin deficiency. Also for anxiety and insomnia due to deficiency conditions such as Heart blood deficiency or Heart yin deficiency. • Invigorates Blood: for pain in the chest due to blood stasis.
Ub-16 **Dushu** *DU - Governing Vessel Shu*	1.5 cun lateral to Du-10, at the level of the lower border of the spinous process of T6.	Cardiac pain; abdominal pain	• Regulates Qi in the chest and abdomen.

Points	Location	Usage	Indications / Functions
Ub-17 **Geshu** *Diaphragm Shu*	1.5 cun lateral to Du-9, at the level of the lower border of the spinous process of T7.	Anemia; chronic hemorrhagic disorders; spasms of the diaphragm; nervous vomiting; constriction of the esophagus; abdominal distension or lumps; good for skin indications (heat in the blood); chronic and acute hepatitis; cholecystitis (Liv/ GB damp-heat); stomach disease (Liv invading ST); eye diseases (ascendant Liv yang); intercostal neuralgia (pathway); irregular menstruation (due to Liv disharmony); emotional aspects of the Liv; measles; night sweats; hiccups	• **Nourishes Blood:** for deficiency of blood in any organ and is combined with other shu points to target blood of specific organs. • **Invigorates Blood and removes blood stagnation:** a general point to remove blood stasis in any organ and from any part of the body. • **Moves Qi in the diaphragm and chest:** for stuffiness and pain of the chest, fullness in the epigastrium, belching and hiccup. • **Pacifies Stomach Qi and Subdues rebellious Stomach Qi:** for hiccup, belching, nausea and vomiting. • **Tonifies Blood and Qi.**
Ub-18 **Ganshu** *Liver Shu*	1.5 cun lateral to Du-8, at the level of the lower border of the spinous process of T9. (Skips T8).	Hepatitis; cholecystitis; gastritis; bitter taste in mouth; dry or bilious vomiting; pain in the flanks; yellowish eyes/ jaundice	• **Benefits the Liver and Gallbladder:** for stagnation of Liver qi or retention of damp-heat in the Liver and Gallbladder causing distension of the epigastrium and hypochondrium, sour regurgitation, nausea, jaundice and cholecystitis. Also for Liver deficiency patterns such as Liver blood deficiency. • **Benefits the eyes:** promotes vision in all eye disorders related to Liver disharmony such as poor night vision, blurred vision, floaters, red and painful and swollen eyes.
Ub-19 **Danshu** *Gall Bladder Shu*	1.5 cun lateral to Du-7, at the level of the lower border of the spinous process of T10.	Jaundice; bitter taste of the mouth; chest and hypochondriac pain; pulmonary TB	• **Resolves Damp-heat in the Liver and Gallbladder:** for jaundice and cholecystitis. • Pacifies the Stomach and Stimulates the Descending of Stomach Qi: for belching, nausea and vomiting. • **Relaxes the diaphragm:** moves qi in the diaphragm for feelings of stuffiness and pain of the chest, fullness in the epigastrium, belching and hiccup due to Liver qi stagnation.
Ub-20 **Pishu** *Spleen Shu*	1.5 cun lateral to Du-6, at the level of the lower border of the spinous process of T11.	Gastritis from deficiency; prolapsed stomach; nervous vomiting; indigestion; edema; weakness or heaviness of the limbs due to damp	• Tonifies Spleen Qi and Yang, Resolves Dampness, Raises Spleen Qi, Regulates and Harmonizes middle jiao.
Ub-21 **Weishu** *Stomach Shu*	1.5 cun lateral to the DU meridian, at the level of the lower border of the spinous process of T12.	Stomach ache; gastric distension; anorexia; regurged vomiting; abdominal pain from cold in ST; diarrhea; nausea	• **Regulates and Tonifies the Stomach:** for subduing ascending Stomach qi causing belching, hiccup, nausea and vomiting. • **Relieves food stagnation:** for food stagnation causing fullness of the epigastrium, sour regurgitation and belching.
Ub-22 **Sanjiaoshu** *Triple Burner Back Shu*	1.5 cun lateral to the Du-5, at the level of the lower border of the spinous process of L1.	Borborygmus; abdominal distention; indigestion; vomiting; diarrhea; dysentery; low back pain (local point); edema from urinary retention	• **Resolves Dampness and Opens the water passages:** for dampness, particularly in the lower burner causing urinary retention, painful urination, edema of the legs and any other manifestation of dampness in the lower burner.

Points	Location	Usage	Indications / Functions
Ub-23 **Shenshu** *Kidney Shu*	1.5 cun lateral to Du-4, at the level of the lower border of the spinous process of the L2.	Low back pain; nocturnal emission; impotence; irregular menstruation; weakness of the knee; dizziness; tinnitus; deafness; edema; diarrhea	• **Tonifies Kidney:** for any chronic Kidney deficiency. • **Nourishes Kidney Essence:** for impotence, nocturnal emissions, infertility, spermatorrhea and lack of sexual desire. Also for chronic asthma due to Kidney not grasping the Lung Qi. Also used as a stimulus.
Ub-24 **Qihaishu** *Sea of Qi Shu*	1.5 cun lateral to the DU meridian, at the level of the lower border of the spinous process of L3.	Low back pain or sprain; irregular menstruation; dysmenorrhea; asthma	• Strengthen low back and unblocks the channels: a local point for low back weakness. • Regulates Qi and Blood: for blood stasis in the lower burner including uterine bleeding and irregular menstruation.
Ub-25 **Dachangshu** *Large Intestine Shu*	1.5 cun lateral to Du-3, at the level of the lower border of the spinous process of L4.	Low back pain; borborygmus; abdominal distention; diarrhea; constipation; numbness and motor impairment of lower extremities; sciatica	• **Promotes Large Intestine Function:** for both constipation and diarrhea and for chronic disease of the Large Intestine. • **Relieves fullness and swelling:** for excess patterns of the Large Intestine with abdominal fullness and distension. • **Strengthens low back:** a local point for acute lower backache.
Ub-26 **Guanyuanshu** *Origin Gate Shu*	1.5 cun lateral to the DU meridian, at the level of the lower border of the spinous process of L5.	Low back pain; abdominal distention; diarrhea; enuresis; urinary incontinence	• Strengthens back, Removes obstructions from the Channels: a local point for low backache.
Ub-27 **Xiaochuangshu** *Small Intestine Shu*	1.5 cun lateral to the DU meridian, at the level of the lower border of the 1st posterior sacral foramen.	Lower abdominal pain and distention; dysentery; nocturnal emission; hematuria; sciatica; low back pain	• **Promotes Small Intestine Function:** for stimulating the receiving and separating functions of the Small Intestine, or any Small Intestine pattern causing borborygmus, abdominal pain and mucus in the stools. • **Resolves dampness, Clears Heat, benefits urination:** also to eliminate damp-heat from the lower burner and benefit urination to treat cloudy urination, difficult urination and burning, painful urination.
Ub-28 **Pangguangshu** *Bladder Shu*	1.5 cun lateral to the DU meridian, at the level of the 2nd posterior sacral foramen.	Incontinence; dark and rough flowing urine; swelling and pain in the genitals; sacral back pain; sciatica; good for UTIs; atonic bladder; prostate problems	• **Regulates the Bladder, Resolves Dampness:** for retention of urine, difficult urination and cloudy urine due to dampness. • **Clears Heat, stops pain:** for painful, burning urine, or pain due to renal stones. • **Opens the water passages:** improves transformation and excretion of dirty fluids in the lower burner and promotes dieresis. • **Strengthens lower back.**
Ub-29 **Zhonglushu** *Central Spine Shu*	1.5 cun lateral to the DU meridian, at the level of the 3rd posterior sacral foramen.	Anal disease; dysentery; stiffness and pain of lower back	• Benefits lumbar region, Dispels Cold, Stops diarrhea.
Ub-30 **Baihuanshu** *White Ring Shu*	1.5 cun lateral to the DU meridian, at the level of the 4th posterior sacral foramen.	Enuresis; pain due to hernia; leukorrhea; dysuria; cold sensation; rectum prolapse; constipation	• Strengthens lumbar region and legs, Regulates menses, Stops leakages: for hemorrhoids, prolapse of the anus, spasm of the anus, and incontinence of feces.
Ub-31 **Shangliao** *Upper Crevice*	In the 1st posterior sacral foramen.	Diseases of the lumbosacral joint; leukorrhea; peritonitis; orchitis; paralysis; paralysis of lower limb; sequelae of infantile paralysis; urinary problems; prolapsed uterus; constipation; infertility	• **Regulates the lower burner:** for genital disorders in men and women causing leukorrhea, prolapse of the uterus and sterility, impotence, orchitis and prostatitis. • **Strengthens the lumbar region and Nourishes the Kidneys:** for benefiting essence, and strengthening the low back and knees.

Points	Location	Usage	Indications / Functions
Ub-32 **Ciliao** *Second Crevice* ↓ 0.8 – 1.2	In the 2nd posterior sacral foramen.	Low back pain; hernia; nocturnal emission; impotence; urinary problems; prolapsed uterus; constipation	• **Regulates the lower burner:** for genital disorders in men and women causing leukorrhea, prolapse of the uterus and sterility, impotence, orchitis and prostatitis. • **Strengthens the lumbar region and Nourishes the Kidneys:** for benefiting essence and strengthening the low back and knees. • Raises the Qi in prolapse of the anus or uterus.
Ub-33 **Zhongliao** *Central Crevice* ↓ 0.8 – 1.2	In the 3rd posterior sacral foramen.	Lower back pain; constipation; diarrhea; dysuria; irregular menstruation	• Regulates the lower burner: for genital disorders in men and women causing leukorrhea, prolapse of the uterus and sterility, impotence, orchitis and prostatitis. • Strengthen the lumbar region and Nourishes the Kidneys: for benefiting essence, and strengthening the low back and knees.
Ub-34 **Xialiao** *Lower Crevice*	In the 4th posterior sacral foramen.	Pain in lower back during menstruation; leukorrhea; impotence; diarrhea; hemorrhoids	• Regulates the lower burner: for genital disorders in men and women causing leukorrhea, prolapse of the uterus and sterility, impotence, orchitis and prostatitis. • Strengthens the lumbar region and Nourishes the Kidneys: for benefiting essence, and strengthening the low back and knees.
Ub-35 **Huiyang** *Meeting of Yang*	On either side of the tip of the coccyx, 0.5 cun lateral to the DU meridian.	Sciatica; paralysis of lower extremity	• Clears Damp-heat, Regulates lower jiao, Treats hemorrhoids.
Ub-36 **Chengfu** *Receiving Support*	In the middle of the transverse gluteal fold. Locate the point in the prone position.	Lower back and gluteal pain; constipation; muscular atrophy	• Opens the channels, Stops pain: used as a local point for sciatica with lower backache and pain radiating down the back of the leg.
Ub-37 **Yinmen** *Huge Gate*	6 cun below Ub-36 on the line joining Ub-36 and Ub-40.	Lower back and thigh pain; muscular atrophy; hemiplegia	• Opens the channels, Strengthens the lumbarspine, Stops pain: used as a local point for sciatica with pain radiating down the back of the leg.
Ub-38 **Fuxi** *Superficial Cleft*	1 cun above Ub-39 on the medial side of the tendon of muscle biceps femoris. The point is located with the knee slightly flexed.	Numbness of gluteal and femoral regions; contracture of popliteal fossa	• Relaxes the sinews, Strengthens the lumbarspine, Clears Heat.
Ub-39 **Weiyang** *Outside of the Crook*	Lateral to Ub-40, on the medial border of the tendon of muscle biceps femoris.	Low back pain; nephritis; cystitis; chyluria (white milky urine); spasms of gastrocnemius; any obstruction of urine flow (especially from dampness)	• Opens the water passages and stimulates the transformation and excretion of fluids in the lower burner: for all excess patterns of the lower burner with accumulation of fluids in the form of dampness or edema causing urinary retention, burning, painful urination, difficult urination, edema of the ankles. Also for lower burner deficiency causing incontinence of urine or enuresis.
Ub-40 **Weizhong** *Supporting Middle* he-sea	Midpoint of the transverse crease of the popliteal fossa, between the tendons of muscle biceps femoris and muscle semitendinosus.	Heat exhaustion; low back pain; arthritis of the knee and other knee pain; paralysis of the knee; skin problems due to heat	• **Clears Heat and Resolves Dampness from the Bladder:** for burning urination. • **Relaxes the sinews and removes obstruction from the channel:** for both chronic and acute low backache, however, used primarily for acute pain. Ub-60 can be used in deficiency cases. Also, best used to treat unilateral or bilateral pain, but not for midline pain. • **Cools the Blood, eliminates blood stagnation:** for skin diseases caused by heat in the blood, and pain in the lower legs due to blood stasis. • **Clears Summer-heat:** for summer-heat attacks with fever, delirium and a red skin rash.

Points	Location	Usage	Indications / Functions
Ub-41 **Fufen** *Attached Branch*	3 cun lateral to the DU meridian, at the level of the lower border of the spinous process of T2, on the spinal border of the scapula.	Back pain; neck pain; shoulder stiffness and pain; elbow and arm numbness	• Opens the channels, Strengthens the lumbarand knees, Cools the blood, Clears Summer-heat, Stops pain.
Ub-42 **Pohu** *Door of the Corporeal Soul*	3 cun lateral to the DU meridian, at the level of the lower border of the spinous process of T3, on the spinal border of the scapula.	Pulmonary TB; cough; asthma; neck stiffness; hemoptysis	• **Regulates the descending of Lung Qi, Stops cough and asthma:** for coughing and wheezing due to rebellious Lung Qi. • For painful obstruction syndrome of the upper back and shoulders. • For emotional problems related to the Lungs causing sadness, grief and worry.
Ub-43 **Gaohuangshu** *Vital Region Shu*	3 cun lateral to the DU meridian, at the level of the lower border of the spinous process of T4, on the spinal border of the scapula.	For late stage chronic deficiency disorders; bronchitis; asthma; TB; neurasthenia (archaic - feeble; neurosis); general weakness caused by prolonged illness; consumptive diseases like HIV; pulmonary TB; poor memory indicating a weakened condition	• **Tonifies Qi, Strengthens Deficient Conditions:** for debilitating, chronic illness. • **Nourishes the Essence:** for Kidney deficiency causing nocturnal emissions, low sexual energy or poor memory. • **Nourishes Lung yin:** in the aftermath of chronic pulmonary disease where the Lung yin has been injured causing chronic dry cough and debility. • **Invigorates the Mind:** stimulates memory after a long-standing disease.
Ub-44 **Shentang** *Mind Hall*	3 cun lateral to the Du-11, at the level of the lower border of the spinous process of T5, on the spinal border of the scapula.	Cardiac palpitation and pain; stuffy chest; back stiffness and pain	• **Calms the Mind:** for emotional and psychological problems related to the Heart causing anxiety, insomnia and depression.
Ub-45 **Yixi** *Sighing Laughing Sound*	3 cun lateral to the Du-10, at the level of the lower border of the spinous process of T6, on the spinal border of the scapula.	Shoulder and back pain; cough; asthma	• Expels Wind, Clears Heat, Descends Lung Qi. • Moves Qi and Blood, Stops pain.
Ub-46 **Geguan** *Diaphragm Pass*	3 cun lateral to the Du-9, at the level of the lower border of the spinous process of T7, approximately level with inferior angle of the scapula.	Dysphagia; hiccups; belching	• Regulates diaphragm, Benefits the middle jiao. • Opens the Channels, Stops pain.
Ub-47 **Hunmen** *Door of the Ethereal Soul*	3 cun lateral to the Du-8, at the level of the lower border of the spinous process of T9.	Chest and hypochondriac pain; back pain; vomiting; diarrhea	• **Regulates Liver Qi:** combined with Ub-18 to eliminate Liver qi stagnation. • **Roots the Ethereal Soul:** for emotional problems related to the Liver manifesting as depression, frustration and resentment over a long period of time.
Ub-48 **Yanggang** *Yang's Key Link*	3 cun lateral to the Du-7, at the level of the lower border of the spinous process of T10.	Abdominal pain; diarrhea; jaundice; borborygmus	• Regulates Gallbladder, Clears damp-heat, Harmonizes the middle jiao.
Ub-49 **Yishe** *Thought Shelter*	3 cun lateral to the Du-6, at the level of the lower border of the spinous process of T11.	Abdominal distension; vomiting; diarrhea; difficult swallowing	• Tonifies Spleen, Stimulates memory and concentration: to tonify the mental aspect of the Spleen.
Ub-50 **Weicang** *Stomach Granary*	3 cun lateral to the DU meridian, at the level of the lower border of the spinous process of T12.	Infantile indigestion	• Harmonizes the middle jiao.
Ub-51 **Huangmen** *Vital Door*	3 cun lateral to the Du-5, at the level of the lower border of the spinous process of L1.	Abdominal pain; constipation; abdominal masses	• Regulates the Triple Burner: spreads the qi in the Heart region when there is a feeling of tightness below the heart.

Points	Location	Usage	Indications / Functions
Ub-52 **Zhishi** *Will Power Room*	3 cun lateral to the Du-4, at the level of the lower border of the spinous process of L2.	Primary for sexual function; nephritis; low back pain; spermatorrhea; infertility (both sexes; but more for men); any sperm related problems; nocturnal emissions; prostatitis; secondary point for urinary dysfunction	• Tonifies Kidney, Strengthens low back: reinforces Ub-23. • Reinforces the will power: for depression that includes disorientation and lack of will power or mental strength to make efforts to get better.
Ub-53 **Baohuang** *Bladder Vitals*	3 cun lateral to the Du-5, at the level of the 2nd posterior sacral foramen.	Sciatica; lower back pain; borborygmus; urine retention; edema; abdominal distention	• Opens water passages: stimulates the transformation and excretion of dirty fluids in the lower jiao when there is retention of urine, difficult urination and burning urination. Spreads the qi in the lower jiao.
Ub-54 **Zhibian** *Order's Limit*	Lateral to the hiatus of the sacrum, at the level of the 4th posterior sacral foramen, 3 cun lateral to Du-2.	Lumbarosacral pain; muscular atrophy; dysuria; external genitalia swelling; hemorrhoids; constipation	• Local point for lower backache radiating to the buttocks and legs (along the bladder line).
Ub-55 **Heyang** *Yang Union*	2 cun directly below Ub-40, between the medial and lateral heads of the gastrocnemius muscle, on a line joining Ub-40 and Ub-57.	Low back pain; lower extremities paralysis and pain	• Opens the channels, Stops pain, Stops uterine bleeding, treats genital pain.
Ub-56 **Chengjin** *Sinew Support*	Midway between Ub-55 and Ub-57, on the line connecting Ub-40 and Ub-57, center of the gastrocnemius.	Pain in lower back and leg; sciatica with UB meridian pain in leg; hemorrhoids; spasms of gastrocnemius; charley horses	• Relaxes sinews, Opens the Channels, Stops pain, Benefits the foot and heel.
Ub-57 **Chengshan** *Supporting Mountain*	Directly below the belly of muscle gastrocnemius, on a line joining Ub-40 and Ub-60, about 8 cun below Ub-40.	Hemorrhoids; pain in lower back and leg with leg weakness; beriberi; rheumatoid arthritis (controversial)	• **Relaxes sinews:** for cramps of the gastrocnemius and muscles of the lower leg. • **Invigorates the Blood:** for menstrual pain or blood in the stools caused by blood stasis. • **Unblocks the Channels:** used as a distal point for lower backache and sciatica. Also frequently used as an empirical distal point for treatment of hemorrhoids.
Ub-58 **Feiyang** *Flying Up* luo-connect	7 cun directly above Ub-60, on the posterior border of the fibula, about 1 cun inferior and lateral to Ub-57.	Headache; hemorrhoids; pain in lower back and leg with leg weakness; rheumatoid arthritis (controversial)	• **Removes obstructions from the channel:** a distal point for lower backache and sciatica. Also an empirical distal point for treatment of hemorrhoids.
Ub-59 **Fuyang** *Instep Yang*	3 cun directly above Ub-60.	Headache; low back pain; paralysis of lower limb; inflammation of ankle joint; heavy sensation in the head	• Unblocks the Channels: a distal point for lower backache, particularly in chronic cases with weakness of the leg and back. It is effective only in unilateral backache.
Ub-60 **Kunlun** *Kunlun Mountains* jing-river	In the depression between the external malleolus and tendo calcaneus.	Pain in ankle and foot; plantar fasciitis (stretch; ice feet; needle other local points all way up to calf); paralysis of lower limb; headache; blurry vision; neck rigidity; difficult labor	• **Expels Wind, Unblocks the Channels:** for painful obstruction syndrome of the shoulder, neck and head due to externally contracted wind or internal wind attacking the upper part of the body. For chronic backache of the deficiency type. Also for headaches of the occiput and head from Kidney deficiency. • **Invigorates the Blood:** for menstrual problems due to blood stasis with painful periods and dark clotted blood.

Points	Location	Usage	Indications / Functions
Ub-61 **Pucan** *Servant's Partaking*	Posterior and inferior to the external malleolus, directly below Ub-60, in the depression lateral to calcaneus at the junction of the red and white skin.	Headache (lateral and midline); Meniere's disease; seizures; psychosis and mania; hemiplegia; arthritis; low back pain; epilepsy	• Relaxes sinews, Opens the Channels, Stops pain.
Ub-62 **Shenmai** *Extending Vessel*	In the depression directly below the external malleolus.	Epilepsy; mania; dizziness; insomnia; backache	• **Unblocks the Channels:** for chronic backache. • **Relaxes the tendons and muscles of the outer leg:** for muscle tension in the outer part of the leg. • **Benefits the eyes:** for dryness of the eyes. • **Clears the Mind and Expels Interior Wind:** for epilepsy with attacks occurring mostly in the daytime.
Ub-63 **Jinmen** *Golden Door* xi-cleft	1 cun anterior and inferior to Ub-62, in the depression lateral to the lower border of the cuboid bone.	Mania; epilepsy; infantile convulsion; motor impairment and pain of lower extremities; sometimes used for bladder incontinence	• Clears Heat, Stops pain: for acute Bladder patterns with frequent and burning urination.
Ub-64 **Jinggu** *Capital Bone* yuan	Below the tuberosity of the 5th metatarsal bone, at the junction of the red and white skin.	Headache; neck rigidity; blurring vision; pain in the lower back	• Clears heat from the Bladder: for burning painful urination. • Eliminates Interior Wind: for epilepsy. • Strengthens back: for chronic lower backache.
Ub-65 **Shugu** *Binding Bone* shu-stream	Posterior to the head of the 5th metatarsophalangeal joint, at the junction of the red and white skin.	Mania; backache; headache; neck rigidity; blurry vision	• **Unblocks the Channels:** used as a distal point for any problem along the Bladder channel particularly if affecting the head. For painful obstruction syndrome of the neck. • **Clears Heat:** for heat in the Bladder, acute cystitis. • **Eliminates Interior Wind:** for epilepsy or the beginning stages of wind-cold attack with headache and stiff neck.
Ub-66 **Zutonggu** *Foot Connecting Valley* ying-spring	In the depression anterior to the 5th metatarsophalangeal joint.	Headache; neck rigidity; blurring vision; mania	• Clears Heat: for Bladder heat in acute cases of cystitis. Also for beginning stages of wind-heat in the defensive qi level with fever, headache and stiff neck.
Ub-67 **Zhiyin** *Reaching Yin* jing-well	On the lateral side of the small toe, 0.1 cun posterior to the corner of the nail	Headaches; malposition of fetus and difficult labor (needle and moxa); feverish sensation in the sole; nasal obstruction; epistaxis	• **Expels Wind:** for both interior and exterior wind, especially when there is headache. • **Unblocks the channel:** for channel disorders causing blurred vision or pain in the eye. • Used empirically for malposition of the fetus (breech). This is done in the 8th month of pregnancy by burning moxa cones on each side once a day for 10 days.

ACUPRESSURE

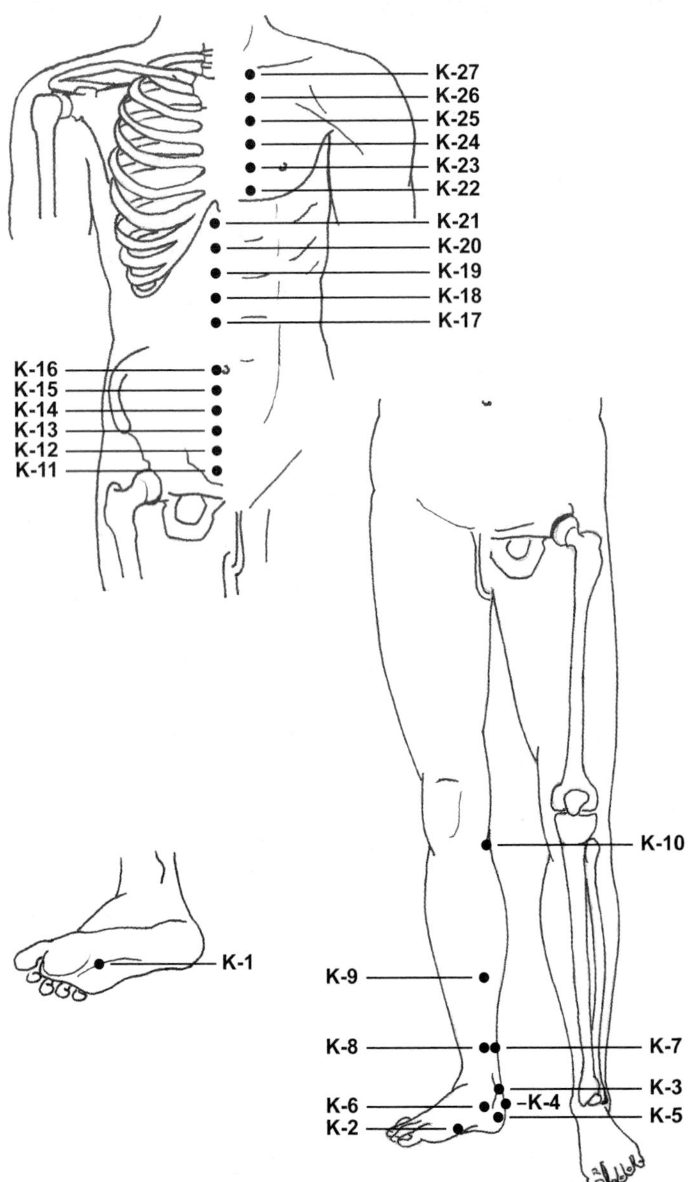

Jing Well	Ying Spring	Shu Stream	Jing River	He Sea
1	2	3	7	10
Yuan	**Luo-connect**	**Xi-Cleft**	**Front Mu**	**Back Shu**
3	4	5	Gb-25	Ub-23

Points	Location	Usage	Indications / Functions
K-1 **Yongquan** *Bubbling Spring* jing-well	On the sole, between 2nd and 3rd toes, in the depression when the foot is in plantar flexion, approximately at the junction of the anterior third and posterior 2/3 of the sole.	Shock; heat exhaustion; stroke; open the orifices and help with loss of voice; hypertension from excess; seizures; infantile convulsions; vertex headache (Liv yang rising); hot soles of the feet; whole body muscle cramping	• **Tonifies Kidney yin, Clears deficiency heat:** for yin deficiency with heat signs. • **Subdue Interior Wind:** for epilepsy, descend liver yang or liver wind. • Restores consciousness.
K-2 **Rangu** *Blazing Valley* ying-spring	Anterior and inferior to the medial malleolus, in the depression of the lower border of the tuberosity of the navicular bone.	Chronic excess and recurring pharyngitis; irregular menstruation due to heat or damp-heat; thirst from diabetes; diarrhea with damp-heat; itching in genital region; plantar fasciitis	• **Clears deficiency heat:** for Kidney yin deficiency heat causing malar flush, feelings of heat in the evening, mental restlessness, thirst without desire to drink and dry throat and mouth at night. Also used to clear excess heat and heat in the blood.
K-3 **Taixi** *Greater Stream* shu-stream, yuan	In the depression between he medial malleolus and tendo calcaneus, at the level of the tip of the medial malleolus.	Nephritis; cystitis; irregular menstruation; spermatorrhea; enuresis; tinnitus; alopecia; impotence; constipation and diarrhea if Kid involved; yin type insomnia; low back pain; knee pain; asthma if Kid deficient	• **Tonifies Kidney, Benefits the Essence:** for any deficiency pattern of Kidney yin, yang, or essence. • **Regulates the uterus:** for irregular periods, amenorrhea and excessive uterine bleeding. • **Strengthens low back and knees.**
K-4 **Dazhong** *Big Bell* luo-connect	Posterior and inferior to the medial malleolus, in the depression medial to the attachment of tendo calcaneus.	Plantar fasciitis; bone spurs	• **Strengthens the back:** for chronic backache from Kidney deficiency. • **Lifts the Spirit:** for exhaustion and depression from chronic Kidney deficiency.
K-5 **Shuiquan** *Water Spring* xi-cleft	1 cun directly below K-3 in the depression anterior and superior to the medial side of the tuberosity of the calcaneus.	Amenorrhea; irregular menstruation; dysmenorrhea; uterus prolapse; dysuria; blurry vision	• **Benefits urination, Stops pain in the Abdomen:** for acute cystitis, urethritis, or pain around the umbilicus. • **Regulates the uterus:** for amenorrhea due to Kidney deficiency.
K-6 **Zhaohai** *Shining Sea*	In the depression of the lower border of the medial malleolus, or 1 cun below the medial malleolus.	Irregular menstruation; uterus prolapse; chronic pharyngitis; tonsillitis; epileptic seizures that occur more at night; deficient yin asthma; constipation; insomnia; dry throat; eye pain from dryness; vaginal discharge like chronic leukorrhea; vaginal dryness (menopause or other); major for yin deficiency	• **Nourishes the Yin:** for any yin deficiency patterns with dry throat and dry eyes. • **Benefits the eyes:** for chronic eye diseases, particularly in the elderly with yin deficiency. • **Calms the Mind:** for restlessness, insomnia, irritability due to yin deficiency. • **Cools the Blood:** for skin diseases caused by heat in the blood. • **Regulates the uterus:** for amenorrhea and prolapse of the uterus due to kidney deficiency. • Opens the chest: for chest pain, circulate qi in the chest when combined with Pc-6.
K-7 **Fuliu** *Returning Current* jing-river	2 cun directly above K-3, on the anterior border of tendo calcaneus.	Leukorrhea; any urinary problems; night sweats; URI sweat or lack of sweat; low back pain; edema with Sp-9; good for ankle edema	• **Tonifies Kidney:** similar to K-3, but is better for Kidney yang. • **Resolves Dampness in the lower jiao**: for edema in the legs. • **Regulates Sweating:** to either promote (with LI-4) or stop sweating (with Ht-6) for night sweats or spontaneous sweats.

Points	Location	Usage	Indications / Functions
K-8 **Jiaoxin** *Exchange Belief*	0.5 cun anterior to K-7, 2 cun above K-3, posterior to the medial border of the tibia.	Irregular menstruation; uterus prolapse; uterine bleeding; diarrhea; constipation; pain and swelling of testis	• Unblocks the Channels, Stops pain, Removes Masses: to eliminate obstructions along the vessel and dissolve abdominal masses due to stagnation of qi or blood, and to stop abdominal pain. • Regulates menses: for menstrual problems due to blood stasis.
K-9 **Zhubin** *Guest Building*	5 cun directly above K-3 at the lower end of the belly of muscle gastrocnemius, on the line drawn from K-3 to K-10.	Mental disorders; hernia; lower leg and foot pain	• **Clears the Mind, Tonifies Kidney yin:** for deep anxiety and mental restlessness caused by Kidney yin deficiency. It also tonifies yin. • **Opens the chest:** for relaxing feeling of oppression in the chest, often with palpitations as with Heart and Kidneys not harmonized.
K-10 **Yingu** *Yin Valley* he-sea	When the knee is flexed, the point is on the medial side of the popliteal fossa, between the tendons of muscle semitendinosus and semimembranosus, level with Ub-40.	Diseases of urogenital system; dysuria; arthritis of knee in medial area; important for water balance	• **Expels Dampness in the lower jiao:** for urinary symptoms such as urinary difficulty, painful urination, and frequency of urination. • Nourishes Kidney yin.
K-11 **Henggu** *Pubic Bone*	5 cun below the umbilicus, on the superior border of the symphysis pubis, 0.5 cun lateral to Ren-2.	Fullness and pain of the lower abdomen; dysuria; enuresis; nocturnal emission; impotence	• Benefits lower jiao.
K-12 **Dahe** *Great Manifestation*	4 cun below the umbilicus, 0.5 cun lateral to Ren-3.	Nocturnal emission; impotence; uterus prolapse; external genitalia pain	• Tonifies Kidney, Nourishes the Essence.
K-13 **Qixue** *Qi Hole*	3 cun below the umbilicus, 0.5 cun lateral to Ren-4.	Irregular menstruation; dysmenorrhea; dysuria; abdominal pain; diarrhea	• Tonifies Kidney, Nourishes the Essence. • Unblocks the Channel: for circulation of Qi and blood in the abdomen, removing masses and obstructions in the abdomen and chest. For excess patterns with abdominal fullness and masses.
K-14 **Siman** *Fourfold Fullness*	2 cun below the umbilicus, 0.5 cun lateral to Ren-5.	Abdominal distension pain; diarrhea; nocturnal emission; irregular menstruation; postpartum abdominal pain	• Strengthens lower jiao, Stops pain. • Regulates Qi, Moves blood stagnation. • Regulates water passages, Promotes urination.
K-15 **Zhongzhu** *Central Flow*	1 cun below the umbilicus, 0.5 cun lateral to Ren-7.	Irregular menstruation; abdominal pain; constipation	• Strengthens lower jiao and Intestines.
K-16 **Huangshu** *Vitals Transporting Point*	0.5 cun lateral to the umbilicus, level with Ren-8.	Habitual constipation with firm and difficult-to-pass stool (need to nourish yin); hiccups; vomiting; dry constipation point	• **Tonifies Kidneys, Benefits the Heart, Calms the Mind:** for Kidney yin deficiency failing to nourish the Heart.
K-17 **Shangqu** *Shang Bend*	2 cun above the umbilicus, 0.5 cun lateral to Ren-10.	Irregular menstruation; abdominal pain; constipation; diarrhea	• Dispels accumulation, Stops pain.
K-18 **Shiguan** *Stone Pass*	3 cun above the umbilicus, 0.5 cun lateral to Ren-11.	Vomiting; abdominal pain; constipation; sterility	• Strengthens lower jiao, Stops pain. • Regulates Qi, Moves blood stagnation, Harmonizes Stomach.
K-19 **Yindu** *Yin Metropolis*	4 cun above the umbilicus, 0.5 cun lateral to Ren-12.	Borborygmus; abdominal pain; constipation; vomiting	• Regulates Qi, Harmonizes Stomach, Stops coughing and wheezing.

Points	Location	Usage	Indications / Functions
K-20 Futonggu *Abdomen Connecting Valley*	5 cun above the umbilicus, 0.5 cun lateral to Ren-13.	Abdominal distension and pain; indigestion; vomiting	• Harmonizes the middle, Unblocks the chest.
K-21 Youmen *Dark Gate*	6 cun above the umbilicus, 0.5 cun lateral to Ren-14.	Abdominal distension and pain; indigestion; vomiting; diarrhea; morning sickness	• Spreads Liver Qi, Benefits the chest, Tonifies Spleen, Harmonizes the Stomach.
K-22 Bulang *Walking Corridor*	In the 5th intercostal space, 2 cun lateral to the Ren meridian.	Cough; asthma; fullness and distension of the chest; vomiting; anorexia	• Unblocks the chest, Subdues rebellious Qi.
K-23 Shenfeng *Mind Seal*	In the 4th intercostal space, 2 cun lateral to the Ren meridian.	Cough; asthma; fullness and distension of the chest; mastitis	• Unbinds the chest, Subdues rebellious Qi, Benefits the breast.
K-24 Lingxu *Spirit Burial Ground*	In the 3rd intercostal space, 2 cun lateral to the Ren meridian.	Cough; asthma; fullness and distension of the chest; mastitis	• Unbinds the chest, Subdues rebellious Qi, Benefits the breast.
K-25 Shencang *Mind Storage* ↘ 0.3 – 0.7 avoid lung, liver, heart, & deep puncture	In the 2nd intercostal space, 2 cun lateral to the Ren meridian.	Cough; asthma; chest pain	• Unbinds the chest, Subdues rebellious Qi, Benefits the breast.
K-26 Yuzhong *Comfortable Chest*	In the 1st intercostal space, 2 cun lateral to the Ren meridian.	Cough; asthma; phlegm accumulation; fullness and distension of the chest	• Unbinds the chest, Benefits the breast, Transforms Phlegm.
K-27 Shufu *Transporting point Mansion*	In the depression on the lower border of the clavicle, 2 cun lateral to the Ren meridian.	Cough; asthma; chest pain	• **Stimulates Kidney Function of Reception of Qi** • **Subdues rebellious Qi:** used to stops cough and calm asthma. • **Resolves Phlegm:** a local point for treatment of asthma due to Kidney deficiency.

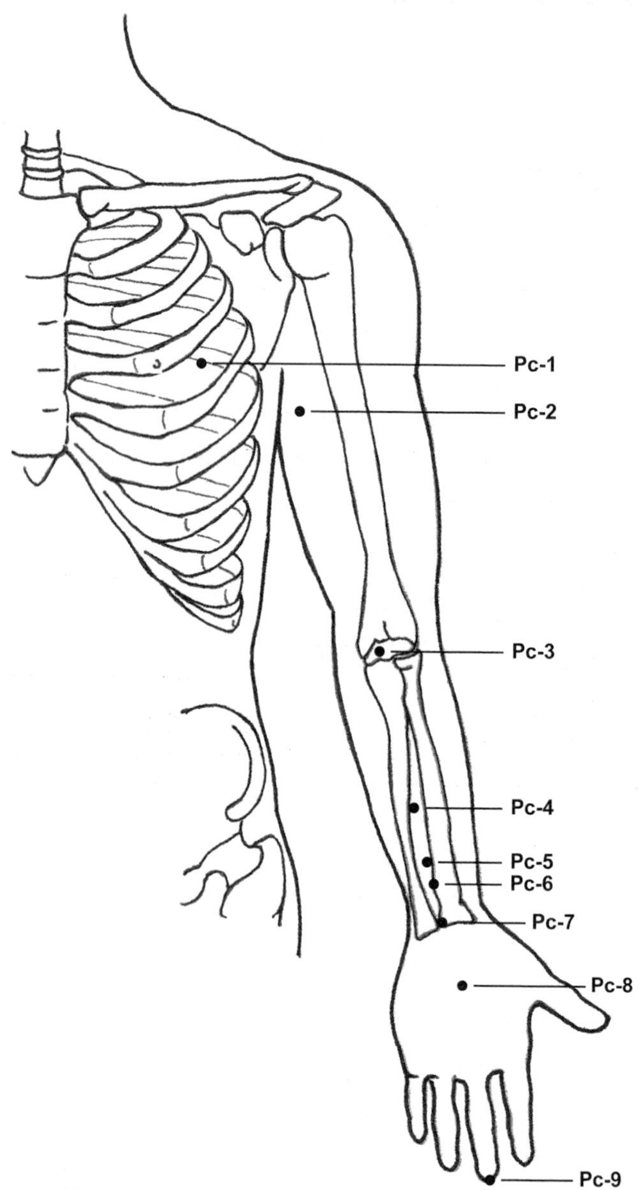

Jing Well	Ying Spring	Shu Stream	Jing River	He Sea
9	8	7	5	3
Yuan	**Luo-connect**	**Xi-Cleft**	**Front Mu**	**Back Shu**
7	6	4	Ren-17	Ub-14

Points	Location	Usage	Indications / Functions
Pc-1 Tianchi *Heavenly Pool*	In the 4th intercostal space, 1 cun lateral to the nipple, 5 cun lateral to anterior midline.	Intercostal neuralgia; pain and swelling under the axilla; mastitis; insufficient lactation	• Local point for distension and pain of the breast caused by Liver qi stagnation.
Pc-2 Tianquan *Heavenly Spring*	2 cun below the level of the anterior axillary fold, between the two heads of the muscle biceps brachii.	Pain along the upper aspect of the arm; local for chest	• Unblocks the chest, Moves blood, Stops pain.
Pc-3 Quze *Marsh on Bend* he-sea	On the transverse cubital crease, at the ulnar side of the tendon of muscle biceps brachii.	Acute gastritis and gastroenteritis; easily startled; pain along the arm; mostly for gastric problems; cardiac pain; palpitation; febrile diseases; tremor of the hand and arm	• **Pacifies the Stomach, Clears Heat, Cools the Blood:** for heat in the Qi level including acute sun stroke and heat in the intestines. Clears heat and cools blood in the blood level including late stages of febrile diseases with skin eruptions and convulsions. Also promotes descending of Stomach qi which is causing nausea and vomiting. • **Opens the Heart:** for loss of consciousness due to heat in the Pericardium obstructing the Heart orifice. • **Invigorates the Blood, Dispels Blood Stasis:** for excessive menstrual bleeding, stagnant blood giving rise to uterine fibroids. • **Calms the Mind:** for severe anxiety caused by Heart fire.
Pc-4 Ximen *Cleft Door* xi-cleft	5 cun above the transverse crease of the wrist, on the line connecting Pc-3 and Pc-7, between the tendons of palmaris longus and flexor carpi radialis	Myocarditis; angina pectoris; palpitations (most are from deficiency); irritability and acute pain in the chest due to emotions; angina; clears the heart channel and stops pain	• **Unblocks the Channels, Regulates Blood, Stop Pain:** for acute arrhythmias and palpitations, and chest pain due to stagnant qi and blood. • **Cools the Blood:** for skin diseases caused by blood heat. • **Strengthens the Mind:** for Heart deficiency causing fear and lack of mental strength.
Pc-5 Jianshi *Intermediate Messenger* jing-river	3 cun above the transverse crease of the wrist between the tendons of palmaris longus and flexor carpi radialis	Cardiac pain; palpitation; stomachache; malaria; mental disorders; contracture of the elbow and arm; seizures with drooling; hysteria; psychosis; clears insubstantial phlegm	• **Resolve Phlegm, Regulate the Heart, Open the Heart Orifice**: for non-substantial phlegm obstructing the Heart and misting the mental faculties resulting in delirium, aphasia and coma often associated with heat in the blood level, also causing mental illness, manic depression, and reckless behavior. Epilepsy with loss of consciousness due to phlegm misting the orifice. • **Regulates Heart Qi:** dispels stagnation of qi in the chest. • Subdues rebellious Stomach qi causing nausea and vomiting. • Clears Heart-fire causing insomnia, tongue ulcers, bitter taste, dry mouth and mental agitation. • **Empirical point for malaria.**
Pc-6 Neiguan *Inner Gate* luo-connect	2 cun above the transverse crease of the wrist, between the tendons of palmaris longus and flexor carpi radialis	Angina pectoris; chest pain; stuffiness in chest; pain in hypochondrium; asthma; nausea or vomiting; opens the chest; stomachache; any kind of upper abdominal pain; spasms of the diaphragm; cough; seizures; hysteria; irritability; insomnia; nervousness; malaria; mental disorders	• **Opens the chest:** for any chest problems. Regulates Qi and blood in the chest to treat stasis of qi and blood causing pain in the chest. • **Calms the Mind:** for irritability due to Liver qi stagnation, especially when there is anxiety due to a Heart pattern. Treats pre-menstrual depression and irritability and promotes sleep. • **Harmonizes the Stomach:** subdues rebellious Stomach qi and stops nausea and vomiting. Also for epigastric pain, acid regurgitation, hiccup and belching. • **Regulates the Triple Burner:** for neck ache on the occiput. • **Regulates Blood:** regulate irregular or painful menses.

Points	Location	Usage	Indications / Functions
Pc-7 **Daling** *Great Hill* yuan	In the middle of the transverse crease of the wrist, between the tendons of muscle palmaris longus and flexor carpi radialis.	Palpitations; gastritis with heat and anxiety; intercostal neuralgia; mental illness	• **Calms the Mind:** for stabilizing emotions. • **Clears Heat:** for Heart-fire causing anxiety and mental restlessness or manic behavior.
Pc-8 **Laogong** *Palace of Toil* ying-spring	On the transverse crease and center of the palm, between the 2nd and 3rd metacarpal bones. When the fist is clenched, the point is just below the tip of the middle finger.	Heat exhaustion; cardiac pain; yin exhaustion; stomatitis; foul breath; ulcerated oral cavity; hysteria and mental illness due to heat; excessive sweating of palms	• **Clears Heart-fire:** for all symptoms of Heart-fire including tongue ulcers, mental symptoms, or high fever and delirium.
Pc-9 **Zhongchong** *Center Rush* jing-well	In the center of the tip of the middle finger.	Shock; apoplectic coma; main jing well point for returning consciousness	• Clears Heat: for chronic conditions with mental symptoms, or in acute cases of exterior heat at the qi or nutritive qi level. • Expels interior Wind and restores consciousness: for wind-stroke.

ACUPRESSURE

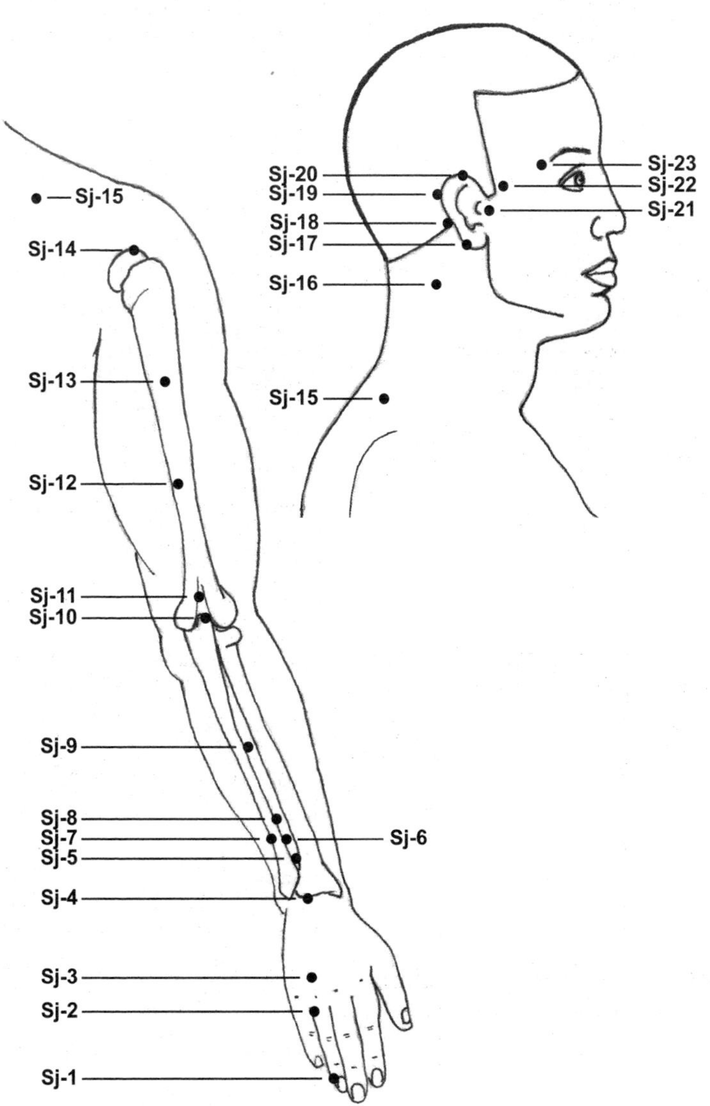

Jing Well	Ying Spring	Shu Stream	Jing River	He Sea
1	2	3	6	10
Yuan	**Luo-connect**	**Xi-Cleft**	**Front Mu**	**Back Shu**
4	5	7	Ren-5	Ub-22

Points	Location	Usage	Indications / Functions
Sj-1 **Guanchong** *Gate Rush* jing-well	On the lateral side of the ring finger, about .1 cun posterior to the corner of the nail.	Headache; red eyes; sore throat; febrile diseases; irritability; stiff tongue	• Clears Heat, Expels Wind: for invasion of exterior wind-heat causing fever, sore throat or earache. For both Taiyang and Shaoyang disorders. • Restores Consciousness: for acute stage of wind-stroke. • For painful and stiff shoulder joint.
Sj-2 **Yemen** *Fluid Door* ying-spring	When the fist is clenched, the point is located in the depression proximal to the margin of the web between the ring and small fingers.	Pain and swelling of the fingers; sudden deafness; sore throat; malaria; headache; red eyes	• Clears Heat, Expels Wind, Benefits the ear: for invasion of exterior wind-heat causing earache due to infection of the middle ear, tinnitus, or deafness due to liver fire. • Unblocks the Channels: for painful obstruction syndrome of the fingers.
Sj-3 **Zhongzhu** *Middle Islet* shu-stream	When the fist is clenched, the point is on the dorsum of the hand between the 4th and 5th metacarpal bones, in the depression proximal to the 4th metacarpophalangeal joint.	Tinnitus; deafness; headache; red eyes; elbow and arm pain	• **Clears Heat, Expels Wind, Benefits the ear:** for invasions of exterior wind-heat causing earache due to infection of the middle ear, tinnitus, or deafness due to liver fire. • **Unblocks the Channels:** for painful obstruction syndrome of the fingers. • **Regulates Qi:** for Liver qi stagnation causing hypochondriac pain and mood swings. Also lifts depression caused by Liver qi stagnation.
Sj-4 **Yangchi** *Yang Pool* yuan	On the transverse crease of the dorsum of the wrist, in the depression lateral to the tendon of muscle extensor digitorum communis.	Pain and diseases of the soft tissues of wrist; carpal tunnel syndrome; malaria; deafness; thirst	• **Relaxes sinews, Unblocks the Channels:** for painful obstruction syndrome of the arm and shoulder. Also for headaches of the occiput due to exterior invasion of wind. • **Regulates the Stomach:** used in combination with St-42, tonifies the Stomach. • Transforms congested fluids. • Benefits Original Qi, Tonifies Penetrating and Directing Vessels: for all chronic diseases when the Kidneys have become deficient and energy is weakened. Also for irregular periods and amenorrhea.
Sj-5 **Waiguan** *Outer Gate* luo-connect	2 cun above Sj-4, between the radius and the ulna.	Common colds; high fever (shao yang); tinnitus; temporal migraines; lateral stiff neck; hemiplegia; pain in joints; controlling point for the hand and opens up qi circulation to the hand; (master point of yang wei)	• **Release the Exterior, Expels Wind-heat:** for fever, sore throat, slight sweating, aversion to cold and a floating, rapid pulse. Used in taiyang wind-heat, Qi level heat, and shaoyang stage disorders with alternating fever and chills, irritability, hypochondriac pain, bitter taste, blurred vision and a wiry pulse. • **Unblocks the Channels:** for painful obstruction syndrome of the arm, shoulder and neck. • **Benefits the ear:** for ear infection from invasion of exterior wind-heat or tinnitus and deafness from liver fire or liver yang rising. • **Subdues Liver yang:** distal point to treat migraine headaches on the temples from liver yang rising.
Sj-6 **Zhigou** *Branching Ditch* jing-river	3 cun above Sj-4, between the radius and the ulna, on the radial side of muscle extensor digitorum.	Intercostal neuralgia; constipation; shingles; herpes zoster; skin disorders	• **Regulates Qi:** used to regulate qi in the three burners and removes stagnation of Liver qi (combine with Gb-34). • Clears Heat: for qi level invasions of heat when there is constipation and abdominal pain. • **Expels Wind-heat:** for wind-heat in the blood affecting the skin and skin diseases from wind characterized by red rashes and hives that come and go or move quickly, including urticaria (combine with Gb-31). Used as a major point for herpes zoster, especially when the eruptions are on the flanks.
Sj-7 **Huizong** *Ancestral Meeting* xi-cleft	At the level of Sj-6, about 1 finger breadth lateral to Sj-6, on the radial side of the ulna.	Ear pain; deafness; arm pain	• For excess patterns to stop pain. It acts on pain in the ears, temples and eyebrows.

Points	Location	Usage	Indications / Functions
Sj-8 **Sanyangluo** *Connecting Three Yang*	4 cun above Sj-4, between the radius and the ulna.	Pain in the arm involving all three arm meridians; pain in forearm inhibiting movement; toothache; deafness; sudden voice loss	• Clears Heat, Unblocks the Channels: for painful obstruction syndrome of the arm, neck, shoulders and occiput. Particularly useful when the pain involves more than one channel on the yang surface of the arm and shoulders. It relaxes sinews and relieves pain and stiffness.
Sj-9 **Sidu** *Four Rivers*	On the lateral side of the forearm, 5 cun below the olecranon, between the radius and the ulna.	Deafness; migraine; forearm pain	• Unblocks the Channels, Stops pain.
Sj-10 **Tianjing** *Heavenly Well* he-sea	When the elbow is flexed, the point is in the depression about 1 cun superior to the olecranon.	Diseases of the soft tissue of the elbow	• **Relaxes tendons:** for painful obstruction syndrome along the channel, especially of the elbow. • **Resolves Phlegm and Dampness, Dispels Masses:** for external invasions of damp-heat causing swelling of glands and tonsils. • **Regulates Nutritive and Defensive Qi:** for invasions of exterior wind-cold to stop sweating and release the exterior.
Sj-11 **Qinglengyuan** *Clear Cold Abyss*	1 cun above Sj-10 when the elbow is flexed.	Shoulder and arm motor impairment and pain; migraine	• Unblocks the Channels, Dispels Wind-Damp, Clears damp-heat.
Sj-12 **Xiaoluo** *Dispersing Riverbed*	On the line joining the olecranon and Sj-14, midway between Sj-11 and Sj-13.	Headache; neck stiffness; arm pain and motor impairment	• Unblocks the Channels, Stops pain.
Sj-13 **Naohui** *Upper Arm Convergence*	On the line joining Sj-14 and the olecranon, on the posterior border of muscle deltoidus.	Goiter; shoulder and arm pain	• Unblocks the Channels, Stops pain, Regulates Qi, Transforms Phlegm.
Sj-14 **Jianliao** *Shoulder Crevice*	Posterior and inferior to the acromion, in the depression about 1 cun posterior to LI-15 when the arm is abducted.	Shoulder and upper arm pain and impairment	• **Dispels Wind-Damp, Stops pain, Benefits the shoulder joint:** for painful obstruction syndrome of the shoulder.
Sj-15 **Tianliao** *Heavens Bone Hole*	Midway between Gb-21 and SI-13, on the superior angle of the scapula.	Shoulder and elbow pain; stiff neck	• Dispels Wind-Damp, Unblocks the channels, Stops pain.
Sj-16 **Tianyou** *Window of Heaven*	Posterior and inferior to the mastoid process, level with mandibular angle, on the posterior border of SCM, almost level with SI-17 and Ub-10.	Tinnitus; deafness; lymphatic swellings around neck	• Benefits the head and sensory organs, Regulates Qi.
Sj-17 **Yifeng** *Wind Screen*	Posterior to the lobule of the ear, in the depression between the mandible and the mastoid process.	All ear problems; tinnitus; parotitis; locked jaw; facial paralysis; most important local point for ear; dizziness involving ear problems	• **Benefits the ears:** for all ear problems of exterior or interior origin. Used in ear infections caused by exterior wind-heat, or for deafness and tinnitus from rising of liver yang or liver fire. • **Expels Wind:** for exterior wind causing trigeminal neuralgia and facial paralysis.
Sj-18 **Qimai** *Spasm Vessel*	In the center of the mastoid process, at the junction of the middle and lower 1/3 of the curve formed by Sj-17 and Sj-20 posterior to the helix.	Tinnitus; headache; deafness; infantile convulsion	• Benefits the ears. • Expels Wind.

Points	Location	Usage	Indications / Functions
Sj-19 **Luxi** *Skull Rest*	Posterior to the ear, at the junction of the upper and middle 1/3 of the curve formed by Sj-17 and Sj-20 posterior to the helix.	Headache; tinnitus; deafness; infantile convulsion	• Benefits the ears, Clears Heat. • Expels Wind.
Sj-20 **Jiaosun** *Angle Vertex*	Directly above the ear apex, within the hair line.	Parotitis; toothache; tinnitus	• Benefits the ears, teeth, gums, and lip. • Clears Heat. • Expels Wind.
Sj-21 **Ermen** *Ear Door*	In the depression anterior to the supratragic notch and slightly superior to the condyloid process of the mandible. The point is located with the mouth open.	Tinnitus; otitis media; pus in ear; temporomandibular joint problems	• **Benefits the ears, Clears Heat:** local point for tinnitus caused by liver yang rising.
Sj-22 **Erheliao** *Ear Bone Hole*	Anterior and superior to Sj-21, level with the root of the auricle, on the posterior border of the hairline of the temple where the superficial temporal artery passes.	Tinnitus; locked jaw; migraine; check for TMJ	• Expels Wind, Stops pain.
Sj-23 **Sizhukong** *Silk Bamboo Hole*	In the depression at the lateral end of the eyebrow.	Redness and pain of the eye; blurry vision; headache; twitching eyelid; facial paralysis	• Expels Wind, Stops pain, Benefits the eye: local point for eye problems and headache around the outer corner of the eyebrow, especially when due to liver yang rising. Also for facial paralysis when there is inability to raise the outer corner of the eyebrow.

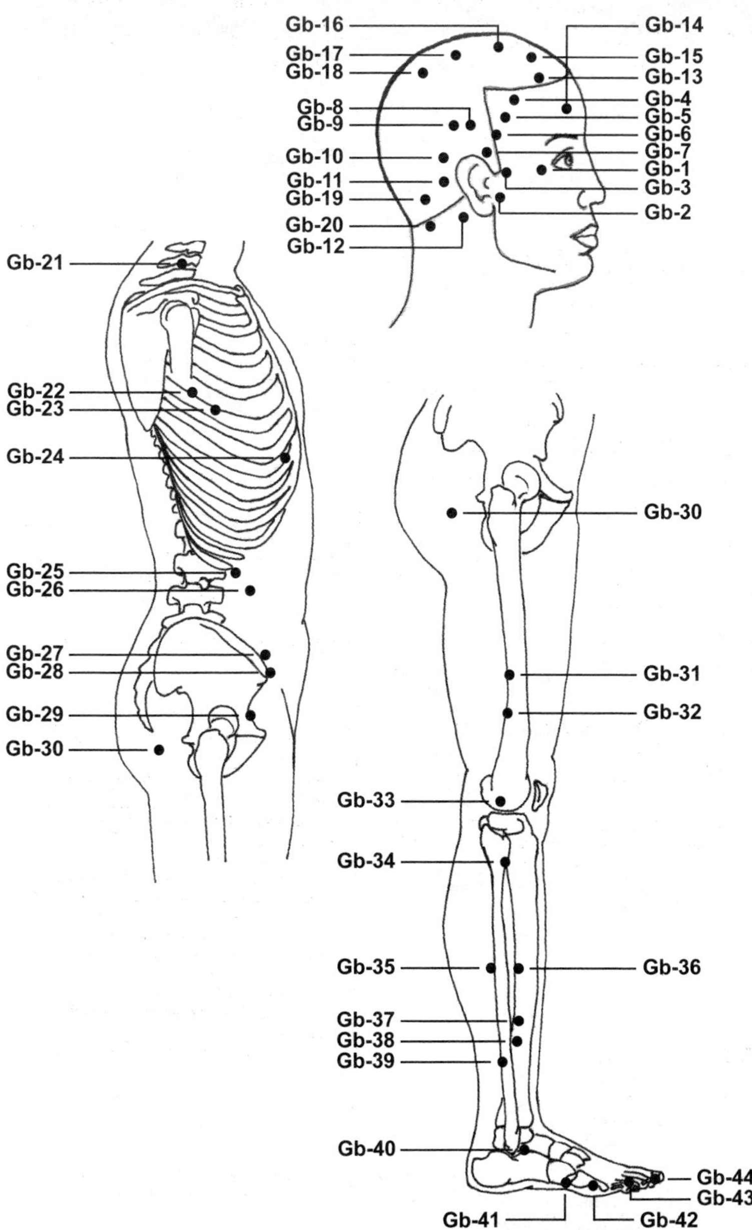

Jing Well	Ying Spring	Shu Stream	Jing River	He Sea
44	43	41	38	34
Yuan	**Luo-connect**	**Xi-Cleft**	**Front Mu**	**Back Shu**
40	37	36	Gb-24	Ub-19

Points	Location	Usage	Indications / Functions
Gb-1 Tongziliao *Pupil Crevice*	0.5 cun lateral to the outer canthus, in the depression on the lateral side of the orbit.	Headache; anything with heat	• **Expels Wind-heat:** for conjunctivitis from wind-heat attack. • **Clears fire:** for liver fire causing red, dry and painful eyes. • Local point for migraine headaches due to liver fire or liver yang rising.
Gb-2 Tinghui *Hearing Convergence*	Anterior to the intertragic notch, at the posterior border of the condyloid process of the mandible. The point is located with the mouth open.	OM; ear pain; tinnitus; facial paralysis; mumps; dislocation or motor impairment of the jaw (TMJ)	• **Unblocks the Channels:** local point for tinnitus and deafness caused by liver-fire or liver yang rising blocking the channels. • **Expels exterior wind-heat:** used for otitis media due to exterior wind-heat.
Gb-3 Shangguan *Above the Joint*	In the front of the ear, on the upper border of the zygomatic arch, in the depression directly above St-7.	Headache; deafness; tinnitus; mouth and eye deviation; toothache	• Expels Wind, Benefits the ears. • Activates the Channels, Stops pain.
Gb-4 Hanyan *Jaw Serenity*	Within the hairline of the temporal region, at the junction of the upper 1/4 and lower 3/4 of the distance between St-8 and Gb-7.	Migraine; vertigo; tinnitus; outer canthus pain; convulsion; epilepsy	• Expels Wind, Clears Heat. • Activates the Channels, Stops pain.
Gb-5 Xuanlu *Skull Suspension*	Within the hairline of the temporal region, at the midpoint of the line joining St-8 and Gb-7.	Migraine; outer canthus pain; convulsion; epilepsy	• Expels Wind, Clears Heat. • Activates the Channels, Stops pain.
Gb-6 Xuanli *Hair Suspension*	Within the hairline, at the junction of the lower 1/4 and the upper 3/4 of the distance between St-8 and Gb-7.	Migraine; outer canthus pain; tinnitus; frequent sneezing	• Expels Wind, Clears Heat. • Activates the Channels, Stops pain: local point for migraine headaches on the side of the head due to liver yang rising, liver fire or liver wind.
Gb-7 Qubin *Turning On the Temple*	Directly above the anterior border of the auricle, 2 cun within the hairline, about .5 cun posterior to Gb-8.	Headache; swelling of the cheek; temporal region pain; infantile convulsion	• Expels Wind, Benefits the mouth and jaw.
Gb-8 Shuaigu *Leading Valley*	Superior to the apex of the auricle, 1.5 cun within the hairline.	Nausea and vomiting with headache; good for migraines	• **Unblocks the Channels, Benefits the ear:** local point for tinnitus and deafness or migraine headache from liver yang rising or liver fire.
Gb-9 Tianchong *Heavenly Rushing*	Directly above the posterior border of the auricle, 2 cun within the hairline, about 0.5 cun posterior to Gb-8.	Headache; epilepsy; pain and swelling of the gums; convulsion	• **Unblocks the Channels, Subdues Rebellious Qi**: local point for migraine headaches due to liver yang rising, liver fire or liver wind. Descends upward rebellious qi. • **Subdues Interior Wind, Alleviates spasms:** for convulsions, epilepsy or contraction of muscles due to liver wind. Also for disturbance of movement such as ataxia and speech originating from disorders of the central nervous system. • **Calms the Mind:** for serious mental disorders such as hypomania.
Gb-10 Fubai *Floating White* sub- ↓ 0.3 – 0.5	Posterior and superior to the mastoid process, junction of middle 1/3 and upper 1/3 on the curved line drawn from Gb-9 to Gb-12.	Headache; tinnitus; deafness	• Clears the Head, Benefits the neck region. • Activates the Channels, Stops pain.
Gb-11 Touqiaoyin *Head-Yin-Orifice* sub- ↓ 0.3 – 0.5	Posterior and superior to the mastoid process, junction of middle 1/3 and lower 1/3 on the line drawn connecting Gb-9 and Gb-12.	Head and neck pain; tinnitus; deafness; ear pain	• Clears the Head, Benefits the sensory organs. • Activates the Channels, Stops pain.

Points	Location	Usage	Indications / Functions
Gb-12 Wangu *Mastoid Process*	In the depression posterior and inferior to the mastoid process.	Headache; insomnia; neck pain	• **Expels Exterior Wind:** used as a local point for otitis media and to subdue interior wind causing epilepsy. • **Subdues Rebellious Qi:** for migraine headaches along the Gall Bladder channel on the posterior side of the head caused by liver yang rising or liver wind. • **Calms the Mind:** for insomnia caused by liver yang rising or liver fire.
Gb-13 Benshen *Origin of the Spirit*	0.5 cun within the hairline of the forehead, 3 cun lateral to Du-24.	Mental disorders; vertigo; seizures; hemiplegia; psychosis; schizophrenia; irrational suspicion and jealousy; rigid thinking; obsessive thought	• **Calms the Mind:** for severe emotional problems such as schizophrenia. Also for anxiety derived from constant worry and fixed thoughts. • **Gathers Essence to the Head:** for calming the mind and strengthening will power when combined with other essence strengthening points. • **Expels internal wind:** for wind stroke and epilepsy.
Gb-14 Yangbai *Yang White*	On the forehead, directly above the pupil, 1 cun directly above the midpoint of the eyebrow.	Supraorbital neuralgia; headache; sinus headache; eye problems	• Benefits the head and eye, Expels Wind, Stops pain.
Gb-15 Toulinqi *Tear Controlling*	Directly above Gb-14, 0.5 cun within the hairline, midway between Du-24 and St-8.	Headache; vertigo; lacrimation; outer canthus pain; nasal obstruction	• Regulates the Mind, Balances the Emotions: for balancing mood swings and manic depressive oscillations.
Gb-16 Muchuang *Eye Window*	1.5 cun posterior to Gb-15, on the line connecting Gb-15 and Gb-20.	Headache; vertigo; red and painful eyes; nasal obstruction	• Benefits the eyes, Expels Wind, Stops pain.
Gb-17 Zhengying *Upright Nutrition*	1.5 cun posterior to Gb-16, on the line connecting Gb-15 and Gb-20.	Migraine; vertigo	• Benefits the Head, Stops pain, Pacifies the Stomach.
Gb-18 Chengling *Spirit Support*	1.5 cun posterior to Gb-17, on the line connecting Gb-15 and Gb-20.	Headache; vertigo; epistaxis; rhinorrhea	• Calms the Mind, Clears the brain: for deep mental problems such as obsessional thoughts and dementia.
Gb-19 Naokong *Brain Depression*	Directly above Gb-20, at the level with Du-17, on the lateral side of the external occipital protuberance.	Headache; stiff neck; vertigo; painful eyes; tinnitus; epilepsy	• Benefits the Head, Stops pain, Clears Wind.
Gb-20 Fengchi *Wind Pool*	In the depression between the upper portion of the SCM and muscle trapezius, on the same level with Du-16.	Common colds including wind-heat or wind-cold; anything with nasal obstruction; vertigo; occipital headache; stiff neck; hypertension; seizures; hemiplegia; very nice insomnia point; opens up whole head	• **Expels Wind:** for both interior and exterior wind including wind-cold, wind-heat, causing headache, stiff neck, dizziness and vertigo due to liver yang rising or liver fire. • **Subdues Liver yang:** for occipital headaches caused by liver yang rising. • **Benefits the eyes:** for eye problems due to Liver disharmony causing blurred vision, cataracts, iritis and optic nerve atrophy. Also can be used for eye problems caused by Liver blood deficiency. • **Benefits the ears:** for tinnitus and deafness due to liver yang rising. • **Clears the brain:** tonifies marrow and nourishes the brain when there are symptoms of poor memory, dizziness and vertigo.

Points	Location	Usage	Indications / Functions
Gb-21 Jianjing *Shoulder Well*	Midway between Du-14 and the acromion, at the highest point of the shoulder.	Hemiplegia due to stroke; any motor impairment of the arm; mastitis; breast abscess; difficult labor	• **Relaxes sinews:** for painful obstruction syndrome of the shoulders and neck. Also relieves stiffness of the neck. • **Promotes Lactation:** empirical point to promote lactation in nursing mothers. • **Promotes Delivery:** empirical point to promote delivery or expulsion of the fetus. For retention of the placenta, post-partum hemorrhage or threatened miscarriage.
Gb-22 Yuanye *Armpit depression*	On the mid axillary line when the arm is raised, in the 4th intercostal, 3 cun below the axilla.	Chest fullness; pain and motor impairment of the arm; hypochondriac pain; swelling of the axillary region	• **Regulates Qi**: unbinds the chest, benefits the axilla.
Gb-23 Zhejin *Flank Sinews*	1 cun anterior to Gb-22, on the 4th intercostal, approximately at the level with the nipple.	Chest fullness; hypochondriac pain; asthma	• Unbinds the chest, Regulates Qi in all three jiaos.
Gb-24 Riyue *Sun and Moon*	Directly below the nipple, in the 7th intercostal space, 4 cun lateral to the anterior midline, one rib below Liv-14.	Intercostal neuralgia; cholecystitis; jaundice; peptic ulcer; hepatitis; heartburn; pain in the hypochondrium; check for herpes zoster; one of main points for gallstones; jaundice; hepatitis; mastitis; for wood attacking earth; good for nausea and vomiting	• **Resolves damp-heat:** for damp-heat in the Liver and Gallbladder causing jaundice, hypochondriac pain, felling of heaviness, nausea and a sticky yellow tongue coating. • **Promotes Qi circulation:** for stagnation of Liver qi causing hypochondriac pain and distension.
Gb-25 Jingmen *Capital Gate*	On the lateral side of the abdomen, on the lower border of the free end of the 12th rib.	Nephritis; serious and/or chronic UTI; intercostal neuralgia; lumbago; Kid stones; back pain from standing long-term	• Tonifies Kidney, Regulates water passages, Strengthens Spleen, Regulates Intestines. • Benefits the lumbar.
Gb-26 Daimai *Girdling Vessel*	Directly below the free end of the 11th rib, where the Liv-13 is located, at the level of the umbilicus.	Stops leukorrhea; main point for vaginal discharges; especially heat or excess type; endometriosis; cystitis; irregular menstruation from damp-heat; profuse uterine bleeding; inguinal hernia	• **Regulates the uterus and the menses:** for irregular periods and dysmenorrhea. • **Resolves damp-heat in the lower jiao:** for chronic vaginal discharges and vaginal prolapse.
Gb-27 Wushu *Pivot of the Five*	On the lateral side of the abdomen, anterior to the superior iliac spine, 3 cun below the umbilicus.	Leukorrhea; lower abdominal pain; lumbar pain; hernia; constipation	• Regulates the girdle vessel and the lower jiao. • Transforms stagnation.
Gb-28 Weidao *Linking Path*	Anterior and inferior to the ASIS, 0.5 cun anterior and inferior to Gb-27.	Prolapsed uterus; pain from intestinal hernia	• Regulates the girdle vessel and the lower jiao. • Transform stagnation.
Gb-29 Juliao *Stationary Crevice*	In the depression of the midpoint between the ASIS and the greater trochanter.	Numbness; paralysis; skin itching; paralysis of lower limb; pain in low back and leg; numbness and stiffness of lower leg; hemiplegia of lower limb	• **Unblocks the Channels:** a local point for painful obstruction syndrome of the hip.

Points	Location	Usage	Indications / Functions
Gb-30 **Huantiao** *Circling Jump*	At the junction of the lateral 1/3 and medial 2/3 of the distance between the greater trochanter and the hiatus of the sacrum (Du-2). When locating this point, put patient in lateral recumbent position with thigh flexed.	Sciatica; Hip, lumbar, and thigh pain; diseases of the hip joint and surrounding tissue; look there for endometriosis as the constricted qi may exacerbate these problems	• **Unblocks the Channels:** local point for painful obstruction syndrome of the hip. Also for atrophy syndrome and sequelae of wind-stroke. For sciatica with pain extending down the lateral side of the leg. • **Tonifies Qi and Blood:** almost as strong as St-36. • **Resolves damp-heat:** for damp-heat in the lower burner causing itchy anus or groin, vaginal discharge and urethritis.
Gb-31 **Fengshi** *Wind Market*	On the midline of the lateral aspect of the thigh, 7 cun above the transverse political crease. When the patient is standing erect with hands at sides, the point is where the tip of the middle finger touches.	Sciatica, especially with lateral leg pain; numbness and paralysis of lower leg; diseases of hip joint and surrounding soft tissue	• **Expels Wind:** for wind-heat moving in the blood causing sudden appearance of red rashes that move from place to place such as in urticaria. Also used to expel wind-heat in herpes zoster (combined with Sj-6). • **Strengthens Bones and sinews:** for atrophy syndrome and sequelae of wind-stroke to relax the sinews and invigorate the circulation of qi and blood to the legs.
Gb-32 **Zhongdu** *Middle Ditch*	On the lateral aspect of the thigh, 5 cun above the transverse popliteal crease, between vastus lateralis and biceps femoris.	Soreness and pain of the thigh and knee; numbness and weakness of the lower limbs; hemiplegia	• Relaxes sinews, Benefits joints, Expels Wind-Damp.
Gb-33 **Xiyangguan** *Knee Yang Gate*	3 cun above Gb-34, with flexed knee, between the tendon of biceps femoris and the femur, in the depression above the lateral epicondyle of the femur.	Diseases of knee and surrounding soft tissue	• Relaxes sinews, Benefits joints, Expels Wind-Damp: local point for painful obstruction syndrome of the knee, especially when there is involvement of the ligaments and tendons of the knee.
Gb-34 **Yanglingquan** *Outer Mound Spring* he-sea	In the depression anterior and in inferior to the head of the fibula.	Major point for musculoskeletal problems; controversial main point for frozen shoulder; important sciatica point; hepatitis; cholecystitis; causes GB contractions and can expel gallstones; hypertension (Liv yang rising type); intercostal neuralgia; herpes	• **Promotes Smooth Flow of Qi:** for Liver qi stagnation causing hypochondriac pain and distention, or pain in the epigastrium. Also for Liver-Stomach disharmony causing vomiting and nausea. • **Resolves damp-heat:** for damp-heat in the Liver and Gallbladder channels. • **Relaxes sinews:** for relaxing tendons whenever there are contractions of muscles, cramps or spasms. • **Unblocks the channels:** for painful obstruction syndrome, atrophy syndrome and sequelae of wind-stroke.
Gb-35 **Yangjiao** *Yang Crossroads*	7 cun above the tip of the lateral malleolus, on the posterior border of the fibula.	Chest fullness; muscular atrophy; leg paralysis	• Unblocks the Channels, Stops pain: for acute pain along the channel with stiffness and cramping of the leg muscles.
Gb-36 **Waiqiu** *Outer Mound* xi-cleft	7 cun above the tip of the lateral malleolus, on the anterior border of the fibula.	Rage; channel excess s/sx like high fever; excess sweating (thought to refer to rabies)	• **Unblocks the Channels, Stops pain, Clears Heat:** for all painful conditions of the Gallbladder channel or organ.
Gb-37 **Guangming** *Bright Light* luo-connect	5 cun directly above the tip of the lateral malleolus, on the anterior border of the fibula.	Main distal point for vision; any eye problems; blurry vision; itching eyes; pain in the eyes	• **Brightens eyes:** improves eyesight and eliminates floaters. • **Conducts fire downwards:** for liver fire affecting the eyes.
Gb-38 **Yangfu** *Lateral Support* jing-river	4 cun above and slightly anterior to the tip of the lateral malleolus, on the anterior border of the fibula, between m. extensor digitorum longus and m. peroneus brevis.	Migraines; hemiplegia; sedation point (but Gb-34 used more); whole body pain of excess type	• **For chronic migraine headaches** caused by liver yang or liver fire.

Points	Location	Usage	Indications / Functions
Gb-39 **Xuanzhong** *Suspended Bell*	3 cun above the lateral malleolus, in the depression between the posterior border of the fibula and the tendons of m. peroneus longus and brevis.	Stiff neck (with Gb-20 and 21 locally); distal for migraines; hemiplegia (flaccid type); sciatica; distal point for knee; any pain in lower leg GB area and pain in all three yang meridians of the leg (such as resulting from hemiplegia); leg qi syndrome; spastic leg; muscular atrophy of lower limbs	• **Benefits the Essence, Nourishes marrow, Expels Wind:** for chronic interior wind with Kidney yin deficiency. Used to prevent wind stroke.
Gb-40 **Qiuxu** *Mounds of Ruins* yuan	Anterior and inferior to the lateral malleolus, in the depression on the lateral side of the tendon of m. extensor digitorum longus.	Pain in chest and ribs; tidal fevers; malaria; cholecystitis; acid reflux; vomiting; distal sciatica point; disease of ankle and surrounding tissues; timidity is often listed as well	• **Promotes Qi circulation:** for hypochondriac pain and distension due to Liver qi stagnation.
Gb-41 **Zulinqi** *Foot Tear-Control* shu-stream	In the depression distal to the junction of the 4th and 5th metatarsal bones, on the lateral side of the tendon of m. extensor digiti minimi of the foot.	HA; migraines; menstrual HA from dai channel connection; vertigo; conjunctivitis (Gb-37 better); mastitis; breast distention; irregular menstruation; scrofula; outer canthus pain; good for pregnancy pain when the tendons and ligaments stretch too early	• **Resolves damp-heat:** for damp-heat in the genital region causing chronic vaginal discharge, cystitis and urethritis. • **Promotes the smooth flow of Liver Qi:** for headaches from Liver qi stagnation of liver fire. • Painful obstruction syndrome of the knee and hip.
Gb-42 **Diwuhui** *Earth Five Meetings*	Between the 4th and 5th metatarsal bones, on the medial side of the tendon of m. extensor digiti minimi of the foot.	Canthus pain; tinnitus; breast distension pain; swelling and pain of the dorsum of the foot	• Spreads Liver Qi, Clears Gallbladder heat.
Gb-43 **Xiaxi** *Narrow Stream* ying-spring	On the dorsum of the foot, between the 4th and 5th toes, 0.5 cun proximal to the margin of the web.	Headache; dizziness and vertigo; outer canthus pain; deafness; tinnitus; breast distension pain; febrile diseases	• **Subdues Liver yang:** for temporal headaches from liver yang rising and migraine headaches affecting the Gallbladder channel on the temples. • **Benefits the ear:** for tinnitus from liver yang rising or otitis media from exterior damp-heat.
Gb-44 **Zuqiaoyin** *Foot Yin Orifice* jing-well	On the lateral side of the 4th toe, about .1 cun posterior to the corner of the nail.	Migraines; headache; intercostal neuralgia; violent nightmares	• **Subdues Liver yang, Benefits the eyes:** for migraine headaches around the eyes caused by liver yang rising. Also for red and painful eyes from liver fire. • Calms the Mind: for insomnia and agitation caused by liver fire.

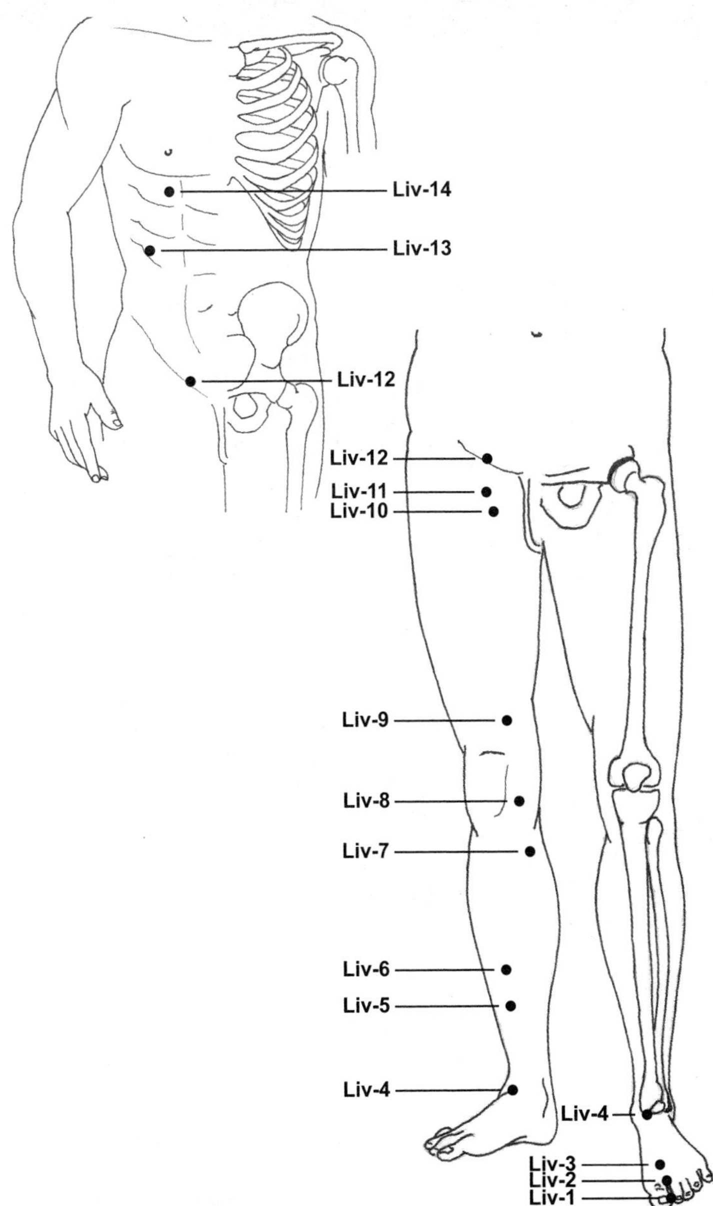

Jing Well	Ying Spring	Shu Stream	Jing River	He Sea
1	2	3	4	8
Yuan	**Luo-connect**	**Xi-Cleft**	**Front Mu**	**Back Shu**
3	5	6	Liv-14	Ub-18

Points	Location	Usage	Indications / Functions
Liv-1 **Dadun** *Big Mound* jing-well	On the lateral side of the terminal phalanx of the great toes, 0.1 cun lateral to the corner of the big toenail.	Abnormal uterine bleeding from hot blood	• **Regulates menses:** stops uterine bleeding due to heat in the blood. • **Resolves damp-heat:** for damp-heat in the lower burner causing difficult urination, retention of urine, enlarged scrotum, itchy scrotum, vaginal discharge or pruritus valvae. • **Promotes the smooth flow of Liver Qi:** for pain on urination with distension of the hypogastrium due to Liver qi stagnation. • **Restores consciousness:** for acute wind-stroke.
Liv-2 **Xingjian** *Temporary In-Between* ying-spring	On the dorsum of the foot, between the 1st and 2nd toes, 0.5 cun proximal to the margin of the web.	Vertex headache; vertigo; dizziness from upsurge of wind (not anything else); intercostal neuralgia from heat; abnormal menstrual bleeding due to heat; cloudy urine or urethra discharge; eyes red and swollen; seizures or convulsions of any type; abdominal distension	• **Clears Liver-fire, Subdues Liver yang:** for patterns including bitter taste, thirst, a red face, headaches, dream-disturbed sleep, scanty dark urine, constipation, red eyes, a red tongue with thick yellow coating, and a rapid-wiry pulse. Used to treat migraine headaches due to Liver-yang rising. Also for liver fire insulting the Lungs and causing coughing accompanied by pain below the ribs and breathlessness. This often is exacerbated by phlegm which combines with fire. • **Expels Interior Wind:** for epilepsy and children's convulsions.
Liv-3 **Taichong** *Bigger Rushing* shu-stream, yuan	On the dorsum of the foot, in the depression distal to the junction of the 1st and 2nd metatarsal bones.	Improves vision; rising Liv yang; Liv wind; vertex and occular headache; dizziness of Liv yang rising and Liv wind type; hypertension (excess or deficient); insomnia; hepatitis; mastitis; major point for irregular menstruation due to stagnation; mouth deviation; uterine bleeding; epilepsy; hernia; urine retention	• **Subdues Liver-yang:** major point for sedating Liver excess patterns, although mostly for subduing liver yang with migraine headaches. • **Expels interior Wind:** calming spasms, contractions and cramps of the muscles, wind in the face (when combines with LI-4) causing facial paralysis and tics. • **Calms the Mind:** for calming tensions, for short temper, anger, irritability, deep frustration and repressed anger, and also for tension from stress. • **Promote Qi circulation:** used with moxibustion to treat genital swelling and orchitis or white vaginal discharge due to cold in the liver channel.
Liv-4 **Zhongfeng** *Middle Seal* jing-river	1 cun anterior to the medial malleolus, midway between Sp-5 and St-41, in the depression on the medial side of m. tibialis anterior.	Genital pain and contraction; hypogastric pain; seminal emission problems; difficult urination; urine retention; lumbar pain; numbness of the body; pain of medial aspect of knee; all ankle problems; difficult defecation; pain and swelling of the lower abdomen; contracted sinews	• Promotes the smooth flow of Liver qi in the lower burner: for urinary symptoms with a feeling of distension in the hypogastrium due to Liver qi stagnation.
Liv-5 **Ligou** *Woodworm Canal* luo-connect	5 cun above the tip of medial malleolus, on the medial aspect and along the medial border of the tibia.	Genital itching like herpes; leukorrhea; irregular menstruation and endometriosis if damp-heat in nature; weakness and atrophy of leg; hernia	• **Promotes Qi circulation:** for any urinary symptom deriving from Liver qi stagnation including distension of the hypogastrium, distension and pain before urination and retention of urine. Also for Liver qi stagnation causing the sensation of a lump in the throat "plum pit". • **Resolves damp-heat:** for vaginal discharge or cloudy urine.
Liv-6 **Zhongdu** *Middle Capital* xi-cleft	7 cun above the tip of the medial malleolus, on the medial aspect and along the medial border of the tibia.	Abdominal pain; diarrhea; hernia; uterine bleeding; prolonged lochia	• Used primarily for acute excess patterns causing pain around the genitalia and deriving from either damp-heat or Liver qi stagnation including cystitis, painful urination, hernia.

Points	Location	Usage	Indications / Functions
Liv-7 **Xiguan** *Knee Joint*	Posterior and inferior to the medial condyle of the tibia, in the upper portion of the medial head of m. gastrocnemius, 1 cun posterior to Sp-9.	Knee pain	• Used as a local point for painful obstruction syndrome of the knee, particularly when caused by wind and with pain on the medial aspect of the knee.
Liv-8 **Ququan** *Spring and Bend* he-sea	When the knee is flexed, the point is located in the depression above the medial end of the transverse popliteal crease, posterior to the medial epicondyle of the tibia, on the anterior part of the insertion of m. semimembranosus and m. semitendinosus.	Genital herpes; vaginitis; local for medial knee pain; nocturnal emissions	• **Benefits the Bladder, Resolves Dampness:** used to eliminate dampness obstructing the lower burner and causing urinary retention, cloudy urine, burning urination, vaginal discharge, pruritus vulvae. Can be used for either damp-heat or damp-cold. • **Nourishes Liver Blood**
Liv-9 **Yinbao** *Yin Wrapping*	4 cun above the medial epicondyle of the femur, between m. vastus medialis and sartorius.	Lumbosacral pain; lower abdominal pain; urine retention; irregular menstruation	• Regulates menses and lower jiao.
Liv-10 **Zuwuli** *Leg Five Miles*	3 cun directly below St-30, at the proximal end of the thigh, below the pubic tubercle and on the lateral border of m. abductor longus.	Lower abdominal fullness and distention; urine retention	• Clears damp-heat, Benefits lower jiao.
Liv-11 **Yinlian** *Yin Angular Ridge*	2 cun directly below St-30, at the proximal end of the thigh, below pubic tubercle and on the lateral border of m. abductor longus.	Irregular menstruation; leukorrhea; lower abdominal pain; thigh and leg pain	• Benefits the uterus.
Liv-12 **Jimai** *Urgent Pulse*	Inferior and lateral to the pubic bone, 2.5 cun lateral to the Ren line, at the inguinal groove, lateral and inferior to St-30.	Cold indications, especially genital area; hernia; lower abdominal pain	• Expels cold from Liver channel, Benefits lower jiao.
Liv-13 **Zhangmen** *Chapter Gate*	On the lateral side of the abdomen, below the free end of the 11th rib.	Liv invading SP is the classic presentation for this point; enlargement of liver and spleen; hepatitis; enteritis; abdominal distension from Liv invading SP; constipation from stagnant Liv qi; pain in hypochondrium; diarrhea due to cold; borborygmus	• **Promotes the smooth flow of Liver Qi, Relieves retention of food.** • **Benefits the Spleen and Stomach:** for Liver qi stagnation patterns when Liver invades Stomach and Spleen, preventing Spleen qi from ascending and causing loose stools and abdominal distension, or preventing Stomach qi from descending causing retention of food, belching and fullness in the epigastrium. Since this is both for strengthening Spleen function as well as for eliminating stagnation, it is the main point for Liver-Spleen disharmony. With moxa it can be used to tonify and warm the Spleen for Spleen yang deficiency.
Liv-14 **Qimen** *Cyclic Gate*	Directly below the nipple, in the 6th intercostal space, 4 cun lateral to the midline.	Main point for intercostal neuralgia; hepatitis; tight chest from anger and frustration; nervous dysfunction of ST (Liv invading the ST); vomiting; hiccups; stuck food; hypochondrium pain and distension; shingles; insufficient lactation	• **Promotes Qi Circulation, Benefits the Stomach:** for Liver qi stagnation patterns when Liver invades Stomach and prevents Stomach qi from descending causing nausea, vomiting, hypochondriac distension and pain, retention of food, belching and fullness in the epigastrium. • **Cools the Blood.**

ACUPRESSURE

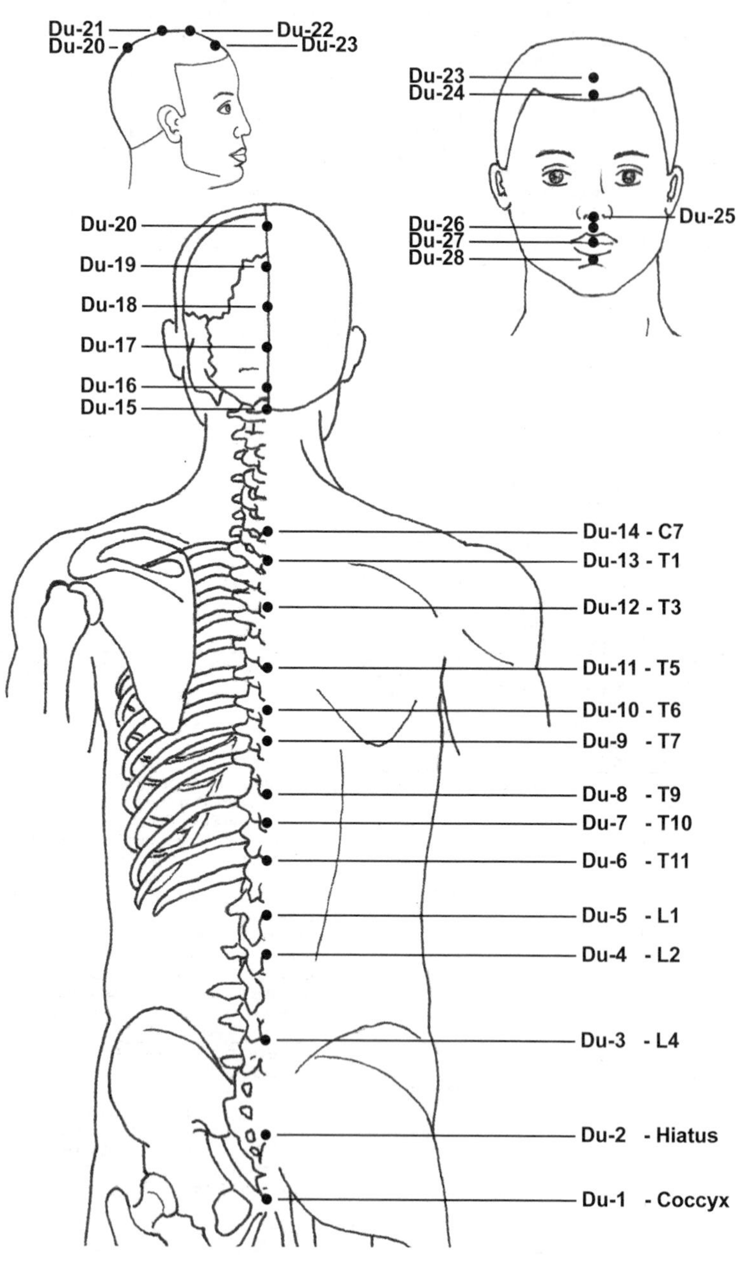
Du-21
Du-20
Du-22
Du-23
Du-23
Du-24
Du-25
Du-26
Du-27
Du-28
Du-20
Du-19
Du-18
Du-17
Du-16
Du-15
Du-14 - C7
Du-13 - T1
Du-12 - T3
Du-11 - T5
Du-10 - T6
Du-9 - T7
Du-8 - T9
Du-7 - T10
Du-6 - T11
Du-5 - L1
Du-4 - L2
Du-3 - L4
Du-2 - Hiatus
Du-1 - Coccyx

Points	Location	Usage	Indications / Functions
Du-1 **Changqiang** *Long Strength* luo-connect	Midway between the tip of the coccyx and the anus, locating the point in prone position.	Diarrhea; constipation; coccyx pain; hemorrhoids; rectal prolapse; rectal bleeding	• **Regulates the Du and Ren:** eliminates obstructions from the channels. It is also a local point for prolapse of the anus. • **Resolves damp-heat:** for hemorrhoids. • **Calms the Mind:** for agitation and hypomania.
Du-2 **Yaoshu** *Lumbar Shu*	On the hiatus of the sacrum.	Hemorrhoids (after DU1); low back pain (local pain; stiffness; and from cold)	• Eliminates Interior Wind: for spasms and convulsions, epilepsy.
Du-3 **Yaoyangguan** *Lumbar Yang Gate*	Below the spinous process of the 4th lumbar vertebrae, level with the iliac crest.	Low back pain; paralysis of lower limbs; muscular atrophy of the legs; impotence; nocturnal emission; epilepsy	• **Strengthens back, Tonifies Yang, Strengthens the legs:** for lower backache, atrophy syndrome.
Du-4 **Mingmen** *Gate of Life*	Below the spinous process of the 2nd lumbar vertebrae.	Low back pain or sprain; 5am diarrhea; enuresis; spermatorrhea; impotence; leukorrhea; irregular menstruation; endometriosis; peritonitis; spinal myelitis; sciatica; nephritis; sequelae of infantile paralysis; asthma due to deficient kidney not grasping lung qi	• **Tonifies Kidney yang:** tonifies and warms the gate of vitality. For Kidney yang deficiency causing chilliness, abundant-clear urination, tiredness, lack of vitality, depression, weak knees and legs, a pale tongue and a deep-weak pulse. • **Benefits Original Qi:** for chronic weakness and both physical and mental. • **Benefits the Essence:** for impotence, premature ejaculation or nocturnal emissions. • **Strengthens lower back and knees:** for chronic backache due to Kidney yang deficiency. • **Expels Cold:** for interior cold due to either Kidney or Spleen yang deficiency causing chronic diarrhea, profuse clear urination, incontinence or enuresis, abdominal pain or dysmenorrhea or infertility.
Du-5 **Xuanshu** *Suspended Pivot*	Below the spinous process of the 1st lumbar vertebrae.	Diarrhea; indigestion	• Strengthens lumbar spine, Benefits lower jiao.
Du-6 **Jizhong** *Spinal Center*	Below the spinous process of the 11th thoracic vertebrae.	Diarrhea; jaundice; epilepsy; stiffness and back pain	• Drains damp, Tonifies Spleen, Benefits lower jiao.
Du-7 **Zhongshu** *Central Pivot*	Below the spinous process of the 10th thoracic vertebrae.	Low back pain; back stiffness; epigastric region pain	• Strengthens lumbar spine, Benefits middle jiao.
Du-8 **Jinsuo** *Tendon Spasm*	Below the spinous process of the 9th thoracic vertebrae.	Epilepsy; gastric pain; back stiffness	• **Expels Interior Wind, Relaxes sinews:** for convulsions, muscle spasms, tremors or epilepsy.
Du-9 **Zhiyang** *Reaching yang*	Below the spinous process of the 7th thoracic vertebrae, approximately at level with the inferior angle of the scapula.	Jaundice; cough; asthma; back stiffness	• **Regulates the Liver and Gallbladder:** promotes the smooth flow of Liver qi when there is hypochondriac pain and distension. • **Opens the chest and diaphragm:** for distension or oppression, hiccup and sighing. • **Resolves damp-heat:** for damp-heat in the Liver and Gallbladder channel causing jaundice.
Du-10 **Lingtai** *Spirits Tower*	Below the spinous process of the 6th thoracic vertebrae.	Back pain; neck rigidity; cough; asthma	• Stops coughing and wheezing, Clears heat and detoxifies poison.
Du-11 **Shendao** *Spirit Pathway*	Below the spinous process of the 5th thoracic vertebrae.	Poor memory; anxiety; palpitation; pain and stiffness of the back	• **Regulates the Heart, Calms the Mind:** clears Heart fire and for other excess Heart patterns.

ACUPRESSURE

Points	Location	Usage	Indications / Functions
Du-12 **Shenzhu** *Body Pillar*	Below the spinous process of the 3rd thoracic vertebrae.	Cough; asthma; pain and stiffness of the back	• **Expels Interior Wind, Relieves spasms:** for spasms, convulsions and tremors or epilepsy. • Tonifies Lung Qi following debilitating illness.
Du-13 **Taodao** *Way of Happiness*	Below the spinous process of the 1st thoracic vertebrae.	Malaria; headache; febrile diseases; stiffness of the back	• **Clears Heat, Release the Exterior, Regulates the Shaoyang:** for beginning stage wind-heat attack. Also for alternating fever and chills and Shaoyang patterns.
Du-14 **Dazhui** *Big Vertebra*	Below the spinous process of the 7th cervical vertebrae, approximately level with the shoulders.	URI; cold; seizures; asthma used with Ding chuan; pain in shoulder; neck pain and rigidity (flexion and extension); any febrile disease; taiyang stage (URI wind-cold) use Du-14 to disperse and cause a sweat; yang ming stage (lung heat) use Du-14 to tonify	• **Clears Heat, Release the Exterior, Expels Wind, Regulates Nutritive and Defensive Qi:** for wind-heat patterns or any heat pattern. • **Tonifies Yang:** with reinforcing method it tonifies the yang and can be used for any yang deficiency pattern. • **Clears the Mind and stimulates the brain.**
Du-15 **Yamen** *Gate of Muteness*	0.5 cun directly above the midpoint of the posterior hairline, in the depression below the spinous process of the 1st cervical vertebrae.	Mental disorders; epilepsy; deafness and muteness; apoplexy after stroke; may not help voice box injury but worth a try	• Clears the Mind, Stimulates speech: for speech impairment.
Du-16 **Fengfu** *Wind Palace*	1 cun directly above the midpoint of the posterior hairline, directly below the external occipital protuberance, in the depression between m. trapezius.	Headache; sore throat; can be used for any of the common wind symptoms; stiff neck; numbness; stroke	• **Expels Wind, Clears the Mind and the Brain:** eliminates both exterior and interior wind causing wind stroke, epilepsy and severe giddiness.
Du-17 **Naohu** *Brain's Door*	On the midline of the head, 1.5 cun directly above Du-16, in the depression on upper border of EOP.	Epilepsy; neck stiffness	• Expels Wind, Clears the brain, Clears the Mind: subdues wind affecting the brain causing epilepsy, wind stroke.
Du-18 **Qiangjian** *Unyielding Space*	On the midline of the head, 1.5 cun directly above Du-17, midway between Du-16 and Du-20.	Headache; neck rigidity; blurry vision; mania	• Expels Wind, Stops pain. • Calms the Mind, Soothes the Liver.
Du-19 **Houding** *Behind the Crown*	On the midline of the head, 1.5 cun directly above Du-18.	Headache; vertigo; epilepsy; mania	• Calms the Mind: for severe anxiety.
Du-20 **Baihui** *Hundred Meetings*	On the midline of the head, 7 cun directly above the posterior hairline, approximately on the midpoint of the line connecting the apexes of the two auricles.	Vertex headache; frontal headache from sinus congestion; dizziness; hypertension; insomnia; seizures (wind); prolapse (lifts energy up); hemorrhoids; diarrhea; vaginal bleeding; tinnitus; nasal obstruction and congestion; stroke; locked jaw; hemiplegia	• **Ascends Yang, Clears the Mind:** for prolapse of the internal organs including stomach, uterus, bladder, anus or vagina. • Eliminates Interior Wind. • Promotes resuscitation and restores consciousness.
Du-21 **Qianding** *In Front of the Crown*	On the midline of the head, 1.5 cun anterior to Du-20.	Epilepsy; dizziness; blurry vision; rhinorrhea; vertical headache	• Expels Wind, Treats convulsions, Benefits the Mind.

Points	Location	Usage	Indications / Functions
Du-22 **Xinhui** *Fontanel Meeting*	2 cun posterior to the midpoint of the anterior hairline, 3 cun anterior to Du-20.	Headache; blurry vision; mental disorders; epistaxis; opthalmalgia	• Benefits the nose, Expels Wind, Benefits the Mind.
Du-23 **Shangxing** *Upper Star*	1 cun directly above the midpoint of the anterior hairline.	Headache; rhinitis; any nose problems involving obstruction	• Opens the nose: for chronic allergic rhinitis or sinusitis.
Du-24 **Shenting** *Mind Courtyard*	0.5 cun directly above the midpoint of the anterior hairline.	Local headache (frontal and sinus); seizures	• **Calms the Mind:** for severe anxiety and fears. Treats schizophrenia.
Du-25 **Suliao** *White Crevice*	On the tip of the nose.	Nasal obstruction; loss of consciousness; epistaxis; rhinorrhea; rosacea	• Benefits the nose.
Du-26 **Renzhong** *Middle of Person*	At the junction of upper 1/3 and lower 2/3 of the philtrum near the nostrils, or upper lip midline.	Loss of consciousness; acute low back sprain; drowning; coma; heat exhaustion; seizures	• **Restores consciousness, Calms the Mind.** • **Benefits the face and nose, Expels Wind.** • **Strengthens lumbar spine.**
Du-27 **Duiduan** *Mouth Extremity*	On the median tubercle of the upper lip, at the junction of the skin and upper lip.	Mental disorders; lip stiffness; lip twitching; pain and swelling of the gums	• Clears Heat, Generates fluid, Benefits the mouth. • Calms the Mind.
Du-28 **Yinjiao** *Gum Intersection*	At the junction of the gum and frenulum of the upper lip.	Mental disorders; pain and swelling of the gums; rhinorrhea	• Clears Heat, Benefits the gums, nose, and eyes.

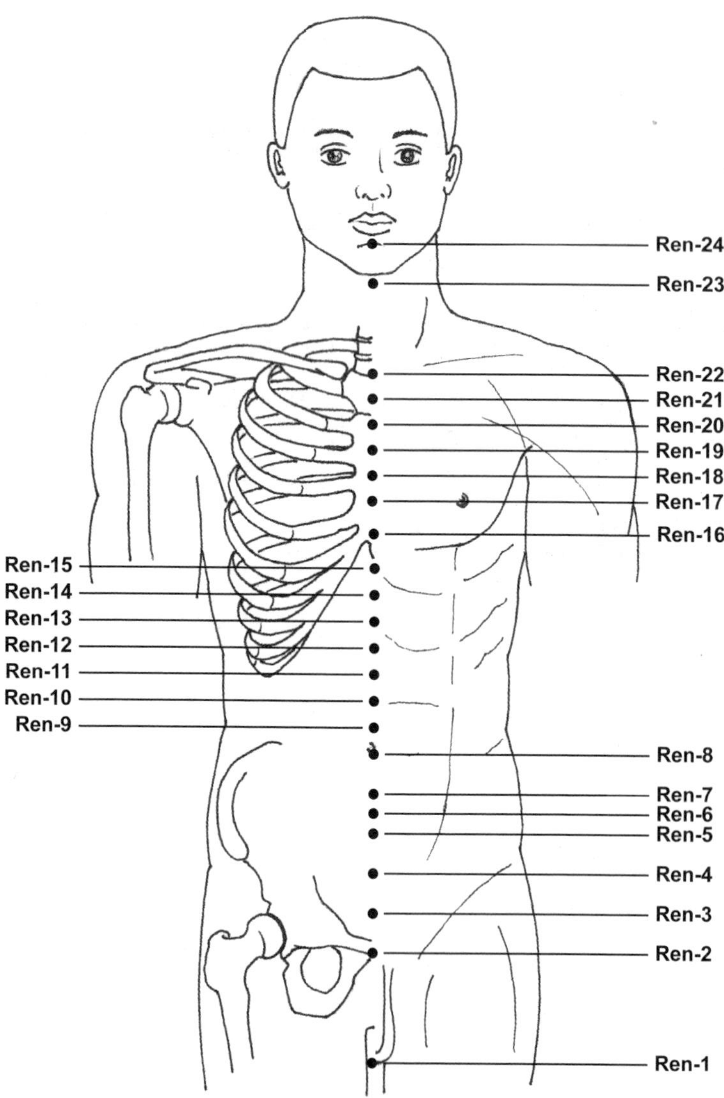
Ren-24
Ren-23
Ren-22
Ren-21
Ren-20
Ren-19
Ren-18
Ren-17
Ren-16
Ren-15
Ren-14
Ren-13
Ren-12
Ren-11
Ren-10
Ren-9
Ren-8
Ren-7
Ren-6
Ren-5
Ren-4
Ren-3
Ren-2
Ren-1

Points	Location	Usage	Indications / Functions
Ren-1 **Huiyin** *Meeting of Yin*	Between the anus and the root of the scrotum in males, and between the anus and the posterior labial commissure in females.	Vaginitis; urine retention; hemorrhoids; nocturnal emission; enuresis; mental disorders	• Nourishes the Yin, Benefits the Essence: for incontinence, enuresis and nocturnal emissions deriving from yin deficiency. • Resolves damp-heat: for damp-heat in the genital area causing vaginal discharge, pruritus vulvae or itching of the scrotum. • Empirical point to promote resuscitation after drowning.
Ren-2 **Qugu** *Curved Bone*	On the midpoint of the upper border of the pubis symphysis.	Urine dribbling and retention; enuresis; nocturnal emission; irregular menstruation; hernia; dysmenorrhea	• Warms and invigorates Kidney, Benefits urination, Regulates lower jiao.
Ren-3 **Zhongji** *Middle Extremity*	On the midline of the abdomen, 4 cun below the umbilicus.	Spermatorrhea; enuresis; retention of urine; leukorrhea; (all due to damp-heat); any urinary tract disorder (90% of the time they are damp-heat related); excessive uterine bleeding; dysmenorrhea (but these are not usually related to damp-heat)	• **Regulates Bladder Function:** for any urinary problem, especially acute. For either excess or deficiency patterns. • **Resolves damp-heat:** for pain and burning on urination and interrupted flow of urine.
Ren-4 **Guanyuan** *Gate to the Original Qi*	On the midline of the abdomen, 3 cun below the umbilicus.	For all Kid problems; abdominal pain; pain from deficiency; cold diarrhea (Kid related); UTI (Ren-3 might be better); urination from cold (clear and copious); deficient types of "rrheas"; can use it to regulate almost any GYN problems	• **Nourishes Yin and Blood:** for any pattern of deficiency of blood or yin. • **Strengthens Yang:** rescue the yang in acute stages of wind-stroke due to collapse of yang. Also for deficiency of Kidney yang. • **Regulates the uterus and menses:** for amenorrhea or scanty periods. • **Tonifies the Kidney and Benefits the Original Qi:** for chronic diseases or for patients with poor constitution or emaciation. • **Calms the Mind**: for anxiety from yin deficiency. • **Roots the Ethereal Soul:** for vague feelings of fear at night due to floating of the ethereal soul.
Ren-5 **Shimen** *Stone Door*	On the midline of the abdomen, 2 cun below the umbilicus.	Abdominal pain; diarrhea; hernia; edema; uterine bleeding; postpartum hermmorhage	• **Benefits the Original Qi:** for Kidney deficiency and a poor constitution. • **Regulates the transformation and excretion of fluids in the lower burner and Opens the water passages:** for edema of the abdomen, urinary retention, difficult urination, diarrhea or vaginal discharge.
Ren-6 **Qihai** *Sea of Qi*	On the midline of the abdomen, 1.5 cun below the umbilicus.	Neurasthenia; abdominal pain and distension related to digestion; impotence; irregular menstruation; intestinal paralysis; all urinary problems like incontinence; infertility spermatorrhea; prolapse rectum; postpartum hemorrhage; diarrhea; (Ren-4 better as it more deeply tonifies the Kid)	• **Tonifies Qi, Yang and Original Qi:** for extreme physical and mental exhaustion and depression. • **Regulates Qi:** for lower abdominal pain and distention due to qi stagnation. • **Benefits Original Qi:** for chilliness, loose stools, profuse pale urination, physical weakness, mental depression, lack of will power. • **Resolves Dampness:** for urinary difficulty, vaginal discharge or loose stool with mucus.
Ren-7 **Yinjiao** *Yin Crossing*	On the midline of the abdomen, 1 cun below the umbilicus.	Abdominal distension; edema; hernia; irregular menstruation	• **Nourishes Yin, Regulates the uterus:** for menstrual problems including amenorrhea, scanty periods or infertility. Also used during menopause to nourish blood and yin.

Points	Location	Usage	Indications / Functions
Ren-8 **Shenque** *Spirit Gateway*	In the center of the umbilicus.	Diarrhea from SP yang deficiency; 5 am diarrhea; apoplexy (flaccid stroke) from yang collapse; any kind of prolapse due to SP yang deficiency	• **Rescues Yang:** for acute stage wind-stroke or the flaccid type characterized by collapse of yang. • **Strengthens Spleen:** for internal cold and extreme weakness, and chronic diarrhea from Spleen deficiency.
Ren-9 **Shuifen** *Water Separation*	On the midline of the abdomen, 1 cun above the umbilicus.	Ascites (retention of fluid in abdomen); edema; retention of urine; diarrhea; general dampness in the body (fluid retention in the body; actual fluid retention in the body as opposed to less material dampness like foggy head)	• **Controls the water passages:** promotes the transportation, transformation and excretion of fluids in all parts of the body. For dampness, phlegm, edema or ascites.
Ren-10 **Xiawan** *Lower Epigastrium*	On the midline of the abdomen, 2 cun above the umbilicus.	Indigestion; food retention after eating; prolapsed stomach	• **Descends Rebellious Qi, Relieves food stagnation:** for stimulating the downward movement of Stomach qi, retention of food in the stomach, abdominal distension, feeling of fullness after eating and sour regurgitation. For treating the pylorus and duodenum.
Ren-11 **Jianli** *Strengthen the Interior*	On the midline of the abdomen, 3 cun above the umbilicus.	Stomachache; vomiting; abdominal distention; borborygmus; edema; anorexia	• Regulates Stomach function, Descend Qi: for feeling of fullness and distension in the epigastrium, nausea, vomiting and epigastric pain.
Ren-12 **Zhongwan** *Middle of Epigastrium*	On the midline of the abdomen, 4 cun above the umbilicus.	Acute or chronic gastritis; gastric ulcers; prolapsed ST; vomiting; nausea; one of the main nausea points and good for any kind; can be used for constipation if chronic or deficient; indigestion; madness from phlegm type of blockage; builds middle energy	• **Tonifies Stomach and Spleen:** for deficiency patterns of the Stomach and Spleen causing lack of appetite, fatigue, and dull epigastric pain relieved by eating. • **Regulates Stomach:** for deficiency cold patterns of the Stomach and Spleen. • **Resolves Dampness.**
Ren-13 **Shangwan** *Upper Epigastrium*	On the midline of the abdomen, 5 cun above the umbilicus.	Stomach pain; nausea; vomiting; abdominal distention	• **Subdues rebellious Stomach Qi:** for hiccup, belching, nausea, vomiting and a feeling of fullness in the upper epigastrium.
Ren-14 **Juque** *Great Palace*	On the midline of the abdomen, 6 cun above the umbilicus.	Mental diseases; seizures; angina pectoris; vomiting; nausea (if more tender than Ren-12); palpitations due to anything; hiatal hernia; strong spirit and mental associations	• **Descends Rebellious Stomach Qi:** for digestive problems with rebellious Stomach qi of emotional origin. • **Clears Heart-fire and Calms the Mind:** for phlegm-heat misting the heart causing mental symptoms.
Ren-15 **Jiuwei** *Dove Tail*	1 cun below the xyphoid process, 7 cun above the umbilicus; locate the point in the supine position with the arms uplifted.	Mental illness; good for fatigue; yang madness; epilepsy	• **Benefits the Original Qi:** nourishes all yin organs and calms the mind when there is anxiety, worry, emotional upsets, fears or obsessions caused by yin deficiency.
Ren-16 **Zhongting** *Center Courtyard*	On the midline of the sternum, at the level of the 5th intercostal space.	Fullness and distension in the chest and intercostal region; hiccups; nausea; anorexia	• Unblocks the chest, Regulates the Stomach, Descends rebellion.

Points	Location	Usage	Indications / Functions
Ren-17 **Shanzhong** *Middle of Chest*	On the anterior midline, at level with the 4th intercostal space.	Asthma; bronchitis; intercostal neuralgia; wheezing; panting; spitting blood; difficulty or inability to swallow food; dilates bronchioles; insufficient lactation; hiccups	• **Tonifies the Qi of the chest, Regulates Qi:** aids the dispersing and descending of qi, dispels stagnation of qi in the chest causing tightness in the chest, breathlessness and pain in the chest. • **Opens the chest:** dispels fullness from the chest and helps breathing. For Lung and Heart qi patterns or obstruction of the chest by phlegm. For chronic bronchitis. • **Benefits the diaphragm:** for hiatal hernia or insufficient lactation from qi and blood deficiency.
Ren-18 **Yutang** *Jade Hall*	On the anterior midline, at the level of the 3rd intercostal space.	Fullness and distension in the chest and intercostal region; hiccups; nausea; anorexia	• Unblocks the chest, Regulates and Subdues rebellion.
Ren-19 **Zigong** *Purple Palace*	On the anterior midline, at the level of the 2nd intercostal space.	Chest pain; cough; asthma	• Unblocks the chest, Regulates and Subdues rebellion.
Ren-20 **Huagai** *Florid Canopy*	On the anterior midline, at the midpoint of the sternal angle, at the level of the 1st intercostal space.	Fullness and distension in the chest and intercostal region; asthma; cough	• Unblocks the chest, Regulates and Subdues rebellion.
Ren-21 **Xuanji** *Jade Pivot*	On the anterior midline, in the center of the sternal manubrium, 1 cun below Ren-22.	Chest pain; cough; asthma	• Descends Stomach Qi, Dispels food stagnation. Unblocks the chest, Descends Lung Qi. • Benefits the throat.
Ren-22 **Tiantu** *Heaven Projection*	In the center of the suprasternal fossa.	Pharyngitis; goiter; hiccups; spasms of the esophagus; diseases of the vocal cords; heavy wheezing; nodules that are phlegm based	• **Stimulates the descending of Lung qi:** for cough and asthma. • **Resolves Phlegm:** for phlegm in the throat and lungs causing acute bronchitis with profuse sputum, or chronic retention of phlegm in the throat. • **Clears Heat:** for Lung heat or wind-heat in the Lungs.
Ren-23 **Lianquan** *Angular Ridge Spring*	Above the Adam's apple, in the depression of the upper border of the hyoid bone.	Loss of voice; paralysis of hypoglossus; excessive salvation; tongue problems	• Descends Qi, Stops cough.
Ren-24 **Chengjiang** *Saliva Receiver*	In the depression in the center of the mentolabial groove.	Facial paralysis; facial edema involving REN meridian; deviated eyes and mouth	• Local point for exterior wind invading the face causing facial paralysis.

Points	Location	Usage	Indications / Functions
E-Anmian *Peaceful Sleep*	Midpoint between Sj-17 and Gb-20	Insomnia; vertigo; headache; palpitation; mental disorders; calms the spirit and clears the brain	• Calms the Mind, Pacifies the Liver.
E-Bafeng *Eight Winds*	On the dorsum of the foot, in the depressions on the webs between toes, 0.5 cun proximal to the margins of the webs, eight points in all.	Beriberi; toe pain; redness and swelling of the dorsum of the foot	• Clears Heat, Reduces swelling.
E-Baichongwo *Shelter of Hundred Insects*	1 cun above Sp-10.	Rubella; eczema; gastrointestinal parasitic diseases	• Clears Heat from the blood, Expels Wind, Drains Dampness.
E-Bailao *100 Labors*	2 cun above Du-14, 1 cun lateral to the midline.	Scrofula; cough; asthma; whooping cough; neck rigidity.	• Transforms Phlegm, Reduce nodules, Stops coughing and wheezing.
E-Baxie *Eight Pathogenic Factors*	On the dorsum of the hand, at the junction of the white and red skin of the hand webs, eight in all, making a loose fist to locate the points.	Excess heat; pain; numbness and swelling of the hands	• Clears Heat, Reduce swelling.
E-Bitong *Nose Passage*	At the highest point of the nasolabial groove.	Rhinitis; nasal obstruction; nasal boils	• Benefits the nose.
E-Bizhong *Middle Of Arm*	On the forearm, midway between the transverse wrist crease and elbow crease, between the radius and the ulna.	Spasm or contracture of the upper extremities; paralysis; pain of the forearm	• Spasm or contracture of the upper extremities; paralysis; pain of the forearm.
E-Dannangxue *Gall Bladder Point*	The tender spot 1-2 cun below Gb-34.	Acute and chronic cholecystitis; cholelithiasis; biliary ascariasis; Giovanni: resolves damp-heat in the GB	• Clears Heat, Drains Damp.
E-Erbai *Two Whites*	On the palmar aspect of the forearm, 4 cun above the transverse wriste crease, on both sides of the tendon of m. flexor carpi radialis.	Hemorrhoids; prolapse of the rectum	• Treats prolapse of rectum and hemorrhoids.
E-Dingchuan *Stop Wheezing*	0.5 to 1.0 cun lateral to Du-14.	Asthma; cough; neck rigid; urticaria; rubella; Giovanni: Expels exterior wind; calms asthma-used to calm an acute attack of asthma	• Stops coughing and wheezing.
E-Erjian *Ear Apex*	Fold of the oracle, the point is at the apex of the auricle (on the helix).	Redness; swelling and pain of the eyes; febrile disease; nebula	• Clears Heat, Reduce swelling, Benefits the eyes.
E-Heding *Crane's Summit*	In the depression of the midpoint of the superior patellar border.	Knee pain; weakness of the foot and leg; paralysis	• Moves Qi and Blood, Strengthens the knees.
E-Huanzhong *Central Round*	Midway between Gb-30 and Du-2.	Lumbar pain; thigh pain	• Moves Qi and Blood: used for lumbar pain and thigh pain.
E-Huatuojiaji *Lining The Spine*	A group of 34 points on both sides of the spinal column, 0.5 - 1.0 cun lateral to the lower border of each spinous process from T1 to L5.	T1-T3 diseases in the upper limbs; T2-T8 diseases in the chest region; T6-L5 diseases in the abdominal region; L1-L5 diseases in the lower limbs	• Regulates and harmonizes zang fu organs.

Points	Location	Usage	Indications / Functions
E-Jiacheng-jiang *Adjacent Container Fluids*	1 cun lateral to Ren-24.	Pain in the face; deviation of the eyes and mouth; spasm of facial muscle	• Expels Wind, Opens the Channels, Stops pain.
E-Jianqian *Front of the Shoulder*	Midway between the top of the anterior axillary crease and LI-15.	Used for shoulder pain or frozen shoulder if pain radiates towards the anterior aspect of the shoulder	• Moves Qi and Blood, Benefits the Shoulder.
E-Jinjin, Yuye *Golden Fluid & Jade Humor*	On the veins on both sides of the frenulum of the tongue,Jinjin is on the left, Yuye is on the right.	Swelling of the tongue; vomiting; aphasia with stiffness of tongue	• Clears Heat, Reduce swelling, Generate fluids, Benefits the tongue.
E-Lanweixue *Appendix Point*	2 cun below St-36. Locate by finding the tender spot between St-36 and St-37.	Acute and chronic appendicitis	• Moves Qi and Blood, Clears excess heat from Large Intestine.
E-Luozhen *Stiff Neck*	On the dorsum of the hand between the 2nd and 3rd metacarpal bones, 0.5 cun posterior to the metacarpophalangeal joint.	Neck pain	• Moves Qi and Blood in the neck region.
E-Naoqing *Clear the Brain Point*	2 cun proximal to St-41 on the St-36-41 line.	Improve memory; clears the brain	• Improve memory; clears the brain.
E-Pigen *Root of Glomus*	3.5 cun lateral to the lower border of L1.	Hepatosplenomegaly; lumbar pain	• Hepatosplenomegaly; lumbar pain.
E-Qianzheng *Pull Aright*	0.5-1 cun anterior to the auricular lobe.	Deviation of the eyes and mouth; ulceration on tongue and mouth	• Deviation of the eyes and mouth; ulceration on tongue and mouth.
E-Qiuhou *Behind the Ball*	At the junction of the lateral 1/4 and 3/4 of the infra orbital margin.	Eye diseases	• Benefits the eyes.
E-Shang-lianquan *Upper Ridge Spring*	1 cun below the midpoint of the lower jaw, in the depression between the hyoid bone and the lower border of the jaw.	Alalia; salivation with stiff tongue; sore throat; difficulty in swallowing; loss of voice	• Alalia; salivation with stiff tongue; sore throat; difficulty in swallowing; loss of voice
E-Shiqizhuixia *Below The 17th Vertebrae*	Below the spinous process of L5.	Lumbar and thigh pain; paralysis of the lower extremities; irregular or painful menses; benefits the lower back and regulates the lower burner	• Tonifies Kidney, Promotes urination, Opens the channels, Stops pain.
E-Shixuan *Ten Diffusions*	On the tips of the ten fingers, about 0.1 cun distal to the nail.	Apoplexy; coma; epilepsy; high fever; acute tonsillitis; infantile convulsion; clear heat; subdue interior wind; open the orifices	• Revives consciousness, Drains Heat, Pacifies Wind.
E-Sifeng *Four Seams*	On the palmar surface, in the midpoint of the transverse creases of the proximal interphalangeal joints of the index, middle, ring and little fingers.	Malnutrition and indigestion syndrome in children; whooping cough	• Tonifies Spleen, Reduce accumulation.

Points	Location	Usage	Indications / Functions
E-Sishencong *Four Alert Spirit*	A group of points, at the vertex, 1 cun respectively posterior, anterior and lateral to Du-20.	Headache; vertigo; insomnia; poor memory; epilepsy; subdue interior wind-used as local point for the treatment of epilepsy	• Calms the Mind, Expels Wind, Benefits the eyes and ears.
E-Taiyang *Greater Yang*	In the depression about 1 cun posterior to the midpoint between the lateral end of the eyebrow and the outer canthus.	Headache; eye diseases; deviation of eye & mouth	• Clears Heat, Expels Wind, Reduce swelling. • Opens channels, Stops pain.
E-Weiguan-xiashu	1.5 cun lateral to the lower border of the spinous process of T8.	Diabetes; vomiting; pain in the chest or abdomen; Note: Considered to be the back shu point of the pancreas	• Clears Heat, Generates fluid.
E-Xiyan/ Xiyuan *Eyes Of the Knee*	A pair of points in the two depressions, medial and lateral to the patellar ligament, locating the point with the knee flexed. Lateral xiyan overlaps with St-35.	Knee pain; weakness of the lower extremities; used for painful obstruction of the knee; needle obliquely upwards or medially with moxa for best results	• Dispels Wind-Damp, Reduce Swelling, Stops pain.
E-Yaoqi *Lumbar Extra*	2 cun directly above the tip of the coccyx	Epilepsy; headache; insomnia; constipation	• Moves Qi and Blood.
E-Yaotongxue *Lumbar Pain Point*	On the dorsum of the hand midway between the transverse wrist crease and metacarpophalangeal joint, between the 2nd and 3rd metacarpal bones, and between the 4th and 5th metacarpal bones, four points in all on both hands.	Acute lumbar sprain	• Moves Qi and Blood in the lumbar region.
E-Yaoyan *Lumbar Eyes*	3.5 cun lateral to the lower border of L4, located in the prone position.	Lumbar pain; frequent urination; irregular menses	• Tonifies Kidney, Strengthens the lumbar region.
E-Yiming *Shielding Brightness*	1 cun posterior to Sj-17.	Eye diseases; tinnitus; insomnia; calms the spirit and brightens the eyes; benefits the ears	• Calms the spirit and brightens the eyes; Benefits the ears.
E-Yintang *Seal Hall*	Midway between the medial ends of the two eyebrows.	Headache; epistaxis; insomnia; head heaviness; frontal headache	• Calms the Mind, Expels Wind, Benefits the nose. • Opens the Channels, Stops pain.
E-Yuyao *Waist Spine*	At the midpoint of the eyebrow, directy above the pupil (in the hair).	Twitching of the eyes; redness; swelling; pain of the eyes; ptosis; cloudiness of the cornea; Giovanni: Used mostly for eye disorders; such as blurred vision or floaters; derived from liver blood deficiency	• Benefits the eyes, Relaxes sinews, Stops pain.
E-Zhongkui *Central Boss*	On the midpoint of the proximal interphalangeal joint of the middle finger at the dorsum aspect.	Nausea; vomiting; hiccups	

Points	Location	Usage	Indications / Functions
E-Zhongquan *Central Spring*	In the depression between LI-5 and Sj-4, on the radial side of the extensor digitorum communis.	Stuffy chest; gastric pain; spitting of blood	• Nausea; vomiting; hiccups.
E-Zhoujian *Tip of the Elbow*	On the tip of the ulnar olecranon when the elbow is flexed.	Scrofula	• Stuffy chest; gastric pain; spitting of blood.
E-Zigongxue *Womb Or Palace Of Child; Uterus Point*	3 cun lateral to Ren-3.	Prolapse of uterus; irregular menses; ovarian cysts; regulates menses; clears heat and transforms damp-heat; raises the middle qi; Giovanni: Used to tonify the kidneys; regulate menses; and for infertility in women	• Raises and regulates Qi, Regulates menses, Stops pain.

BIG PICTURE

Zang – Yin Channels		Wood Jing Well	Fire Ying Spring	Earth Shu Stream	Metal Jing River	Water He Sea	Fu – Yang Channels		Metal Jing Well	Water Ying Spring	Wood Shu Stream	Fire Jing River	Earth He Sea
Tai	Lu	11	10	9	8	5	Yang	LI	1	2	3	5	11
Yin	Sp	1	2	3	5	9	Ming	St	45	44	43	41	36
Shao	Ht	9	8	7	4	3	Tai	SI	1	2	3	5	8
Yin	K	1	2	3	7	10	Yang	Ub	67	66	65	60	40
Jue	Pc	9	8	7	5	3	Shao	Sj	1	2	3	6	10
Yin	Liv	1	2	3	4	8	Yang	Gb	44	43	41	38	34

	Yuan	Luo-connect	Xi-Cleft	Front Mu	Back Shu
Lu	9	7	6	Lu-1	Ub-13
LI	4	6	7	St-25	Ub-25
St	42	40	34	Ren-12	Ub-21
Sp	3	4	8	Liv-13	Ub-20
Ht	7	5	6	Ren-14	Ub-15
SI	4	7	6	Ren-4	Ub-27
Ub	64	58	63	Ren-3	Ub-28
K	3	4	5	Gb-25	Ub-23
Pc	7	6	4	Ren-17	Ub-14
Sj	4	5	7	Ren-5	Ub-22
Gb	40	37	36	Gb-24	Ub-19
Liv	3	5	6	Liv-14	Ub-18
Ren		Ren-15			
Du		Du-1			

8 Influential Points	
Zang	Liv-13
Fu	Ren-12
Qi	Ren-17
Blood	Ub-17
Sinews	Gb-34
Marrow	Gb-39
Bones	Ub-11
Vessels	Lu-9

4 Command Points	
Abdomen	St-36
Head & Neck	Lu-7
Back	Ub-40
Face & Mouth	LI-4

Lower He Sea Points		
3 Arm Yang	LI	St-37
	SI	St-39
	Sj	Ub-39
3 Leg Yin	St	St-36
	Ub	Ub-40
	Gb	Gb-34

Group Luo Points	
3 Arm Yang	Sj-8
3 Arm Yin	Pc-5
3 Leg Yang	Gb-39/35
3 Leg Yin	Sp-6

4 Sea Points	
Blood	Ub-11, St-37, St-39
Qi	Ren-17, Ub-10, St-9
Bone	Du-15, Du-16, Du-19, Du-20
Nourishment	St-30, St-36

Window of Sky	
Ub-10	Pc-1
St-9	Ren-22
Sj-16	Du-16
LI-18	SI-16
Lu-3	SI-18

Muscle Meridian Points	
3 Arm yang	Gb-13
3 Arm yin	Gb-22
3 Leg yang	SI-18 or St-3
3 Leg yin	Ren-3

8 Extra Meridian Points				
	Master	Xi-Cleft	Luo	Indications
Ren	Lu-7		Ren-15	Abdomen, chest, lungs, throat, face
Yin Qiao	K-6	K-8		
Du	SI-3		Du-1	Back of legs, back, spine, neck, head,
Yang Qiao	Ub-62	Ub-59		eyes, brain
Dai	Gb-41			Outer aspect of leg, sides of body,
Yang Wei	SJ-5	Gb-35		shoulders, side of neck
Chong	Sp-4			Inner aspect of leg, abdomen, chest ,
Ying Wei	Pc-6	K-9		heart, stomach

Jing Well	Ying Spring	Shu Stream	Jing River	He Sea
Mental illness, stifling chest, fullness under the heart	Febrile complexion, hot sensations	Bi, wind, damp, heaviness, joint pain	Asthma, cough, hot/cold sensations, change of voice	Fu organs, stomach, intestines, rebellious Qi, diarrhea

Twelve Officials of the Court		
Ht	King	Source of Shen and clear insight
Lu	Minister to the King	Receives the pure Qi from Heaven
Liv	General	Sets strategy
Gb	Judge	Decisions of courage & wise judgment
Pc	Messenger to the King	Protects the King
Sp	Official	Grainery, transform & transport
St	Official	Grainery, rotting & ripening
LI	Official	Drainage
SI	Receiving Official	Separates pure from the impure
Kid	Minister of Health	Strength of body, controls water
Sj	Irrigation Official	Water channels, balance & harmony
Ub	Minor district Official	Controls storage of water & excretes fluids

Five Element Acupressure

Understanding the relationships of the five elements in an individual provides clues for better health and treatment with acupressure. The Five Elements: wood, fire, earth, metal and water have their own characteristics that correspond to energies of the individual and are divided into two distinct cycles of creation and control. In Traditional Chinese Medicine, the body is regarded as a microcosm of the universe. Five element concerns the process of transformation from one phase of a cycle into another. Each element corresponds with particular organs and processes (such as digestion, respiration, circulation, elimination, etc.) in the body. The treatment of organ system can be treated by determining which organ is out of place and selecting acupressure points based on disharmonies to bring balance back into the body.

Step One: Determine which organ system is out of balance
Step Two: Determine whether the imbalance is excess or deficiency
Step Three: See Below

Deficiency Conditions

- Tonify the horary point on the mother organ's channel.
- Tonify the mother organ's element point on the affected channel.
- Sedate the horary point on the "controlling" organ's channel.
- Sedate the controlling organ's element point on the affected organ.

Tonification prescriptions for conditions of deficiency

Meridian	Tonify		Sedate	
	Horary Pt	Son Pt.	Horary Pt.	Control Pt.
Lung	Sp-3	Lu-9	Ht-8	Lu-10
Large Intestine	St-36	LI-11	SI-5	LI-5
Stomach	SI-5	St-41	Gb-41	St-43
Spleen	Ht-8	Sp-2	Liv-1	Sp-1
Heart	Liv-1	Ht-9	K-10	Ht-3
Small Intestine	Gb-41	SI-3	Ub-66	SI-2
Urinary Bladder	LI-1	Ub-67	St-36	Ub-40
Kidney	Lu-8	K-7	Sp-3	K-3
Pericardium	Liv-1	Pc-9	K-10	Pc-3
San Jiao	Gb-41	Sj-3	Ub-66	Sj-2
Gallbladder	Ub-66	Gb-43	LI-1	Gb-44
Liver	K-10	Liv-8	Lu-8	Liv-4

Excess Conditions

- Tonify the horary point on the controlling organ's channel.
- Tonify the controlling point on the affected channel.
- Sedate the horary point on the "son" channel.
- Sedate the son point on the affected channel.

Sedation prescriptions for conditions of excess

Meridian	Tonify		Sedate	
	Horary Pt	Control Pt.	Horary Pt.	Son Pt.
Lung	Ht-8	Lu-10	K-10	Lu-5
Large Intestine	SI-5	LI-5	Ub-66	LI-2
Stomach	Gb-41	St-43	LI-1	St-45
Spleen	Liv-1	Sp-1	Lu-8	Sp-5
Heart	K-10	Ht-3	Sp-3	Ht-7
Small Intestine	Ub-66	SI-2	St-36	SI-8
Urinary Bladder	St-36	Ub-40	Gb-41	Ub-65
Kidney	Sp-3	K-3	Liv-1	K-1
Pericardium	K-10	Pc-3	Sp-3	Pc-7
San Jiao	Ub-66	Sj-2	St-36	Sj-10
Gallbladder	LI-1	Gb-44	SI-5	Gb-38
Liver	Lu-8	Liv-4	Ht-8	Liv-2

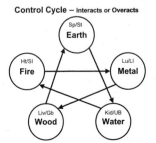

Control Cycle – Interacts or Overacts

Sp/St Earth
Ht/SI Fire
Lu/LI Metal
Liv/Gb Wood
Kid/UB Water

Mother-Son Cycle

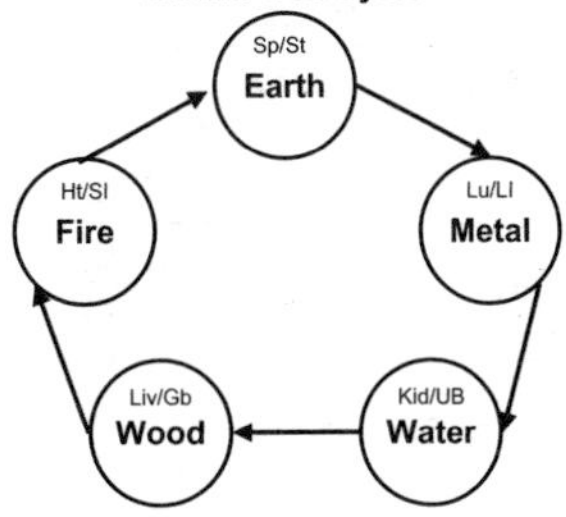

FIVE ELEMENTS

Elements	Wood	Fire	Earth	Metal	Water
Yin	Liver	Heart	Spleen	Lung	Kidney
Yang	Gallbladder	Small intestine	Stomach	Large intestine	Bladder
Color	Green/blue	Red	Yellow	White	Black, deep blue
Flourishes/ manifests	Nails	Complexion	Lips	Body hair, skin	Head hair
Sense organ	Eyes	Tongue	Mouth	Nose	Ears
Tissue dominated/ rules over	Ligaments, tendons, tissues, sinews	Blood & vessels	Muscles	Skin, mucous membranes	Bones, teeth, marrow, nerves
Orifice/ opens into	Eyes	Tongue	Mouth	Nose	Ears
Physiognomy	Eyes	Nose, tongue	Tongue, mouth	Cheeks & nostrils	Ears
Eye	Iris	Canthus	Lids	Sclera	Pupil
Tongue	Sides	Tip	Center	Posterior of tip	Root
Secretion	Tears	Sweat	Saliva	Mucous	Urine
Pulse	Stringy, wiry	Large, rapid	Slippery	Floating, slow	Sunken, deep
Emotion	Anger, jealousy	Joy	Anxiety, pensiveness, sympathy, desire	Sorrow, worry, grief	Fear & depression
Odor/smell	Rancid (cheese), goatish, fetid	Scorched (burnt)	Fragrant	Rotten (fish), rank	Putrid (urine), rotten
Flavor	Sour & acid	Bitter & sharp	Sweet	Pungent & spicy	Salty
Strained by	Reading	Walking	Sitting	Lying	Standing
Sound emitted to emotion	Shouting	Laughter & talkative	Singing	Weep, wail, cry	Groan & complain
Sound emitted in illness	Talking	Belching	Swallowing	Coughing	Yawning
Direction	East	South	Center	West	North
Climate	Windy	Hot	Moisture & thunder	Dryness & cold	Cold & wet
Season	Spring	Summer	Late summer, Indian summer	Autumn	Winter
Development	Birth	Growth	Change	Decline	Death
Granted power	Control	Sadness, grief	Belching	Cough	Trembling
Sense	Vision	Speech	Taste	Smell	Hearing
Instinct	Emotion	Spirit	Conscience	Health	Will
Thought	Relaxed	Enlightened	Careful	Energetic	Quiet
Motion	Clench	Anxiety	Hiccup	Cough	Tremble
Heavens	Stars	Sun	Earth	Zodiac	Moon
Planet	Jupiter	Mars	Saturn	Venus	Mercury
Number	8 & 3	7 & 2	10 & 5	9 & 4	6 & 1
Tendency	Up	Periphery	Balance	Down	Center
Ministries	Agriculture	War	Capital	Justice	Works
Classes	Fish	Birds	Man	Mammals	Invertebrate
Instruments	Compasses	Weights & measures	Plumb lines	T-square	Balances
Covering	Scales	Feathered	Naked	Hairy	Shelled
Wild animal	Tiger	Stag	Bear	Bird	Monkey
Grain	Wheat, rye, barley	Corn, beans	Rice, millet	Rice, oats	Peas, millet, buckwheat
Vegetable	Short green	Round	Leafy green	Tall green	Bushy
Fruit	Plum	Apricot	Date	Peach	Chestnut
Animal food	Sheep	Fowl	Beef, ox	Horse, dog	Wild pig
Cooking	Steam	Raw	Stew	Bake	Sautéed

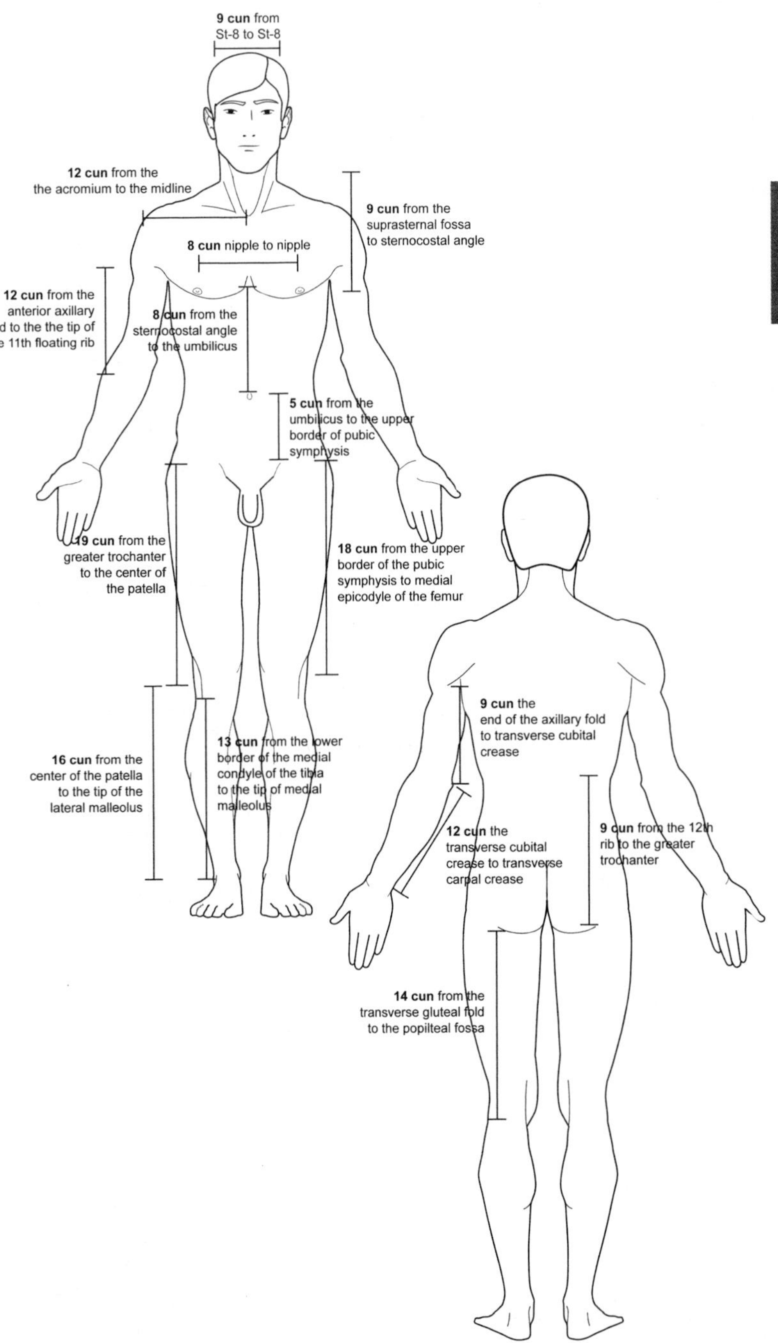

9 cun from St-8 to St-8
12 cun from the the acromium to the midline
9 cun from the suprasternal fossa to sternocostal angle
8 cun nipple to nipple
12 cun from the anterior axillary fold to the the tip of the 11th floating rib
8 cun from the sternocostal angle to the umbilicus
5 cun from the umbilicus to the upper border of pubic symphysis
19 cun from the greater trochanter to the center of the patella
18 cun from the upper border of the pubic symphysis to medial epicodyle of the femur
9 cun the end of the axillary fold to transverse cubital crease
16 cun from the center of the patella to the tip of the lateral malleolus
13 cun from the lower border of the medial condyle of the tibia to the tip of medial malleolus
12 cun the transverse cubital crease to transverse carpal crease
9 cun from the 12th rib to the greater trochanter
14 cun from the transverse gluteal fold to the popilteal fossa

Swedish Massage

Swedish, or classical, massage is the style that comes to mind when most people think of massage. It is among the first styles of massage that new massage therapists practice during their training. It was developed centuries ago by University of Stockholm physiologist Henri Peter Ling, who was in awe of Chinese massage techniques and benefits. Swedish massage is considered to be the basis for other types, such as Western massage, aromatherapy, sports massage and deep-tissue massage. It is also used to reduce pain and joint stiffness, increase circulation and oxygen flow, and release toxins (especially lactic acid) from the muscles. It can aid in muscle recovery because it helps the body release lactic acid, uric acid, and other metabolic wastes more quickly. It is used to relieve stress and improve mood, providing overall physical wellness and mental well-being.

There are five techniques used in administering Swedish massage. These techniques are as follows:

- **Effleurage.** Effleurage technique is the most versatile and most used technique commonly associated with general massage and Swedish massage. The effleurage session usually begins with the application of oil and lotion. It involves long, sweeping and light, gliding strokes. The therapist uses palms, thumbs and/or fingertips to help connect one part of the body to others that cover more than just one area of the body. Though it makes the client feel as if his muscles are being broken down, the purpose of effleurage is used for connecting and transitioning strokes.

- **Friction.** Friction involves repetitive surface rubbing to generate heat. It warms the treated area and prepares and relaxes the muscles for deeper work. The therapist uses palms of the hands, thumbs and/or fingertips in a friction technique by rubbing vigorously on the surface of the client's skin. Friction can be applied by rubbing palms together and laying them on the skin, using palms, thumbs and/or fingertips, knuckles in a constant brisk manner to create heat.

- **Petrissage.** Petrissage is the act of kneading, lifting, rolling, squeezing, pressing, or rolling the tissue under or between the hands. The therapist uses palms, thumbs and/or fingertips in a constant "milking" alternating manner from one area of the body to another. Petrissage does not target or focus on any particular part of the body, but the process of kneading the body's muscles separates muscles fibers and allows for deeper and more penetrating effects of massage.

- **Tapotement.** Tapotement is strokes that aim to energize the area of the body through brisk striking, tapping, beating, and percussion movements in a rhythmic fashion. This is done by chopping the area with the sides of the hands. It can also be done by hitting the area being treated rhythmically with cupped or fisted hands. Tapotement is aimed towards energizing the area being treated, stimulating the nerves, muscles, and circulation through tapping, yet at the same time making it loosened and relaxed

- **Vibration.** The vibration technique is a quick, oscillating, quivering, trembling, or rocking motion to shake up the area mechanically or manually. This is done by moving the heel of the hand, sides of the hand, or even the fingertips, forward and backward across the skin to loosen the muscles of that particular area.

Deep-Tissue Massage

Deep-tissue massage (also known as myofascial release) is a type of massage that seeks to release the myofascial restrictions of the deeper muscles, tendons and ligaments of the body. It uses the same principles and strokes of effleurage, friction, petrissage, tapotement, traction, and vibration similar to that of Swedish, with slight variations on the focus and depth. The primary focus of deep tissue massage is to address specific tight muscles and to correct postural distortion caused by these tight muscles. There is a misconception that deep tissue simply means classical massage with heavier pressure. A practitioner may use very deep pressure without really addressing postural problems. Conversely, a practitioner may sometimes use light pressure in a precise manner to facilitate deeper muscle relaxation, with little or no effort. More importantly, the idea of deep tissue is not necessarily focused on pressure but should be focused on realigning the deeper layers of muscles and connective tissues.

The primary stroke of deep tissue massage is linear friction– sustained, slow and deliberate strokes along the muscles fibers to unblock adhesions. Some practitioners use little or no oil for better control in realigning the deeper layers of the connective tissues. This stroke activates the stretch receptors of the muscle, giving it a signal to release. A deep-tissue massage may also use static pressure in one spot to release muscles. Some clients may experience a slight tingling or burning sensation in the skin or describe deep tissue as a balance of pain and pleasure. Others may describe deep tissue as a gentle to deep stretch on the area being treated. When skillfully applied to a group of muscles, deep-tissue massage can "educate" the body to overcome dysfunctional muscle patterns and adopt a more balanced and healthier posture.

Deep-tissue massage also has wonderful health benefits. The release of habitually tight muscles relieves chronic pain and speeds the healing of injuries. Balanced posture improves organ function and athletic performance as well as addressing chronic pain. Relieving the stress and energy drain of chronically tight muscles improves general health as well.

It is important that practitioners be exposed to the range of myofascial techniques in order to effectively tailor their treatment to the needs of each individual client. In general, myofascial release is used to improve the health of the muscles and fascia, improve circulation and restore good posture. Before we learn about myofascial release, it would be helpful to learn what this therapy actually treats. It is critical to understand from the outset that there is a wide variety of techniques employed in deep-tissue myofascial release. Other schools that have origins in realigning deeper layers of muscle and connective tissues include: Rolfing, Structural Integration, Neuro-Muscular Therapy, CranioSacral Therapy, Polarity Therapy, Travell's Trigger point therapy, Pfrimmer Deep Tissue, Postural Integration, Soma Neuromuscular Integration, Thai Massage, and Trager.

While there are various competing theories regarding proper technique and application, it is generally understood by practitioners of deep-tissue massage that:

- Blocked circulation is a detriment to overall health. As such, myofascial release techniques can be administered in order to eliminate these harmful blocks (often caused by muscle tightness). Furthermore, deep-tissue techniques can be administered in order to enhance the circulation of blood, lymph, interstitial fluids and cerebro-spinal fluids.
- A healthy lifestyle requires regular physical activity. To be sure, the muscles of the body are interconnected with other bodily functions and physiological processes. Thus, exercise and vigorous physical activity is an important part of a healthy lifestyle and should be pursued in tandem with massage therapy.
- Connective tissue is integral to maintaining overall health. It is widely known that connective tissue plays a critical role in most bodily systems and, as such, it is important to nurture strong, robust connective tissues through massage. Indeed, when these tissues fail to function properly due to restrictions, the body can be put at systemic risk. It is thus imperative that these tissues are maintained through deep-tissue massage in conjunction with other means.

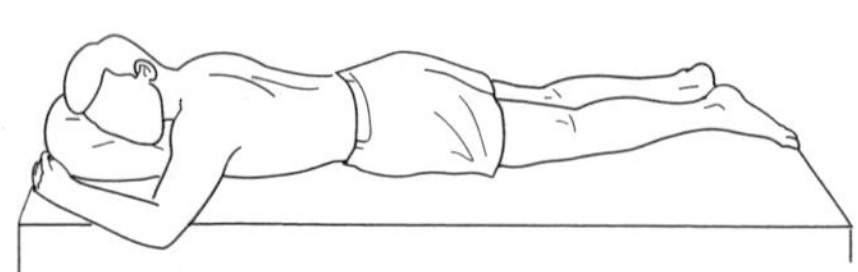

Prone Start
Position the subject on their stomach with their head resting comfortably in a headrest or pillow.

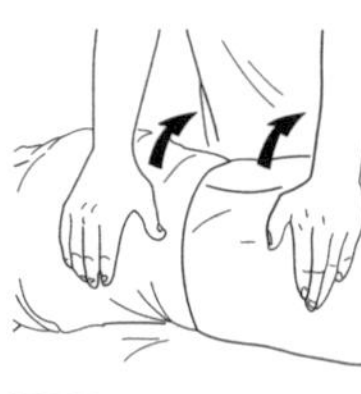

Rocking
Move side to side in a soothing, rhythmic method using both hands gently placed on either side of the torso to rock the subject back and forth. This is known to have a calming effect and to initiate parasympathetic mechanism.

Single or Double Hand Effleurage
Begin in a static resting position by applying a light touch followed by the application of lotion or oil evenly with a butterfly effleurage. Using both hands, apply effleurage, petrissage pressure to the upper back and glide the palms down the surrounding muscles with bilateral and transverse strokes. Long strokes can be applied up and down the muscles of the back and gradually increase pressure if desired.

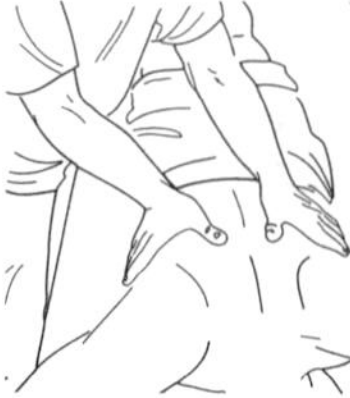

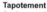

Double Hand Effleurage
Using both hands, glide in the direction of the muscle fibers from the lower back up to the shoulders. Petrissage, friction, kneading and effleurage can be applied to trapezius, latissimus dorsi and erector spinae muscles of the back.

Tapotement
Apply open-handed hacking percussion wherein only the little finger or the ulnar side of the hand is used to strike the surface of the body. Heavy percussion is *not* indicated over the kidneys or areas of pain or discomfort.

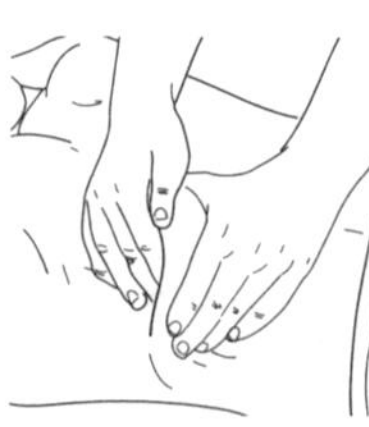

Petrissage of the Back
Using both hands apply petrissage pressure to the subject's back using kneading, picking up, wringing, rolling and pinching strokes on the back to the top of the shoulders with fingers and thumbs. Kneading can be applied with hand lifting and squeezing with fingers and thumbs.

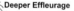

Deeper Effleurage
Apply gradual effleurage and petrissage pressure to the subject's back and, using both hands in long, alternating strokes, lengthen the muscles from the lower back to the top of the shoulder. Deeper friction can be applied with forearm erector spinae muscles and ligaments along the spine.

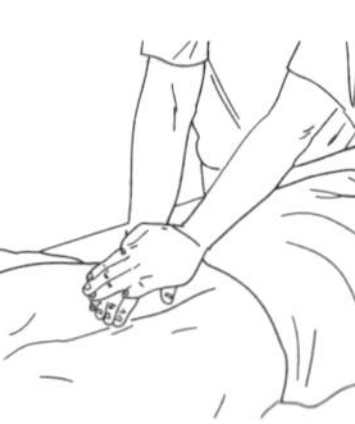

Effleurage of the Back
Starting from the hips and lower back with one hand on top of the other hand, gradually apply a deeper effleurage pressure to the desired area of the back by leaning your body weight into subject's body. Apply a deeper stroke with the forearms and fist, if desired.

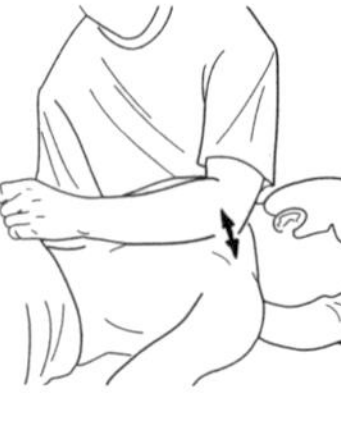

Forearm Friction of the Shoulder
Using the forearm, create a transverse and bilateral movement across the trapezius and erector muscles of the back. Deeper friction can be applied over the ridge of the upper trapezius and carefully circle around each scapula. You can also position the hand above the subject's head to elevate the scapula for better access.

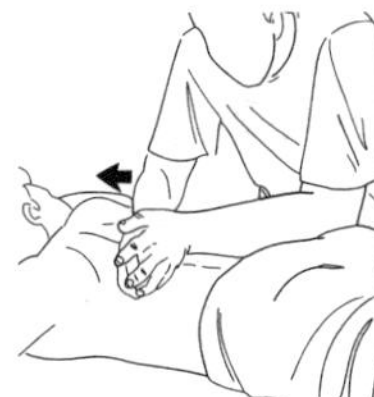

Double Forearm
Using both forearms, glide smoothly in the direction of the muscle fibers from the lower back to the shoulders to lengthen the erector muscles.

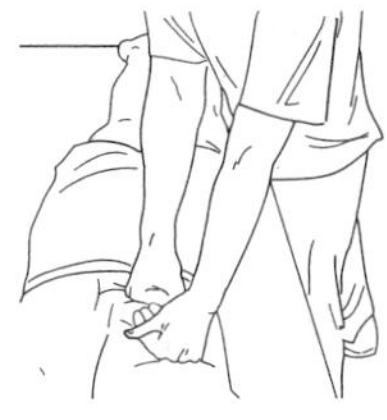

Double Hand Ironing
With the elbow and wrists held straight, use both hands simultaneously to glide along the length of the muscle to elongate and relax the muscle. The other hand can be used to guide the stroke. Apply different strokes up and down erector muscles of the back if desired.

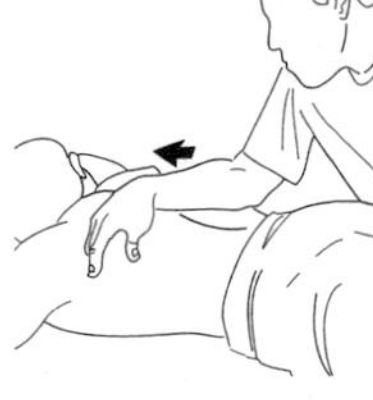

Deeper Forearm
Using one forearm, apply a deep stroke with the ulnar border of the forearm, gliding smoothly in the direction of the muscle fibers from the lower back up to the shoulders and trapezius. Contour your forearm to the subject's back and adjust pressure accordingly.

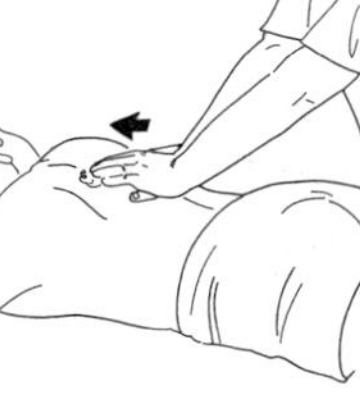

Reinforced Hand
Using one hand on top of the other hand, glide smoothly in the direction of the muscle fibers to lengthen the muscles from the lower back to the shoulders.

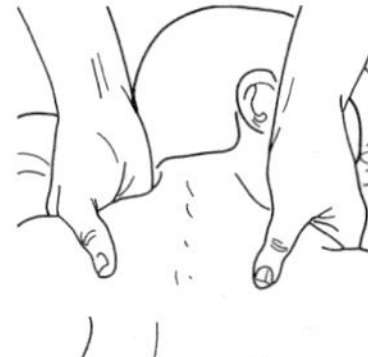

Kneading of the Trapezius
Apply kneading, picking up, wringing, rolling and friction strokes around the trapezius and upper shoulders.

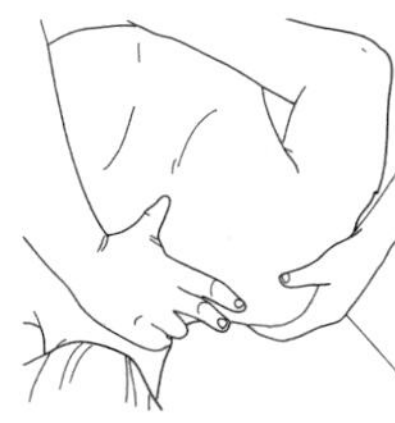

Kneading of the Scapula
Apply kneading, picking up, wringing, rolling and friction strokes around the edges of the scapula.

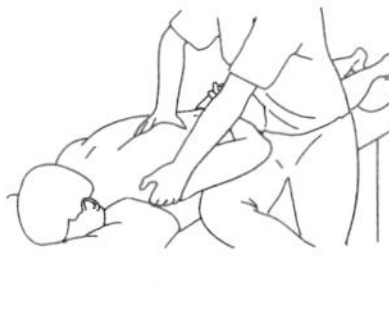

Scapula Lifting and Shoulder Pull
With one hand, grasp the subject's shoulder as the other hand lifts the scapula away from the body. Use the fingers to press against the lower edge of the scapula and raise the medial border of the shoulder. Deep friction, stroking and thumbing of rhomboid muscle and shoulder can be guided along the edges.

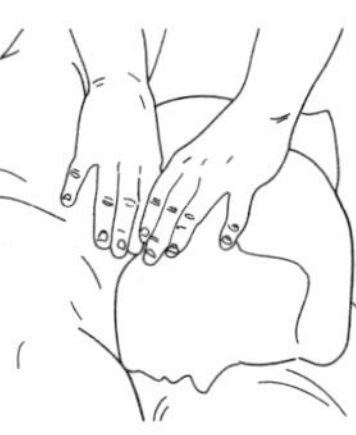

Neck Traction
Stroke, stretch and friction the upper trapezius away from the back of the neck.

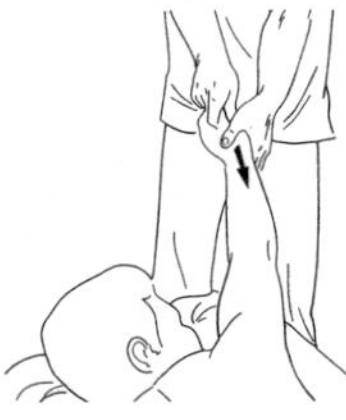

Arm Traction
Hold the arm away from the body and apply gentle traction on the wrist by leaning backwards. Using the opposite hand, stroke from the subject's hand towards the elbow. Wave like arm shaking can be applied if desired.

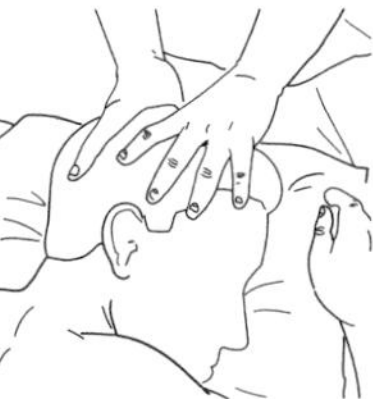

Head Compression
Head compression and pressure points can be applied to the top and back of the head to complete the prone position.

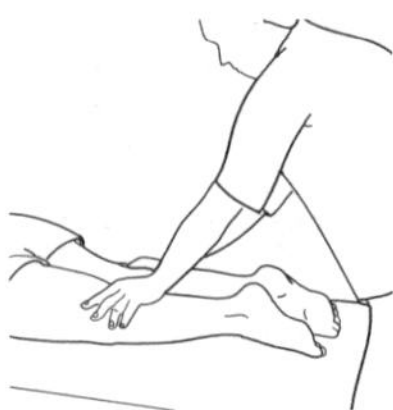

Effleurage of the Legs
Apply effleurage and petrissage strokes to the backs of both legs simultaneously so as to create a feeling of evenness and to lengthen the muscles of the leg.

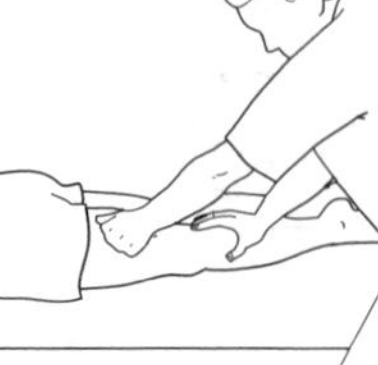

Ironing of the Hamstrings
Apply a stabilized gliding technique by gliding with one fist with the elbow and wrist held straight. Apply light to deep strokes while using the opposite hand to stabilize the leg. Deeper stroking with a forearm glide or thumb friction can be applied if desired.

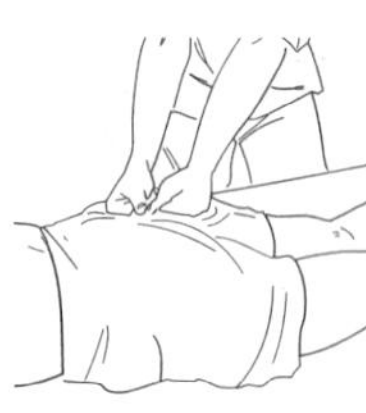

Petrissage of the Glutes
Use both fists to knead the gluteal muscle, to loosen tissue, and to break up adhesions in the muscle and surrounding connective tissue. Compression, deep friction, and deep pressure can be applied to the posterior thigh and glutes.

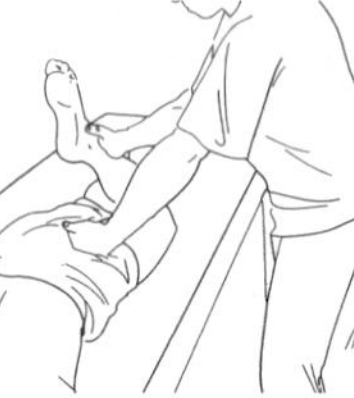

Kneading with Flex Leg
Flex the subject's knee towards the midline of the body and towards the buttocks to allow relaxation of the gluteal muscles and to open the hip joint. Use your fist to knead the gluteal muscles. Apply compression or thumb friction and deeper strokes simultaneously with the stretch, if desired.

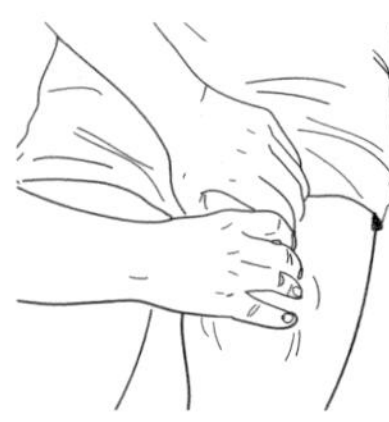

Kneading of the Hamstring
Apply kneading, picking up, wringing, rolling and friction strokes of the hamstring and upper leg.

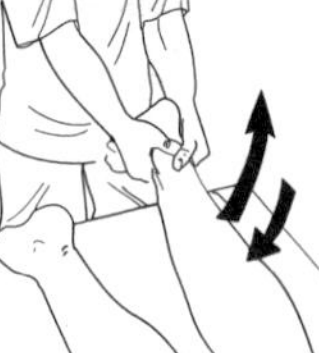

Leg Shaking
Using both hands, grasp the subject's ankle and pull out the slack in the tissue. Apply abrupt pressure to lift the leg off the table and then allow it to return to its original position

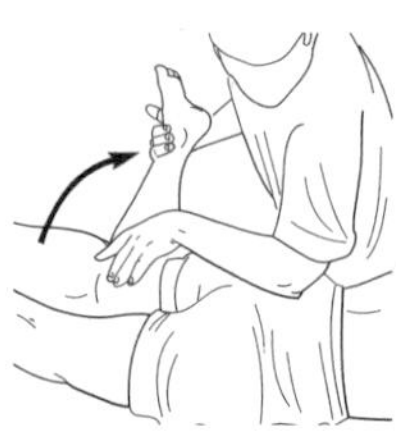

Compression with Flex Knee
Flex the subject's knee to allow relaxation of the gluteal muscles. Use your elbow to compress the gluteal pressure points and piriformmis origins.

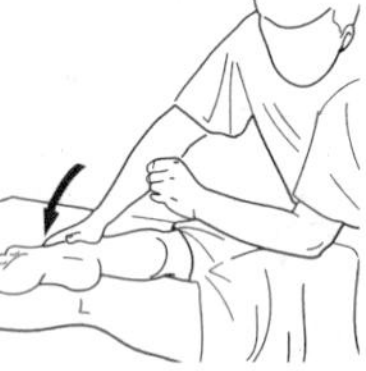

Compression with Flex Knee 2
Flex the subject's knee towards the midline of the body to allow relaxation of the gluteal muscles and to open the hip joint. Use your elbow to compress the gluteal pressure points.

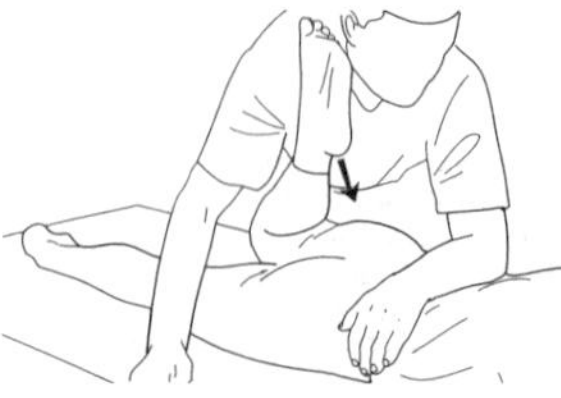

Quadriceps Stretch
Flex the subject's knee and position the bent knee so that it rests on your shoulder and gradually lean forward to stretch the leg. Position your forearm across their torso to secure the hips and maintain balance as you use your body weight to stretch the quadriceps.

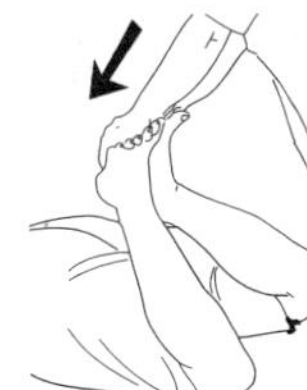

Knee Flex
Place both hands to press the subject's heel towards the buttocks, using your body weight to stretch the shin and quadriceps.

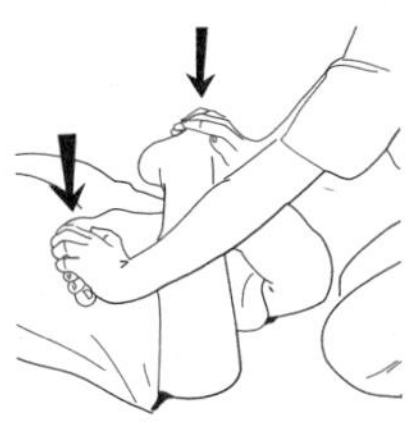

Cross Double Knee Flex
Cross both the subject's knees and press the heel towards the buttocks using your body weight to stretch the shin and quadriceps for a deep stretch.

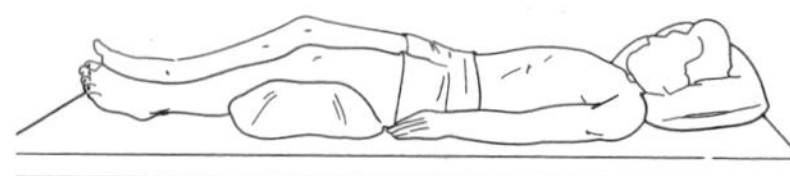

Supine Position
Have the subject lie on their back, with support under their head and knees.

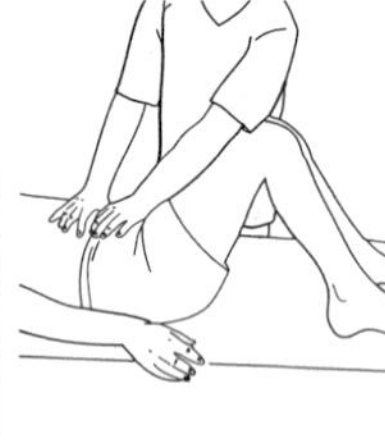

Abdomen
A light and superficial stroke to the abdomen area is a helpful introduction of touch. Apply effleurage and petrissage strokes to the abdomen in a clockwise direction following the path of large intestines using one, two or alternating hands. Transverse inward and outwards strokes to the abdominal region can also be applied.

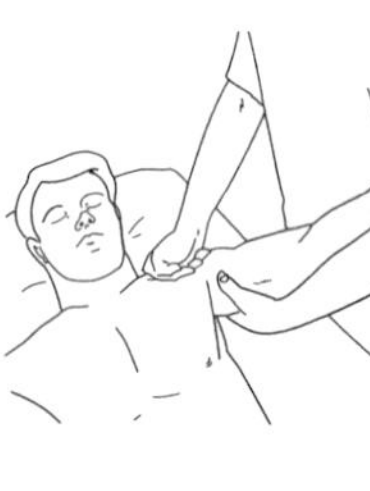

Chest, Abdomen, and Shoulder Petrissage
Without losing contact, knead the subject's chest, shoulder and abdomen to lengthen and elongate the muscle fibers. Work generously on the upper torso of the subject's body with varying petrissage, effleurage with double, single and alternating hand strokes.

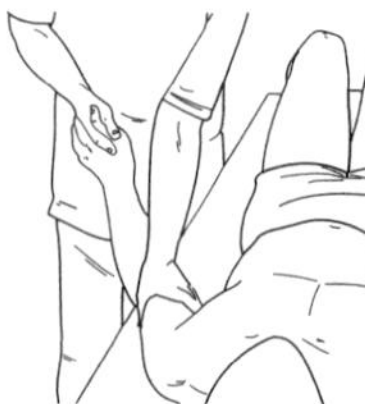

Arm Kneading
Use both hands to simultaneously knead the subject's bicep, forearm and hand. Alternating hand strokes and slight traction can be applied by gently leaning away from the body. Apply slight downward pressure if desired.

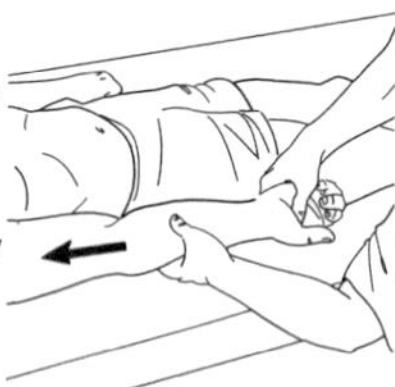

Arm Milking
Use both hands to knead the subject's bicep, forearm and hand by applying squeezing sustained pressure up the forearm and towards the heart.

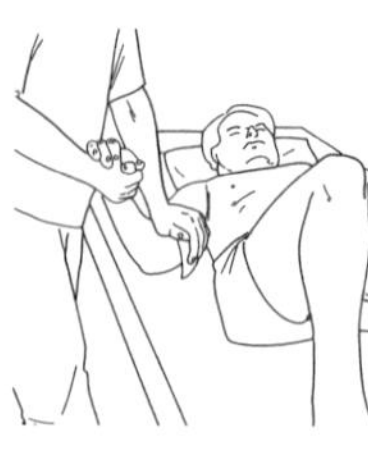

Flex Elbow Kneading
Use one hand to hold the subject's upper arm in place. Use the opposite hand to gently flex, extend, and circle the subject's elbow joint. Apply joint movement to the shoulder by moving the elbow in a circular motion.

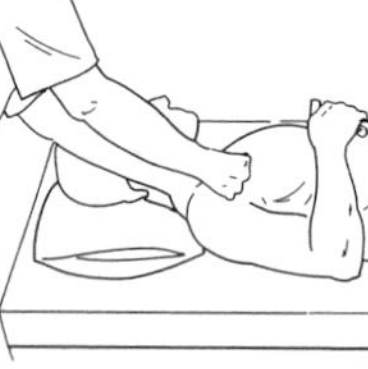

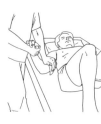

Chest Kneading
Apply effleurage and petrissage strokes using open handed, alternating hand strokes and loose fists. Work generously over and around the shoulders and up the neck and in between the ribs and pectoral muscles of the chest and shoulder muscles.

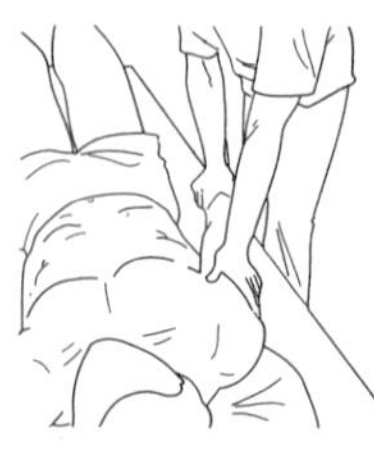

Arm Kneading
Use one hand to hold the subject's arm in place. Use the opposite hand to glide from the subject's elbow to the shoulder. Apply light to deep pressure to the hands, arm and forearm with friction and kneading if desired.

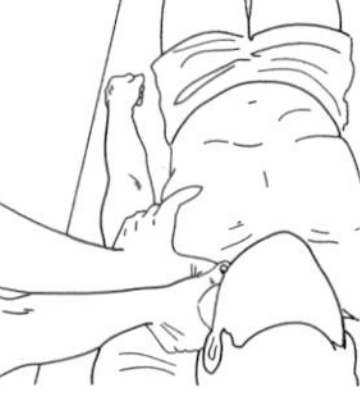

Shoulder Kneading
Apply effleurage and petrissage strokes using open handed, alternating hand strokes and loose fists to the sides of the neck and shoulder.

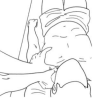

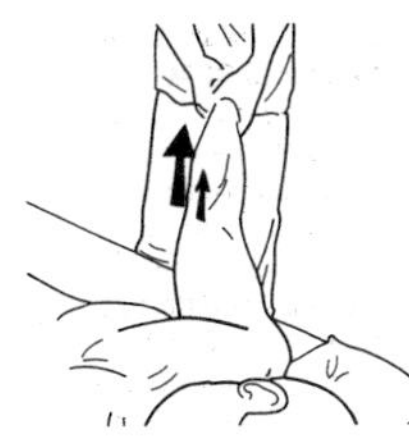

Arm Shaking
Using both hands, grasp the arm around the wrist and pull out the slack in the tissue. Apply abrupt pressure, lifting it off the table, and then return it to its original position.

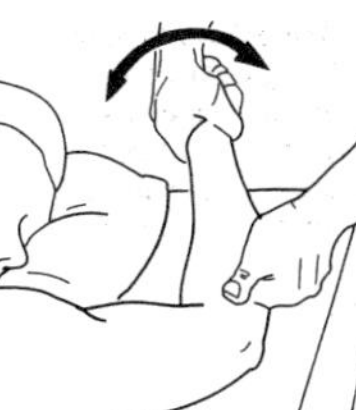

Wrist Rotation
Gently rotate the wrist with one hand while kneading the forearm with the other. Rotation of the arm can be applied simultaneously, if desired.

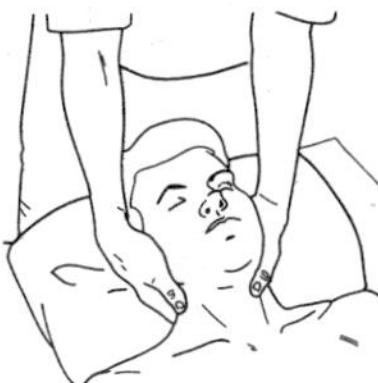

Neck Traction
Using both hands, pull gently on the subject's head to move it away from the shoulders, stretching and elongating the muscles of the neck. Circle and knead the sides of the neck. Apply strokes to scalene muscles and alongside the levator scapulae if desired.

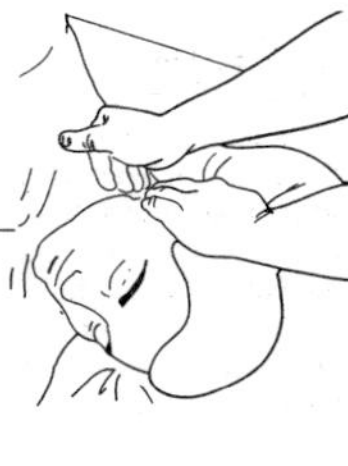

Side Neck Traction
Turn the head slightly to the side, stroke, stretch, kneading, and friction techniques are applied to the upper trapezius away from the sides of the neck. Slowly secure the shoulder with a loose fist while simultaneously stretching the neck and the exposed muscles of the sternocleidomastoid muscle.

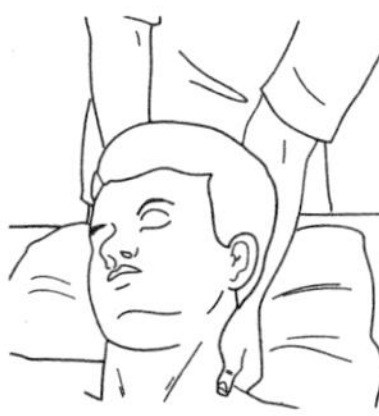

Neck Stretch and Kneading
Using one hand, turn the subject's head slightly to one side and support its weight. Using the opposite hand, knead the neck muscles of the side being stretched. Apply stroking and friction to scalene muscles and alongside the levator scapula if desired.

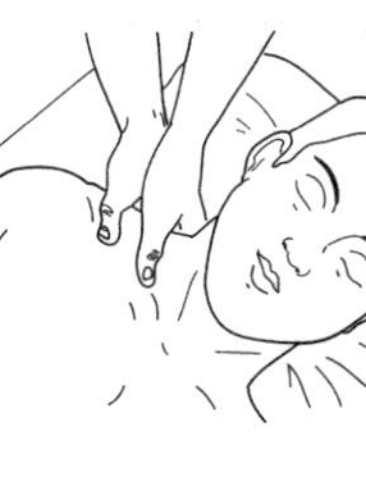

Shoulder and Neck Kneading
Knead the shoulder, neck muscles and scalene muscles, using the weight of the subject's body to provide pressure against your fingers. Stroking or friction can be applied to the scalene, trapezius, and sternocleidomastoid of desired.

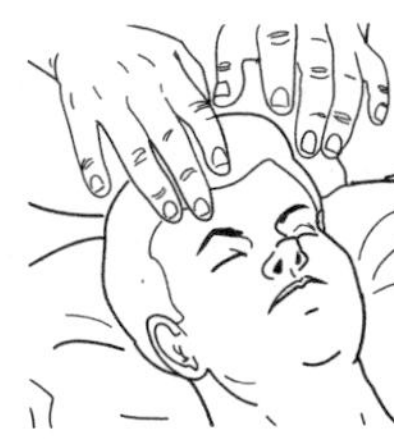

Head Tapping
Apply a gentle finger tapping technique to the subject's forehead and surrounding pressure points.

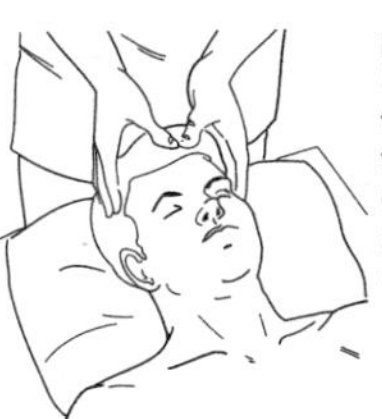

Head Friction
Using both thumbs, apply friction to the scalp or finger and palm spot compression to the pressure points on the scalp and forehead.

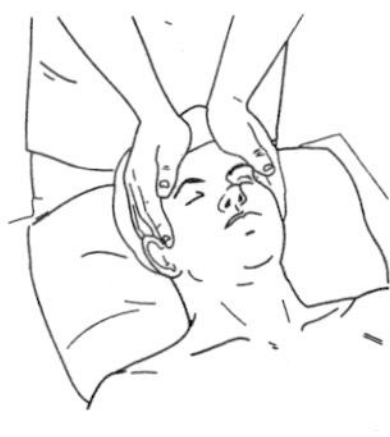

Forehead Strokes
Using the palm side of both hands, apply strokes, friction, and palm compression from the middle of the subject's forehead to the ears.

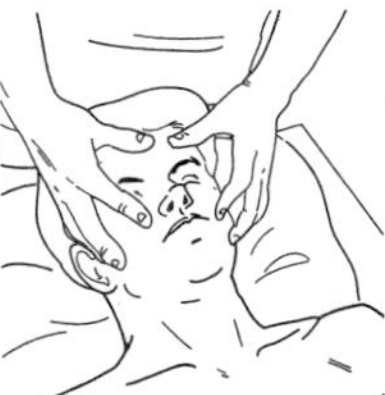

Face Compression
Using the tips of the thumbs and fingers, apply finger compression on the pressure points throughout the face. Compression can be applied to the center of the forehead, cheek, nose eyebrow, jawbone and cheek by moving from region to region, covering the entire face.

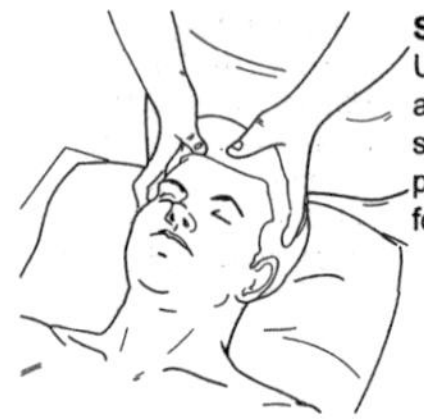

Scalp Compression
Using both the thumbs and the fingertips, apply spot compression to pressure points on the forehead and scalp.

Occipital Lift
Using both hands, carefully cup the back of the subject's head. Hook your fingers under the occipital ridge, allowing the subject's neck to slowly fall into your fingers and gradually lift the head with a slight rocking motion in your hands to encourage a release of the neck and surrounding muscles.

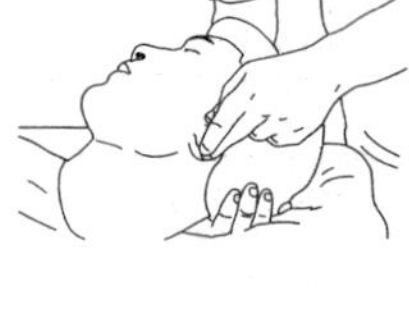

Deep Friction of the Neck and SCM
With one hand, grasp and stabilize the subject's head just above the neck. Using the other hand, apply gradual traction to the head and neck, taking care not to overstretch any of the surrounding muscles. Deep thumb friction can be applied to tender points along the sides and base of the neck.

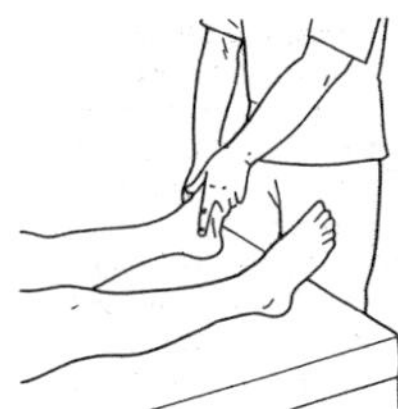

Leg Traction
Lightly and superficially stroke the foot to introduce touch. Grasp the subject's ankle and gently pull the leg away from the body by leaning back with your body weight to loosen the hip joint.

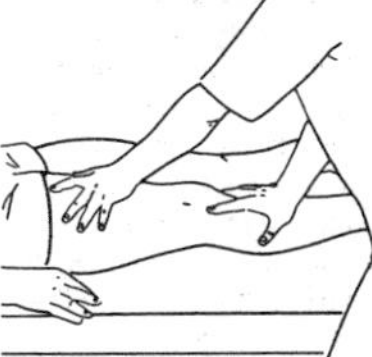

Effleurage of the Legs
Apply effleurage and petrissage strokes to the front of both legs. Glide slowly up around the thighs, knee and hip joint as to create a feeling of evenness and to lengthen the muscles of the leg.

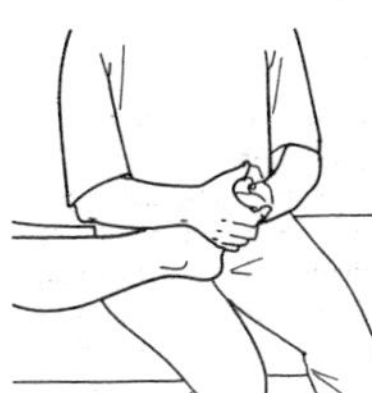

Effleurage of Foot
Apply effleurage and kneading to both the tops and bottoms of the foot, working in between the digits of each foot.

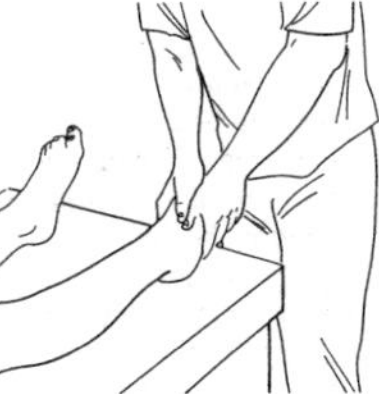

Foot Stripping
Strip the foot, using both thumbs to apply even pressure to the thin muscles that extend from the ankle to the toes. Apply friction between the toes and all surfaces of the foot.

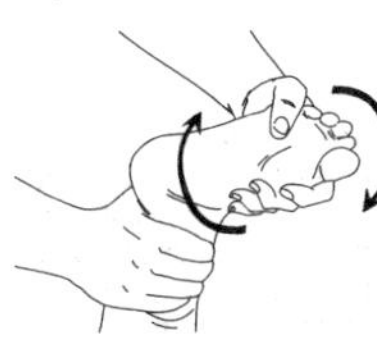

Foot Rotation
Rotate and stretch the tarsals and metatarsals of the foot in both directions, taking care not to overstretch the ankle.

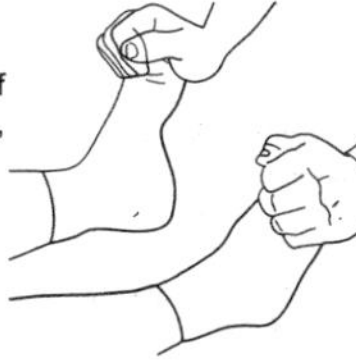

Foot and Ankle Stretch
Using both hands, grasp the subject's feet around the toes. Gradually apply pressure by either leaning forward to stretch the ankle or kneading the tissue with the fingertips. Alternatively, lean backwards to stretch the subject's feet away from the body.

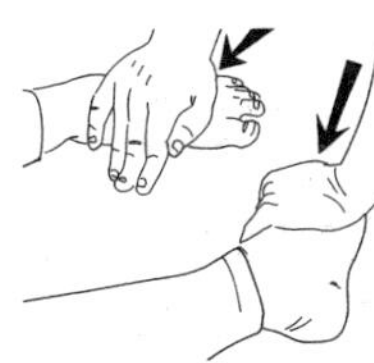

Foot Stretch and Ankle Inversion
Using the palms of both hands, apply gradual downward pressure to the subject's feet. Lean forward to generate more pressure if desired.

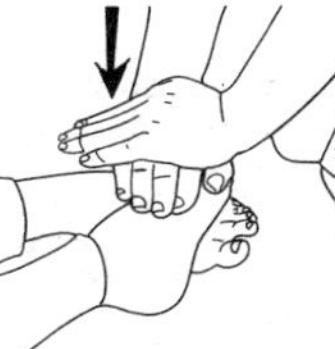

Cross Feet Stretch
Using the palms of both hands, cross one foot over the other foot and apply gradual pressure to the subject's feet. Lean forward to generate more pressure if desired.

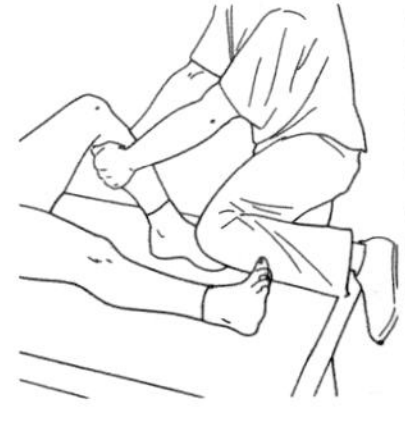

Calf Pull
Flex one knee and apply gentle traction on the calf using interlaced fingers. Gradually work your way around the calf. Lean backwards to generate more pressure if desired.

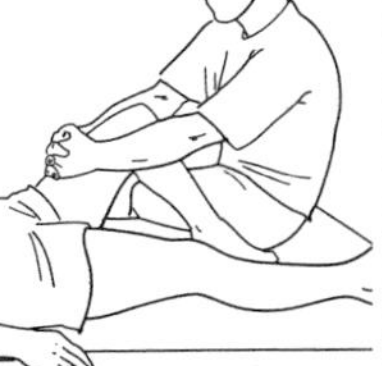

Assisted Stretch of Hip
Place the subject's foot under your knee to stabilize the leg and using both hands form an interlocking grip just below the knee. Lean backwards to generate pressure to stretch the hip.

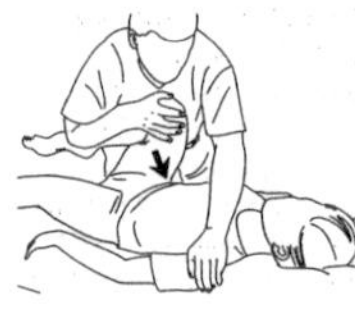

Knee Flex and Hamstring Stretch
With one knee straight, move the subject's other knee to the chest to stretch the hip and lower back. Use your shoulder to flex the subject's hip for a deep stretch. The other hand should be pressed downward lightly on the subject's leg to prevent pelvic movement.

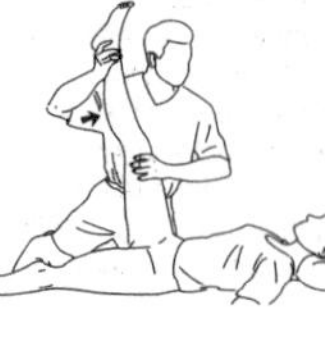

Hamstring Stretch
Stretch the hamstring by lifting the foot towards the ceiling with one leg extended straight outwards. Apply pressure to the subject's lower leg with your knee and secure the subject's leg. With the other hand, raise the leg to stretch the muscle. Keep the outer leg stabilized to prevent the pelvis from moving.

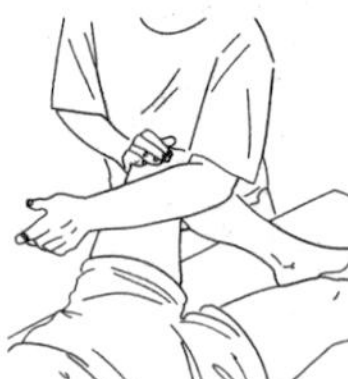

Kneading of the Inner Thigh
Use your body and arm to support the subject's bent knee. Use the other hand to knead the inner thigh. Light and deep forearm strokes can be applied to the adductor muscle group and inner thigh of the leg. Be careful not to apply too much pressure to the area directly behind the knee.

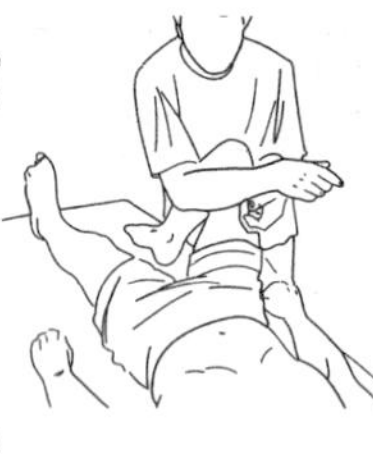

Forearm Kneading of the Thigh
Flex one knee and place one hand on the subject's thigh and simultaneously use the other forearm to guide the subject's knee towards your chest so as to stretch the thigh.

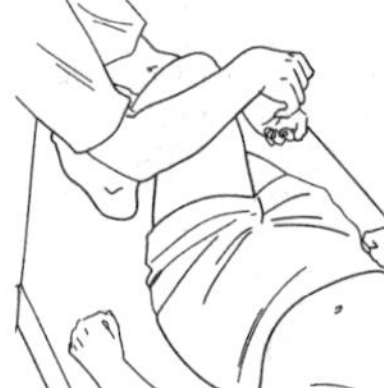

Forearm Kneading of the Outer Thigh
Use your body and arm to support the subject's bent knee. Use the other forearm to apply light or deep gliding strokes to the subject's outer thigh.

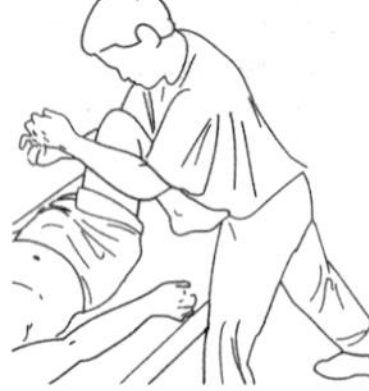

Knee to Hip Stretch
Flex one knee and place one hand on the subject's thigh and simultaneously lean forward to generate pressure and stretch the subject's thigh and hip.

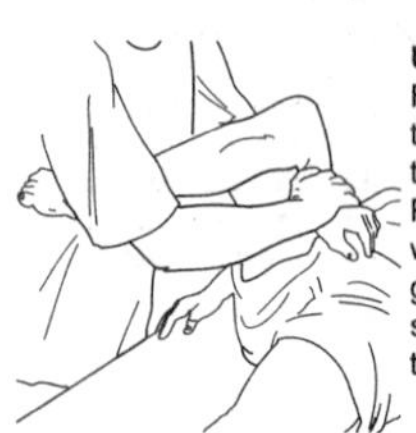

Upper Leg Stretch
Flex one leg and securely tuck one arm just behind the subject's bent knee. Push towards the subject with the other hand to generate pressure and stretch the hamstring and thigh.

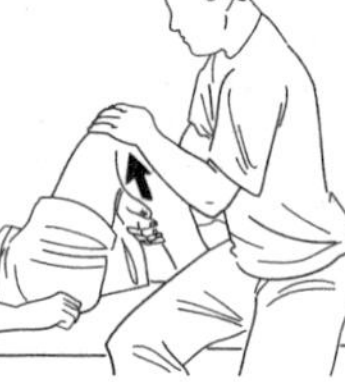

Kneading the Calf
Using one hand or both hands, apply kneading, picking up, wringing, rolling and friction strokes from the ankle up to the knee. The opposite arm should support the subject's bent knee.

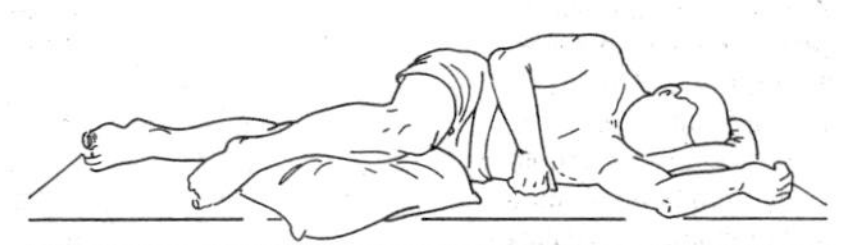

Side-Lying Position
Position the subject on their side with a pillow under their head and another supporting their top leg.

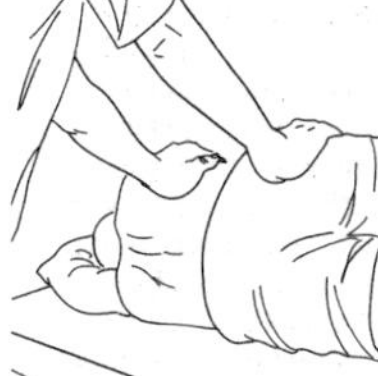

Rocking
Gently rock the subject's body back and forth.

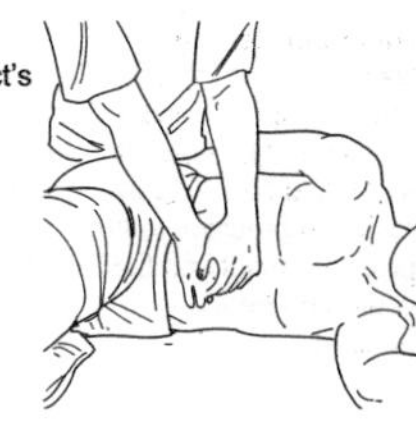

Kneading the Abdomen
Using both hands in an overlaying grip, gently apply superficial pressure to the subject's belly. Apply kneading, picking up, wringing, rolling and friction strokes to the abdomen.

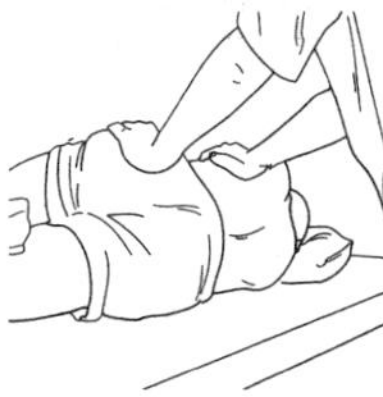

Traction and Rocking of the Back
Using both hands apply gentle pressure to push the hip away and pull the shoulder towards the practitioner.

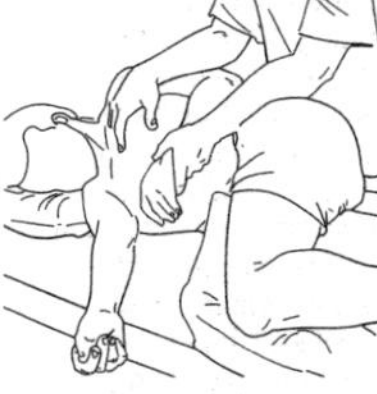

Arm Kneading
Stabilize the subject's upper arm with your forearm while simultaneously gliding the subject's forearm with the other hand. Apply kneading, picking up, wringing, rolling and friction strokes to the arm.

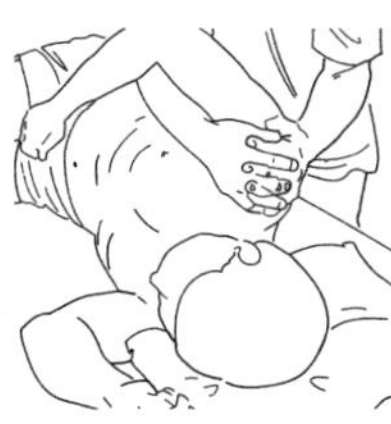

Shoulder Girdle Rotation and Pulling
Using an interlacing grip around the subject's upper shoulder, gradually apply pressure by shifting your weight backwards to rotate the shoulders.

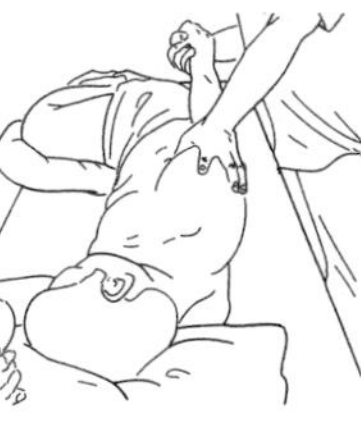

Bicep Kneading
Use one hand to hold subject's arm steady use the other hand to knead the subject's bicep. Apply kneading, picking up, wringing, rolling and friction strokes to the biceps of the arm.

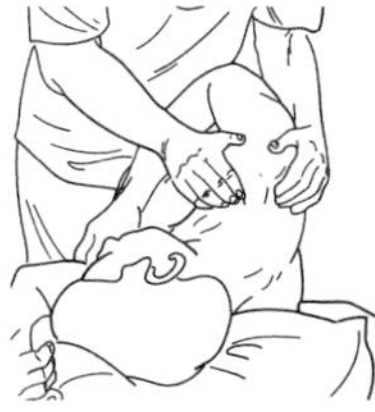

Shoulder Vibration and Friction
Using both hands grasp the subject's shoulder and tremble rapidly to vibrate the surrounding muscles. Apply deep penetrating friction strokes with thumbs and fingers to the shoulders and upper trapezius.

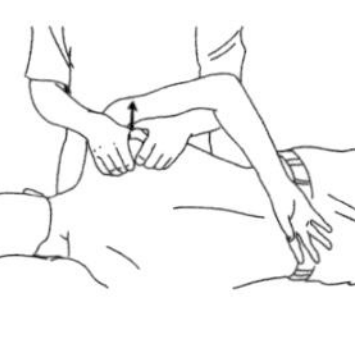

Scapula Lift
Grasp the subject's scapula by scooping fingers under the underneath and lift scapula upward and away from the body.

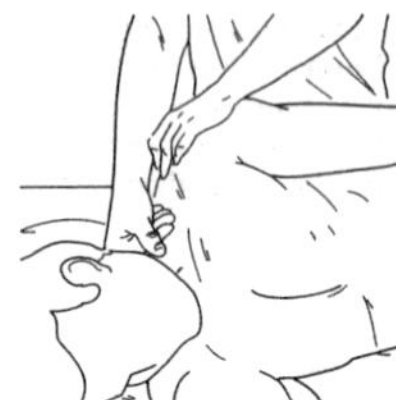

Kneading of the Neck
Use loose fists to knead the muscles of the neck. The opposite hand can pull the subject's shoulder away from head to stretch and elongate the muscles if desired.

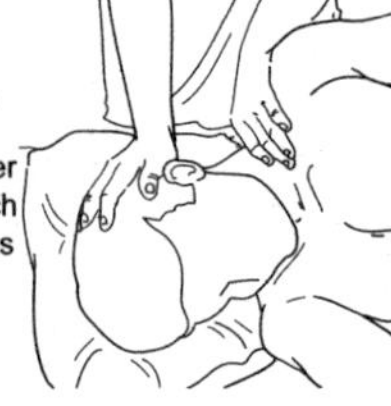

Neck Traction
While one hand gently pushes the head away, the other pulls the shoulder towards the practitioner. Stretch and elongate the muscles in the neck and shoulders.

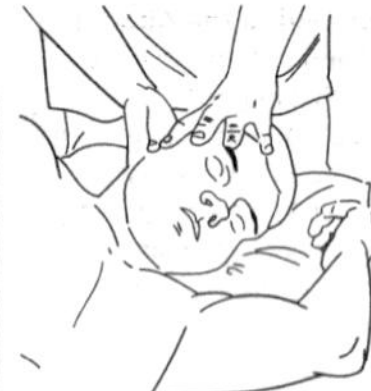

Head Scratching
Using the fingertips and thumbs, apply circular friction to the subject's scalp and head. Apply spot compression to the pressure points on the scalp and forehead, if desired.

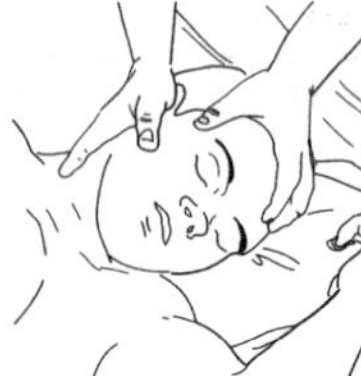

Face Compression
Use one hand to steady the subject's head. Using the tips of the thumbs and fingers, apply finger compression on the pressure points throughout the face. Compression can be applied to the center of the forehead, cheek, nose, eyebrow, jawbone and cheek by moving from region to region, covering the entire face.

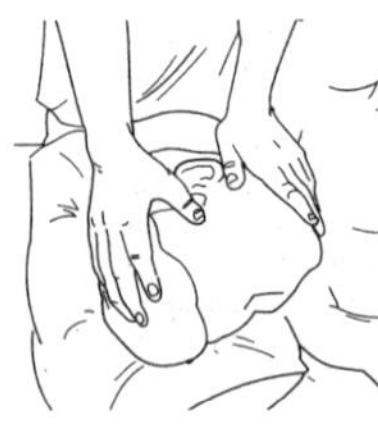

Face Friction
Using the tips of the thumbs and fingers, apply light friction to the face or spot compression on the pressure points throughout the face. Light friction can be applied to the center of the forehead, cheek, nose, eyebrow, jawbone and cheek by moving from region to region, covering the entire face.

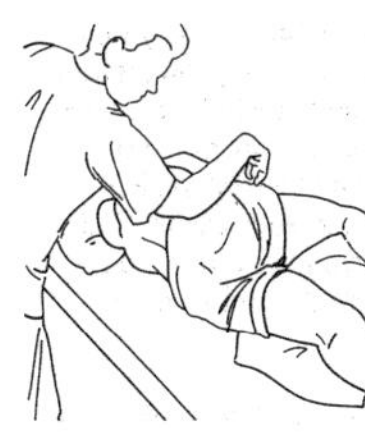

Compression with Flex Knee
Position the subject on their side with a pillow providing support between the legs. Use your elbow to compress the gluteal pressure points and piriformis origins.

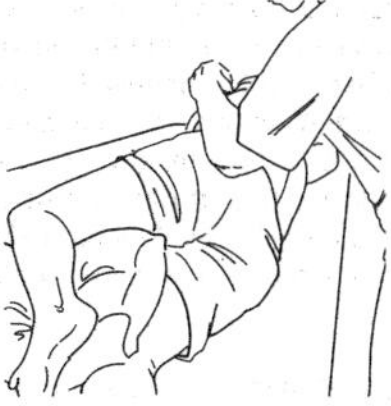

Gluteal Compression
Use your elbow to compress the pressure points in the hips and gluteals. Be sure to keep the knees in line with hips.

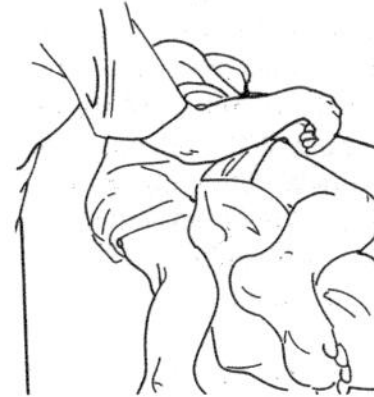

Kneading the Outer Thigh
Use broad, flat, long strokes with your forearm on the subject's outer thigh. Use your elbow to work piriformis muscles and glutes of desired.

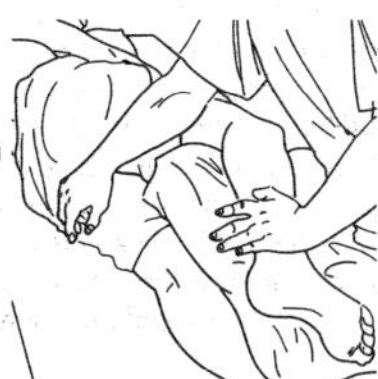

Forearm Outer Leg
Using an open palm, gradually apply pressure to the subject's upper leg by leaning forward. Work your way across the leg, if desired.

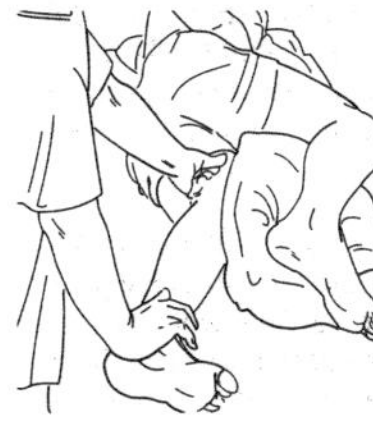

Kneading the Inner Leg
Using one hand, stabilize the lower leg near the ankle. Simultaneously apply direct pressure on either side of the subject's knee with the thumb and palm of the other hand. Apply kneading, picking up, wringing, rolling and friction strokes around the inner leg.

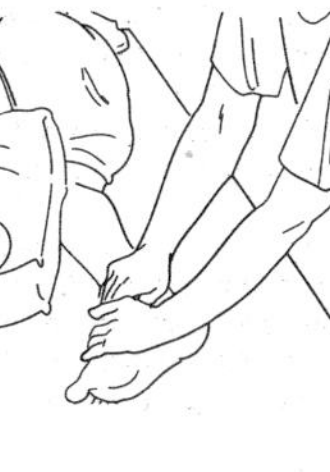

Kneading the Lower Leg
Using both hands, massage either side of the ankle of the subject's lower leg. Apply kneading, picking up, wringing, rolling and friction strokes around the lower leg.

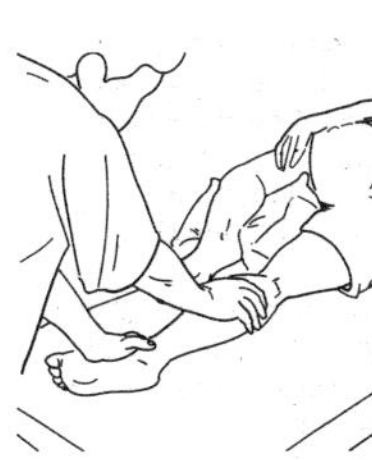

Kneading the Calf
Stabilize the lower leg around the ankle with one hand while simultaneously gliding down the calf, apply kneading, picking up, wringing, rolling and friction strokes with the palm to calf and lower leg.

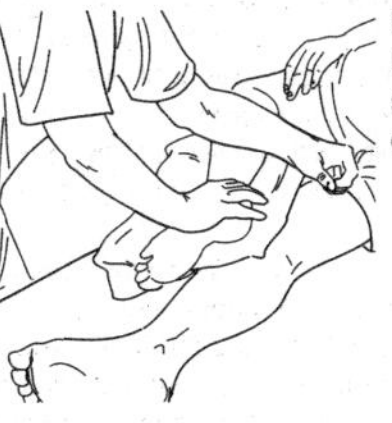

Forearm Lower Leg
Use broad, flat, long strokes with your forearm on the subject's lower leg.

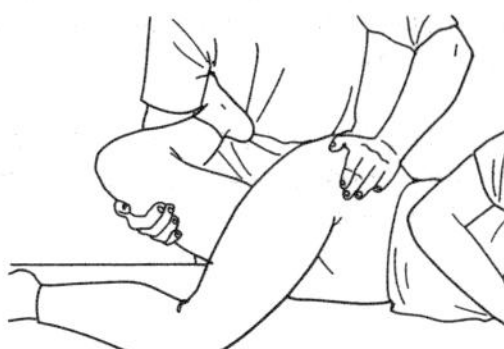

Pivoting Side Stretch
Firmly grasp the lower leg of the subject and pull leg backwards towards you while using the other hand to stabilize the hips. Stretch and hold position, if desired.

Thai Massage

The history of traditional Thai massage is interwoven within the cultural imprint that dates back 2500 years, with influences coming from China, India, Burma and Tibet. Thai massage, also known as Thai yoga therapy, Nuad phaen boran or Nuat Thai, is a therapeutic technique and one of the oldest massage techniques being used today. It is one of four branches of traditional medicine in Thailand, along with herbs, nutrition, and spiritual practice. Its precise origins are unknown, but practitioners traditionally trace their lineage to Jivaka Komarabhacca (also called Jivaka Kumar Bhaccha or Shivago Kumarpaj) the source and authority of Thai massage throughout Thailand and also the founder of Buddhist Thai medicine. Dr. Shivago Kumrpaj was a personal physician to the Sangha, a friend and physician of Buddha who was renowned as a healer in Buddhist tradition.

It evolved within the context of Buddhist monasteries and temples, a natural, holistic approach to health and well-being, with a goal of treating the body, mind, and spirit. Traditional Thai medicine included nutrition, physical exercise, the use of medicinal herbs and therapeutic massage. The medical knowledge developed by Thai people through many generations has come to be known as the ancient wisdom of Thailand. Ancient medical texts were carved in stone in attempts to preserve the tradition of Thai massage and passed along in teachings to their children and family. Stone inscriptions with diagrams etched within the walls of the Wat Pho temple in Bangkok parallel traditional Chinese medicine principles and illustrate energy flows along ten major channels or sen lines through the body. This life force is believed to run along approximately 72,000 sen lines, roughly equivalent to the meridians of Chinese acupuncture and to the Ayurvedic channels. When this energy flow is blocked or restricted, it creates pain, sickness or disease. In this sense, traditional Thai medicine is similar to many other ancient healing systems, which believe that illnesses are caused by an imbalance or obstruction within the individual, or by an imbalance between an individual and his environment.

In Thailand, there are many agricultural people who do a lot of physical work through the day and their muscles become very sore. So children are taught to massage their parents– a tradition which was passed down as an oral teaching from generation to generation. Thai massage is based on the belief that all disease is due to an imbalance of the body's energy. Its goal is to promote this balance and therefore assist in the healing of the entire person. To do this, Thai massage employs several techniques. The first technique is the application of pressure through leaning into the area being treated, produced with hands, thumbs, elbows, forearms, feet and knees similar to that of acupressure/shiatsu meridian system with manipulation, adjustment and muscle stretching into a full bodywork. The only difference is Thai massage treats these channels in both directions, while shiatsu moves in only one direction.

Reflexology is also an important aspect of Thai massage. Reflexology is based on the belief that points on the hands and feet can be used to treat the entire body. There is a lot of attention paid to the feet and legs in Thai massage because getting energy moving in these areas helps to better connect the client to the earth, causing them to be more "grounded and balanced." A considerable amount of time is spent treating the body through reflexology and working along the sen lines of the feet and extremities of the body during a traditional Thai massage.

Another technique of Thai massage is blood stopping. This is achieved by putting pressure on a major artery in the arm or leg for an extended period of time from 15 seconds up to about a minute. The theory behind this technique is that cutting off a major source of circulation to an area will initially result in increased pressure, which will cause the heart muscle to slow its contractions in order to bring the pressure down. When the pressure on the artery is released, a fresh supply of blood rushes into the area, causing it to relax more deeply. This technique is contraindicated for anyone with heart or circulatory problems or with diabetes.

Thai massage is an interactive form of bodywork that is often compared to dance in which the bodies of both the practitioner and client merge in a continuously flowing motion or mediation in motion. The influence of yoga is apparent from the positions and stretching movements. Thai massage also employs a type of passive stretching. This means that the client does not participate in the stretching, and the practitioner does all the work. Thai massage combines assisted asanas, or yoga postures, facilitated by the practitioners to create a physical and spiritual healing process. Stretching is done in stages with rest periods between, working gradually up to as much range of motion as possible, incorporating rocking, compressions and pressure in between each movement. It is also done slowly to avoid the muscle shortening – or spasm – that can occur when a muscle is stretched too far, too fast.

Thai massage offers benefits that are multi-level by removing the obstructions that cause illness within the body, the most notable effects being an opening of tight joints, pain relief, a lengthening of muscles, and a very deep sense of well-being and relaxation.

Techniques of Traditional Thai Massage

Thai massage practitioners operate on the theory that the body is permeated with energy, "prana, qi, air, lom" which is inhaled into the lungs and which subsequently travels throughout the body along pathways or by pressing certain points along the sen lines. While there are some similarities to Chinese meridian theory, the Thai system is markedly different, as the sen are unconnected from the internal organs, and channels along sen lines can be moved in both directions. The sen lines originate at the navel and spread throughout the body to terminate at the orifices. A significant part of the practice of Thai massage includes yoga, meditation, reflexology, acupressure and healing arts. During these assisted asanas, or yoga-like stretches, which are intended to stimulate the movement of "lom" through the body via a pumping action which is connected with the client's breathing. You should play close attention to your body mechanics and breathe calmly during the session and, as always, use good judgment during passive stretching movements. Never overstretch or force the movement, as it can cause more harm than benefit.

There are variations of Thai massage, ranging from university-driven or supported programs of Thai massage with lineages that trace back to different tribes or royal families in Thailand. Some parts of Thailand, including the schools in Chiangmai, are closer to mainland China, where you will see more Chinese- and Laotian-influenced massage technique similar to those of Chinese Tui na and acupuncture. Some Thai massage schools are more focused on prayer, others on mechanics and repetition, and some on breath work. Over the years, massage schools in the United States have begun offering Thai massage courses with instructors who are influenced by direct lineages tracing back to royal families or tribes. Regardless of the lineage of Thai massage, they all practice common techniques. It is important to have an understanding of these basics of Thai massage techniques.

Massage can affect people differently, with some being more sensitive than others. To clear these blockages, Thai massage combines the application of pressure (produced with hands, thumbs, elbows, forearms, feet and knees) with manipulation, adjustment and muscle stretching in bodywork, which improves overall health and well-being. Energy pathways are cleared, muscles are elongated, mind is quieted, blood is oxygenated, posture is aligned, joints are freed, breathing is balanced, internal organs and all bodily functions are stimulated into moving towards a more balanced state. All techniques should begin with gentle pressure, with gradual increase to avoid injury. Always observe and receive feedback from the client, especially during stretching and or on deeper pressure.

We have organized the following techniques:

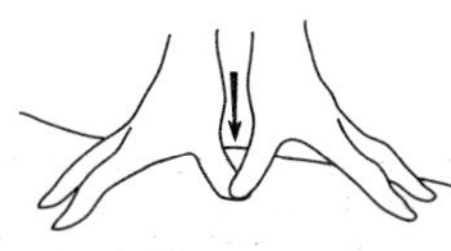

Thumb Pressing
Use the thumb pad, not the tip. Press down very gently, gradually increasing the force directly in line with your arm (adjust the force and pressure accordingly). Use circular motion rather than direct pressure. This technique can be combined with the stretching.

- Variations of thumb press include: single, double thumbs, double thumb facing each other, double thumb walking, double thumb parallel to each other, double thumb overlapping, palm and thumb overlapping

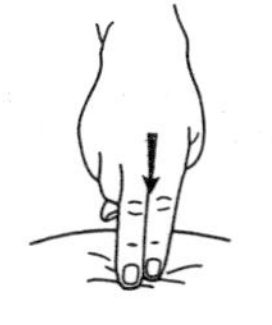

Finger Pressing
Use the finger tip, press down very gently, gradually increasing the force directly in line with your arm (adjust the force and pressure accordingly). Use direct pressure. This technique can be combined with the stretching.

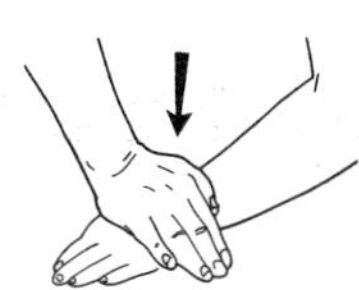

Palm Pressing
Use the palms of the hand, press down very gently, directly in line with your arm, gradually increasing pressure using body weight on the arm without force (adjust the force and pressure accordingly). Pressure can be applied and maintained and increased without fatigue. This technique can be combined with a rocking motion.

- Variations of palm press include: single, double palms, and butterfly palms

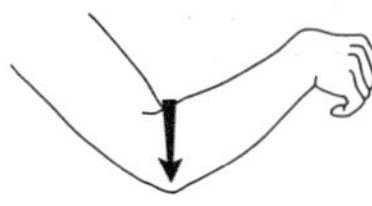

Elbow Pressing
Use this technique for deeper pressure. Press down very gently, gradually increasing the force (adjust the force and pressure accordingly). Use the tip of the elbow pressed straight down or spiraling usage of the elbow. Use on thighs, buttocks, upper shoulders or areas with thick muscles. This technique can be combined with revolving of the elbow.

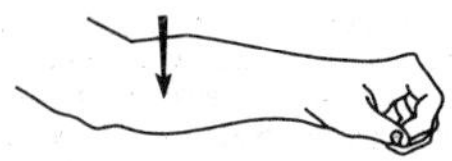

Forearm Pressing
Use the edge of the forearm. Press down very gently, gradually increasing the force and simultaneously rolling the forearm (adjust the force and pressure accordingly). Roll and press rhythmically and repeatedly. This technique can be combined with rolling of the forearm.

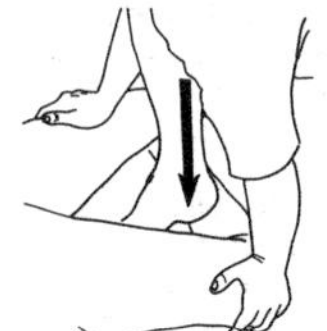

Foot Pressing
Use the foot press for applying pressure over large areas. Use on thighs, buttocks, and areas with thick muscles, gradually increasing the force (adjust the force and pressure accordingly). Use the front of the sole of the foot, arches or the heels. Foot press can be strong and penetrate deeply into the muscles. This technique can be combined with stretching some parts of the body while pulling on the feet.

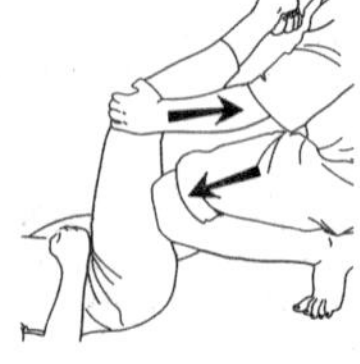

Knee Pressing
Using the knee, press gradually, increasing the force (adjust the force and pressure accordingly). Use on buttocks and back of the legs. Pressure can be applied and maintained and increased without fatigue. This technique will give deep pressure while freeing the hand with a more controlled stretch.

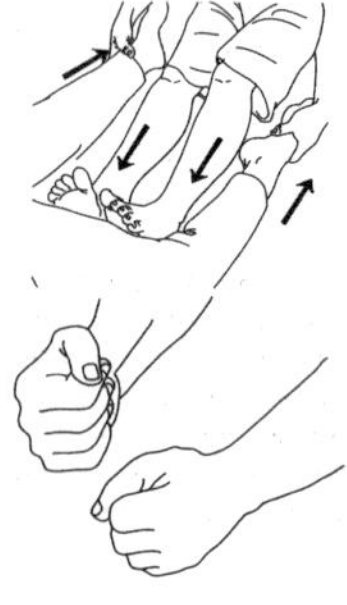

Pressing / Pulling Technique
Use the pressing and pulling technique (adjust the pulling and pressing technique accordingly). Use all four fingers of both hands to pull and press simultaneously. Use on calf and back of the legs. This technique can be combined with the other techniques.

Fist Hitting
Use clenched hands in a loose fist, striking with the base or butt of the fists in a percussive manner. Hit along the points or the sen lines of the body. Hit rhythmically and repeatedly. This technique is usually combined with other techniques.

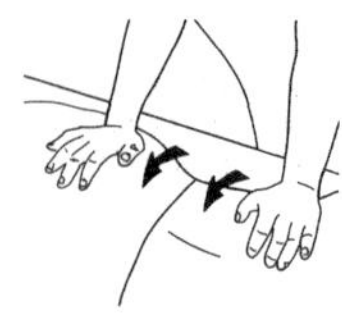

Rocking
Use the thumb and fingers of both hands to grasp the muscles while rocking forward and back. Rock rhythmically and repeatedly.

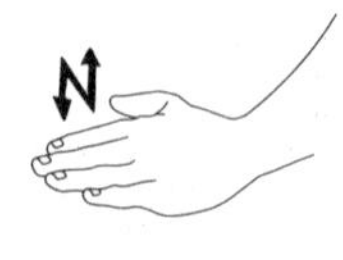

Patting
Use the flat palm with very light force applied to area. Use to spread force after using direct force. Pat rhythmically and repeatedly. This technique is lighter than the fist-hitting technique.

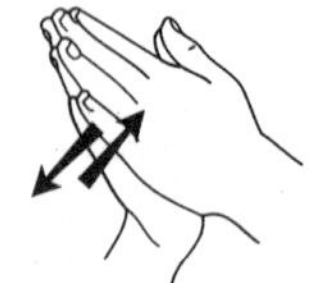

Hand Chopping
Use both hands with palms joined together and fingers stretched out and separated. Chop with the outer edge of the hands. Apply quick repetitive up-and-down chopping motion to desired area. Use on all parts of the body.

Sen Lines

Thai massage is based on the idea that there are energy lines or sen lines that run throughout the body. These sen lines are the passages for energy and it is now known that the lines correspond with blood vessels in the body which have similarities to meridian lines in Shiatsu and acupuncture. Palm press, thumb press, butterfly press and massage are applied to sen lines throughout acupressure, shiatsu and Thai treatments. When these Sen lines become blocked, the energy becomes stagnant and the body loses its balance.

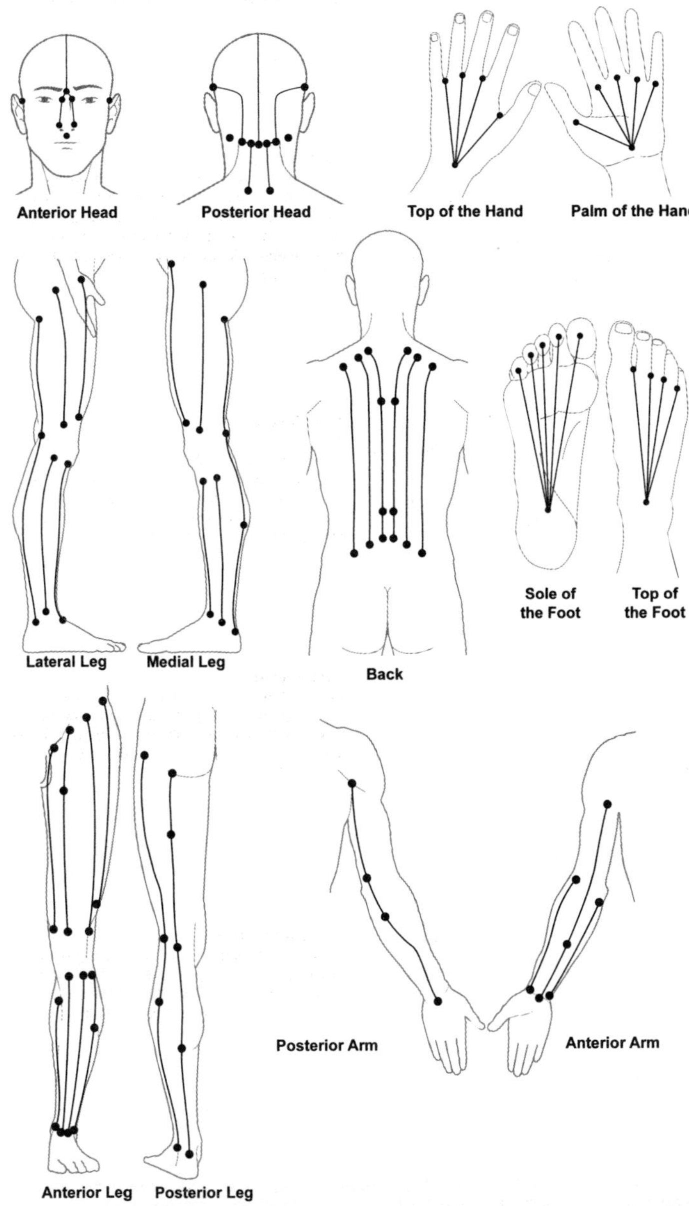

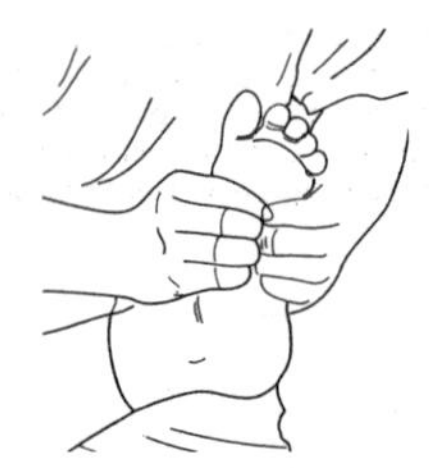

Foot Kneading
Position the subject on their back. Using both hands, grasp the bottom of the subject's foot and apply pressure with the fingertips. Apply finger press, kneading, squeezing to the sen lines of the foot. Work your way around the foot, if desired.

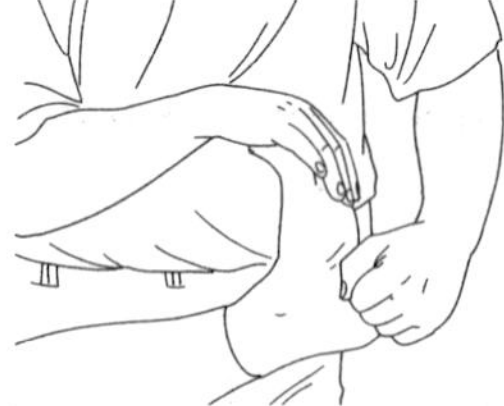

Foot Pummeling
Position the subject on their back. Using one hand, grasp the top of the subject's foot and draw it towards the subject's body to stretch around the toes. Form a fist with the other hand and simultaneously knead and pummel the bottom of the subject's foot.

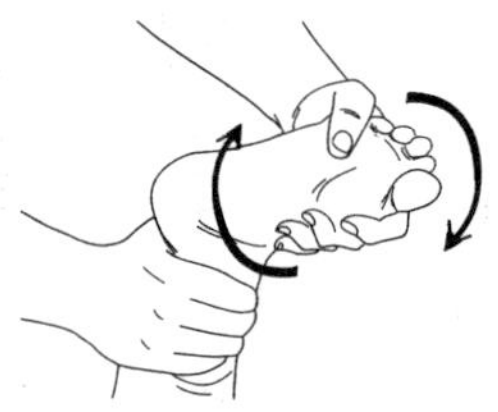

Foot Rotation
Position the subject on their stomach with one leg raised and bent at the knee. With one hand, grasp the subject's raised leg just above the ankle. Using the other hand, grasp the subject's foot and simultaneously rotate the foot in both directions, taking care not to overstretch the ankle.

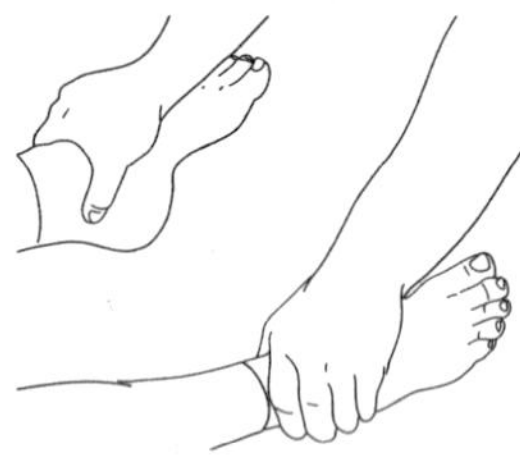

Foot Squeeze
Position the subject on their back. Using both hands, grasp the subject's feet just below the ankles. Gradually apply thumb pressure and work your way around the margins and heels of each foot.

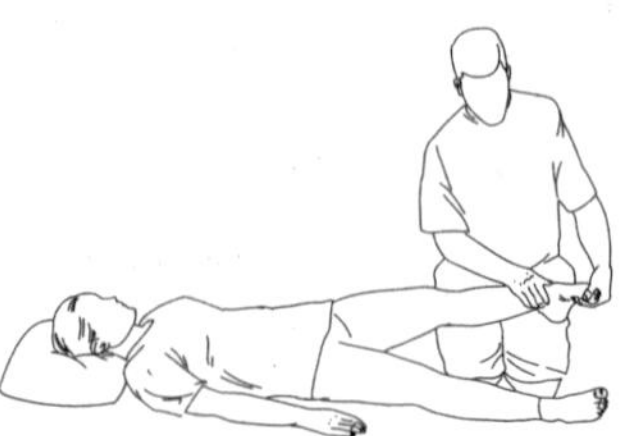

Rotate & Pull Toes
Position the subject on their back. Using both hands, grasp the subject's feet and rotate gently. Work your way up to the toes and pull on the toes as you continue to rotate around the ankle.

Caution: Some of the Thai massage movements require practice under experienced supervision to be safely performed. Please see the cautions and contraindications on massage as they are applicable to Thai massage.

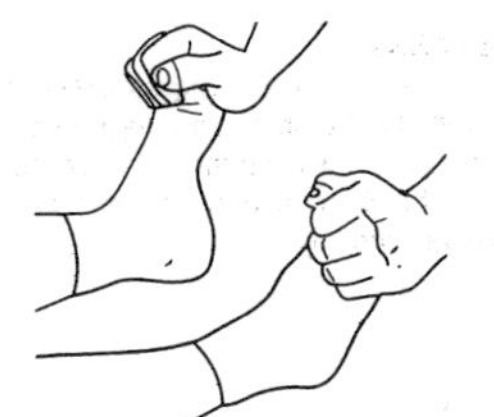

Stretch Feet & Ankles
Position the subject on their back. Using both hands, grasp the subject's feet around the toes. Gradually apply pressure by either leaning forward to stretch the ankle or kneading the tissue with the fingertips. Alternatively, lean backwards to stretch the subject's feet away from the body.

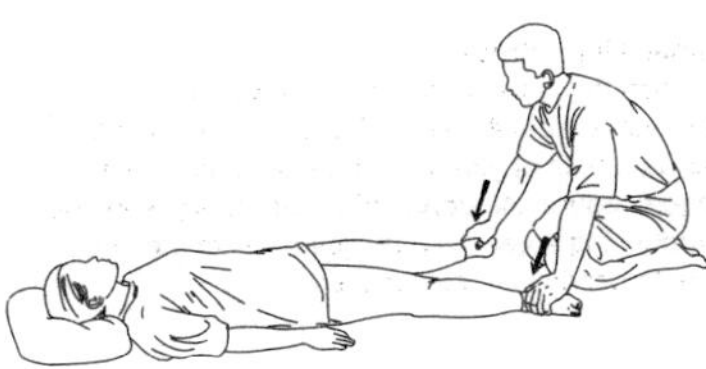

Feet & Ankle Press
Palm Feet Walk & Leg Press
Position the subject on their back. Using both hands, apply even traction sideways and downwards, inverting and everting both feet once or twice. Continue to apply pressure as you work your way across the feet. Apply palm press, thumb press and stretching to applicable sen lines of the leg.

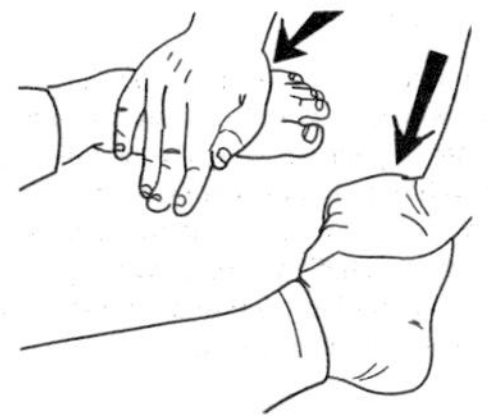

Stretch Feet & Ankles Inversion
Position the subject on their back. Using the palms of both hands, apply gradual downward pressure to the subject's feet. Lean forward to generate more pressure if desired.

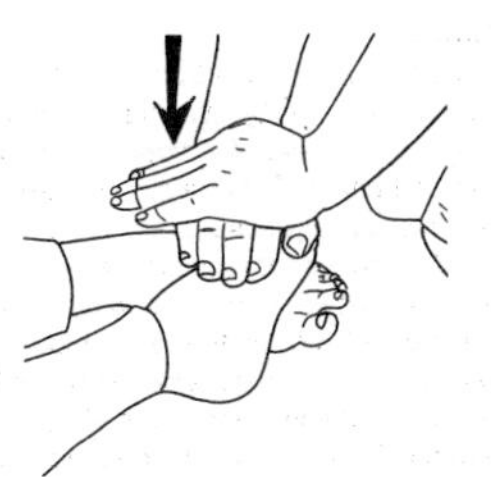

Cross Feet Stretch
Position the subject on their back. Using the palms of both hands, cross one foot over the other foot and apply gradual pressure to the subject's feet. Lean forward to generate more pressure if desired.

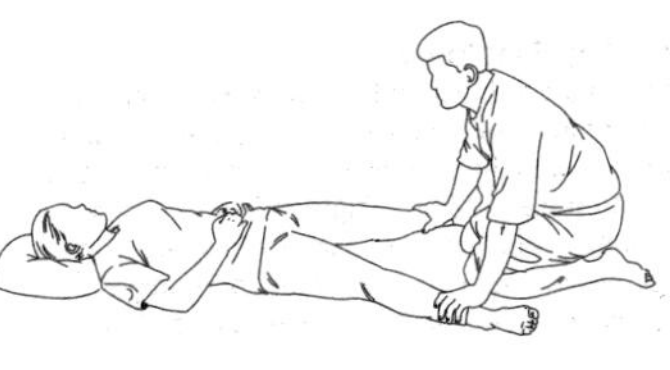

Inner Feet & Leg Press
Palm Feet Walk & Leg Press
Palm Press Inner & Outer Leg
Position the subject on their back with their legs shoulder width apart. Apply pressure to the feet and ankles by gently transferring your body weight through the arms from side to side. Gradually work your way across the toes, foot, and ankle up the inner legs and back with applied even pressure. Apply palm press, palm walk, thumb press and stretching to applicable sen lines of the leg.

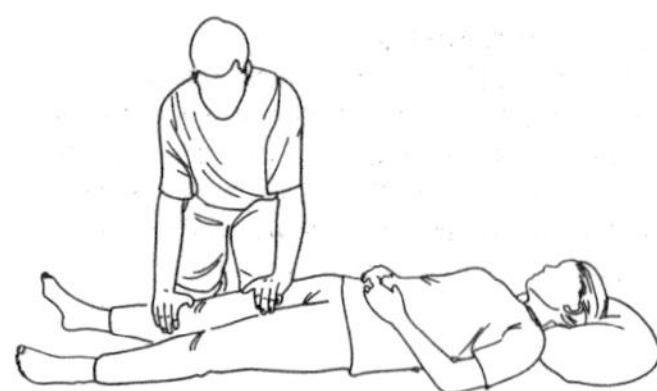

Outer Leg Press
Position the subject on their back. Apply even pressure with the thumb and the palm of each hand, working your way up the outer leg. Apply palm press, thumb press and stretching to applicable sen lines of the leg.

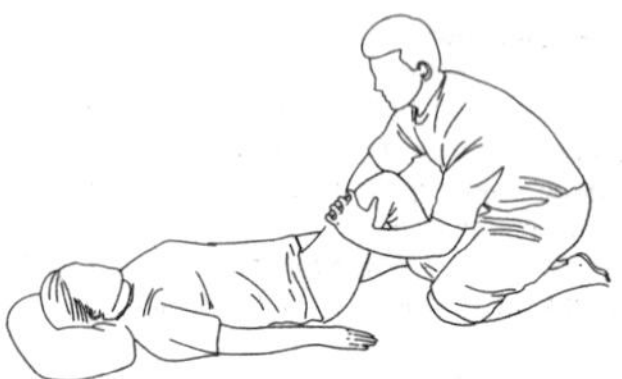

Upper Thigh Press
Position the subject on their back with one leg bent upwards at the knee. Securely place the leg between both of your knees and interlace your fingers around the upper thigh. Gradually work the surrounding areas as you squeeze with the heels of both hands to apply pressure.

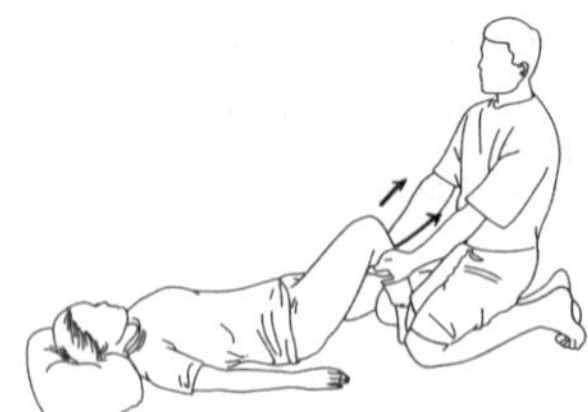

Calf Pull
Position the subject on their back with one leg bent upwards at the knee. Securely place the leg between both of your knees and grasp the back of the calf with both hands just below the knee. Gradually work your way around the calf as you stretch the leg by shifting your body weight away from the subject and apply pressure and stretching to applicable sen lines of the upper leg.

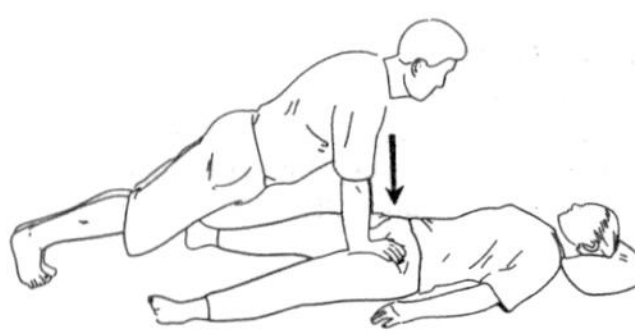

Blood Stop
Position the subject on their back. Position both of your hands on the subject's thighs and push yourself upwards, feeling for blood flow and subject's heart beat in your palms. Be careful not to put any excessive pressure on the hip bone. Press for 30 seconds to a minute. May press their palms, knees, elbows, forearms, shins, or feet over the big blood vessels that bring blood to legs and arms, or over any major arteries of the body that conduct blood flow. Blood stop should not be performed on clients with high blood pressure, heart or circulatory problems or pregnant.

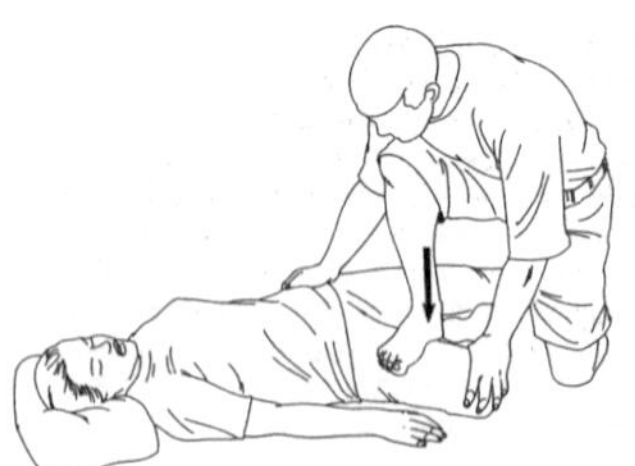

Inner Leg Foot Press
Position the subject on their back with one leg bent at the knee in half lotus/tree position. Apply pressure with the foot while balancing your body weight on the subject's thigh and knee. Press carefully to applicable sen lines of the leg and thigh. Work your way across the inner thigh, applying pressure with the entire foot and toes.

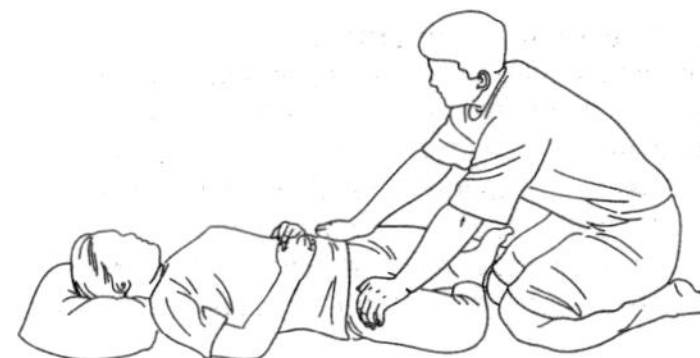

Half Tree/Lotus Leg Press
Hip Stretch
Position the subject on their back in a half lotus/ tree position with one leg bent inward at the knee. Place one hand on the subject's thigh and apply pressure while balancing with the other hand placed at the hip/pelvic area. Progressively lean forward in a rocking motion. Apply palm press, palm walk, thumb press and stretching to applicable sen lines of the leg as you continue to gradually increase pressure on the subject's thigh by securing the hips to the mat.

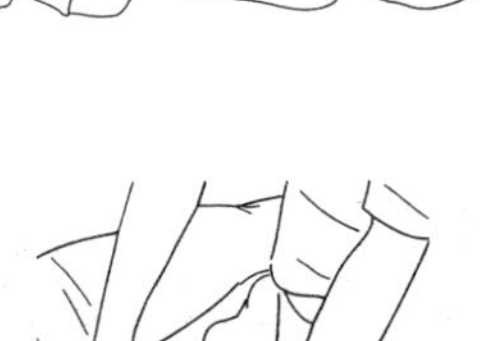

Palm & Thumb Press Inner Leg
Position the subject on their back in a half lotus/ tree position with one leg bent inward at the knee. Apply palm press, palm walk, thumb press and stretching to applicable sen lines of the leg.

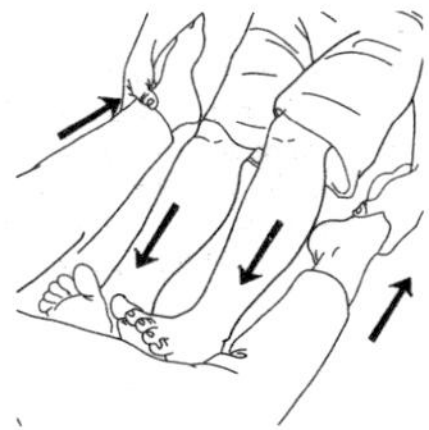

Thigh Press
Paddleboat
Position the subject on their back with one leg bent outwards at the knee. Tuck both legs snugly under the subject's lower leg and grasp the thigh with both hands. As you leverage the lower leg with your feet, gradually pull the thigh in the opposite direction so as to simultaneously massage the lower leg with the feet and stretch the upper leg with both hands.

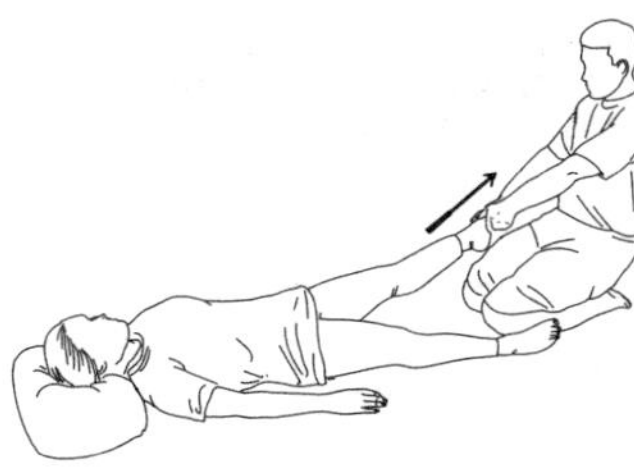

Feet Stretch
Position the subject on their back with one foot arched and extended outwards. Grasp the foot with both thumbs near the front of the ankle. Gradually work your way down the foot, applying pressure with the thumbs as you glide the traction down the foot.

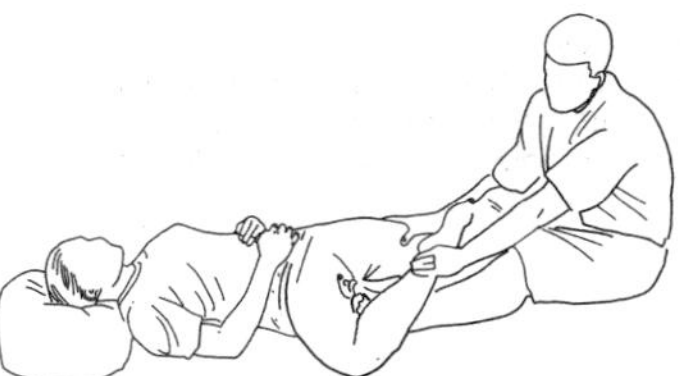

Inner Leg Press
Position the subject on their back with one leg extended outwards and bent at the knee. Securely tuck one leg behind the subject's knee and apply pressure on the hamstring. With one hand, grasp the subject's foot extended straight outwards. With the other hand, gently bend the knee and grasp the back of the ankle. As you apply pressure with your feet, gradually pull the subject's leg away from the body and apply pressure and stretching to applicable sen lines of the leg.

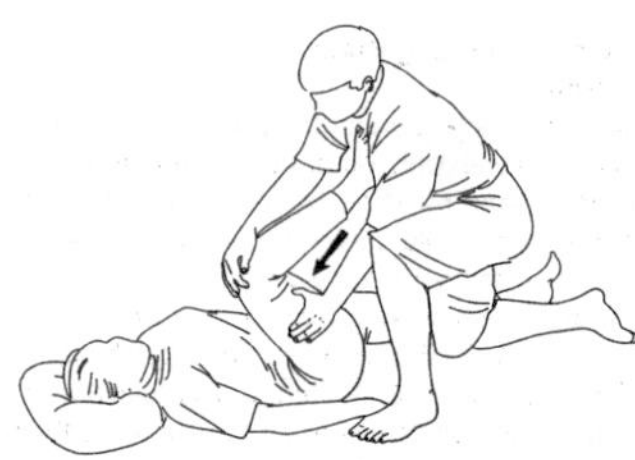

Chest to Thigh to Foot Press
Position the subject on their back with one arm raised and bent at the knee. Position the raised leg so that it rests on your shoulder and, using both hands, grasp the subject's leg at the knee and the thigh. Rock forward and backward, gradually leaning to press up and down the thigh muscle to stretch the subject's leg, taking care not to cause any discomfort.

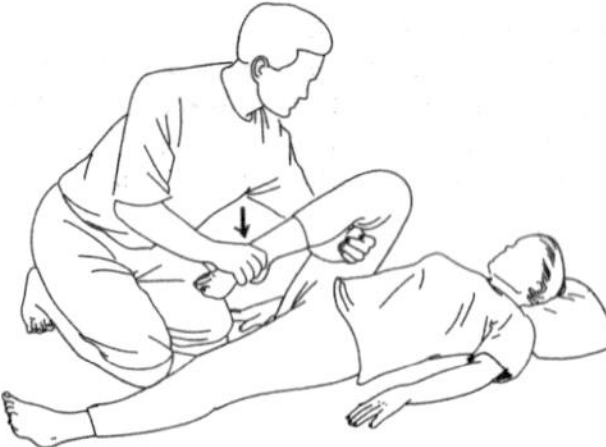

Flex Leg Stretch
Place the subject on their back with one leg extended upwards and bent at the knee. Snugly tuck one arm into the inside of the knee joint and place the opposite hand near the ankle. Apply pressure downwards as you use the opposite arm to keep the upper leg in place.

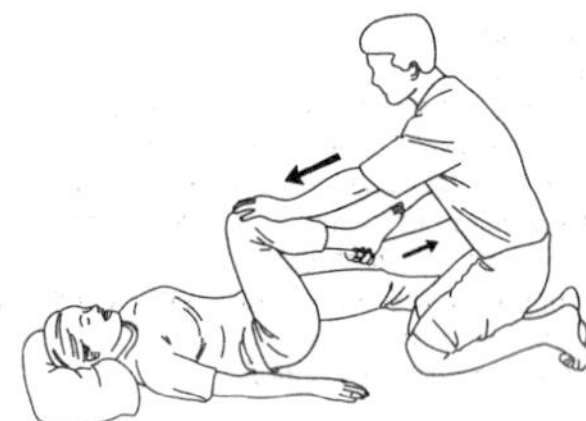

Flex Leg Stretch
Place the subject on their back with one leg extended upwards and bent at the knee. Grasp the knee with one hand and lean towards the subject so as to stretch the hamstring. Simultaneously grasp the back of the ankle with the other hand and pull it in the opposite direction.

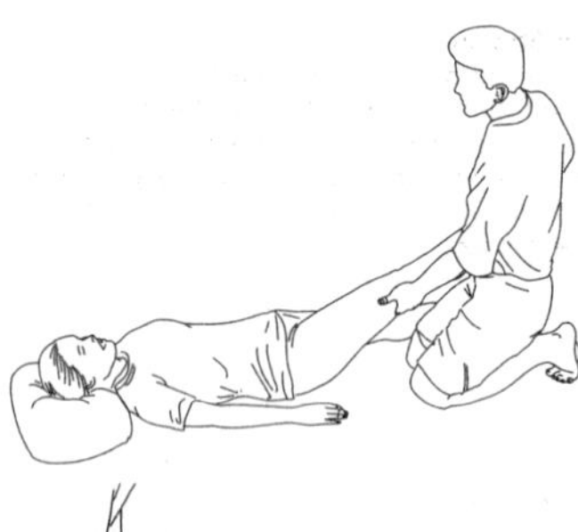

Leg Stretch
Relax the leg by releasing the pressure and extending it forward. Repeat the stretch, if desired.

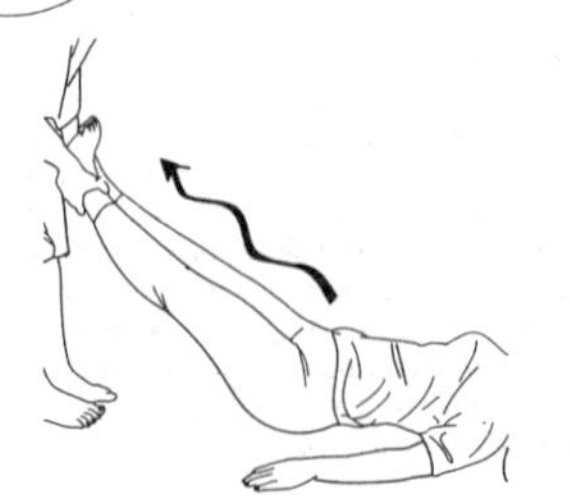

Shake Leg
Position the subject on their back. Using both hands, grasp the subject's leg around the knee and ankle. Shake gently approximately 10-15 times.

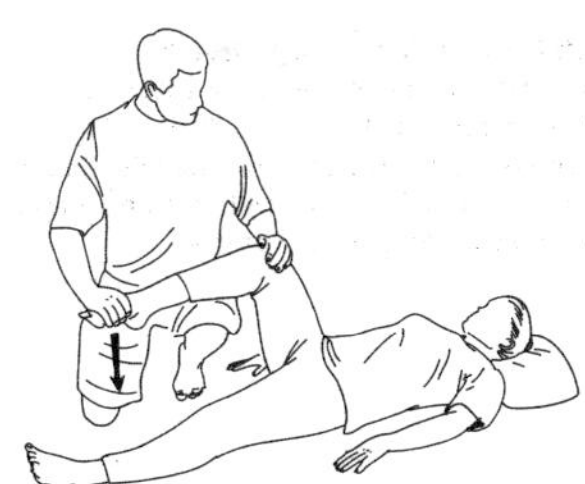

Thigh to Calf Press
Place the subject on their back with one leg extended upwards and bent at the knee. Place your leg under the extended limb and apply pressure with one hand around the ankle so as to create a fulcrum-like stretching effect downwards on the knee and foot.

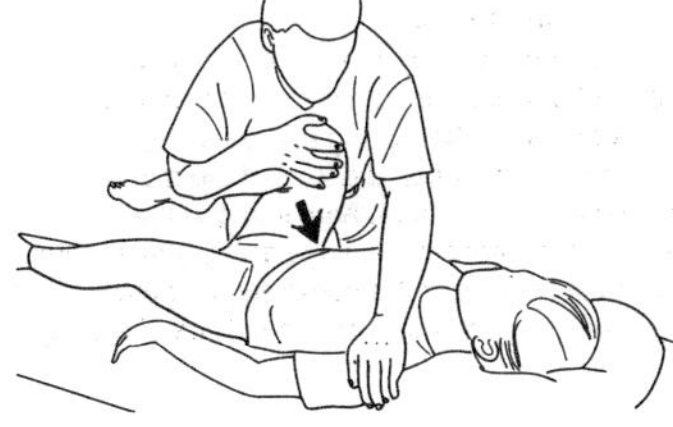

Knee Flexion & Hamstring Stretch
Position the subject on their back. Use your shoulder to flex the subject's hip. The other hand presses downward lightly on the subject's shoulder and your body over the leg to prevent pelvic movement.

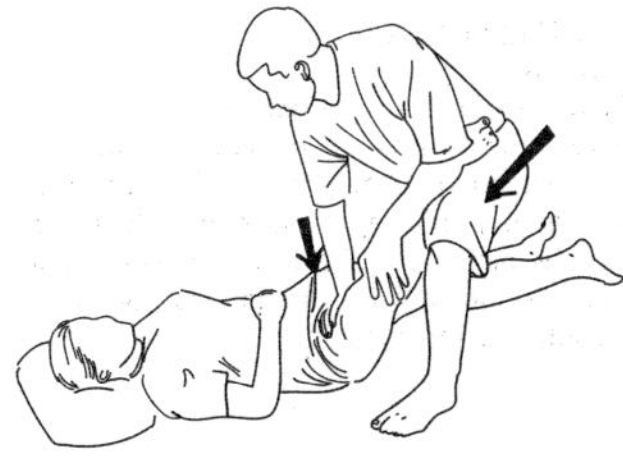

Praying Mantis & Hip Stretch
Position the subject on their back with one leg lifted upwards and placed snugly into your groin area. Place one hand on the subject's inner thigh and gently apply pressure. Grasp the subject's knee with the other hand and progressively apply pressure downward by shifting your weight towards the subject. Apply palm press, thumb press and stretching to applicable sen lines of the inner thigh.

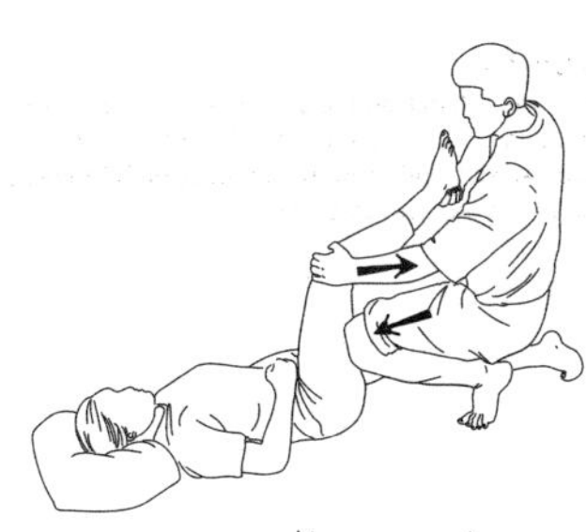

Kneeing the Thigh
Place the subject on their back with one leg extended upwards and bent at the knee. Grasp the extended leg at the knee and the ankle. Gently apply pressure with the knee around the hamstring. Gradually knee the entire length of the hamstring and back thigh in a pulling motion against your knee.

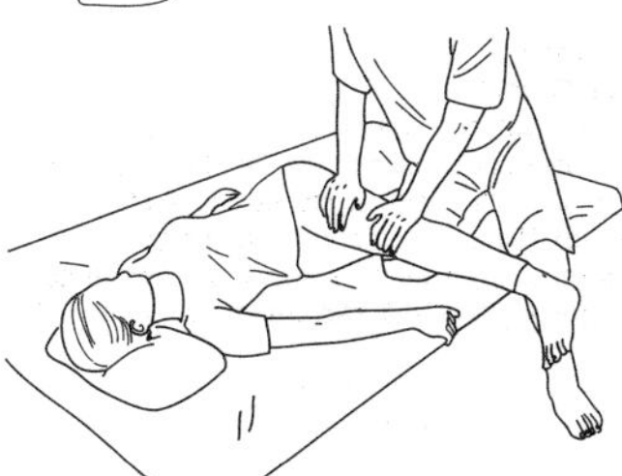

Hip Abductor Stretch
Position the subject on their back with one leg extended straight outwards crossing the torso. Position the subject's leg so that it rests on your knee and, using both hands, apply pressure on either side of the knee. Gradually lean forward to increase pressure as you leverage the subject's leg against your own knee. Apply palm press, thumb press and stretching to applicable sen lines of the outer thigh.

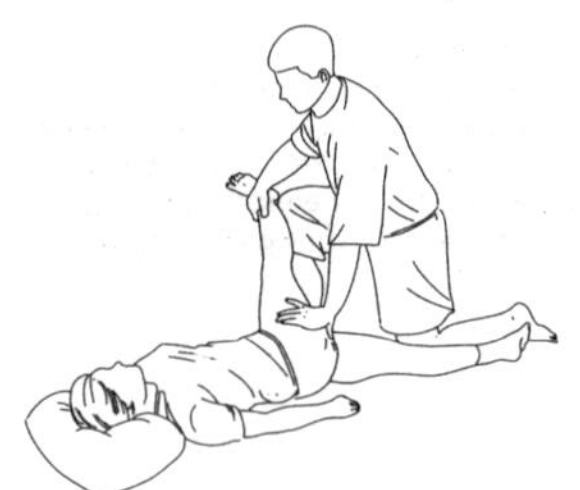

Thumb Press & Cross Leg Stretch
Position the subject on their back with one leg extended across the torso. Stabilize the leg with one hand as you apply pressure with the thumb of the other hand to the subject's hamstring. Apply thumb press to the glutes, if desired.

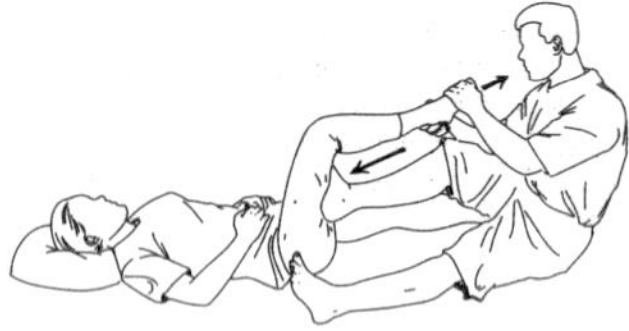

Foot to Thigh Press
Place the subject on their back with one leg extended upwards and bent at the knee. Place one foot near the hamstring and gently apply pressure with the heel and toes of the foot. Simultaneously use both hands to grip the subject's foot around the ankle and gradually lean back so as to stretch the hamstring and thigh. Apply foot press to applicable sen lines of the leg.

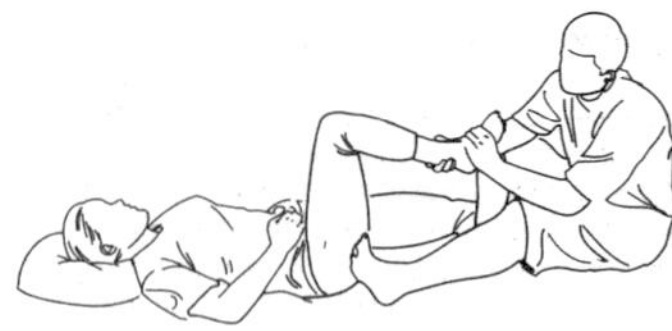

Foot to Thigh Press 2
Leg Traction
Position the subject on the floor with one leg extended upwards and bent at the knee. Gradually push the subject's knee forward while simultaneously applying pressure with the feet and toes on the buttocks and pelvis. Reposition your feet as you lean back in order to massage the back thigh and sen lines.

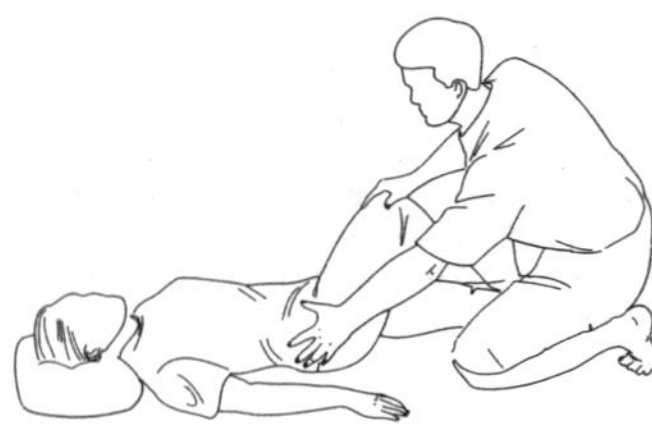

Hip Stretch
Place the subject on their back with one leg bent at the knee and crossed over the other. Apply pressure with both hands as you stretch the hip by rocking the leg and torso gently.

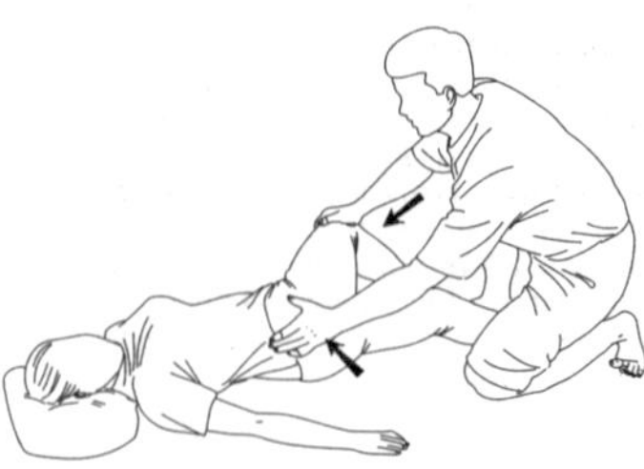

Hip Stretch
Spinal Stretch
Place the subject on their back with one leg bent at the knee and crossed over the other. Position one hand on the upper buttocks and apply pressure. Place the other hand around the knee and progressively lean forward in order to stretch the upper leg and buttocks areas across the body.

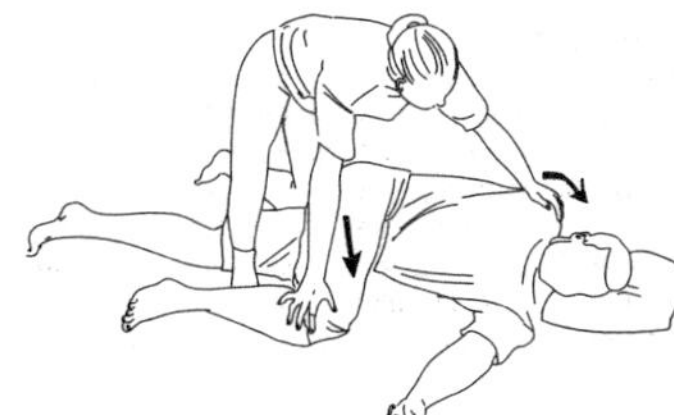

Spinal Twist
Place the subject on their side with one leg bent at the knee. Apply pressure with one hand around the knee and simultaneously guide the shoulder away in the opposing direction from the leg so as to stretch the upper leg and torso. Hold for 5-10 seconds.

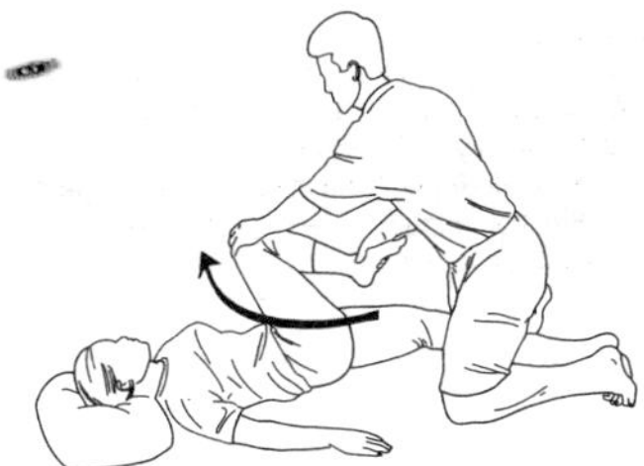

Hip Rotator
Place the subject on their back with one leg extended upwards and bent at the knee. Using both hands, grasp the knee and the upper ankle while simultaneously rotating the thigh in small circular movements. Progressively stretch the extended knee by guiding it across the torso through the entire range of motion.

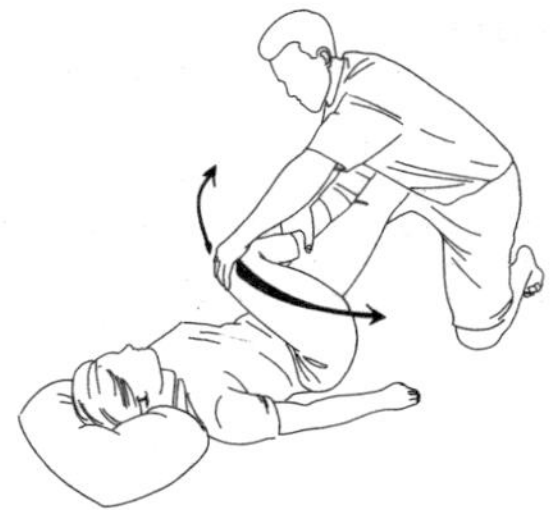

Half Lotus & Hip Rock
Place the subject on their back with one leg snugly placed between your knee and torso in a half lotus position. Wrap the subject's other knee around the extended leg. Place one hand at the knee and the other hand near the ankle. Rock the knee back and forth as you firmly grasp the subject's leg with your hands and leveraged body.

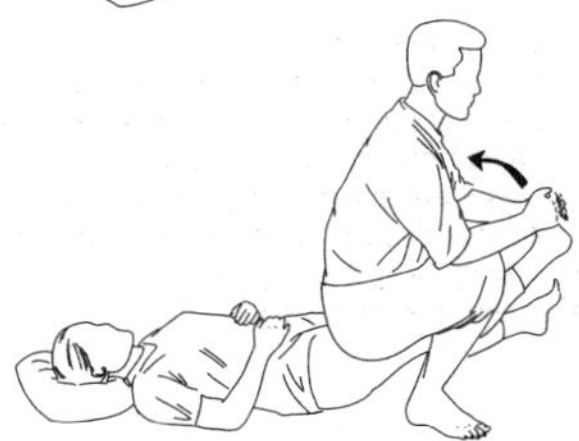

Buttock Press & Stretch
Place the subject on their back and gently rest your buttocks on their upper thigh as you carefully assume a straddle position. Grasp the heel and toes of one foot and lift it upwards as you lightly pull the foot towards the body, making sure to gently shift weight to the feet and knees. Work your grip across the entire foot and then switch feet. Increase pressure gradually if desired.

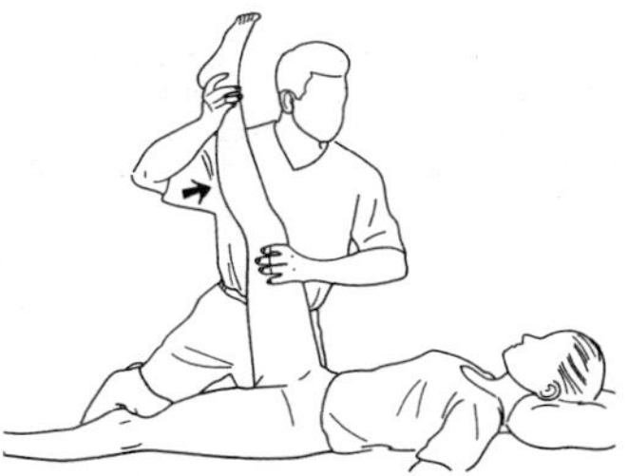

Hamstring Stretch
Position the subject on their back with one leg extended straight outwards and lifted. Apply pressure to the subject's lower leg with your knee and secure the subject's leg. With the other hand, raise the leg to stretch the muscle. Keep the outer leg stabilized by hooking your knee across the subject to prevent the pelvis from moving.

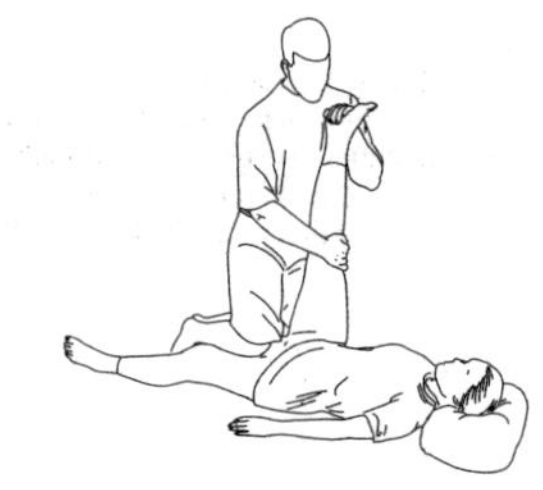

Leg Stretch
Position the subject on their back with one leg extending upwards towards the ceiling. With one hand on the knee and the other grasping the foot, lean forward to apply pressure. Simultaneously place a knee on the subject's other leg to secure the leg while applying light pressure to stretch the hamstrings. Consult with the subject so as not to overstretch the hamstring, lower back, and gluteal muscles.

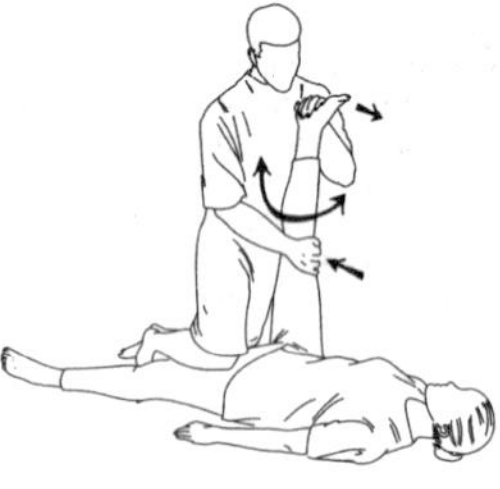

Leg Stretch 2
Place the subject on their back with one leg extended straight upwards. Place one hand near the knee and lightly pull the leg away from the body while simultaneously pushing the foot in the opposite direction. Lightly rotate the leg back and forth as you apply pressure.

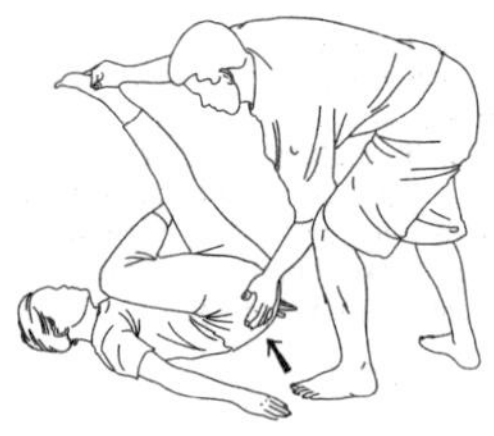

Half Lotus Lift
Place the subject on their back with one leg extended straight upwards and the other in a half lotus position. Push the leg forward with one hand and simultaneously support the subject with the other hand placed on the buttocks. Gradually rock the subject back and forth in the position so as to stretch both legs and the lower back.

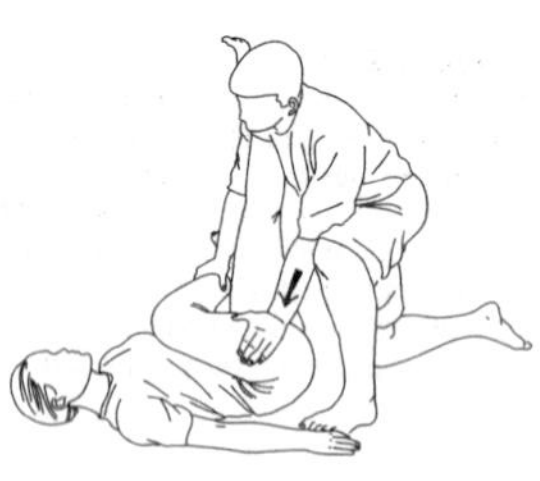

Half Lotus Thigh Press
Place the subject on their back with one leg extended straight upwards and the other wrapped around in a half lotus position. As you rest the extended leg on your shoulder, place one hand on the hamstring and apply light pressure downwards using your body weight. Apply palm press to applicable sen lines of the leg if desired.

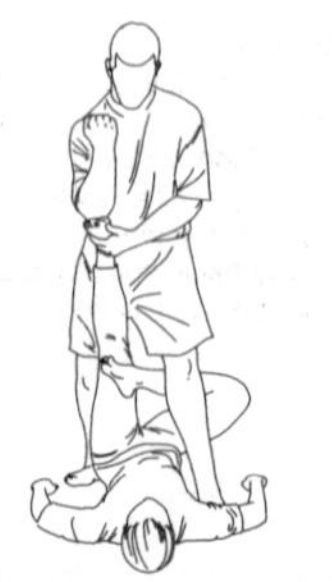

Elbow Press
Position the subject on their back with one leg extended straight upwards and the other in a half-lotus position. With one hand grasp the top of the extended foot as you knead the bottom of the foot with your elbow.

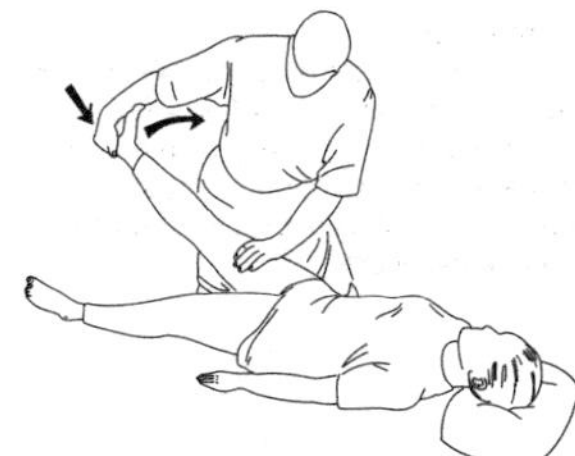

Straight Leg Stretch
Place the subject on their back with one leg raised. Grasp the heel of the raised foot and place your other hand near the top of the thigh to straighten the leg. As you apply light pressure downward, simultaneously stretch the heel with your forearm for a deeper stretch.

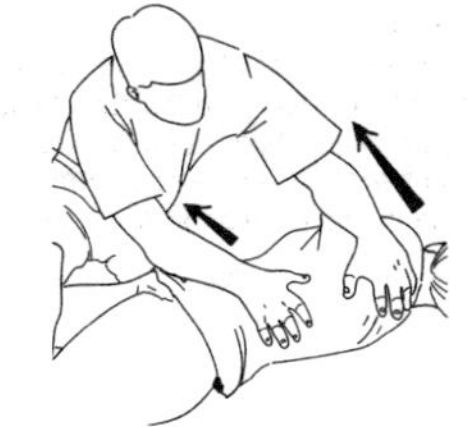

Torso Twist
Place the subject on their back. Using both palms, grasp the subject's side around the hips and upper back and gently roll them towards you.

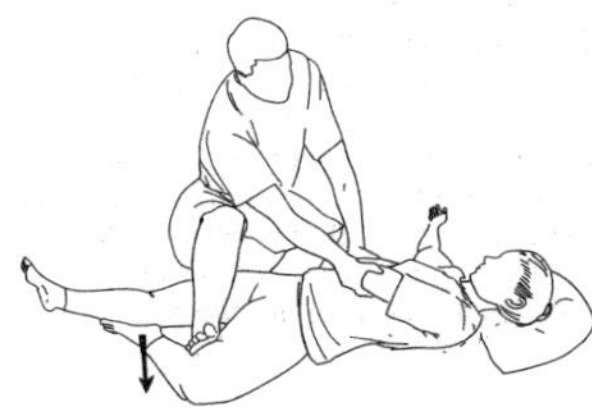

Spinal Twist
Place the subject on their back with one leg bent at the knee and extended outwards. Securely place your heel behind the flexed knee joint to secure the leg and use both hands to grasp the forearm as you pull it towards you in a twisting stretch.

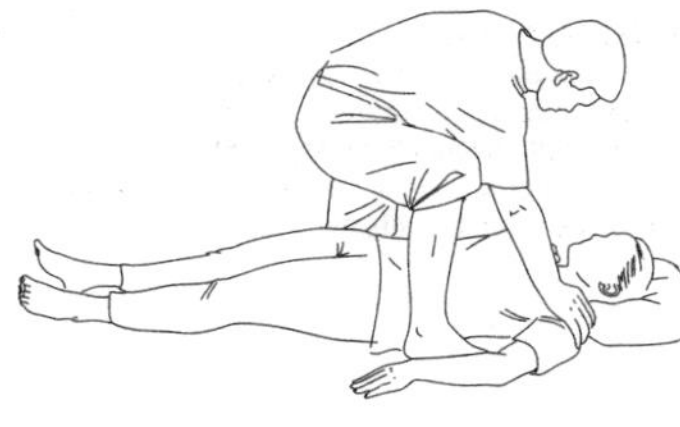

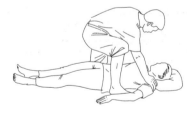

Chest & Shoulder Press
Place the subject in a comfortable resting position on their back. Using your palms, apply even pressure along the shoulders, chest, and arms of the subject, increasing pressure in desired areas. Continue this palming motion down to the arms and fingers, if desired.

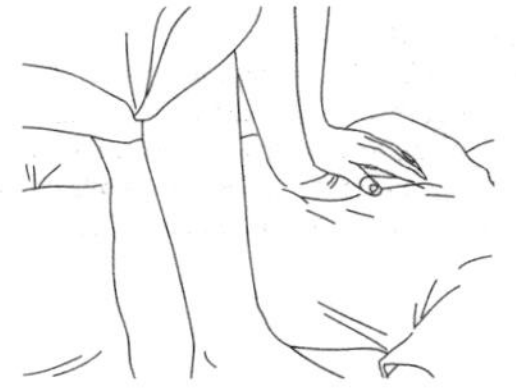

Chest Press
Position the subject on their back. Carefully straddle the subject and, using both palms, progressively apply pressure to the subject's chest.

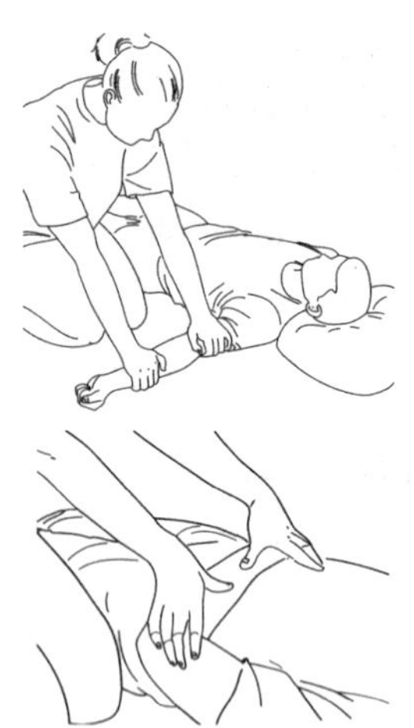

Inner Arm Press
Position the subject on their back with the arm extended outwards at a 90-degree angle and the palm facing upwards. Using both hands with a straight arm, apply palm press, thumb press, thumb walk to sen lines of the inner arm and either side of the elbow.

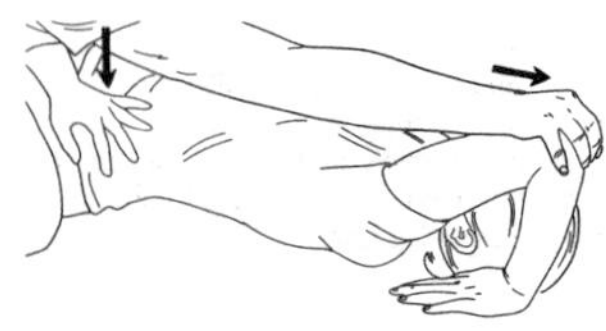

Outer Arm Press
Position the subject on their back with one arm folded over the belly. Using the thumbs of both hands, apply pressure to points on the subject's arm. Work your way across the outer arm applying a thumb and palm press to the sen lines of the arm.

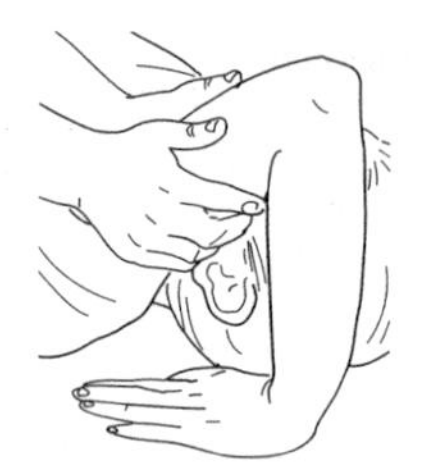

Triangle Arm Stretch
Position the subject on their back with their arm bent backwards and the hands placed on the ground pointed towards the body in a triangle-like formation. Using one hand, apply gradual pressure to the subject's bent arm by pushing the elbow away from the body. Simultaneously push down on the subject's elbow with the other hand to fully stretch across the trunk and arm.

Triangle Arm Stretch 2
Position the subject on their back with the arm bent backwards and the hands placed on the ground pointed towards the body in a triangle-like formation. Butterfly palm the back of the exposed area from the armpit to the elbow.

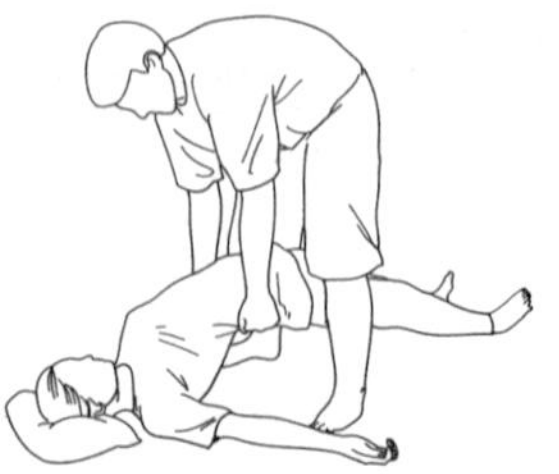

Lift Under the Back
Position the subject on their back. Carefully straddle the subject and place your hands on either side of the lower back. Assist the subject as they gradually arch their back and gently lift them upwards so as to stretch the entire back.

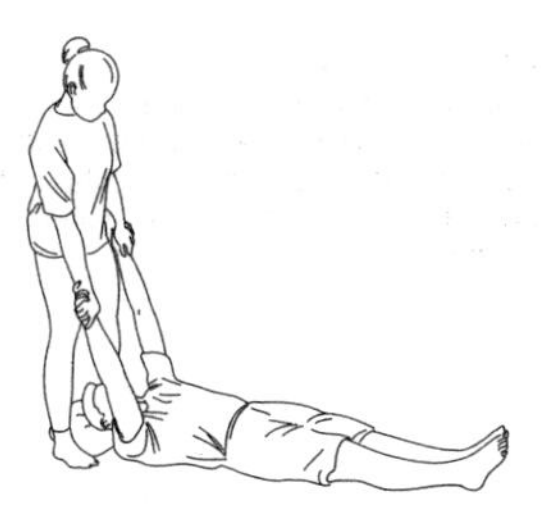

Alternate Arm Pull
Position the subject on their back with both arms lifted upwards towards the ceiling. While standing, straddle the subject's head and grasp both hands by interlocking the wrists. Pull lightly, alternating the shoulders to stretch the arms and upper back.

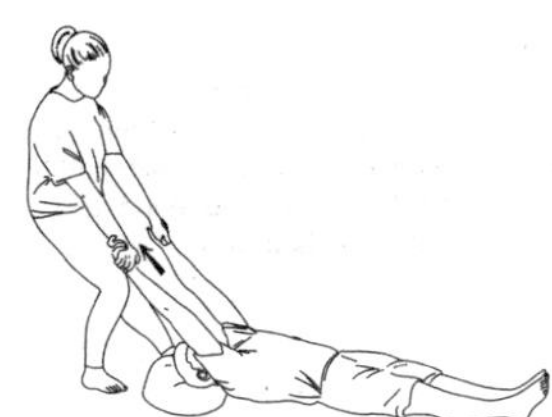

Arm Pull 2
Position the subject on their back with both arms extended upwards. Grasp both hands while interlocking the wrists. Progressively lean back with your body weight so as to stretch the arms and hold.

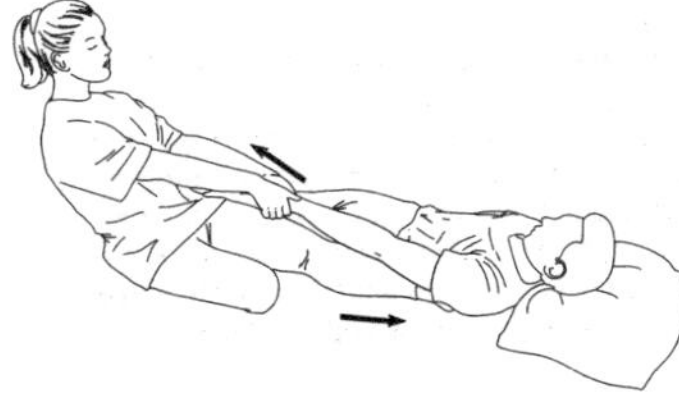

Foot to Armpit Stretch
Position the subject on their back. Securely tuck your foot into the armpit of the subject and firmly grasp the corresponding hand. As you apply pressure with your foot and toes, pull the arm away from the body and hold.

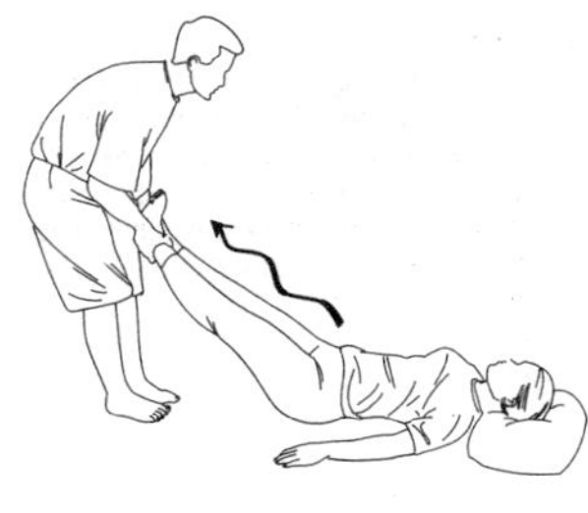

Leg Shake
Place the subject on their back. Grasp both legs at the ankles and shake up and down rapidly to create a wave-like effect. Shaking should go right into the hip and the rest of the body.

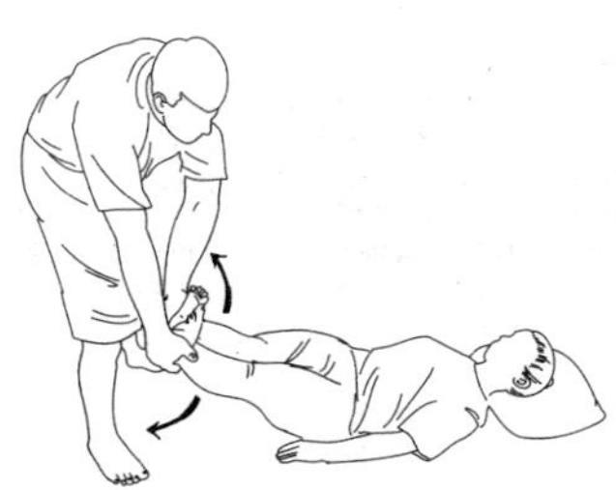

Leg Swing
Position the subject on their back. Grasp both legs at the ankles and rotate from side to side, varying the range of motion of the swings as you go.

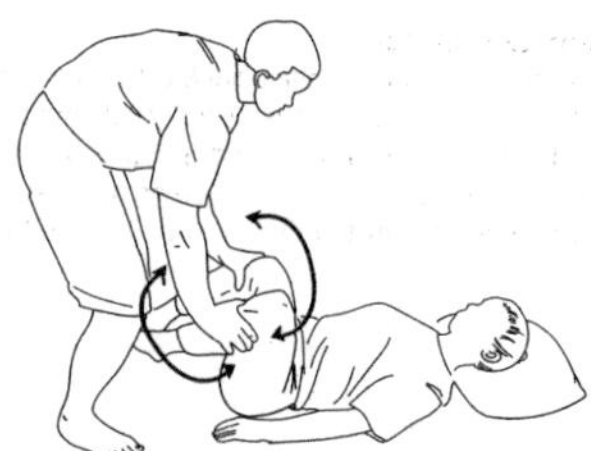

Hip Rotator
Place the subject on their back. Grasp the subject's legs just below the knees. Keep both knees together, rotate the legs in a circular motion as you gradually increase in speed and amplitude of the rotation.

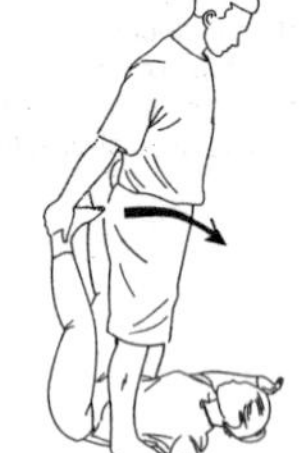

Plough 1
Place the subject on their back. While standing, straddle the subject and grasp both legs just behind the ankles and tuck your feet slightly below the armpits. Gradually lean forward in order to stretch the legs and buttocks.

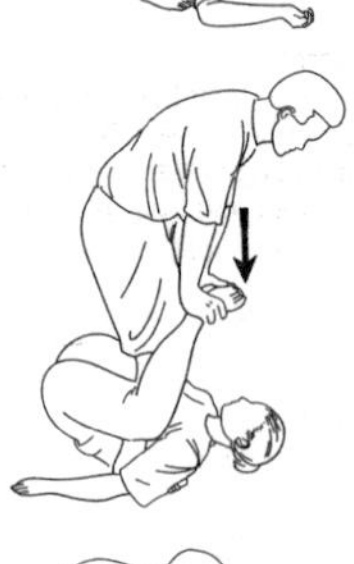

Plough 2
Position the subject on their back with both legs wrapped around your own at knee level. Tuck your feet under the armpits and press the subject's feet together, pushing downward gently. Slowly guide the legs further towards the body and hold, so as to stretch the lower back and legs. Be sure to check the comfort level of the subject as you increase pressure and leverage.

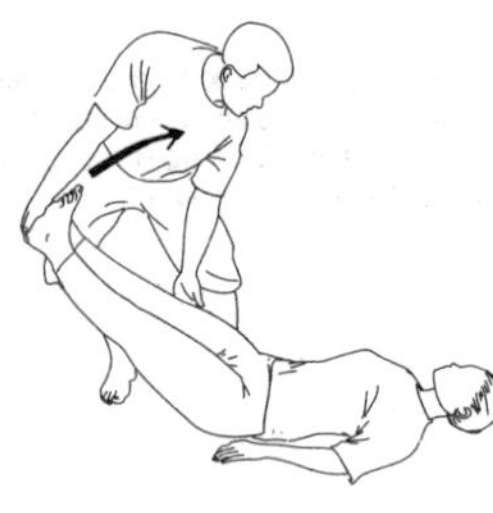

Rock & Roll Back
Position the subject on their back. Securely grasp the heels of both feet and lift upwards. Push the subject's feet over the head to lift the subject's buttocks with a supported hand under the thigh. Roll back to the extent possible and continue to rock back and forth in a smooth manner in order to stretch the back and legs.

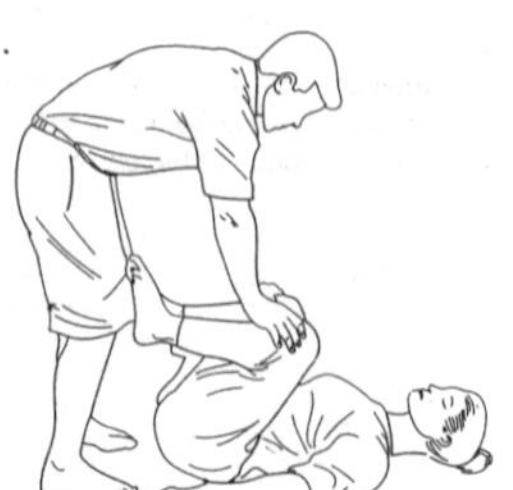

Back Stretch
Position the subject on their back with both legs bent at the knee and the arches of the foot resting on your knees. Gently press the subject's knees towards the stomach and, if desired, simultaneously bend your knees to apply additional pressure and hold.

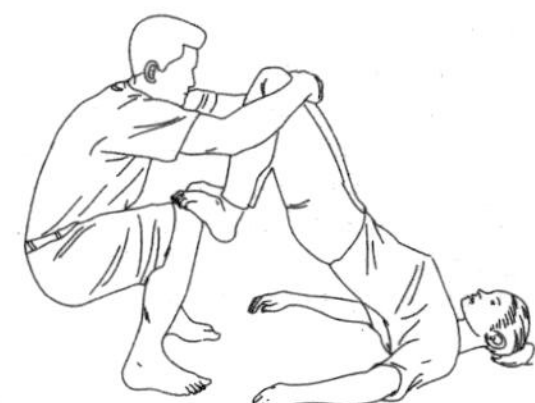

Half Bridge Shoulder Stand
Carefully position the subject on their shoulders with the arches of their feet resting securely on your knees. Wrap your arms just below the subject's knees and gradually lean back so as to generate pressure on the upper back, abdomen, and legs while pulling the pelvis off the ground. Only perform this stretch with limber, physically fit subjects.

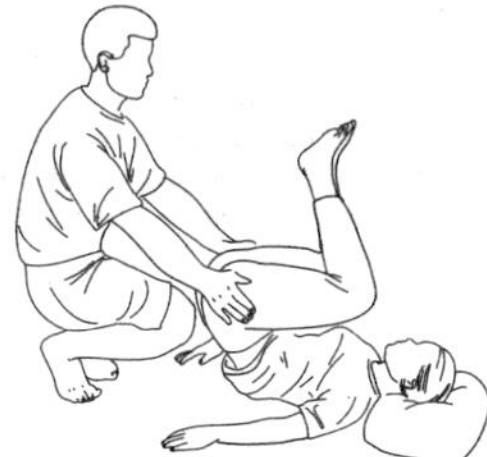

Knee to Buttocks
Carefully position the subject on their shoulders and assist them as they extend both feet upwards in a headstand-like position. Lift the subject's buttocks off the ground and support with both hands as they stretch the lower back.

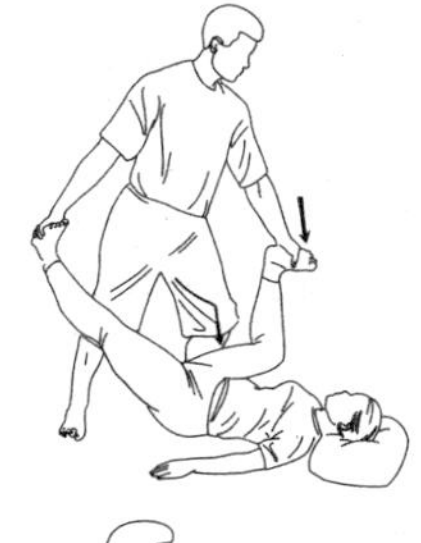

Knee & Shinning Thighs
Position the subject on their back with both legs extended in opposite directions with one leg at right angle against the subject's stomach. Hold the outer leg outwards while simultaneously applying pressure with the shin and knee to the subject's hamstring. Gradually increase pressure, if desired.

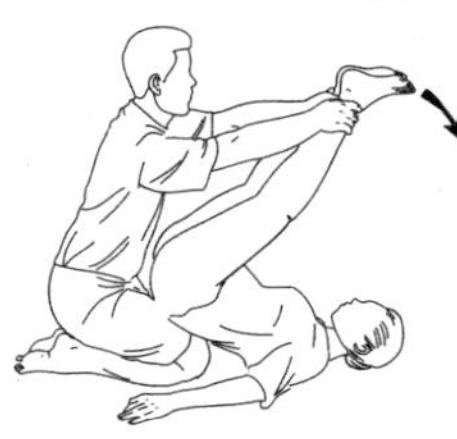

Back Stretch
Position the subject on their back with their buttocks resting on your thighs. Grasp both ankles and gradually lean into the subject so as to stretch the hamstring and buttocks.

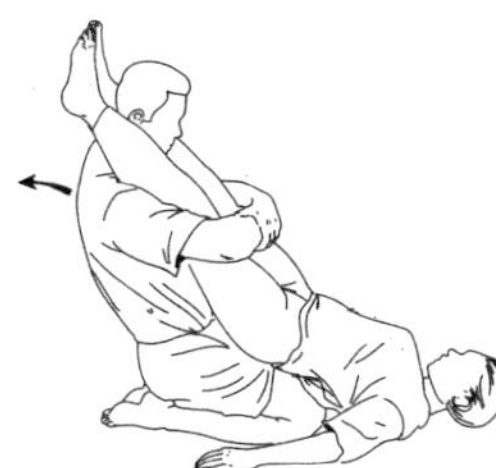

Back Stretch 2
Position the subject on their back with their buttocks resting comfortably on your thighs. Place their legs on either side of your head and securely wrap your arms around them. Progressively lean backwards at a near 45-degree angle to stretch their upper back and shoulders.

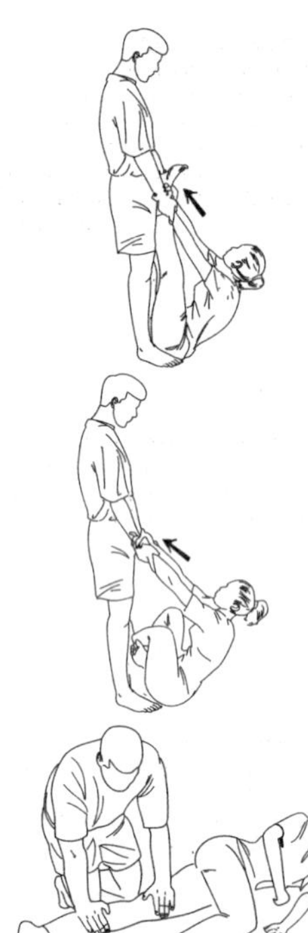

Straight Leg Lift
Position the subject with their legs extended straight upwards or to a comfortable angle, propped up against your own. Lock hands with the subject and bring them towards you in order to stretch their back and leg muscles. Use your body weight instead of muscle to lift. Be sure to consult with the subject so as not to overstretch their comfort zone.

Cross Leg Lift
Position the subject with both legs crossed in a sitting position, propped up against your own. Lock hands and pull the subject into a rocking position in order to stretch the arms and back. Use your body weight instead of muscle to lift.

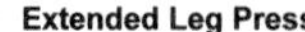

Extended Leg Press
Position the subject on their side with one leg extended straight outwards, resting on the mat, with both hands at a 90-degree angle. Use your body weight to thumb walk, palm, and butterfly palm the inner sen lines of the leg. Apply pressure to either side of the knee and inside lower leg in a rhythmic rocking motion.

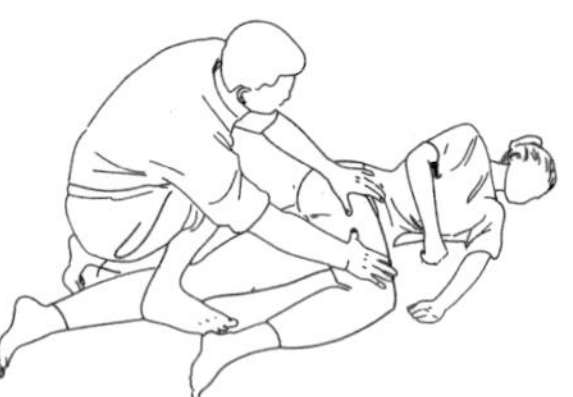

Flex Leg Press
Position the subject on their side with one leg extended straight outwards and the other flexed at the knee. Using both the palms and the thumbs, lightly knead the outer thigh and sen lines of the bent leg and increase in intensity, if desired.

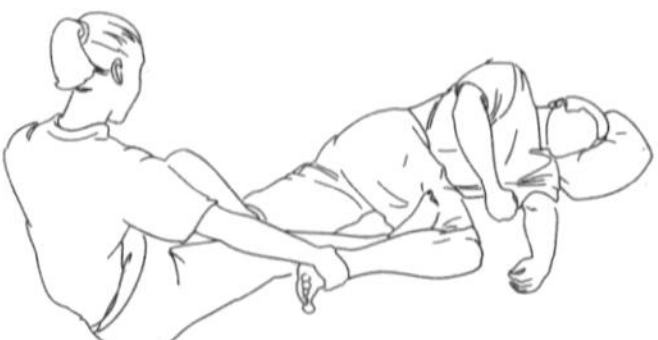

Side Leg Press
Position the subject on their side with one leg flexed at the knee. Grasp both ankles and place one foot on the subject's inner thigh. Gradually lean back to apply pressure on the sen lines of the leg. Work your foot across the thigh and hamstring if desired.

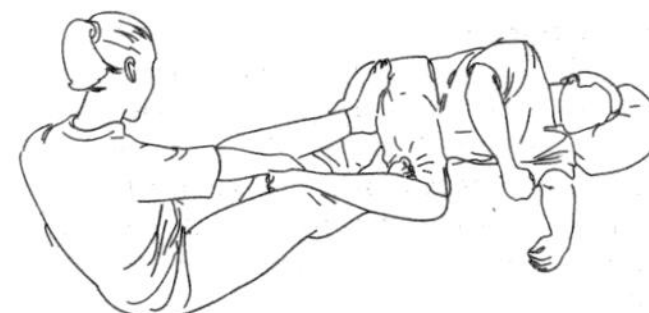

Side Leg Paddleboat Press
Position the subject on their side with one leg flexed at the knee. As you tuck one leg into the back of the subject's thigh, snugly place their corresponding leg behind your own knee. Grasp the subject's leg near the ankle. Place your other leg just below the buttocks. Gradually lean back to apply pressure.

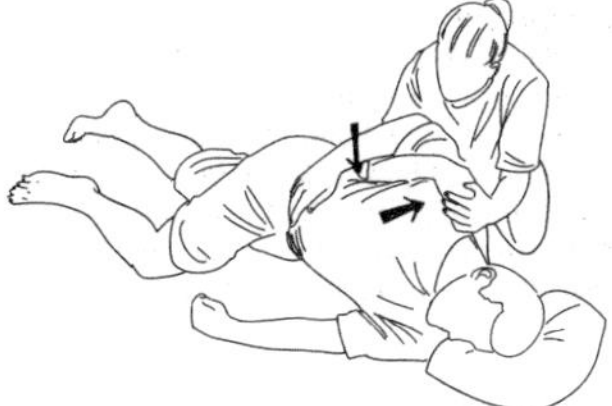

Shoulder Rotator
Position the subject on their side with one leg flexed at the knee. Hook your forearm under their arm and grasp with interlocking fingers the subject's shoulder. Rotate the shoulder slowly, starting with small movements and gradually increasing rotation at a comfortable level. Push and pull as you feel resistance from the subject. Two equalizing forces can be applied in opposing direction helps flex joints and increase mobility.

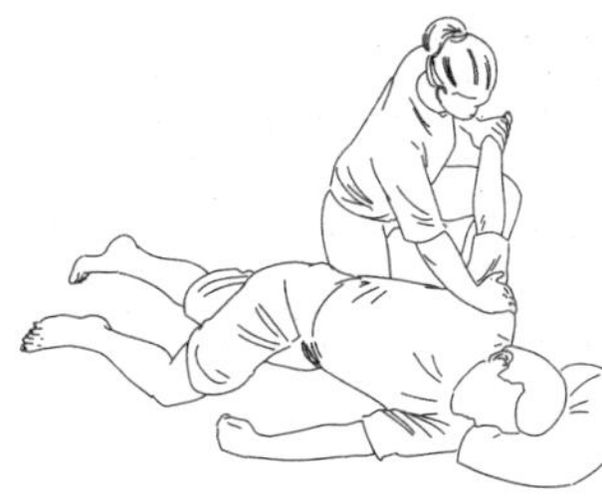

Knee Supported Arm Press
Position the subject on their side with one arm extended and resting comfortably on your knee. Apply pressure to the shoulder by gently pulling the arm backwards against your knee. Palm up and down the entire arm if desired.

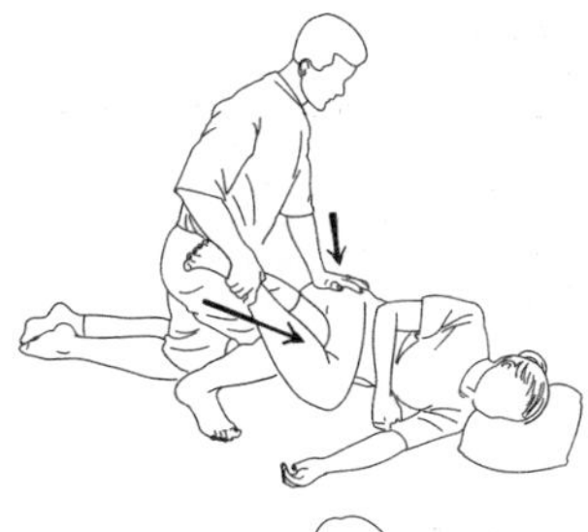

Knee to Knee Hip Flexor
Position the subject on their side with one leg flexed at the knee. Grasp the lifted leg around the ankle and snugly tuck your knee behind theirs. Simultaneously apply downward pressure with the other hand to their hip and gradually lean forward to generate pressure in the flexed knee.

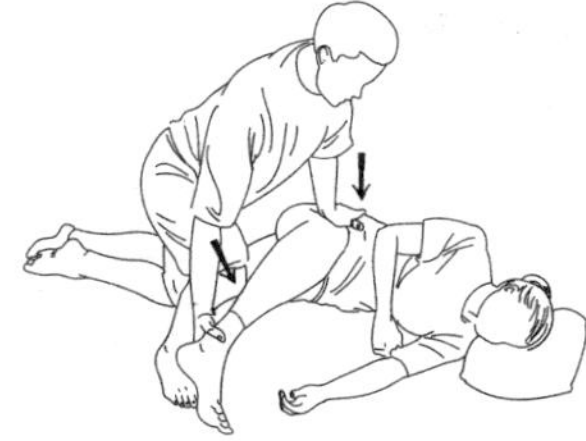

Horizontal Cross Leg Stretch
Position the subject on their side with one leg flexed at the knee. Grasp the lifted leg around the ankle and place your knee just behind their calf. Simultaneously apply downward pressure with the other hand to their thigh and gradually lean forward to generate pressure in the flexed leg.

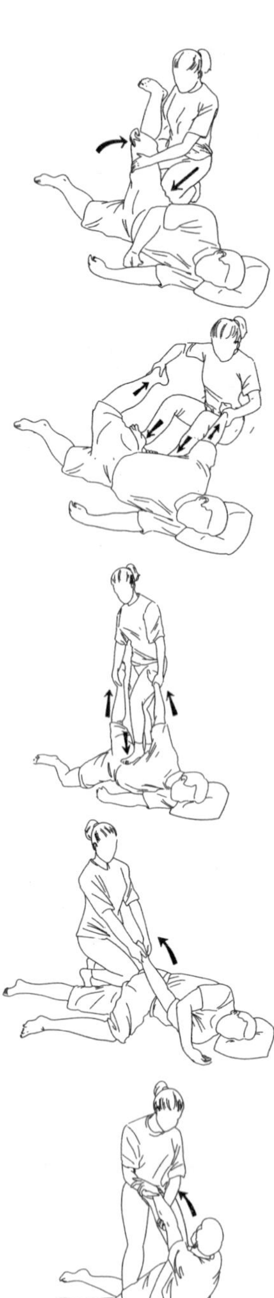

Pivot Hip Stretch
Position the subject on their side with one leg lifted into the air. Firmly grasp the raised leg on either side of the knee and pull their leg towards you and simultaneously apply pressure with your knee just below the subject's buttocks in a pivoting motion as you stretch the front of the hip and thigh.

Scissor Stretch
Position the subject on their side. With one hand, grasp the subject's upper leg just below the ankle. Using the other hand grasp their wrist. As you gradually lean back to generate pressure, simultaneously apply pressure to the buttocks, lower back, and pelvic arch with both feet by stretching the quadriceps and psoas.

Scissor Stretch 2
Position the subject on their side. With one hand, grasp the subject's upper leg just below the ankle. Using the other hand, securely grasp the corresponding arm around the wrist. While maintaining slight tension on the arm, pull both limbs upwards simultaneously to apply pressure downwards with one foot near the subject's waist. Stretch and hold the position.

Cross Arm Pull
Position the subject on their side with the upper leg flexed at the knee and both arms crossed at the chest. Using both hands, grasp the subject's lower arm and lean back to generate a crossed arm stretch towards you while simultaneously applying pressure to the upper buttocks with one knee. Stretch and hold the position.

Lifting Spinal Twist
Position the subject on their side with the upper leg bent at a 90-degree angle at the knee. Snugly tuck one leg under their bent knee and the other leg behind the subject. Using both hands, securely grasp the lower arm and lift the subject off the floor so as to stretch the arm and back by leaning backwards with your body weight. Be sure to consult with the subject on their comfort level.

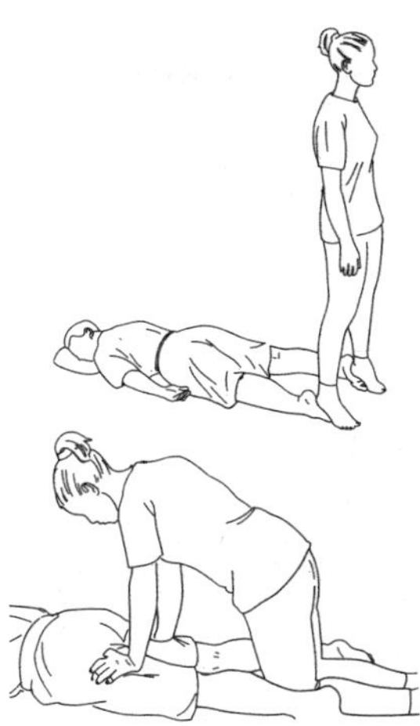

Standing Feet Press
Position the subject on their stomach in a relaxed position. Gently place the heels of both feet against the subject's and gradually lower your heels onto the soles of the subject's feet to the floor so as to apply gentle rocking motion pressure across the subject's feet.

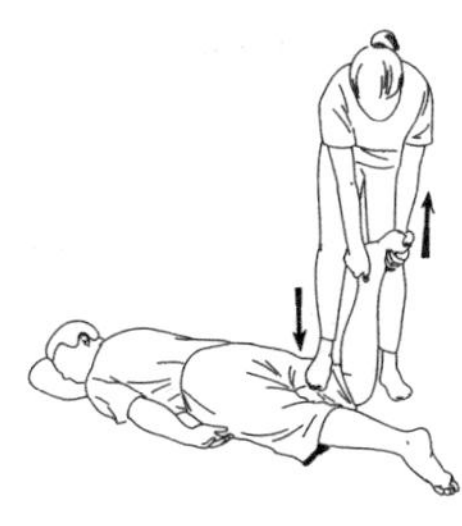

Leg, Buttock and Back Press
Position the subject on their stomach. Using the palms of both hands, gently palm press and knead the lower buttocks, and hamstring. Apply palm press, butterfly press, and kneading to sen lines of the back leg. Work your way across the hamstring and gluteal folds in a rocking motion as your move down the leg.

Heel to Buttock Press
Position the subject on their stomach. Using both hands, grasp one leg on either side of the ankle. Lift the leg to form a near 90-degree angle. As you gradually pull up on the leg, simultaneously apply pressure with one foot across the hamstring. Apply foot pressure to the sen line of the back leg.

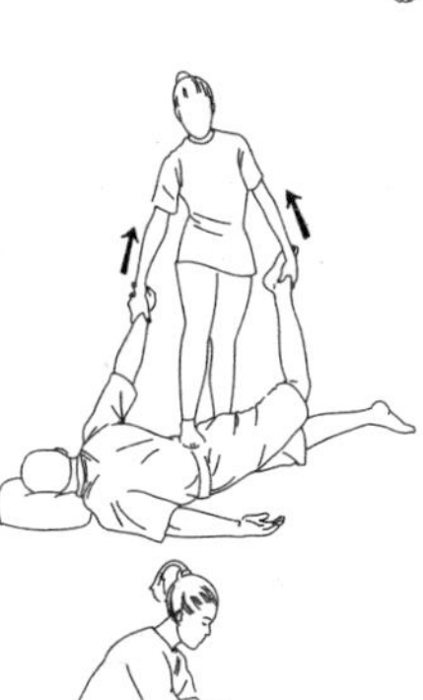

Reverse Half Lotus Leg Lift
Position the subject on their stomach. With one hand grasp the subject's leg just below the ankle, grasp the opposite arm around the wrist with the other hand. As you gradually pull on both limbs simultaneously apply pressure to the lower back with one foot. Be sure that the placement of your foot is on the lower back and not on the spine.

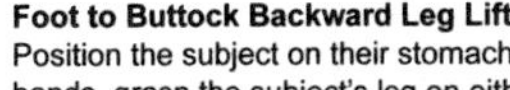

Foot to Buttock Backward Leg Lift
Position the subject on their stomach. Using both hands, grasp the subject's leg on either side of the ankle and lift it upwards. As you gradually lean back pull up on the leg to simultaneously apply pressure to the lower back using one foot.

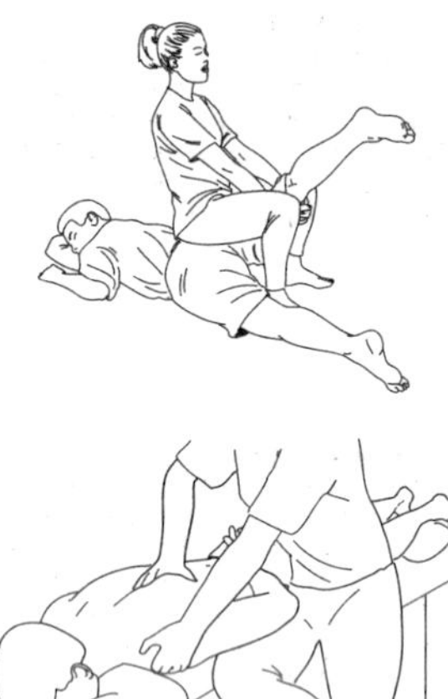

Backward Leg Lift
Position the subject on their stomach and carefully straddle the subject's torso, using the buttocks as a resting place. With an interlocking grip, grasp the subject's thigh just above the knee as you lean back and pull the leg upwards and hold.

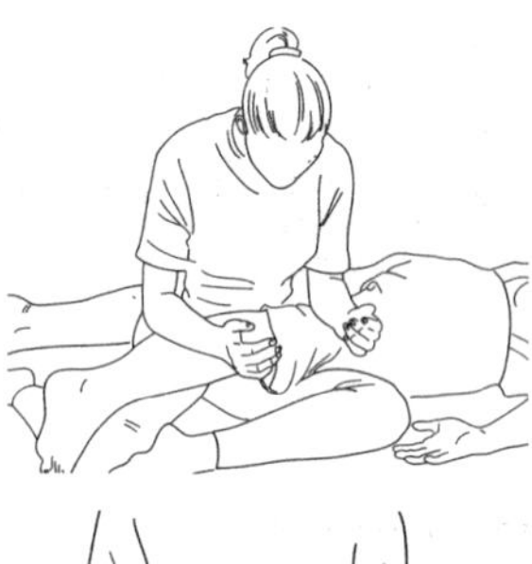

Scapula Lift & Shoulder Pull
Position the subject on their stomach. With one hand, grasp the subject's shoulder as the other hand lifts the scapula away from the body. Use the fingers to press against the lower edge of the scapula and raise the medial border of the shoulder. Deep friction, stroking and thumbing of rhomboid muscle and shoulder can be guided along the edges.

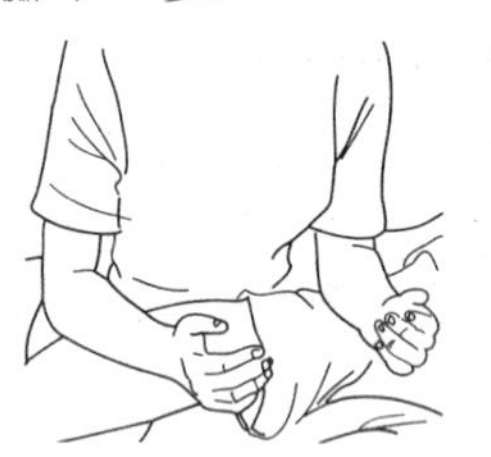

Forearm Calf &Thigh Press
Position the subject on their stomach. Assume a sitting position between the subject's legs and place one leg just above your knee. Using both forearms, apply pressure to either side of the knee with a forearm roll. Apply forearm presses on the sen lines of the leg. Gradually work your way across the entire leg, hamstring, gluteals, and lower back, if desired.

Double Forearm
Position the subject on their stomach. Assume a seated position between the subject's leg and place one leg so that it rests on your thigh. Using both forearms gradually apply pressure to either side of the knee and work your way around the leg.

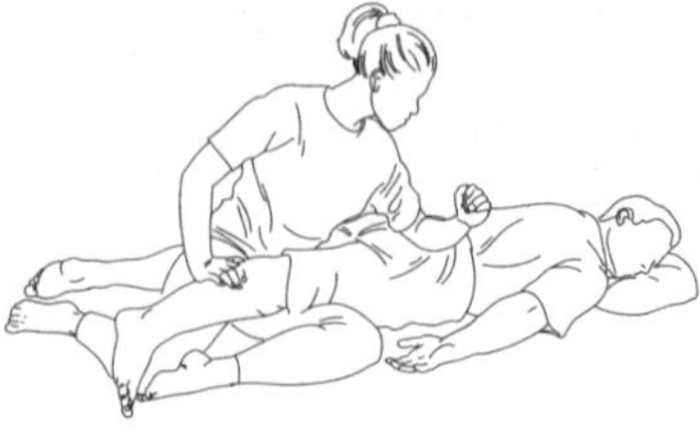

Forearm Calf &Thigh Press 2
Position the subject on their stomach. Assume a sitting position between the subject's legs and place one leg just above your knee. Use elbow and forearm to roll the sen lines of the back leg. Knead the tissue of the lower buttocks and hamstring and work your way across the area. You can also work on the sacrum, femur and iliac crest with a pointed elbow.

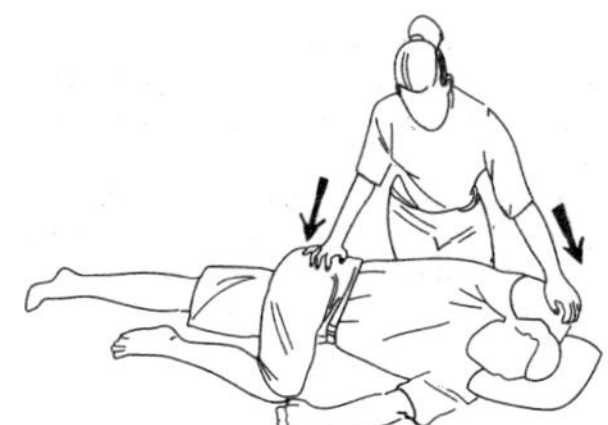

Triangle Arm Stretch
Position the subject on their side with the upper arm tucked behind the head and the upper leg bent at the knee. Place one hand on the subject's thigh and gradually lean forward to apply pressure to the hips and the side of the body. With the other hand, simultaneously apply pressure just above the raised elbow.

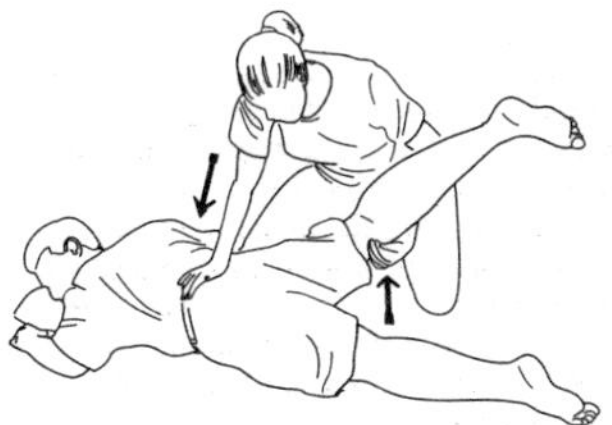

Knee to Buttock Backward Leg Lift
Position the subject on their stomach. Wrap one hand around the subject's leg just above the knee and gradually lift upwards. Using the other hand, simultaneously apply pressure downwards to the subject's lower back and sacrum and hold.

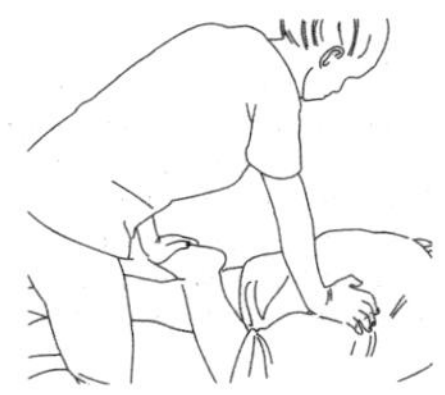

Frog Position
Position the subject on their stomach. Using one hand guide the subject's leg so that it folds across the other leg near the knee into a frog position. Apply pressure to the hamstring and buttocks of the flexed leg with the other hand by gradually leaning forward.

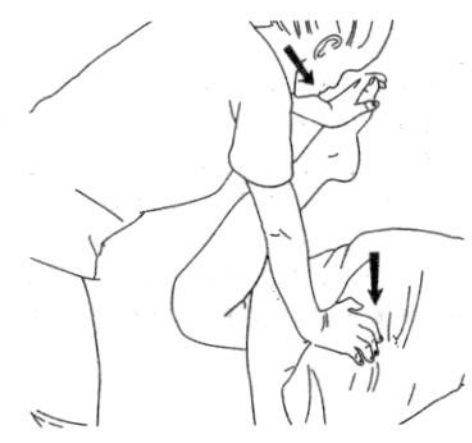

Cross Double Knee Flex
Position the subject on their stomach with one leg crossed and tucked snugly into the knee joint of the other. With one hand, grasp the foot of the subject's raised leg below the ankle and apply pressure downwards. Simultaneously place one hand on the other leg's hamstring and gradually lean forward to apply pressure.

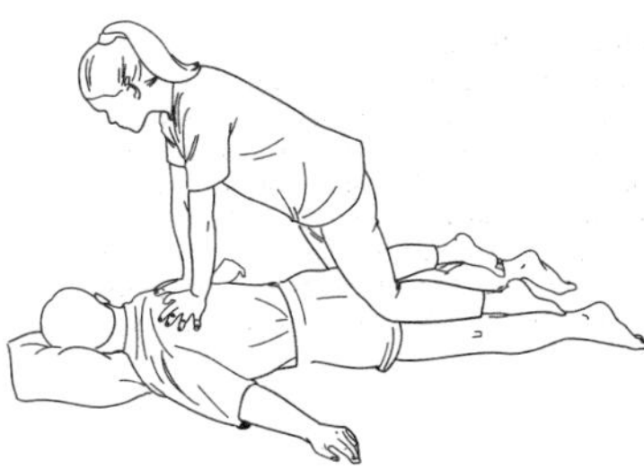

Palm & Back Press from Kneeling
Position the subject on their stomach. Place your palms with the core directly over your subject as you direct your body weight through the shoulder, elbow and wrists, checking with the subject that the placement is comfortable. Position your hands in a butterfly palm press that can be applied to the back, buttocks and legs. As you move to other areas, distribute your body weight evenly and in a balanced manner.

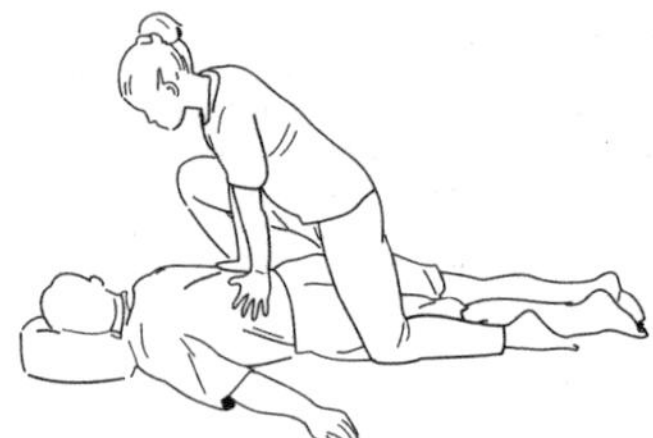

Back Press from Kneeling 2
Position the subject on their stomach. Carefully straddle the subject and place both hands on the lower back. Keep arms straight as you apply downward pressure. Apply palm press, butterfly palm press and kneading to the sen lines of the back as you gradually lean forward with your body weight evenly with both hands.

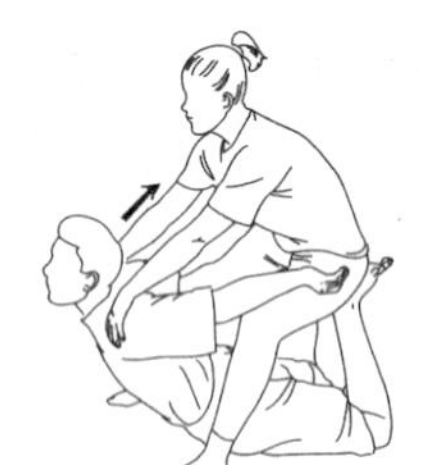

Sitting King Cobra
Position the subject on their stomach with both feet raised in a cobra-like position. Bend the subject's knees to 90 degrees while sitting on their feet. Lift subject's arm and place on your thigh. Carefully lean back on both feet, using them to prop yourself up. Place your hands on the subject's shoulder and lean back using body weight. Take care not to overstretch the subject's back as you lean back to assume a bow-like position. Gradually pull upwards to further stretch the back, if desired.

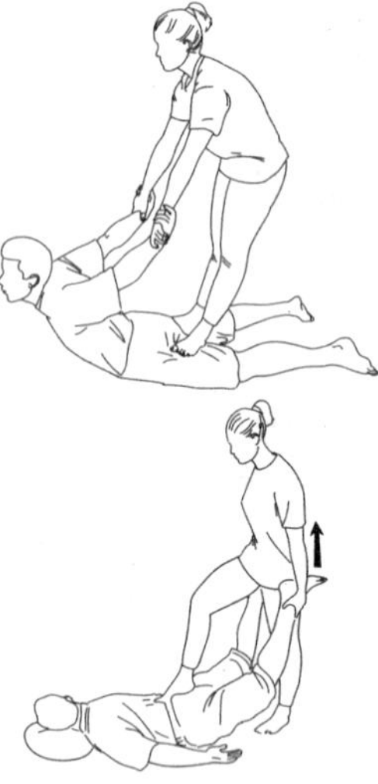

Standing King Cobra
Position the subject on their stomach. Place both feet between the hamstring, toes outward and arches of the feet at the lower edges of the buttocks, taking care not to apply too much pressure to one specific area. Grasp both hands and assist the subject by pulling upwards as they raise their upper body to form a cobra-like position.

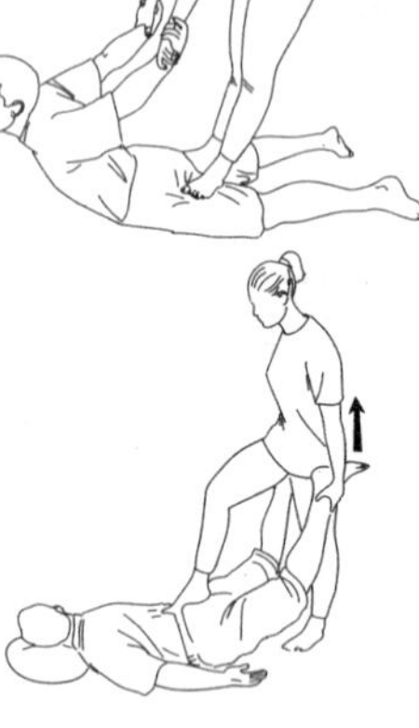

Single Leg Locust
Position the subject on their stomach. Using both hands, grasp the subject's feet around the ankles and lift upwards as you simultaneously apply gentle pressure to the lower back with one foot by anchoring the pelvis to the mat to hold the stretch. Be sure that the placement of the foot is on the lower back or sacrum and not directly on the spine.

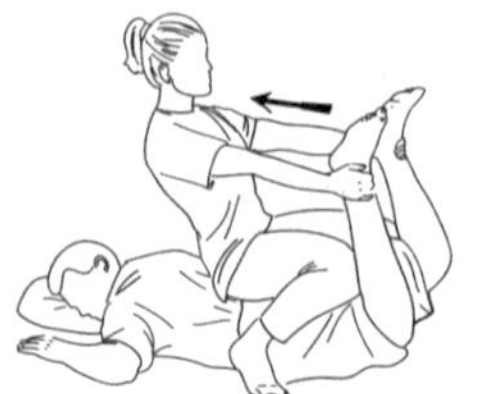

Knee to Calf Press
Position the subject on their stomach with both knees bent upwards. Straddle the subject and carefully assume a sitting position near their buttocks. Using both hands, grasp the subject's feet around the ankles and gradually lean backwards to generate pressure. Simultaneously use both knees to apply pressure to the back of the subject's calves as you lean backwards and hold.

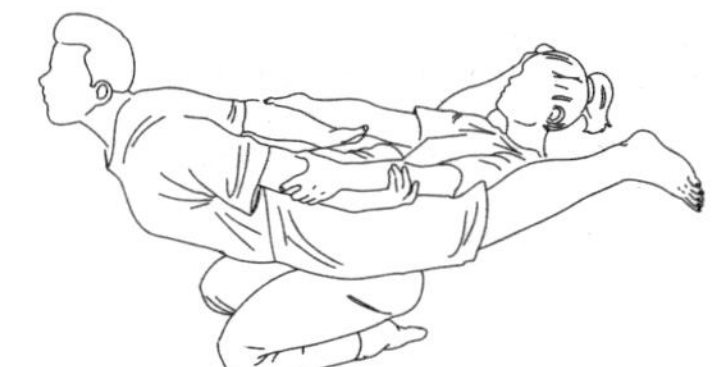

Intimate Cobra
Position the subject on their stomach. Slide between the subject's legs, resting their quads on yours and interlocking the arms around the elbows. Carefully lift the subject off the ground and assume a comfortable position. Gradually lean backwards to stretch the subject's arms and back and hold.

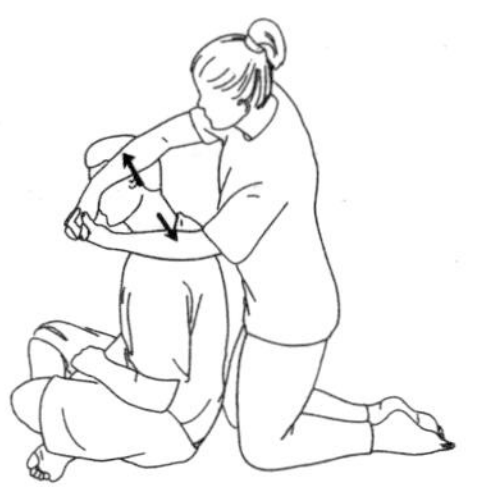

Neck & Trapezius Stretch
Position the subject in a comfortable cross-legged seated position. Assume a kneeling position just behind the subject and clasp your hands together. Using both the elbows and forearms, apply gentle pressure to the neck and shoulders by rolling your arms away from each other.

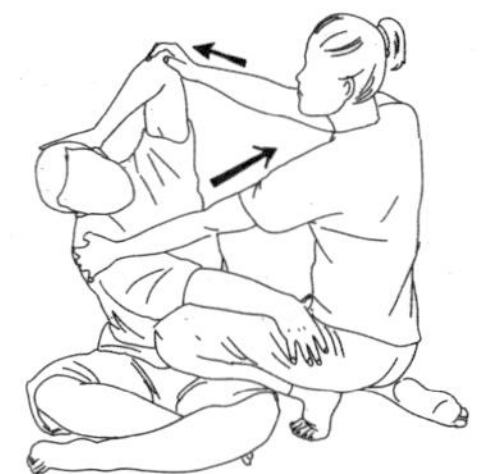

Seated Arm Lever
Position the subject in a cross-legged seated position with one arm bent in order to rest on the side of the head. Kneel next to the subject and, using one hand, grasp the subject's far shoulder and pull it towards you. Using the other hand simultaneously grasp the elbow of the subject's other arm and gradually push it in the opposite direction.

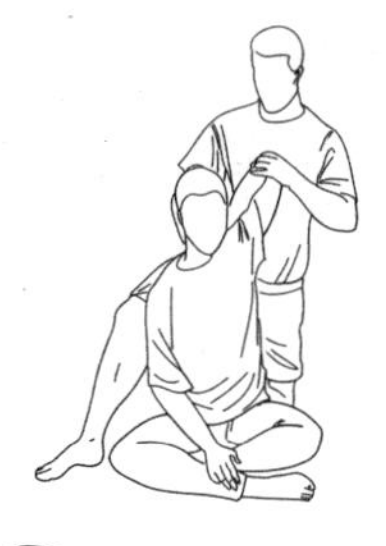

Backward Arm Lever
Position the subject in a seated position with one arm raised and bent at the elbow. Assume a kneeling position behind the subject and grasp the raised arm near the elbow. Gradually stretch the arm away from the body using a lever-like motion, taking care not to cause any discomfort.

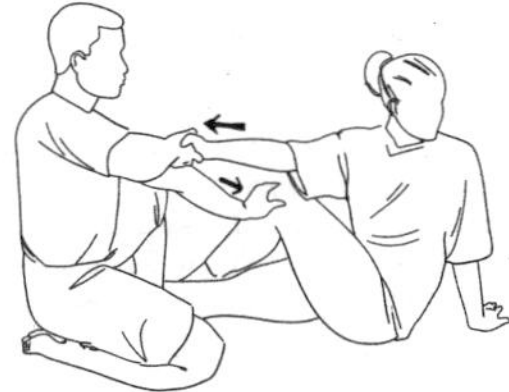

Sitting Spinal Twist
Position the subject in a seated position with one leg extended forwards and the other crossed over it. Kneel next to the subject and, using one hand, apply gradual pressure to the subject's crossed knee. Use the other hand to grasp the subject's hand and simultaneously pull the opposite arm away from the body and hold the stretch.

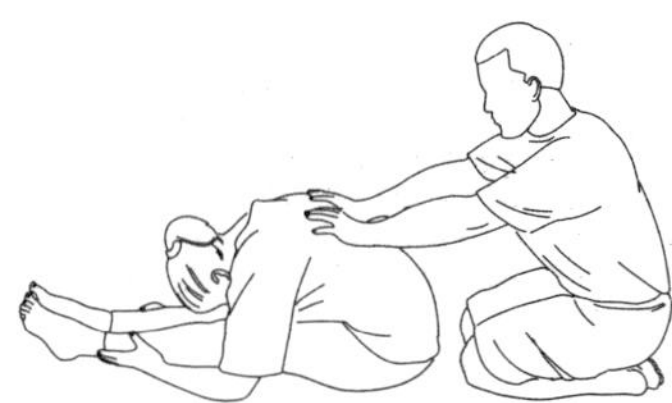

Head to Knee Press
Position the subject in a seated stretching position with both legs extended straight in front of them. Place both hands on the upper back and gently assist the stretch by gradually leaning forward if necessary.

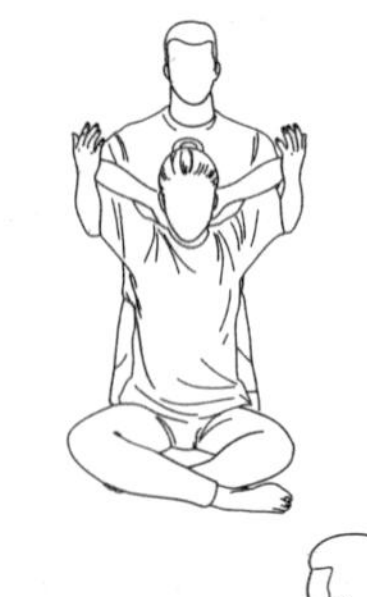

Butterfly Shoulder Stretch
Position the subject in a cross-legged seated position with both hands interlaced behind the neck. Assume a kneeling position behind the subject and, using both forearms, gradually draw the subject's arms towards your chest to hold the stretch.

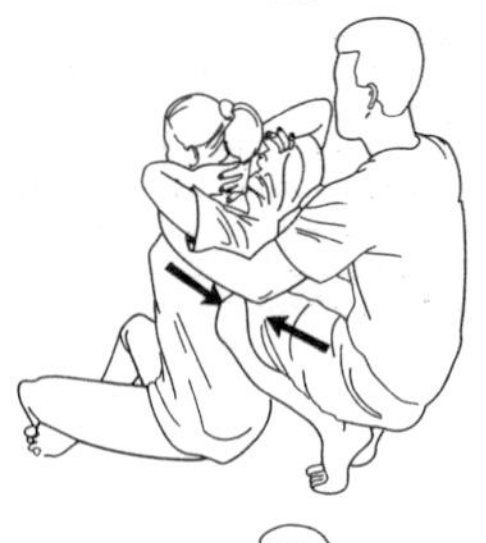

Backward Butterfly
Position the subject in a cross-legged seated position with both hands interlaced behind the neck. Place your knee against the subject's back and slightly below the shoulder blades. As you use both of your arms to draw the subject's towards your chest, simultaneously apply pressure to the subject's lower back using both knees.

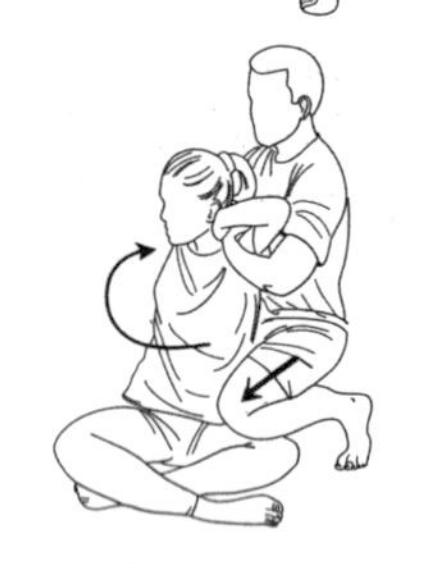

Butterfly Spinal Twist
Position the subject in a cross-legged seated position with both hands interlaced behind the neck. Wrap both arms around the subject's and gently rotate the subject at the torso. Use your knee to brace the subject while rotating the torso smoothly with a planted knee in a spinal twist and hold.

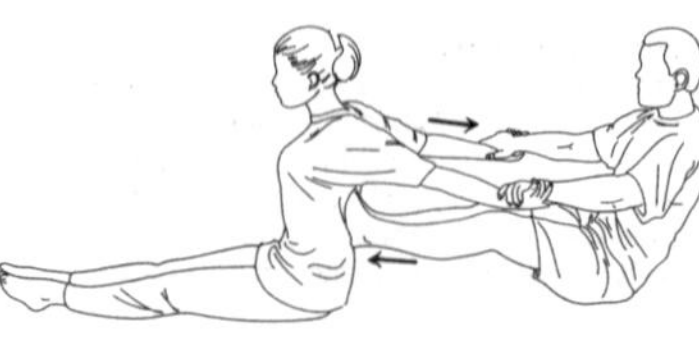

Walking on Back Feet Stretch
Position the subject in a seated position with both legs extended straight outwards and both arms extended in the opposite direction. Using both hands, grasp the subject's hands around the wrist and gradually lean backwards for gentle stretch. Simultaneously apply slight pressure from the balls of feet to the subject's lower back and sen lines with your body weight.

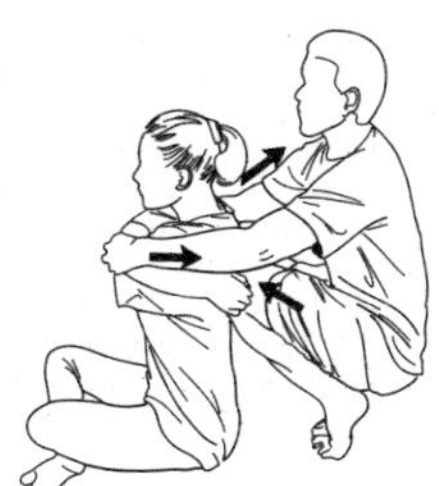

Upper Cross Arm Stretch
Position the subject in a cross-legged seated position with both arms crossed at the chest. Carefully place both knees against the subject's upper back and apply gradual pressure. Using both hands, simultaneously grasp the subject's elbows and pull upwards and backwards to apply the desired pressure.

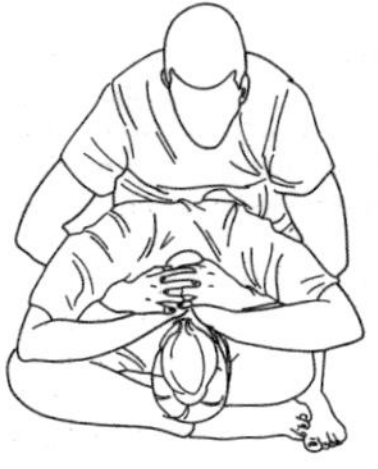

Butterfly Stretch
Position the subject in a forward-leaning, cross-legged seated position with both hands interlaced behind the neck. Assume a position behind the subject and weave your arms behind their own so as to interlace your fingers over the subject's. Gradually lean forward to stretch the neck and back while holding the position.

Tui na

Tui na uses Chinese taoist and martial arts principles to bring the body to balance. "Tui na" literally translates to "push pull" and is the name given to Chinese Medical Massage. Based on Traditional Chinese Medicine, (TCM) Tui na may actually predate the practice of acupuncture, with origins going back to Shennong era, 3000 B.C. and famous Chinese physician Jiu Daiji. It incorporates techniques that are similar to Western and Asian massage, chiropractic, osteopathic, and western physical therapy. Tui na uses a variety of hand massage techniques and passive and active stretching to restore correct anatomical musculo-skeletal relationships, neuromuscular patterns, and to increase the circulation of qi and blood to remove biochemical irritants. It works not just on the muscles, bones, and joints, but also with the energy of the body at a deeper level. Its objective is to keep the body's energy in balance, preventing injury and maintaining good health. Tui na uses rhythmic compression along energy channels of the body and a variety of techniques that manipulate and lubricate the joints. The therapist directly affects the flow of energy by holding and pressing the body at acupressure points.

Tui na balances the eight principles of TCM in which practitioners work on the areas between each of the joints, or "eight gates," to open the body's defensive qi, move the energy through the meridians, and get the muscles working. Brushing, kneading, rolling/pressing and rubbing are used to open the qi; then range of motion, traction, massage, and stimulation of acupressure points are used to treat the musculoskeletal physical conditions. In China, Tui na is used in hospital settings and is closer to the work of osteopaths, chiropractors and physical therapists. It may include some form of bone setting and manipulation. It is often used in conjunctive therapies in TCM with acupuncture, cupping, Chinese herbs, tai chi and qigong.

The following section focuses on basic hand techniques in Tui na and has been organized to illustrate techniques that are commonly used in traditional Western massage. Use good judgment when performing these techniques as "manual therapy" and not as "manipulation and bone setting" as they are not covered under the massage therapist's scope of practice in certain regions and states. Some external herbal poultices, compresses, liniments, and salves can also be used to enhance the other therapeutic methods. See page 36 for a listing topical applications used with manual therapy.

In China, the concept of Tui na is part of the rigorous TCM training. The main schools in China include the rolling method school which emphasizes manual therapy soft tissue techniques and specializes in joint injuries and muscle sprains. Rolling uses the back of the hand and knuckles against the body at a rapid pace, using relaxed forearm and flexed wrist. The one-finger pushing method school emphasizes techniques for acupressure and the treatment of internal diseases that have many parallels that to Shiatsu. Another school is the Nei Gung method, which emphasizes the use of qi gong energy generation exercises and specific massage methods for revitalizing depleted energy systems. Practitioners of the qi gong school use exercises to increase their ability focus, control, and emit their body's energy. With proper training, these skills allow the practitioner to feel, diagnose, and heal injuries and energetic imbalances in the client. The bone-setting method school emphasizes manipulation methods to realign the musculoskeletal issues, joint injuries, and nerve pain which have similarities to chiropractic, physical therapy, and osteopathic manual therapy.

Tui: pushing/pulling
Na: pulling/grasping
Tao: strong pinching pressure
Nie: kneading
Moa: rubbing
An: rapid, rhythmic pressing
Rou: kneading

Dian: finger pressing
Ca: rubbing
Gun: rolling
Zhen: vibrating
Cuo: twisting/rubbing
Mo: wiping
Tina: lifting and grasping

Anrou: pressing
Boyun: forearm kneading
Ji: beating or drumming
Pai: tapping/patting
Dou: shaking
Yao: rotating
Ban: pulling
Bashen: extending

Recommended reading and resources on Tui na Therapy:

Jinxue Li, Chinese Manipulation and Massage: Chinese Manipulative Therapy, Elsevier Science, London, England, 1990.

Maria Mercati, The Handbook of Chinese Massage: Tui Na Techniques to Awaken Body and Mind, Healing Arts Press, Rochester, VT, 1997.

Sarah Pritchard, Chinese Massage Manual: The Healing Art of Tui Na, Sterling, New York, NY, 1999.

Shen Guoquan & Yan Juntao, Illustrations of Tuina Manipulations, Shanghai Scientific & Technical Publisher, Shanghai, China, 2004.

Sun Chengnan, Chinese Bodywork: A Complete Manual of Chinese Therapeutic Massage, Pacific View Press, Shanghai, China, 2000.

Sun Shuchun, Atlas of Therapeutic Motion for Treatment and Health: A Guide to Traditional Chinese Massage and Exercise Therapy, Foreign Languages Press, Beijing, China, 1989.

Wang Fu, Chinese Tuina Therapy, Foreign Languages Press, Beijing, China, 1994.

Xu Xiangcai, Chinese Tui Na Massage: The Essential Guide to Treating Injuries, Improving Health & Balancing Qi, YMAA Publication Center, Jamaica Plains, MA, 2002.

Wei Guikang, Illustrated Therapeutic Manipulation in TCM Orthopedics and Traumatology, Shanghai Scientific and Technical Publishers, Shanghai, China 2003.

Zhang Enqin, Chinese Massage: A Practical English-Chinese Library of Traditional Chinese Medicine, Publishing House of Shanghai College of Traditional Chinese Medicine, Shanghai, China, 1992

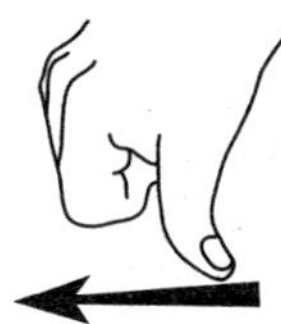

Kneading / Pushing with Thumbs
Press your thumb to the desired spot and knead/push in a straightforward direction. Use all of your fingers, if desired.

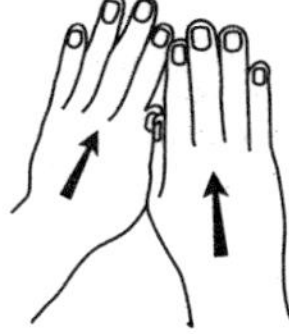

Pushing with Both Hands
Using the palm of one hand or both hands, apply pressure to the desired area and work the surrounding muscles in a straightforward direction. Modify in intensity to the needs of the subject.

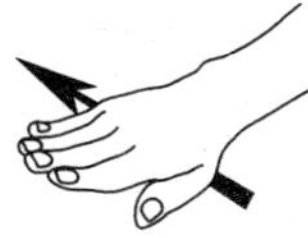

Kneading / Pushing with Thenar Eminence
Using the entire hand, press your palm to the desired spot in a straight forward direction. Work your hand around the designated area and modify the intensity if desired.

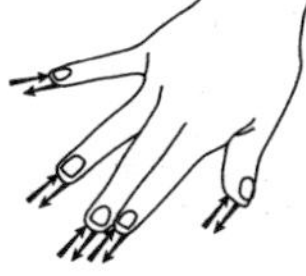

Rubbing with Fingers
Press your thumb and fingers against the skin and rub back and forth. If you desire, use both hands simultaneously.

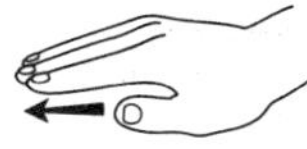

Flat Palm Pushing
Using the heel of the hand and flat palm, apply pressure to the desired area in a straight forward direction. Work your hand around the designated area and modify the intensity if desired.

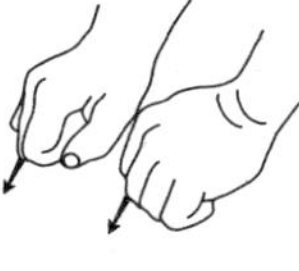

Pushing with Both Fists
Using a loose fist palm down, apply pressure to the desired area and work the surrounding muscles. Modify in intensity to the needs of the subject.

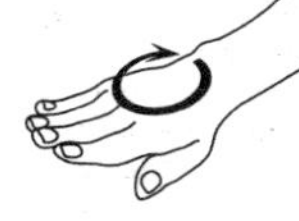

Round Rubbing with Palm
Using the entire hand, press your palm to the desired spot in a circular motion. Work your hand around the designated area and modify the intensity if desired.

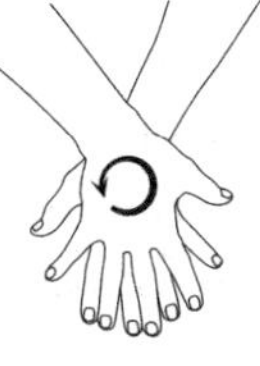

Round Rubbing
Using one hand on top of the other hand, apply pressure to the desired area and work the surrounding muscles in a circular motion. Modify in intensity to the needs of the subject.

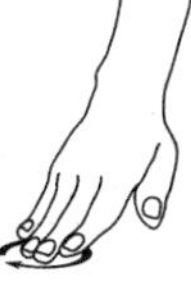

Round Rubbing with Fingers
Using the tips of all four fingers to the desired spot in a circular motion. Work your hand around the designated area and modify the intensity if desired.

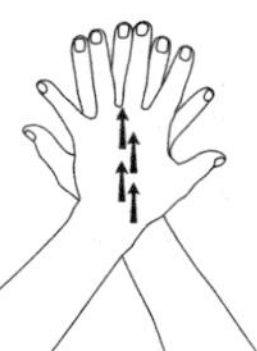

Intermittent Pushing
Using one hand on top of the other hand, apply pressure to the desired area and work the surrounding muscles in an intermittent pushing motion. Modify in intensity to the needs of the subject.

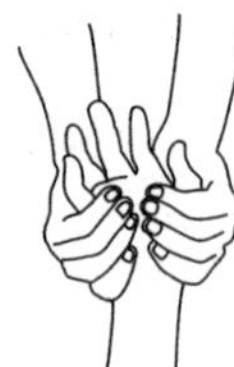

Palm Opening
Grasp the hand with your fingers and thumbs by squeezing and stretching the hands away by opening the palms.

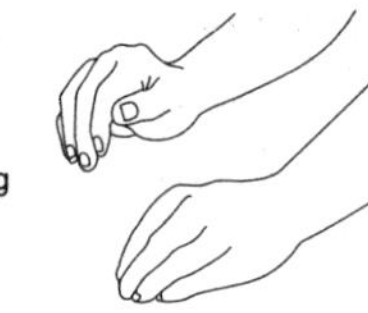

Cupping
Using a cupped palm, knock the desired area and gradually increase in intensity, if desired. Knock rhythmically and repeatedly with both hands down.

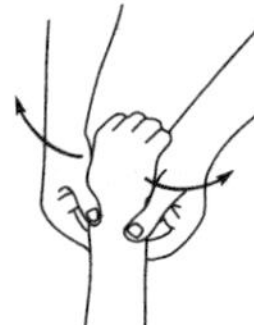

Hand Rotating
Grasp the wrist with your fingers and thumbs and apply rotating circular strokes to the hands and wrist area in a to and fro motion.

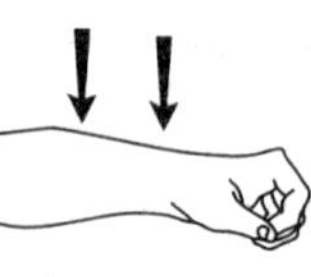

Deep Forearm Pressure
Using the forearm, apply pressure to the desired area of the subject. Rock back and forth to work the area. Or hold forearm to reinforce pressure, if desired.

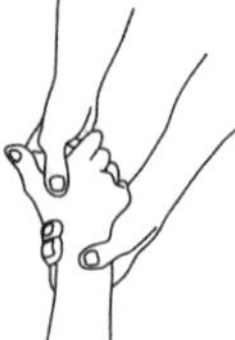

Wrist Cleaning
Support the wrist with your hands, and use your thumb and fingers to apply stokes in between the bones and grooves of the hands, wrists and webs of each finger.

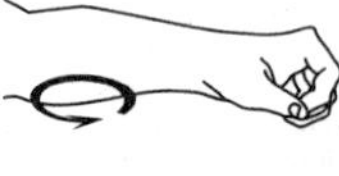

Forearm Revolving
Using your forearm, apply long, revolving strokes to the desired area. Consult with the client on the intensity and area of application. Continue until the area is warmed up.

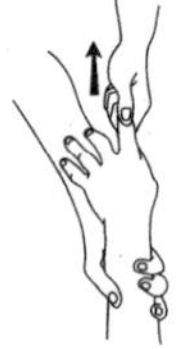

Finger Pulling / Finger Wringing
Enclose the thumb of each finger as you gently pull, stretch and twist each finger. Slide your hand down and off the each finger tip. Release and repeat on each individual finger.

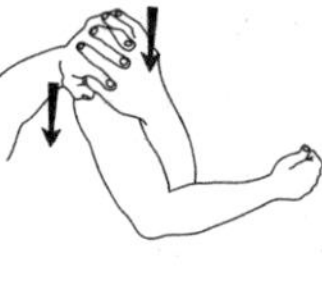

Interlocking Hand Squeeze/ Straight Pulling
Using both hands, grasp and interlock fingers over the top and squeeze from heels of the hand. Pull the desired area in a straight downward motion. Release and repeat, if desired.

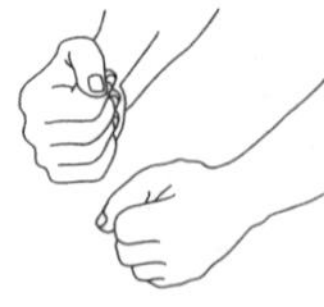

Pummeling
Using a loose clenched fist, apply alternating and simultaneous fists up and down to the desired area and increase in intensity, if desired.

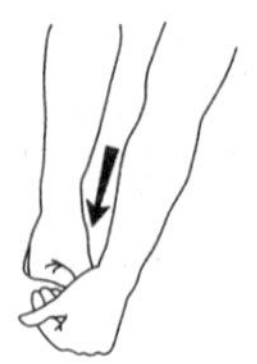

Deep Compression / Ironing
Using closed fists with both hands and locked elbows directly in line with your arm, apply direct fist pressure to the desired area of the subject. Release and repeat, if desired.

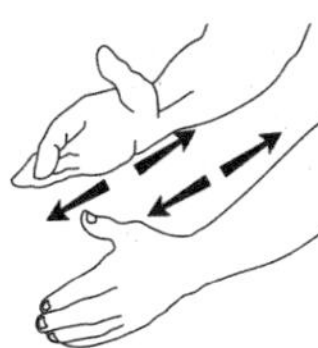

Chafing
Using both hands with palms facing each other, apply direct contact to the desired area and apply quick repetitive back and forth sawing motion, creating friction and increase in intensity if desired.

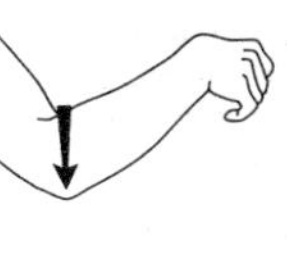

Elbow Pressing
Using a bent elbow, apply gradual to heavy pressure to the desired area using the tip of the elbow as a focal point. Work your elbow around the desired area, if desired.

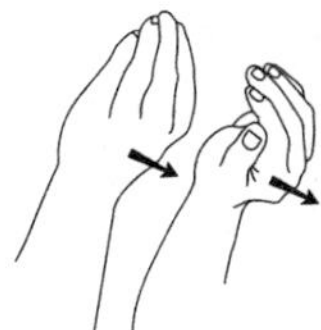

Knocking with Back Hands
Using the back of the hand, knock the desired area and gradually increase in intensity, if desired. Knock rhythmically and repeatedly.

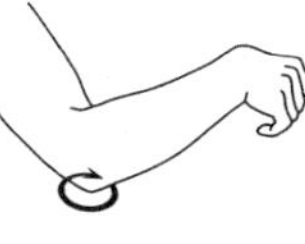

Elbow Revolving
Using your elbow, apply long, revolving strokes to the desired area. Modify in intensity to the needs of the subject.

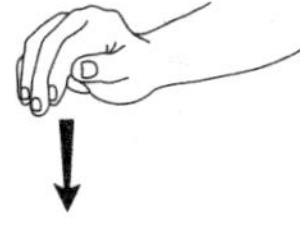

Knocking with Cupped Palm
Using a cupped palm, with all fingers slightly bent, knock the desired area and gradually increase in intensity, if desired. Knock rhythmically and repeatedly.

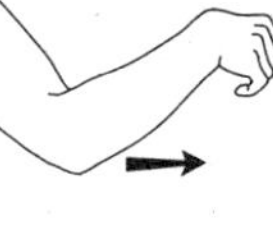

Elbow Pushing
Using your elbow, with a relaxed, flexed wrist, apply long, deep strokes to the desired area, pushing forward with the elbow, taking care not to cause any discomfort.

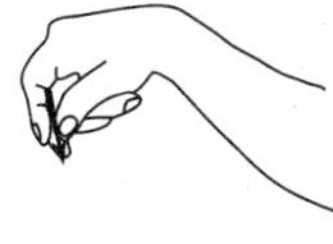

Dotting / Tapping / Pecking
Using the tips of the fingers, tap and peck the desired area. Modify intensity, if desired. Using the middle finger, tap the desired area.

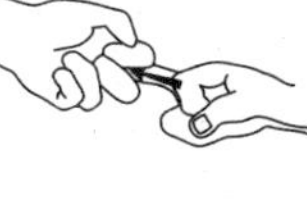

Rectifying Finger Pulling
Using the knuckles of your bent index and middle fingers, hold, compress or stroke the fingers, applying a pulling stretch from the root to the tip. Release and repeat on each finger and gradually increase in intensity if desired.

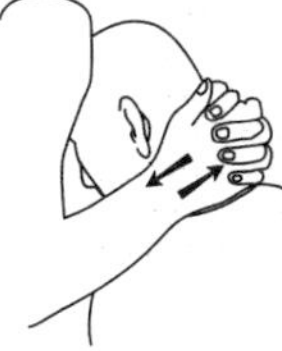

Rubbing with Joined Hands
Using both hands in an interlaced grip, apply pressure to the desired area of the subject's body. Work your grip across the area and repeat until you achieve the desired effects.

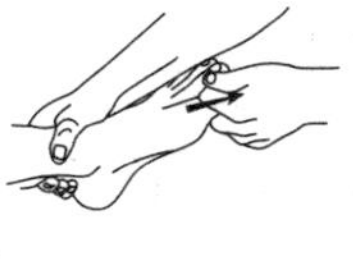

Rectifying Toe Pulling
Using the knuckles of your bent index and middle fingers, hold, compress or stroke the toes, applying a pulling stretch from the base to the tip of the toe. Tug and twist from side to side as your fingers slide off and down each toe tip. Release and repeat on each toe and gradually increase in intensity, if desired.

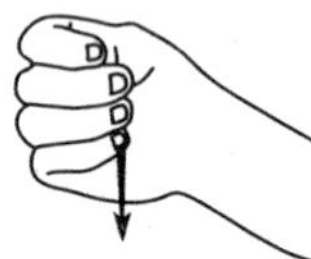

Open Fist Pounding
Using an open fist, gently pound the desired area rhythmically and repeatedly. Gradually increase in intensity, if desired.

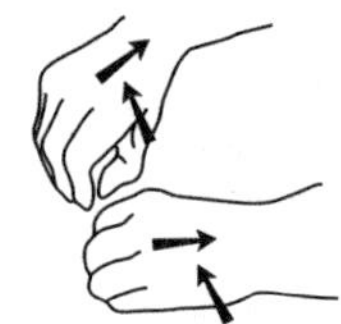

Plucking / Grasping
Using both hands, apply a pluck-like pressure to the designated area and repeat rhythmically.

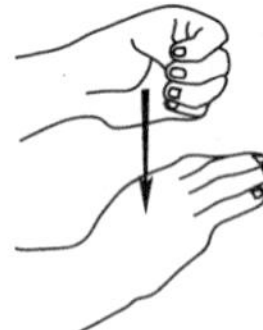

Padded Pounding
Using a cupped palm grip, gently pound the desired area with the fist. Gradually increase in intensity, if desired.

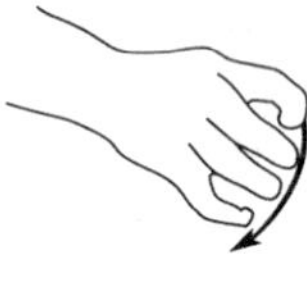

Nipping / Grasping
Using both hands in a hook-like fashion, work the subject's joints and other designated areas. Work your way across the body, if desired.

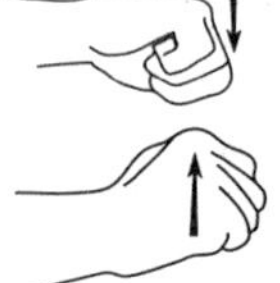

Prone Fist Pounding
Using a fist with the fingers clenched and facing downwards, gently pound the desired area rhythmically and repeatedly. Gradually increase in intensity, if desired.

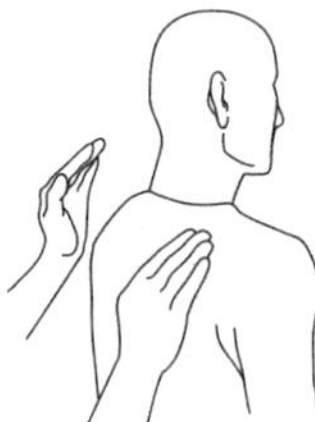

Palm Cupping / Patting
Using a cupped palm, pat the desired area and gradually increase in intensity, if desired. Pat rhythmically and repeatedly.

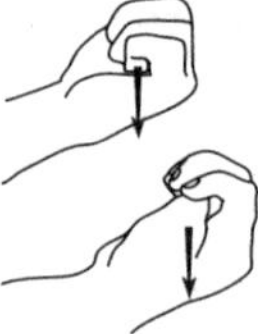

Knocking with Back Hands/ Supine Fist Pounding
With the fingers facing up, gently pound the desired area with the back of the fist. Gradually increase in intensity, if desired.

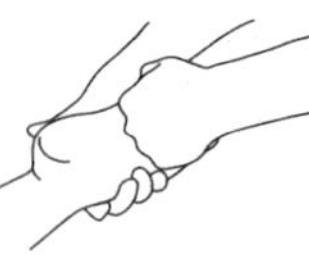

Knuckle Rolling
Using a closed tighten fist, apply knuckle pressure and strokes to the desired area and work the surrounding muscles. Modify in intensity to the needs of the subject.

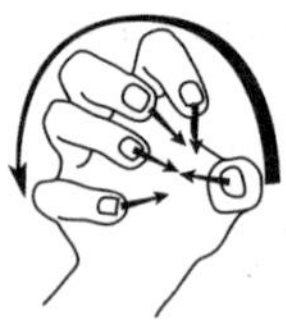

Grabbing / Grasping
Grasp the desired area with one or both hands and pull it away from the subject's body. Quickly release the tissue and repeat in a rhythmic pattern. Increase in intensity, if desired.

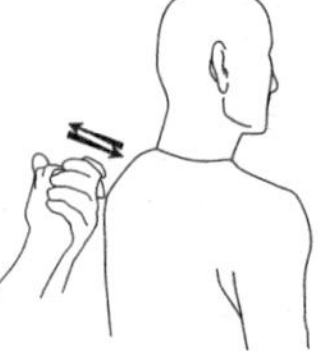

Double Cupping
Using a cupped palm to cushion the air with cupped hands, knock the desired area and gradually increase in intensity, if desired. Cupped rhythmically and repeatedly.

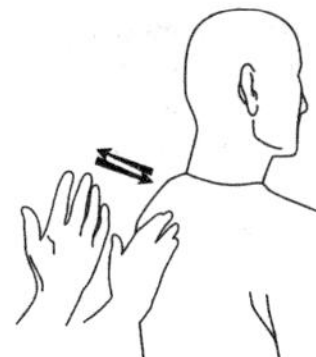

Loose Finger Chopping
Using both hands, apply alternate or simultaneous chops, knock the desired area and gradually increase in intensity, if desired. Chop rhythmically and repeatedly.

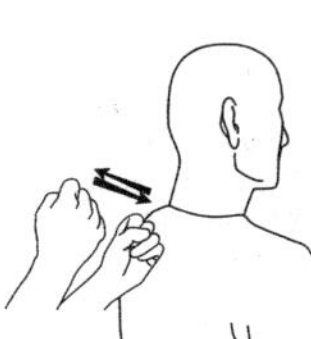

Loose Fist Pummeling
Using loose closed fist, apply alternate or simultaneous chops, knock the desired area and gradually increase in intensity, if desired. Pummel rhythmically and repeatedly.

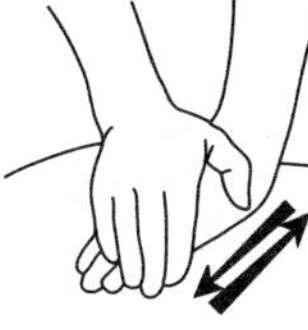

Rocking / Vibrating
Using one hand on top of the other hand, apply pressure to the desired area and work the surrounding muscles in a back-and-forth motion. A continuous trembling motion can be applied with the hands or fingers. Modify in intensity to the needs of the subject.

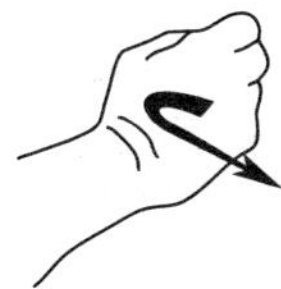

Palm Rolling
Using a loose fist, roll your hand out back and forth across the designated area with flexion and extension of the wrist. Adjust the fingers so that they stretch when the fist rolls out and contract when it is brought in.

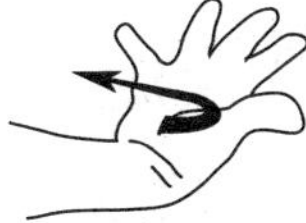

One Hand Rolling
With the fingers stretched outwards, roll your hand out back and forth across the designated area with flexion and extension of the wrist. Adjust the fingers so that they stretch when the fist rolls out and contract when it is brought in. Continue to roll your hands back and forth to work the surrounding areas.

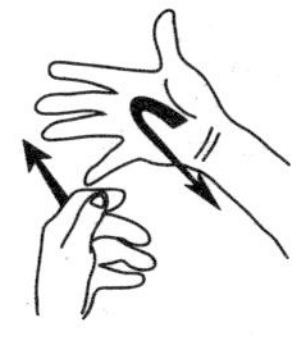

Two Palms Rolling
With two hands alternate palms rolling outwards, rolling your hand and palms back and forth across the designated area with flexion and extension of the wrist. Adjust the fingers so that they stretch when the fist rolls out and contract when it is brought in. Continue to roll your hands back and forth to work the surrounding areas.

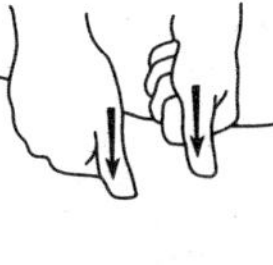

Closed Hand Thumb Pressing
Using an extended thumb directly in line with your arm, apply direct pressure with thumbs supported against index finger with a closed hand. Gradually increase in intensity, if desired.

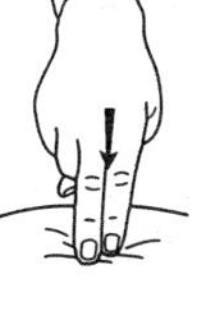

Two Fingers Pressing
Using the two middle fingers directly in line with your arm, apply direct pressure with the fingers supported against index finger with a closed hand. Gradually increase in intensity, if desired.

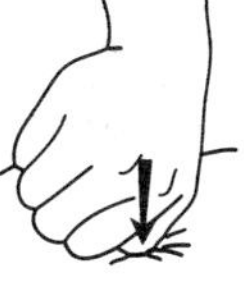

Joint Thumb Pressing
Using interphalangeal joint of the thumb with a hollow fist directly in line with your arm, apply direct pressure with the joint of the thumbs. Gradually increase in intensity, if desired.

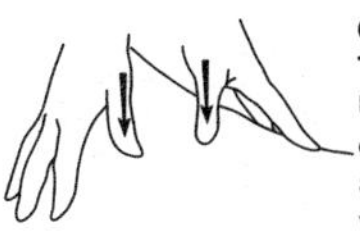

Open Hand Thumb Pressing
Using an extended thumb directly in line with your arm, apply direct pressure with four fingers spread with an open hand. Gradually increase in intensity, if desired.

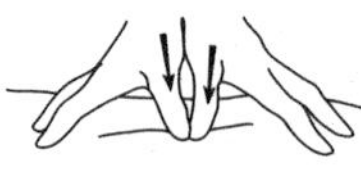

Open Hand Adjacent Thumb Pressing
Using an extended thumb directly in line with your arm, apply direct pressure with thumbs side by side supported against each other with an open hand. Gradually increase in intensity, if desired.

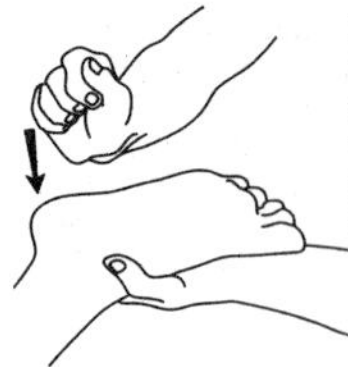

Foot and Heel Pummeling
Using an open fist, gently pound the sole of the foot rhythmically and repeatedly. Gradually increase in intensity, if desired.

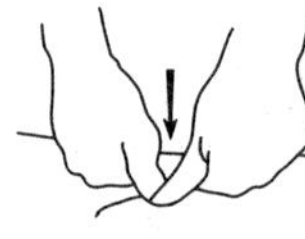

Closed Hand Overlap Thumb Pressing
Using an extended thumb directly in line with your arm, apply direct pressure with thumbs on top of each other with a closed hand. Gradually increase in intensity, if desired.

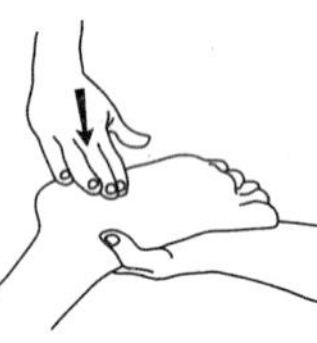

Foot Slapping
Using a relaxed wrist, gently slap the sole of the foot rhythmically and repeatedly. Gradually increase in intensity, if desired.

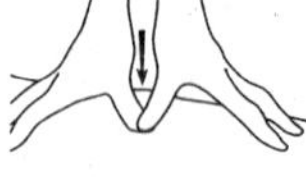

Open Hand Overlap Thumb Pressing
Using an extended thumb directly in line with your arm, apply direct pressure with thumbs on top of each other with an open hand. Gradually increase in intensity, if desired.

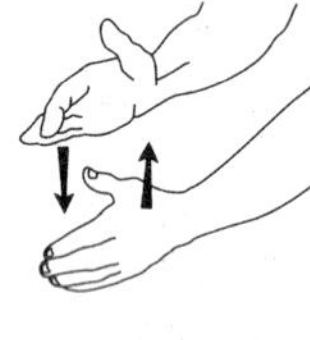

Hacking
Using both hands with palms facing each other, apply alternating and simultaneous chops up and down to the desired area and increase in intensity, if desired.

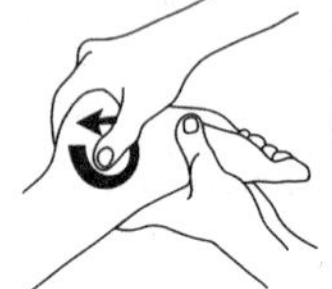

Heel Kneading
Hold the foot firmly and apply circular strokes with your thumbs to the heels of the foot.

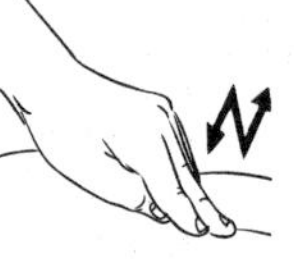

Vibrating
Using one or more fingers, apply pressure to the desired area and vibrate. Work your way around the area, if desired.

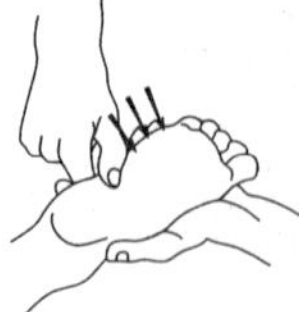

Foot Pinching
Hold the foot firmly and apply direct pressure with thumbs to the insides and outside edges of the foot.

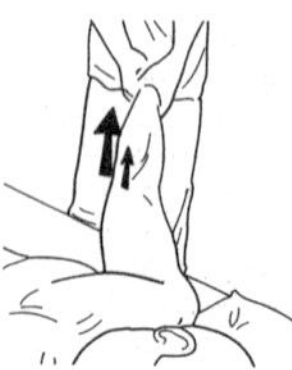

Arm Shaking
Using both hands, grasp the wrist firmly. Pull gently with slight traction to stretch the arm and simultaneously shake the arm up and down with small movements.

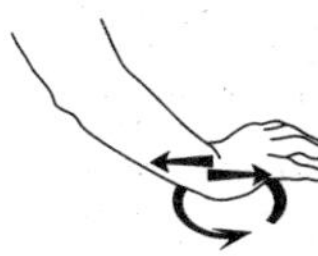

Palming with Vibrating
Using the thenar eminence of the palm, apply pressure to the desired area and work the surrounding muscles in an alternating circular and vibrating motion to generate pressure. Modify in intensity to the needs of the subject.

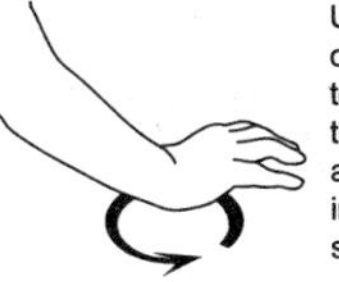

Revolving
Using the thenar eminence of the palm, apply pressure to the desired area and work the surrounding muscles in a circular motion. Modify in intensity to the needs of the subject.

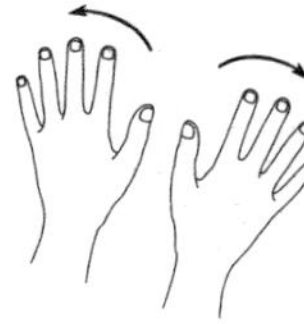

Double Hand Whisking
Apply pressure with both hands to the desired area and, in a sweep-like motion, brush and glide the hands across the tissue to generate pressure, gradually increasing in speed and intensity.

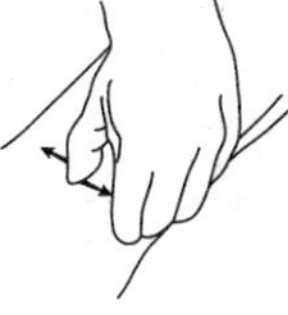

Finger Plucking
Nip the selected point with one or more fingernails. Nipping with the thumbnail alone is called a single-finger method and moving the fingernail back and forth is called plucking. Modify in intensity to the needs of the subject.

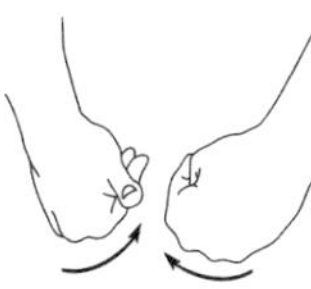

Knuckling
Using a closed tight fist, apply knuckle pressure to the desired area and work the surrounding muscles. Modify in intensity to the needs of the subject.

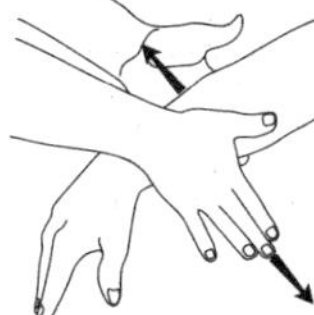

Arm Rolling
Support arm between your hands, roll your hands back and forth rapidly. Roll hands loosely from wrist up to elbow and shoulders.

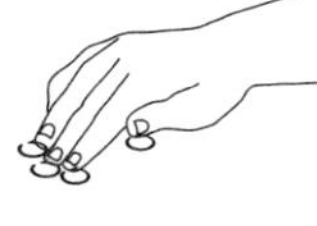

Round Rubbing with Fingers
Using the tips of all fingers, apply pressure to the desired area and work the surrounding muscles in small circular strokes. Modify in intensity to the needs of the subject.

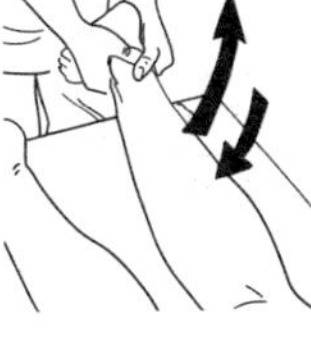

Leg Shaking
Using both hands, grasp the ankle firmly. Lift the leg off the table, pull gently with slight traction to stretch the leg and simultaneously shake the leg up and down with small movements into the hip and the rest of the body.

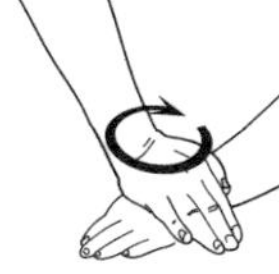

Cross Palm Revolving
Using one hand on top of the other hand, apply pressure to the desired area and work the surrounding muscles in a circular motion. Modify in intensity to the needs of the subject.

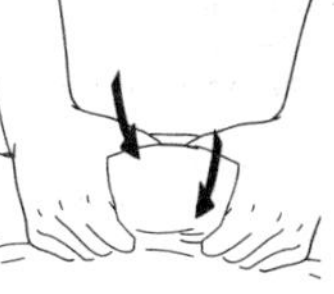

Wringing / Grasping and Lifting
Using both hands, grasp and lift desired area symmetrically to desired area. Gradually increase in intensity, if desired.

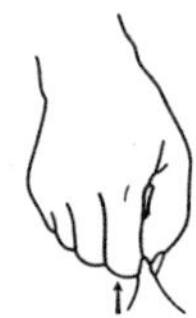

Tearing / Twisting
Grasp and pinch between thumb and fingers in a twisting manner. Gradually increase in intensity, if desired.

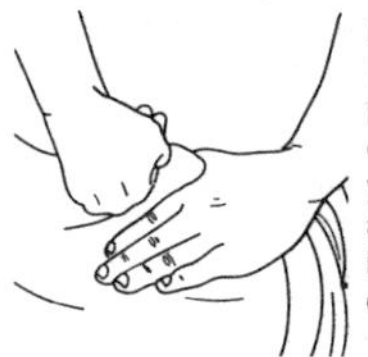

Petrissage / Kneading 2
Using two hands with fist pushing into grasping hand on the desired spot. Move your fingers and hands in a to-and-fro motion, which includes rolling, squeezing, or pressing the muscles.

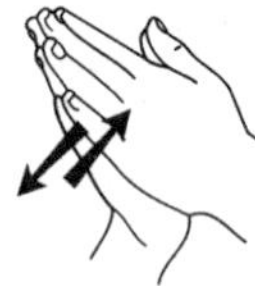

Double Hand Chopping
Using both hands with palms joined together with fingers stretched out and separated, apply quick repetitive up-and-down chopping motion to desired area. Gradually increase in intensity, if desired.

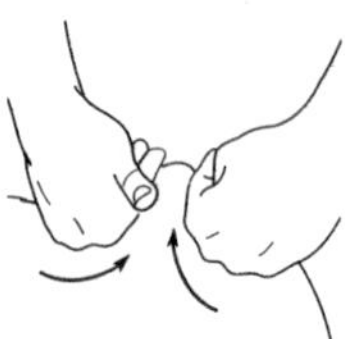

Petrissage / Kneading 3
Using two loose fists, lift and grasp the desired spot. Move your fingers and hands in a to and fro motion which includes rolling, squeezing, or pressing the muscles.

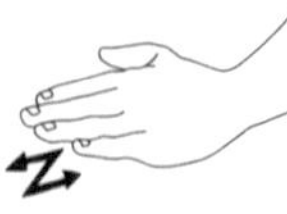

Vibrating Palms
Using the heel of the hand and flat palm apply pressure to the desired area and vibrate vigorously. Work your way around the area, if desired.

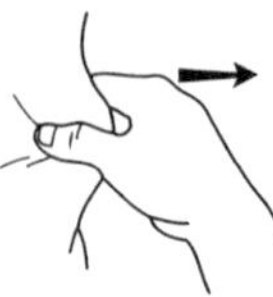

Plucking
Grasp and pull the desired area with tip of the thumb and fingers as if you are playing a guitar. Gradually increase in intensity, if desired.

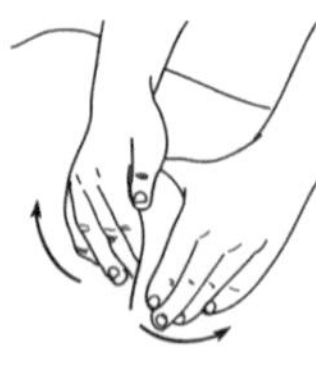

Petrissage / Kneading 1
Press the fingers or your hand on the desired spot as if you are kneading dough. Move your fingers and hands in a to-and-fro circular motion which includes rolling, squeezing, or pressing the muscles.

While in acupuncture school, I had the opportunity to study under Wei Guikang, who was the former president of Guangxi College of TCM and director of Guangxi International Association of Manipulation Medicine. The following section is dedicated to Professor Wei who was a source of inspiration in my development and education in Chinese Massage Therapy.

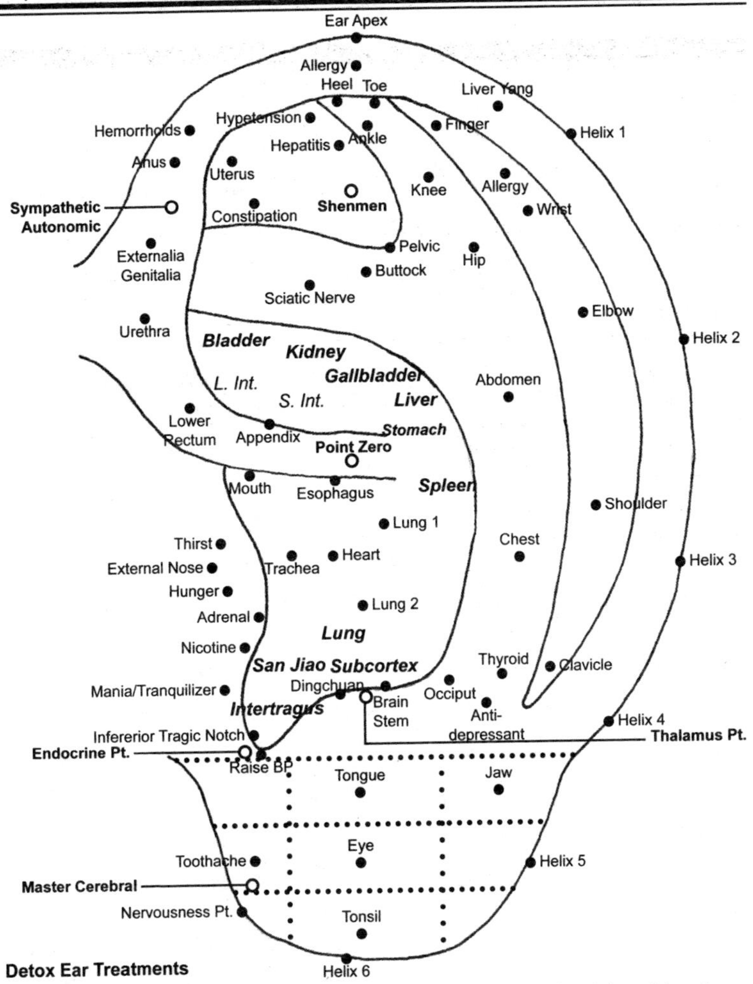

Detox Ear Treatments

Auricular therapy without needles can be as effective tool for massage therapist. Stimulating points on the ear with ear probes, seeds, tacks, and pellets can alleviate a variety of conditions in any part of the body. The National Acupuncture Detoxification Association **(NADA)** and American College of Addictionology and Compulsive Disorders **(ACACD)** auricular acupuncture protocol are used around the world to help people deal with and recover from substance abuse. The **NADA** and **ACACD** protocol has been shown in a variety of clinical settings to be beneficial in the process of detoxification from substance abuse as well as to help with the emotional, physical and psychological attributes involved in addictions.

NADA Protocol

Lung 2	Addiction-related lung issues
Shen Men	Stress, anxiety, excessive sensitivity
Autonomic	Balance sympathetic and parasympathetic nervous systems, blood circulation
Liver	Hepatitis, cirrhosis
C. Kidney	Kidney disorders, urination issues

ACACD Protocol

Point Zero	General homeostatic balance
Shen Men	Stress, anxiety, excessive sensitivity
Autonomic	Balance sympathetic and parasympathetic nervous systems, blood circulation
C. Kidney	Kidney disorders, urination issues
Brain	Pituitary gland, endocrine glands, addictions, sleep
Limbic System or *Master Cerebral*	Aggressiveness, compulsive behavior

Condition	Protocols
Acne	Face, Skin, Lung 1 & 2, Point Zero, Shenmen
Alcoholism	Alcoholic Point, Liver, Lung 1, Lung 2, Brain, Occiput, Forehead, Kidney, Point Zero, Shenmen, Lesser Occipital Nerve
Allergy	Apex of the Ear, Allergy Point, Omega 2, Inner Nose, Asthma, Point Zero, Shenmen, Sympathetic, Endocrine
Anxiety	Nervousness, Master Cerebral, Tranquilizer Point, Heart, Point Zero, Shenmen, Sympathetic
Back Pain	Thoracic Spine, Lumbosacral Spine, Buttock, Sciatic Nerve, Lumbago, Lumbar Spin, Pint Zero, Shenmen, Thalamus Point
Cancer	Corresponding body area, Thymus Gland, Vitality Point, Heart, Point Zero, Shenmen, Thyroid Gland
Carpal Tunnel	Wrist I-III Forearm, Hand, Thoracic Spin, Point Zero, Shenmen, Thalamus
Chronic fatigue	Vitality Point, Antidepressant, Brain, ACTH, Adrenal Gland, Point Zero, Shenmen, Master Oscillation
Common Cold	Inner Nose, Throat, Forehead, Lung 1 & 2, Asthma, Prostaglandin 1 & 2, Ear Apex
Constipation	Constipation, Large Intestines, Rectum, Omega 1, Abdomen
Cough	Asthma, Antihistamine, Point Zero, Adrenal Gland, Throat 1 & 2, Lung 1 & 2
Depression	Antidepressant, Brain, Excitement Pint, Pineal Gland, Master Cerebral, Shenmen, Sympathetic
Diarrhea	Small Intestines, Large Intestines, Point Zero, Shenmen, Sympathetic
Dizziness	Dizziness, Inner Ear, Cerebellum, Occiput, Lesser Occipital Nerve, Point Zero,
Drug Addiction	Lung 1, Lung 2, Shenmen, Sympathetic, Endocrine, Liver, Kidney, Brain
Fibromyalgia	Thoracic Spine, Lumbosacral Spine, Muscle Relaxation, Antidepressant, Point Zero, Shenmen, Thalamus
Headaches	Temples, Lesser Occipital Nerve, Vagus Nerve, Shenmen, Kidney, Thalamus Point, Cervical Spine
Hypertension	Hypertension 1 & 2, Heart, Sympathetic, Point Zero, Shenmen
Hyperthyroidism	Thyroid Gland, Point Zero, Shenmen, Endocrine, Brain, Master Oscillation, Apex of the Ear
Infertility	Uterus, Ovary, Shenmen, Point Zero, External Genitalia, Endocrine, Adrenal, Kidney, Abdomen, Brain
Insomnia	Insomnia 1 & 2, Pineal Gland, Heart, Master Cerebral, Point Zero, Shenmen, Thalamus Point, Forehead, Occiput, Brain, Kidney
Memory Loss	Frontal Cortex, Hippocampus, Memory 1 & 2, Master Cerebral, Heart, Point Zero, Shenmen
Multiple Sclerosis	Corresponding body area, Brainstem, Medulla Oblongata, Master Oscillation, Point Zero, Thalamus Point, Thymus Gland, Vitality
Muscle Sprain	Corresponding body area, Heat Point, Point Zero, Shenmen, Thalamus Point, Adrenal Gland, Liver, Spleen, Kidney
PMS	Uterus, Ovary, Endocrine, Shenmen
Rheumatoid Arthritis	Corresponding body area, Omega 2, Prostaglandin 1 & 2, Allergy Point, Adrenal Gland, Point Zero, Shenmen, Thalamus Point, Endocrine Point
Sciatica	Sciatica Nerve, Buttocks, Lumbago, Lumbar Spin, Hip, Thigh, Calf , Point Zero, Shenmen, Thalamus Point, Adrenal, Kidney, Bladder
Shoulder Pain	Shoulder, Shoulder Phase II, Master Shoulder, Clavicle, Cervical Spine, Thoracic Spine
Sinusitis	Inner Nose, Frontal Sinus, Forehead, Occiput, Point Zero, Shenmen, Adrenal
Smoking	Nicotine, Lung 1, Lung 2, Mouth, Point Zero, Shenmen, Sympathetic, Brain
Sore throat	Throat, Mouth, Trachea, Tonsil 1-4
Stress	Adrenal Gland, Tranquilizer Point, Point Zero, Shenmen, Master Cerebral, Muscle Relaxation
Stroke	Corresponding body area, Brain, Adrenal Gland, ACTH, Shenmen, Sympathetic, Master Cerebral, Endocrine
Tennis Elbow	Elbow Phase I-III, Forearm, Thoracic Spine, Point Zero, Shenmen, Thalamus Point, Muscle Relaxation Point, Adrenal, Kidney, Occiput
Tinnitus	Inner Ear, External Ear, Auditory Nerve, Kidney, Point Zero, Shenmen, San Jiao
TMJ	TMJ, Upper Jaw, Lower Jaw, Cervical Spine, Trigeminal Nerve, Occiput
Toothache	Toothache 1-3, Upper Jaw, Lower Jaw, Trigeminal Nerve, Shenmen
Weight Control	Appetite, Stomach, Mouth, Esophagus, Small Intestines, Shenmen, Point Zero

Source: Oleson, Terry, *Auriculotherapy Manual 3rd Edition*, 2003, Churchill Livingston, London, England.

REFLEXOLOGY

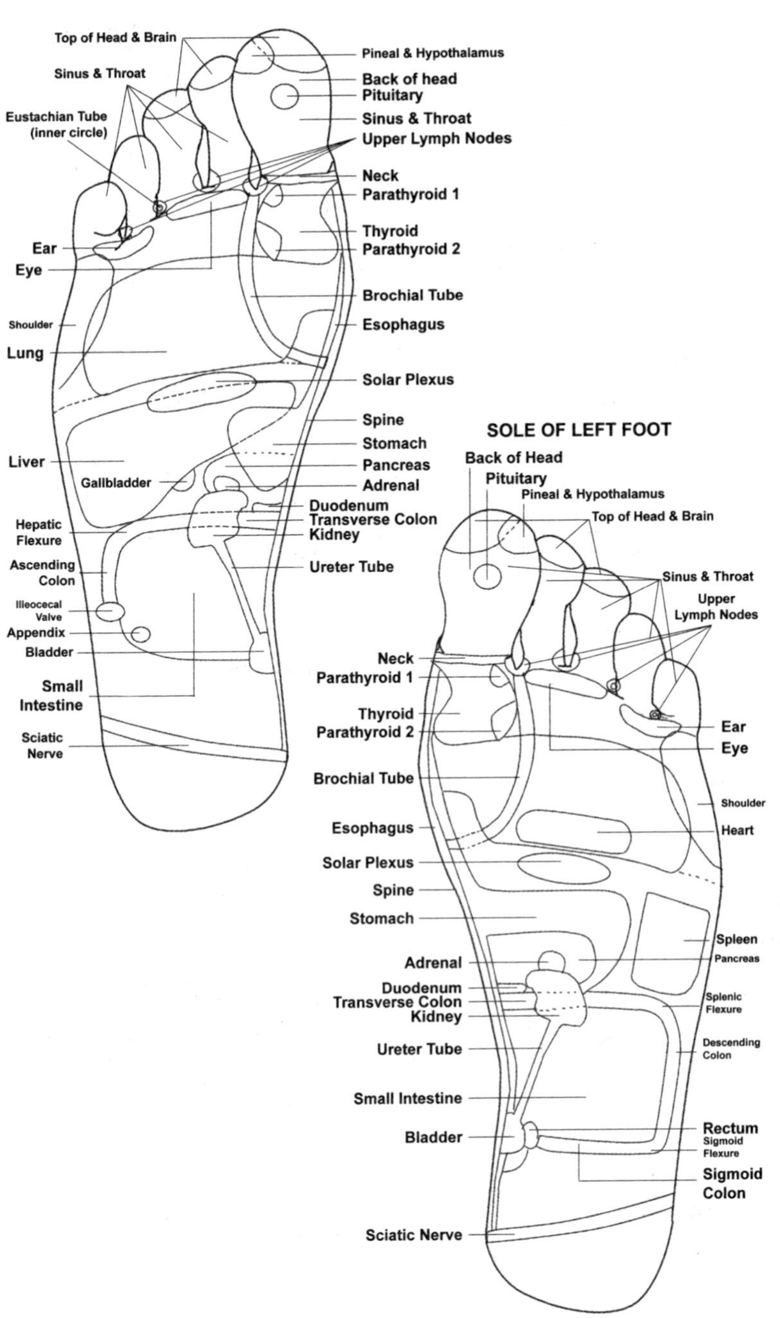

REFLEXOLOGY

MEDIAL FOOT

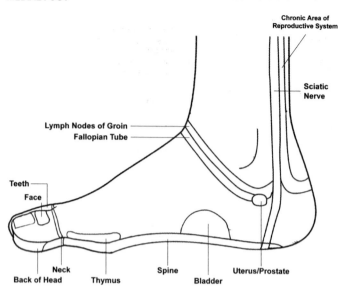

Chronic Area of Reproductive System
Sciatic Nerve
Lymph Nodes of Groin
Fallopian Tube
Teeth
Face
Neck
Back of Head
Thymus
Spine
Bladder
Uterus/Prostate

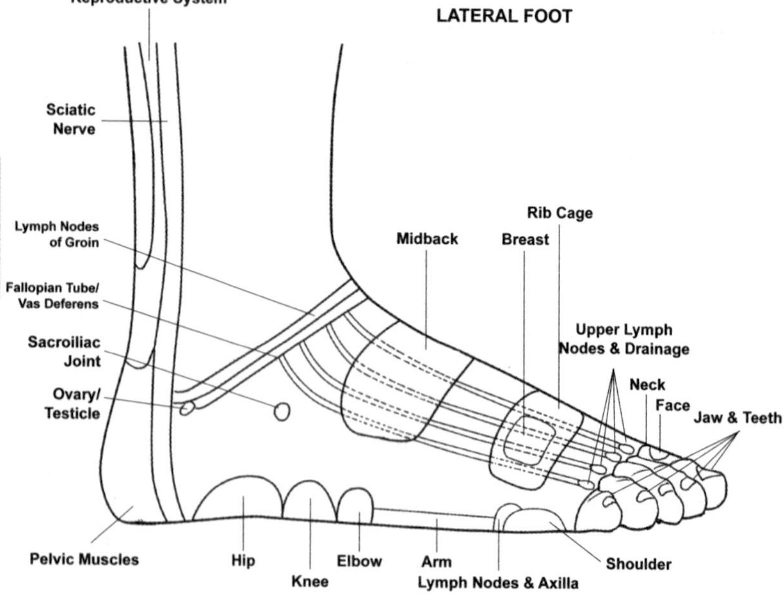

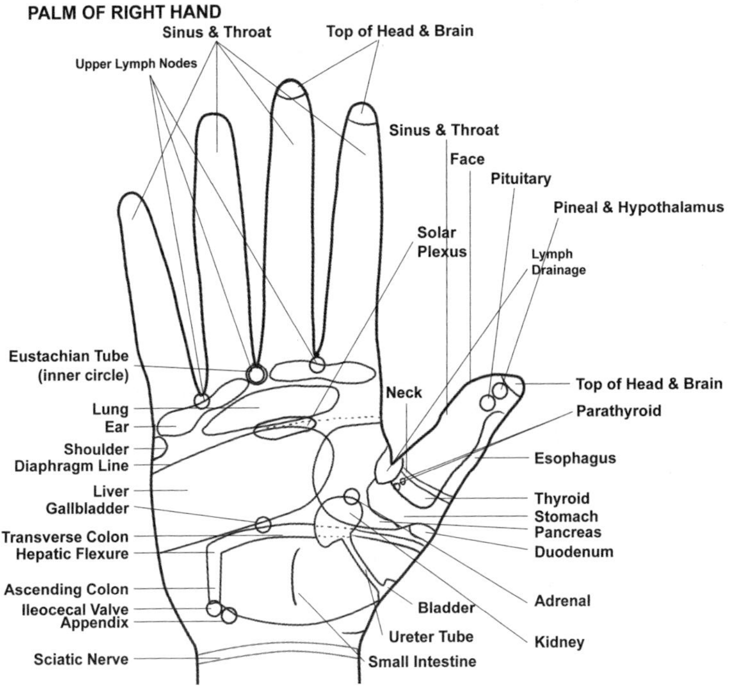

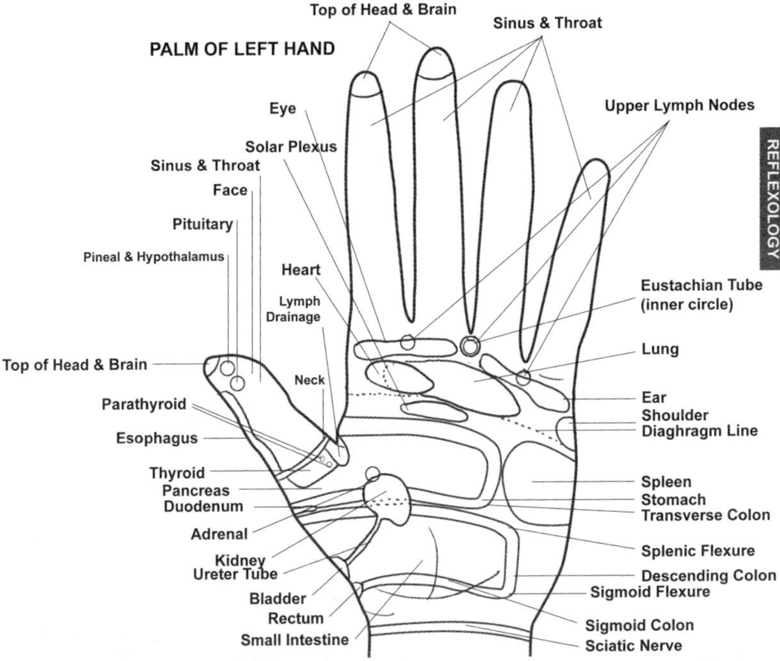

PALM OF RIGHT HAND

Sinus & Throat
Top of Head & Brain
Upper Lymph Nodes
Sinus & Throat
Face
Pituitary
Pineal & Hypothalamus
Solar Plexus
Lymph Drainage
Eustachian Tube (inner circle)
Lung
Ear
Shoulder
Diaphragm Line
Neck
Top of Head & Brain
Parathyroid
Esophagus
Liver
Gallbladder
Thyroid
Stomach
Transverse Colon
Pancreas
Hepatic Flexure
Duodenum
Ascending Colon
Ileocecal Valve
Appendix
Bladder
Adrenal
Ureter Tube
Kidney
Sciatic Nerve
Small Intestine

PALM OF LEFT HAND

Top of Head & Brain
Sinus & Throat
Eye
Upper Lymph Nodes
Solar Plexus
Sinus & Throat
Face
Pituitary
Pineal & Hypothalamus
Heart
Lymph Drainage
Eustachian Tube (inner circle)
Top of Head & Brain
Neck
Lung
Parathyroid
Ear
Shoulder
Esophagus
Diaghragm Line
Thyroid
Spleen
Pancreas
Stomach
Duodenum
Transverse Colon
Adrenal
Splenic Flexure
Kidney
Ureter Tube
Descending Colon
Sigmoid Flexure
Bladder
Rectum
Sigmoid Colon
Small Intestine
Sciatic Nerve

REFLEXOLOGY

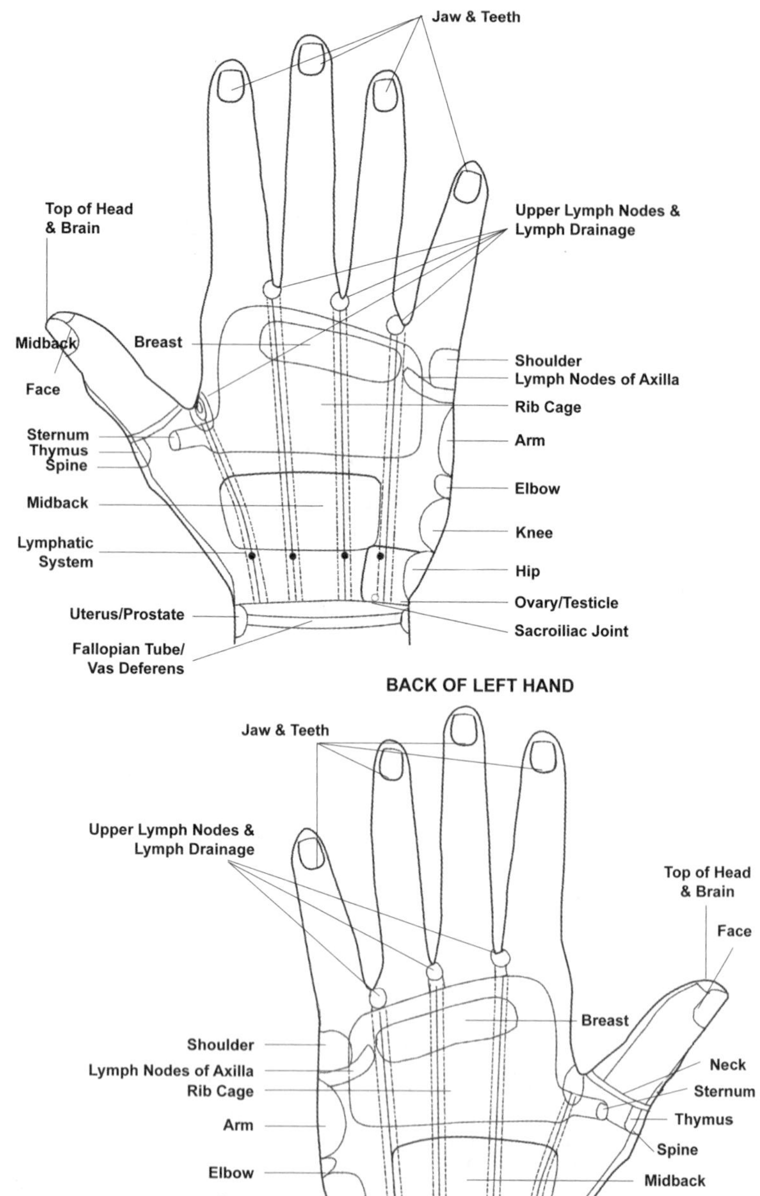
BACK OF RIGHT HAND
Jaw & Teeth
Top of Head & Brain
Upper Lymph Nodes & Lymph Drainage
Midback
Breast
Face
Shoulder
Lymph Nodes of Axilla
Rib Cage
Sternum
Thymus
Spine
Arm
Midback
Elbow
Knee
Lymphatic System
Hip
Ovary/Testicle
Uterus/Prostate
Sacroiliac Joint
Fallopian Tube/ Vas Deferens
BACK OF LEFT HAND
Jaw & Teeth
Upper Lymph Nodes & Lymph Drainage
Top of Head & Brain
Face
Breast
Shoulder
Lymph Nodes of Axilla
Rib Cage
Neck
Sternum
Thymus
Arm
Spine
Elbow
Midback
Knee
Lymphatic System
Hip
Ovary/Testicle
Uterus/Prostate
Sacroiliac Joint
Fallopian Tube/ Vas Deferens

Manual Lymphatic Drainage is rhythmic pumping which stimulates movement of lymph through the lymph vessels. It is a gentle method of promoting lymphatic drainage - activates lymph function and circulation, drains waste, and stimulates immune system as it carries useful white blood cells and lymphocytes to the circulatory system. It helps stimulate parasympathetic nervous system by relaxing the body, increasing muscle tone and stimulating C-fiber mechanoreceptors which reduce chronic pain. Vessels for the drainage of lymph fluid exist directly underneath the skin, so very light pressure is needed to reroute lymphatic flow. The technique uses short, light, rhythmical strokes, which are non-gliding in the direction of lymphatic flow without the use of lubrication.

Application

- Use 1 to 4 oz of pressure- pressure is deep enough so you do not slide over skin, but light enough so that you don't feel tissue below the skin
- Always push fluid towards the direction of the node
- Perform 3 rhythmic patterns to allow for initial lymphatic ducts to open, shut, and release
- Start closest to the draining point, working down the extremity
- Short strokes 1/4 to 1/2 inch are ideal for harder and tighter tissues
- Longer strokes 3/4 to 1 inch are ideal when tissues become more pliable and mobile

Indications	Contraindications	
• Congestion of lymph flow due to tissue injury • Lymphoedema • Removes toxins in the body • Post surgery recovery and pre surgery preparation • Chronic pain • Stimulates parasympathetic system	• All malignant diseases • Major heart problems • Asthma • Lymph node affected by tuberculosis • Edema from right-sided heart failure	• Recent thrombosis • Abdominal treatment during menstruation • Acute inflammation

Physiologic Effects

- Removes blockages along vessels and within nodes
- Stimulates the immune system
- Helps to clear cellulite
- Reduces chronic pain
- Encourages lymph to flow more freely
- Removes harmful toxins
- Fats evacuate through lymphatic vessels more quickly
- Improves scars, stretch marks, wrinkles, and fracture or surgical-incision sites
- Improves circulation of lymph, blood capillaries, veins, interstitial and liquids
- Activates cerebrospinal and synovial fluids indirectly
- Helps to clear lymphedema and fluid retention

Main Lymph Areas

- Mastoid and sub occipital nodes of the head
- Cervical lymph nodes of the neck
- Axillary lymph nodes under the arms
- Popliteal nodes behind the knee
- Inguinal lymph nodes of the groin area

Draining Patterns

- The main lymphatic system flows into the left side of the body and left lymphatic duct
- The thoracic duct located on the left side of body and from the right side of the body below the chest and empties under left clavicle
- The right lymphatic duct on the right side of the head, neck, upper chest and right arm empties under right clavicle
- Drain axillary area first before draining the arm
- Drain inguinal area first before draining the leg

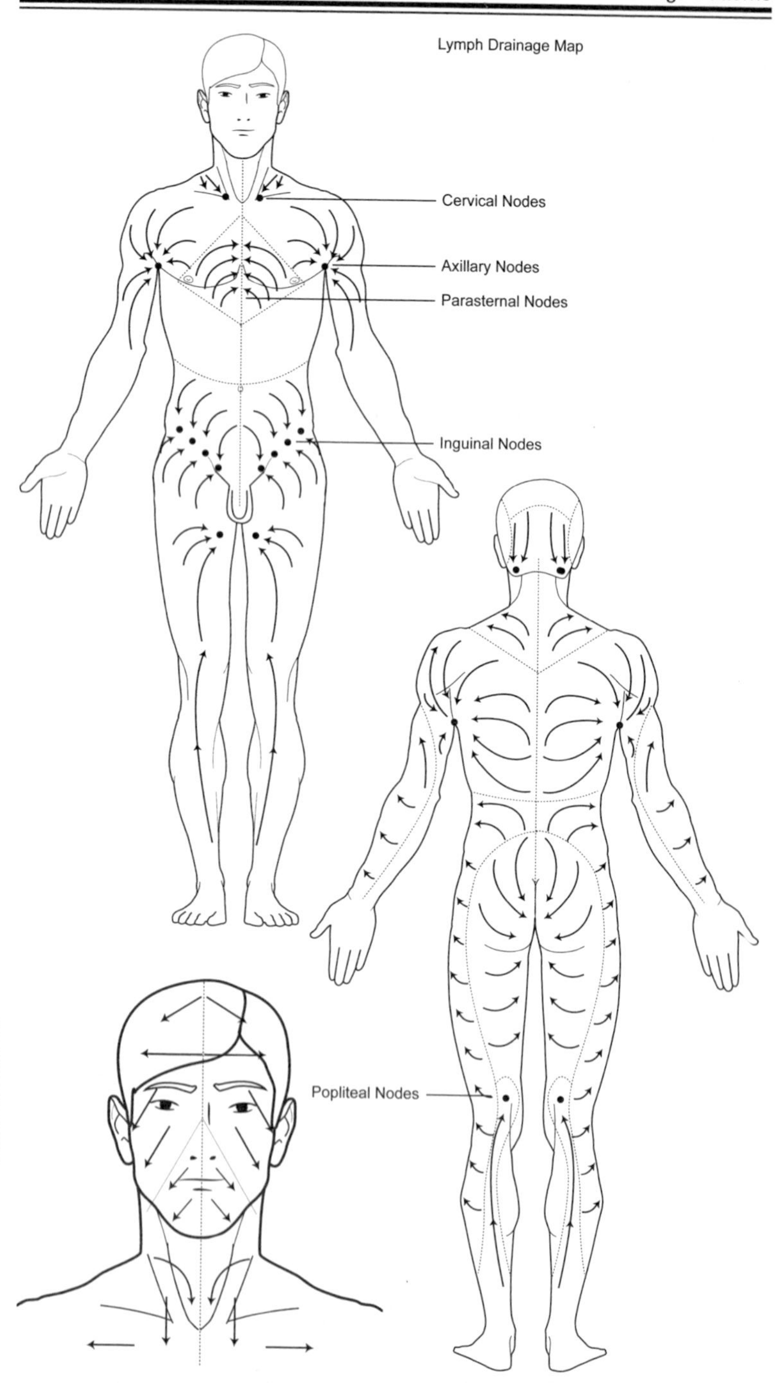
Lymph Drainage Map
Cervical Nodes
Axillary Nodes
Parasternal Nodes
Inguinal Nodes
Popliteal Nodes

Endocrine System

The endocrine system normalizes the secretion of many hormones, or chemical messengers, in the body. It consists of the pituitary gland, adrenal gland, thyroid, hypothalamus, pineal gland, kidney, pancreas, ovaries, testes, and other ductless glands (tissues that secrete hormones that diffuse into blood vessels). The glands discharge these hormones, each of which affect specific body processes. The adrenal gland, for example, releases chemicals that adjust water balance, tissue metabolism, and cardiovascular and respiratory activity. The thyroid gland controls tissue metabolic rate and also regulates calcium levels. The thymus manages the maturation of lymphocytes, cells that are part of the lymphatic system and which play a role in immune health and waste excretion. The pancreas releases several hormones that add to hunger and digestion. Some major hormones that are made by glands in the endocrine system are adrenaline, insulin, growth hormone, and thyroid-stimulating hormone. Sex hormones, such as follicle-stimulating hormone and prolactin, are also created by endocrine organs.

The endocrine system uses the blood vessels as channels of communication. The glands are regulated by feedback control – information about hormone levels or their effects is returned to the gland to either increase or decrease the release of the hormone. The hypothalamus, a gland in the brain, connects the nervous and endocrine systems and regulates much endocrine activity. It secretes inhibiting and releasing hormones that influence the activity of the other endocrine glands, in particular the pituitary gland, which in turn controls many other endocrine organs. Hormones regulate many functions in an organism, including growth and development, metabolism, tissue function, puberty and reproduction, internal environment (temperature, water balance, ion balance), and mood. For endocrine glands to be able to do their work, they are reliant on the existence of specific receptor cells on the target organ. Some chemicals that are released by endocrine glands have only a certain type of cell that is a receptor for the chemical.

Urinary System

The urinary system's function is to rid the body of excess water, salts, and waste products. It consists of the kidneys, ureters, bladder, and urethra. The urinary system operates with the lungs, skin, and intestines to harmonize the chemicals in the body by getting rid of this waste and keeping necessary fluids. Urine is formed in the kidneys, travels through the ureters to be stored in the bladder, and ultimately exits the body through the urethra. The kidneys are two bean-shaped organs situated close to the vertebral column at the small of the back. Each kidney contains 1.2 million nephrons, which are filtering units. One end of the nephron enlarges into the glomerulus (essentially a filter), which surrounds a group of blood capillaries. Blood containing waste products enters the glomerulus, where water and waste products are extracted as the blood exits through the outgoing glomerular blood vessel. This filtration separates out wastes such as urea, which is created when protein is broken down. The blood leaving the glomerulus (the "filtrate") goes through a network of capillaries that surrounds each tubule, where water and certain salts that the body still needs are reabsorbed into the blood. After the body has removed the nutrients it needs from food, waste products remain in the urine.The urine flows from the ends of the tubules to the kidney pelvis, a collecting chamber in the center of the kidney.

Here it leaves through the ureters and goes to the bladder. Muscles in the ureter walls continually contract and relax to push urine away from the kidneys into the bladder. As the bladder fills, it motivates sensory nerves that cause a person to need to urinate. As the bladder becomes more swollen, the sensory stimulation rises and the desire to go increases. When urinating, the brain sends signals to the bladder muscle to contract; at the same time, it sends signals to the sphincter to rest and allow the passage of urine. The male urethra is about eight inches (20 cm) long and ends at the tip of the penis; through the urethra, urine, as well as ejaculatory fluid, are released. The female urethra is less than two inches long and ends just to the front of the vaginal orifice. Only urine exits the body through the female urethra. Adults purge about a quart and a half of urine each day, but that amount can vary depending on many factors, including fluids and food consumed, sweat loss, and water loss through breathing.

Nervous System

The nervous system assists in monitoring the five senses and acts as a liaison between incoming information and control or response of the body. It consists of the brain, spinal cord, nerves, and sense organs. The nervous system is seen as having two parts: the central nervous system; and the peripheral nervous system. The central nervous system (the brain and spinal cord) is the "control center," where information is processed and decisions are made. The spinal cord sends information to and from the brain and directs simple involuntary activities. The brain is the integration center, where voluntary (and many involuntary) behaviors and functions have their foundation. The peripheral nervous system (the cranial nerves, spinal nerves and sense organs) connects the brain to other body systems and to the sense organs. Peripheral nerves are either afferent (sensory neurons which bring information to the spinal cord and brain) or efferent (motor neurons which bring information from the spinal cord and brain). The peripheral nervous system is additionally subdivided into the somatic and autonomic nervous systems. The somatic nervous system is made of the sense organs and the afferent nerves; it is concerned with changes in the outside environment and bringing information to the central nervous system. It is allied with the bones, muscles, and skin. The autonomic nervous system is primarily the efferent nerves and controls sympathetic ("fight or flight") and parasympathetic ("rest and digest") responses to stimuli. It is related to the internal glands, organs, blood vessels, and mucous membranes.

The basic cell of the nervous system is the neuron, which links the CNS to the rest of the body by transmitting impulses via chemicals called neurotransmitters. Neurons are assisted by glial cells, which help repair neurons and perform other protective operations. Concentration of neurotransmitters between neurons can either excite or inhibit cells, leading to an increase or decrease of particular behaviors. The PNS receives stimuli from its internal environment and from its external environment and relays information about these stimuli to the brain. The information is integrated, processed, and responded to, and nerve cells then send impulses back to the origin of stimulus or to other areas of the body to direct response to the stimulus. This process produces an organism's perception of the world, including emotions, physical states and sensory perception. Therefore, behavior is regulated by the nervous system's integration of and response to stimuli.

Skeletal System

The skeletal system acts as a support system for soft body tissues and provides attachment points for muscles and ligaments. It protects internal organs such as the brain, heart, lungs, and spinal cord. It stores calcium, phosphorus, and other minerals, as well as lipids in the bone marrow; when the quantity of these minerals within the blood is low, it will be taken from the bones to replenish the supply. It also acts as the site of new blood cell production (in the red marrow). The skeletal system supplies protection for organs and supports the muscles of the body, acting as levers that transmit muscular forces; it also acts as storage for minerals and creates new blood cells. The skeletal system is composed of the bones, cartilage, and ligaments. The axial skeleton includes the 80 bones that make up the skull, vertebrae, ribs, sternum, and sacrum. The appendicular skeleton includes the 126 bones that make up the limbs, the shoulder girdle, and the pelvic girdle.

There are six shapes of bone: flat (ribs, skull), long (femur, tibia), short (metacarpals), irregular (vertebrae, scapula), cube-shaped (wrist, ankle), and sesamoid (patella). The bones are kept together by connective tissue to produce the structure of the body. Muscles are connected to bones by tendons. Bones are connected to each other at joints by ligaments. Bony landmarks can be used as reference points for various organs and muscles in the body. The basic cell of the skeletal system is the osteocyte. Bone cells are produced through a two-step process that begins with the creation of a cartilage model of bones. Osteoblasts (cells that build bone) develop bone tissue from the cartilage model. The bone calcifies, or hardens, soon after birth. There are two types of tissue that make up bone. Compact, or dense bone, has little space between its tissues. This bone is very solid and forms the protective exterior portion of all bones. Spongy bone has greater space between its cells, and some of these spaces are filled with red or yellow marrow. This type of bone tissue is found in most bones, especially flat and long bones.

Integumentary System

The integumentary system covers and protects the body, and keeps it from losing water. It is made up of the skin, hair, nails, and sweat glands, and is considered to be the largest organ system. The different layers of the skin play various roles in protecting the body. Sensory receptors on the skin inform the body about the environment, sensing heat, pain, pressure or cold, for example. This information helps the nervous system to determine if the environment is suitable for the body; then the individual can modify behavior as needed. The epidermis covers the surface of the skin and protects deeper tissues. It is mostly made up of keratinocytes, which are the structural cells of skin. Keratinocytes produce keratin, which is a protein that provides strength to the skin, hair, and nails. Melanocyte creates the skin's pigment, which protects against the damaging effects of ultra-violet rays of light. They also produce hair and eye color. The epidermis contains Langerhans cells, which are the skin's first immune defense. Beneath the epidermis is the dermis, which feeds the epidermis and gives it strength. The dermis contains exocrine glands which produce perspiration. The collagenous tissues also give the skin strength and protect it against damage. The subcutaneous layer stores lipids, buffers the body, and attaches the skin to deeper structures.

The integumentary system has a number of mechanisms that maintain body temperature. Sweat glands produce perspiration for evaporative cooling, as well as excreting some byproducts and ridding the body of waste. When the body is warm, blood flow in skin capillaries increases, allowing heat to be released. When the body is cold, blood flow slows down in skin capillaries, retaining heat. Hair on the skin protects it and keeps warmth in. Sebaceous glands supply another defensive function for the body. They are located mostly at the hair follicles and produce an oily matter called sebum that lubricates the hair shaft and waterproofs the epidermis. This defends the hair and skin and thwarts drying and inflammation of membranes. Skin also has a vitamin D antecedent that helps to develop the vitamin when exposed to sunlight.

Respiratory System

The respiratory system's functions are to transport oxygen from the air into the body, and to excrete carbon dioxide and water back to the air. It is made up of the nose, mouth, nasal cavities and paranasal sinuses, larynx, pharynx, trachea, bronchi, and lungs. Air enters the body through the nose and mouth and is filtered, warmed and humidified by the nasal cavities and paranasal sinuses. The pharynx (the throat), which is shared with the digestive tract, moves the air to the larynx, which protects the opening to the trachea and houses the vocal cords. The epiglottis keeps food from entering the trachea during chewing and swallowing. The air then goes to the trachea and bronchi, which filter it and trap particles in mucus. Finally, air arrives at the lungs, where gas exchange can take place. The lungs are made up of millions of tiny sacs named alveoli. Alveoli are the sites of the carbon dioxide-oxygen exchange, using the blood that moves in the capillaries from the pulmonary veins and arteries as the medium for gas exchange. This intimate relationship between the respiratory and cardiovascular system is vital for efficient gas exchange. The respiratory system can be separated into two functional divisions: the conducting zone, which is composed of all of the passageways and transports air between the lungs and the outside of the body; and the respiratory zone, which is where gas exchanges in the lungs.

Respiration takes place through four individual steps. Pulmonary ventilation refers to the action of breathing, which transports air into and out of the lungs in a constant flow. Then, external respiration, or gas exchange that happens between the blood and the gas-filled chambers of the lungs (alveoli), takes place. Next, respiratory gases must be moved between the site of gas exchange in the lungs and the respiring tissue in the body (the connection to the cardiovascular system). Finally, the gas exchange must take place between the blood and the respiring tissues (internal respiration). Depth of respiration is regulated by variations in pressure on the lungs. When the diaphragm contracts, it moves down, so the chest cavity enlarges, which decreases the pressure on the lungs and allows for inhalation. When the diaphragm relaxes, the pressure increases and the chest cavity decreases in size, causing exhalation. The respiratory rate is regulated by the brain in response to the amount of carbon dioxide in the blood.

Digestive System

The digestive system takes consumed food and processes it into usable energy for the body. The four major processes of the digestive system are: ingestion of food; digestion or breakdown of food into smaller pieces; absorption of digested food; and elimination of waste from the body. The digestive system consists of the digestive tract (the mouth, pharynx, esophagus, stomach, small and large intestines, rectum, and anus) and the accessory organs that release chemicals that help the body digest. Food enters the body through the mouth, where it is chewed into smaller pieces and covered with saliva. The saliva provides enzymes that begin digestion and lubricate the food so it can move without difficulty through the esophagus. The pharynx conducts solid foods and liquids from the mouth to the esophagus. The epiglottis keeps food from passing from the pharynx into the trachea, which is part of the respiratory system. The chewed and saliva-coated food goes down the esophagus into the stomach, which secretes acids and enzymes that start to chemically digest the food. The stomach also automatically digests food (breaks larger pieces into smaller ones) through contractions. Boluses of food repeatedly exit the stomach and enter the small intestine as a thick liquid called chyme. Since the chyme is extremely acidic, only a little can leave the stomach at a time to enter the duodenum (the first part of the small intestine), where it is neutralized with bicarbonate.

The small intestine, which secretes many enzymes, buffers, and hormones, is the place where most chemical digestion and nutrient absorption take place. The pancreas and gall bladder secrete chemicals (for example, bile) into the small intestine; these chemicals help break down the food into nutrients that can be absorbed into the bloodstream. What is left are waste products and water. The absorbable nutrients pass through the lining of the small intestine and are transported to the blood, which carries them to other parts of the body. What remains passes through the large intestine; this is the site of most of the water reabsorption that will occur during digestion, as well as a little more nutrient absorption. The final waste product, feces, passes through the rectum and anus to exit the body. The entire digestive tract has a layer of smooth muscle that surrounds it and helps break down food and move it along the tract. It is considered an external body system since it is one tube that is continuous with the external body and opens to the outside on both ends.

Cardiovascular / Circulatory System

The cardiovascular system transports oxygen, gases, blood cells, and nutrients (like amino acids and electrolytes) to all parts of the body. It is made up of the heart, blood, and blood vessels (arteries, veins, and capillaries), and, combined with the lymphatic system, is part of the circulatory system. Arteries carry blood away from the heart, while veins carry blood to the heart. Deoxygenated blood exits the heart through the pulmonary artery and goes to the lungs to exchange carbon dioxide for oxygen. The carbon dioxide will exit the lungs as waste. The now-oxygenated blood goes back to the heart via the pulmonary vein, where it is pumped into the body via the systemic arteries, bringing oxygen and nutrients everywhere. As the arteries get further away from the heart, they branch out and become smaller and smaller until they become capillaries. Capillary walls are very thin and allow for gas, nutrient and waste exchange between the blood and the respiring tissue. The blood flows through the capillaries into veins, which are little and merge into successively larger vessels as they get closer to the heart. Blood flows through the arteries because of the pressure from the heart beating. Blood flows through veins due to a valve system that needs the help of skeletal muscle contraction to work.

The average adult has five to six quarts of blood, which contains plasma, red blood cells, white blood cells, and platelets. Blood is a form of connective tissue that transports nutrients to the individual cells and removes waste products. Red blood cells form 90 percent of the formed elements in blood. They transport oxygen to the cells and carbon dioxide away from the cells to the lungs for excretion. The heart constantly pumps the blood through the cardiovascular system. It receives both sympathetic and parasympathetic innervations, which alter the rate of the heartbeat. The contraction itself is controlled by autorhythmic cells. The heart has cardiac muscle which is striated, or striped. The heart contains four chambers – two atria and two ventricles. The chambers are separated by valves that prevent backflow. The cardiac cycle consists of diastole and systole, which is the sequence of events in one heartbeat. Blood pressure is the amount of pressure created by the blood on the walls of the blood vessels.

Muscular System

The muscular system operates directly with the skeletal system to aid humans in movement, steady joint structures, pump blood, produce heat, and assist passage of internal materials. Muscle tissue needs ATP and calcium to contract and relax. Calcium is released from its storage into the sarcomere when a muscle is stimulated to contract. The calcium uncovers the actin-binding sites, allowing for binding and contraction to occur. When the muscle finishes contracting, the calcium ions are restored to the sarcoplasmic reticulum for storage. The three types of tissue that compose the muscular system are cardiac, smooth and skeletal. Cardiac muscle is in the walls of the heart. It is striated ("striped") but contracts involuntarily. Smooth muscle is located in the walls of the digestive tract, uterus, blood vessels, and other internal organs. Smooth muscle fibers are not striated and are involuntary. Muscle stores glycogen, oxygen, and calcium.

Skeletal muscles connect to bones through tendons and have cylindrical, tapered cells. Each of the muscles has an origin and an insertion. The origin is the least movable part, or the part that attaches closest to the center of the body, while the insertion is the more movable section that attaches farther from the center. Skeletal muscle is voluntary muscle that is striated in appearance and multinucleated. A sarcomere is the smallest cross-section of skeletal muscle and is the functional unit within the cell. When motivated by an action potential, the sarcomere shortens and contraction occurs. Skeletal muscles work in couples, with one muscle contracting as the other relaxes. To create the antagonistic movement, the opposite occurs. The two types of skeletal muscle fibers include: fast-twitch (white) fibers, which contract quickly and forcefully and create quick, powerful movement, but are quick to fatigue; and slow-twitch (red) fibers which contract at a slower pace and are weaker, creating more delicate or specific movement.

Lymphatic System

The primary functions of the lymphatic system are removing interstitial fluid from the tissues, absorbing fat and fatty acids for the circulatory system, and transporting immune cells to and from lymph nodes. The lymphatic system consists of lymph, thymus, spleen, bone marrow, and lymphoid tissue related to digestive system. Every part of the body, except the central nervous system, contains lymphatic tissue.

As blood is moved through the body, rather than making direct contact with the tissues or the functional cells of the body, the nutrients and water from the blood diffuse through the capillaries to become interstitial fluid, which then comes into contact with the functional tissue cells. When the interstitial fluid enters the initial vessels of the lymphatic system, it becomes lymph, whose composition is similar to blood, except that it does not have red blood cells, platelets, or much protein. Roughly 90 percent is returned to the venous capillaries and continues through blood circulation. The remainder of the lymph moves along the lymphatic vessel network either by contractions of the vessels or by contraction of skeletal muscle causing compression of the lymphatic vessels. The extra interstitial fluid in this way can be returned to the blood, bringing dissolved materials, nutrients, wastes, and gases. Lymph moves immune cells and other immune factors throughout the body. These lymphocytes are immune cells that protect the body from viruses, bacteria, and other micro-organisms that invade it. Lymphocytes are created as precursor cells in the bone marrow. Then they mature either in the bone marrow (B-cells) or in the thymus (T-cells). If a foreign object (antigen) is discovered, the lymph transports antigen-presenting cells to the lymph nodes, which stimulates an immune response.

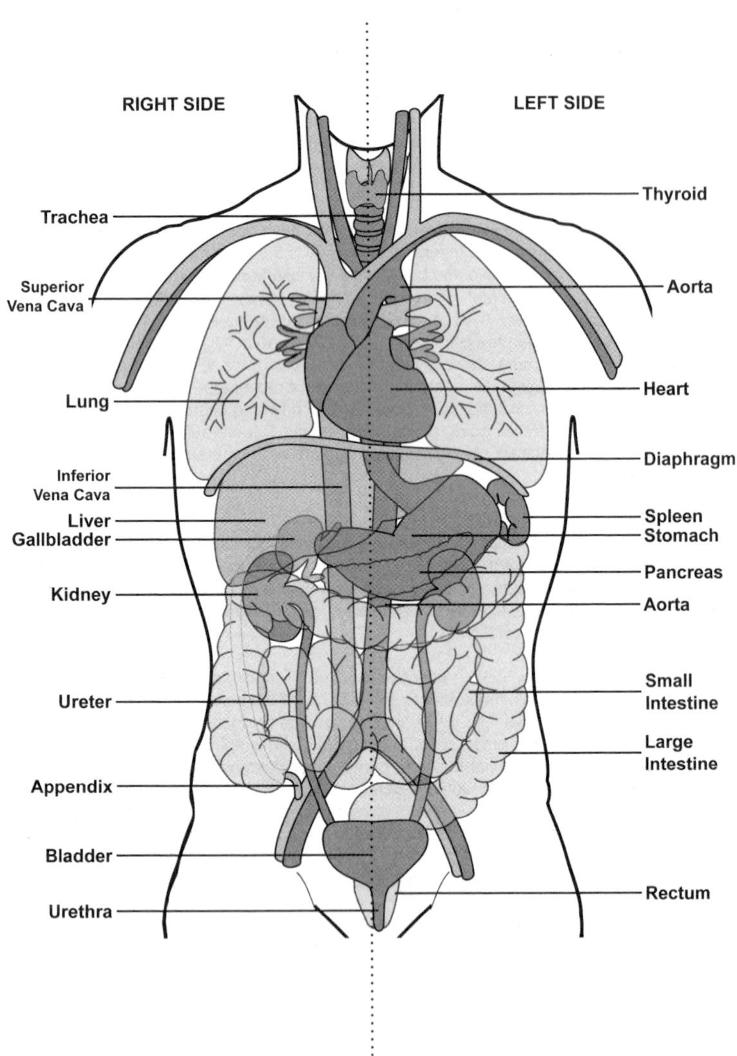
RIGHT SIDE
LEFT SIDE
Thyroid
Trachea
Superior Vena Cava
Aorta
Heart
Lung
Diaphragm
Inferior Vena Cava
Spleen
Liver
Stomach
Gallbladder
Pancreas
Kidney
Aorta
Small Intestine
Ureter
Large Intestine
Appendix
Bladder
Rectum
Urethra

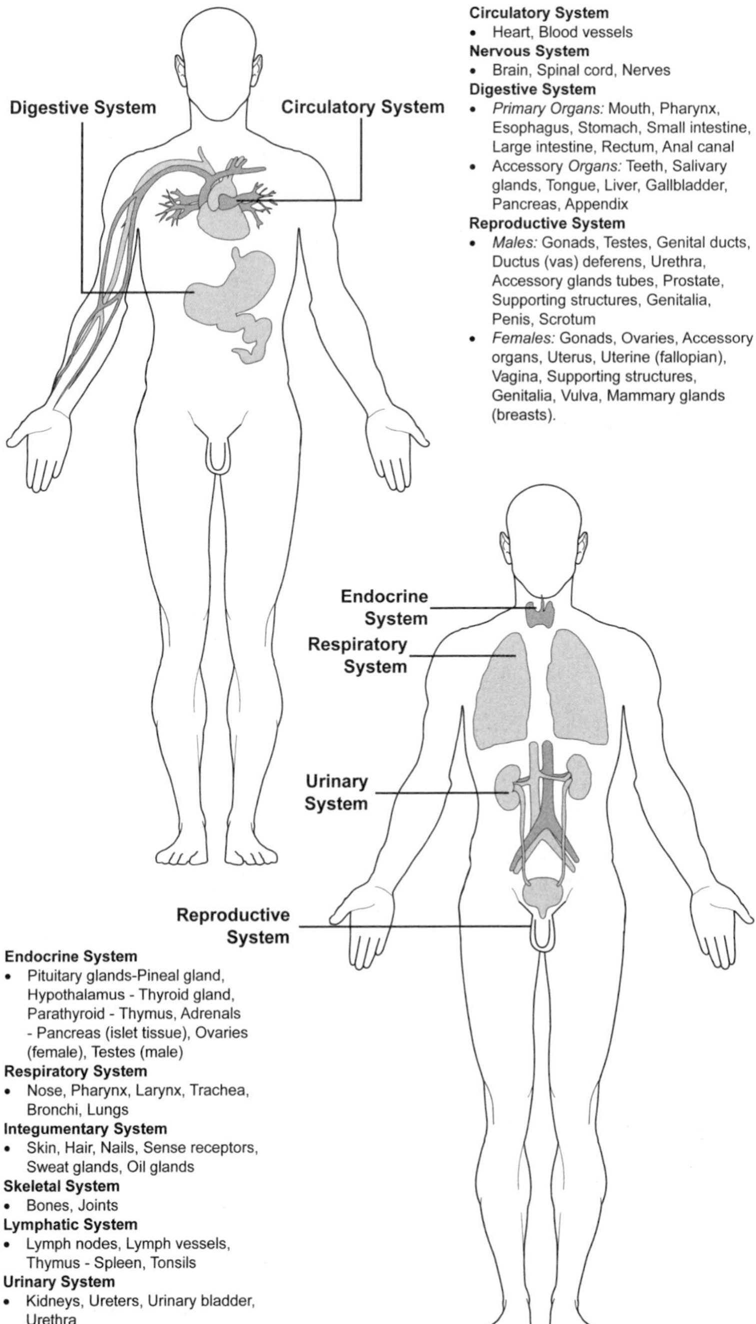

Circulatory System
- Heart, Blood vessels

Nervous System
- Brain, Spinal cord, Nerves

Digestive System
- *Primary Organs:* Mouth, Pharynx, Esophagus, Stomach, Small intestine, Large intestine, Rectum, Anal canal
- Accessory *Organs:* Teeth, Salivary glands, Tongue, Liver, Gallbladder, Pancreas, Appendix

Reproductive System
- *Males:* Gonads, Testes, Genital ducts, Ductus (vas) deferens, Urethra, Accessory glands tubes, Prostate, Supporting structures, Genitalia, Penis, Scrotum
- *Females:* Gonads, Ovaries, Accessory organs, Uterus, Uterine (fallopian), Vagina, Supporting structures, Genitalia, Vulva, Mammary glands (breasts).

Endocrine System
- Pituitary glands-Pineal gland, Hypothalamus - Thyroid gland, Parathyroid - Thymus, Adrenals - Pancreas (islet tissue), Ovaries (female), Testes (male)

Respiratory System
- Nose, Pharynx, Larynx, Trachea, Bronchi, Lungs

Integumentary System
- Skin, Hair, Nails, Sense receptors, Sweat glands, Oil glands

Skeletal System
- Bones, Joints

Lymphatic System
- Lymph nodes, Lymph vessels, Thymus - Spleen, Tonsils

Urinary System
- Kidneys, Ureters, Urinary bladder, Urethra

Muscular System
- Muscles

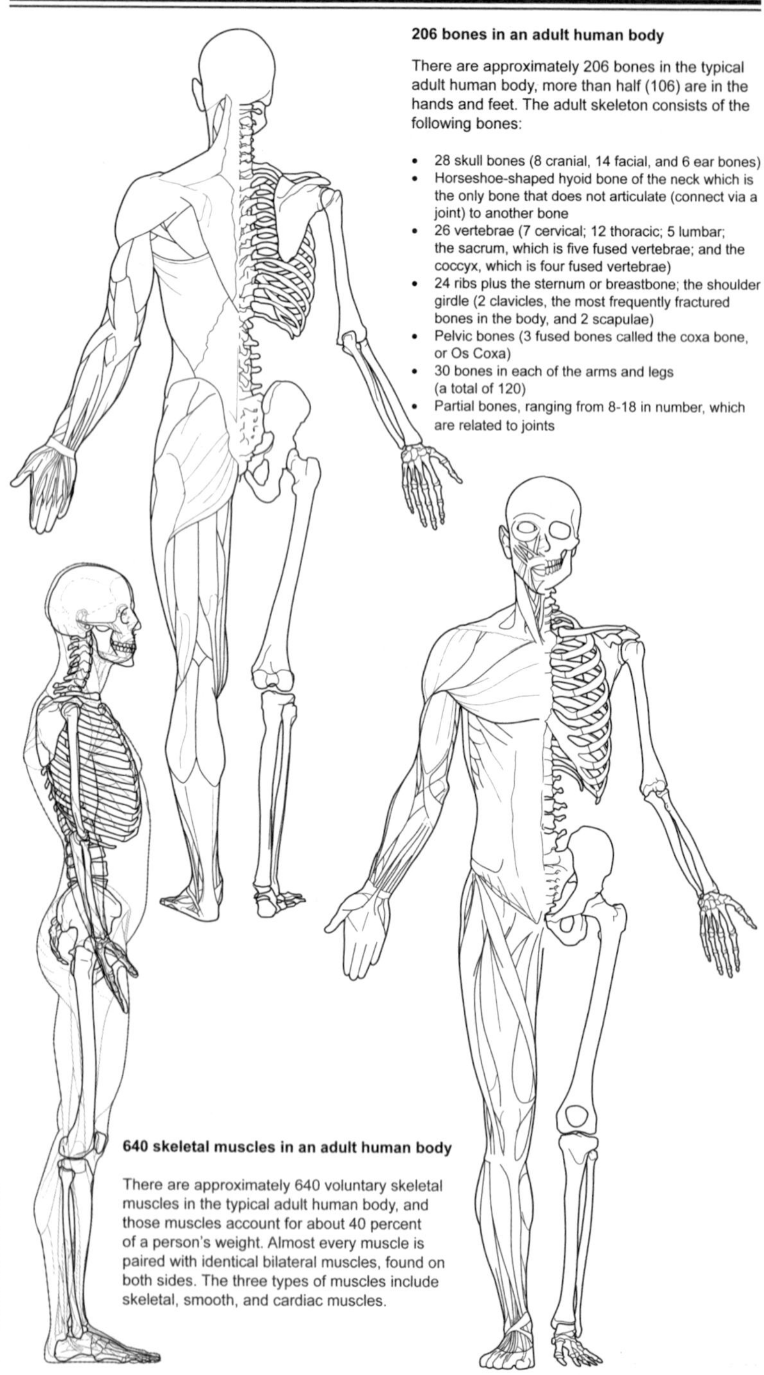

206 bones in an adult human body

There are approximately 206 bones in the typical adult human body, more than half (106) are in the hands and feet. The adult skeleton consists of the following bones:

- 28 skull bones (8 cranial, 14 facial, and 6 ear bones)
- Horseshoe-shaped hyoid bone of the neck which is the only bone that does not articulate (connect via a joint) to another bone
- 26 vertebrae (7 cervical; 12 thoracic; 5 lumbar; the sacrum, which is five fused vertebrae; and the coccyx, which is four fused vertebrae)
- 24 ribs plus the sternum or breastbone; the shoulder girdle (2 clavicles, the most frequently fractured bones in the body, and 2 scapulae)
- Pelvic bones (3 fused bones called the coxa bone, or Os Coxa)
- 30 bones in each of the arms and legs (a total of 120)
- Partial bones, ranging from 8-18 in number, which are related to joints

640 skeletal muscles in an adult human body

There are approximately 640 voluntary skeletal muscles in the typical adult human body, and those muscles account for about 40 percent of a person's weight. Almost every muscle is paired with identical bilateral muscles, found on both sides. The three types of muscles include skeletal, smooth, and cardiac muscles.

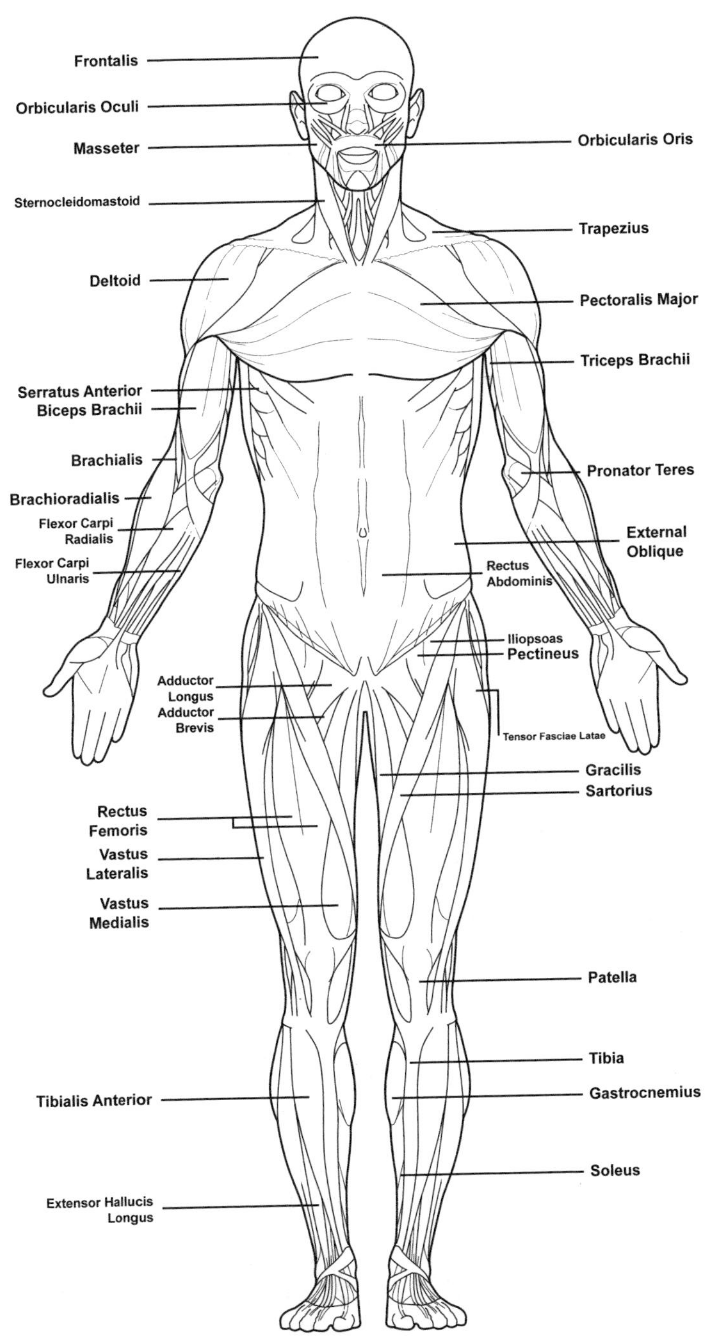
Frontalis
Orbicularis Oculi
Masseter
Sternocleidomastoid
Deltoid
Serratus Anterior
Biceps Brachii
Brachialis
Brachioradialis
Flexor Carpi Radialis
Flexor Carpi Ulnaris
Adductor Longus
Adductor Brevis
Rectus Femoris
Vastus Lateralis
Vastus Medialis
Tibialis Anterior
Extensor Hallucis Longus
Orbicularis Oris
Trapezius
Pectoralis Major
Triceps Brachii
Pronator Teres
External Oblique
Rectus Abdominis
Iliopsoas
Pectineus
Tensor Fasciae Latae
Gracilis
Sartorius
Patella
Tibia
Gastrocnemius
Soleus

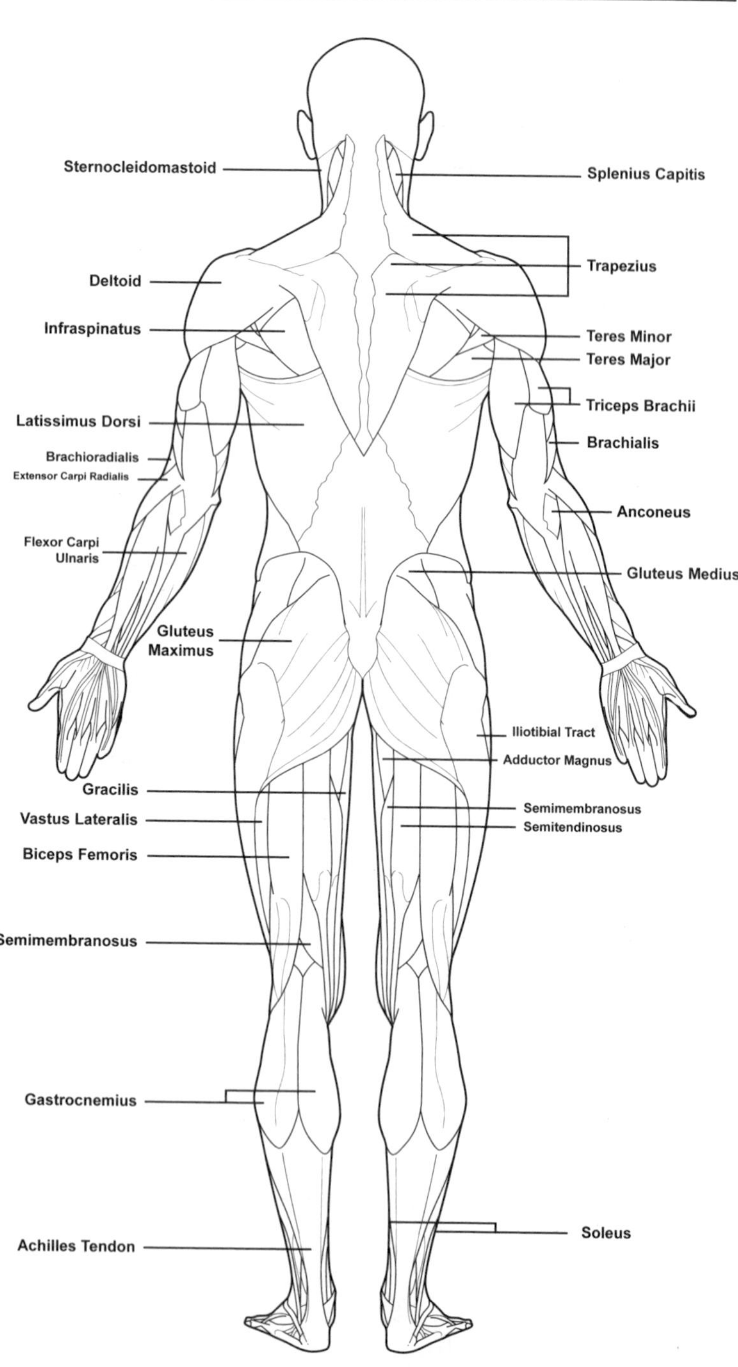
Sternocleidomastoid
Splenius Capitis
Trapezius
Deltoid
Infraspinatus
Teres Minor
Teres Major
Triceps Brachii
Latissimus Dorsi
Brachialis
Brachioradialis
Extensor Carpi Radialis
Anconeus
Flexor Carpi Ulnaris
Gluteus Medius
Gluteus Maximus
Iliotibial Tract
Adductor Magnus
Gracilis
Semimembranosus
Vastus Lateralis
Semitendinosus
Biceps Femoris
Semimembranosus
Gastrocnemius
Soleus
Achilles Tendon

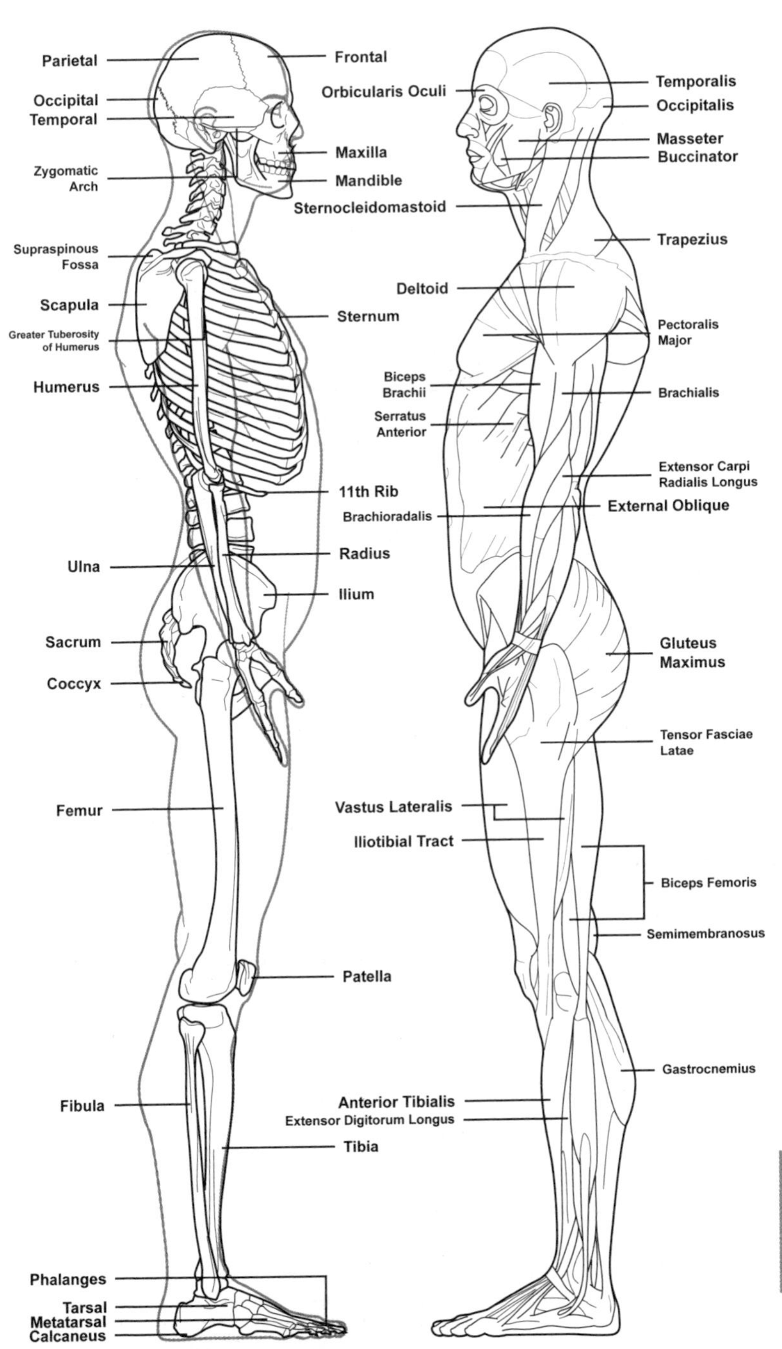
Parietal
Occipital
Temporal
Zygomatic Arch
Supraspinous Fossa
Scapula
Greater Tuberosity of Humerus
Humerus
Ulna
Sacrum
Coccyx
Femur
Fibula
Phalanges
Tarsal
Metatarsal
Calcaneus
Frontal
Orbicularis Oculi
Maxilla
Mandible
Sternocleidomastoid
Deltoid
Sternum
Biceps Brachii
Serratus Anterior
11th Rib
Brachioradalis
Radius
Ilium
Vastus Lateralis
Iliotibial Tract
Patella
Anterior Tibialis
Extensor Digitorum Longus
Tibia
Temporalis
Occipitalis
Masseter
Buccinator
Trapezius
Pectoralis Major
Brachialis
Extensor Carpi Radialis Longus
External Oblique
Gluteus Maximus
Tensor Fasciae Latae
Biceps Femoris
Semimembranosus
Gastrocnemius

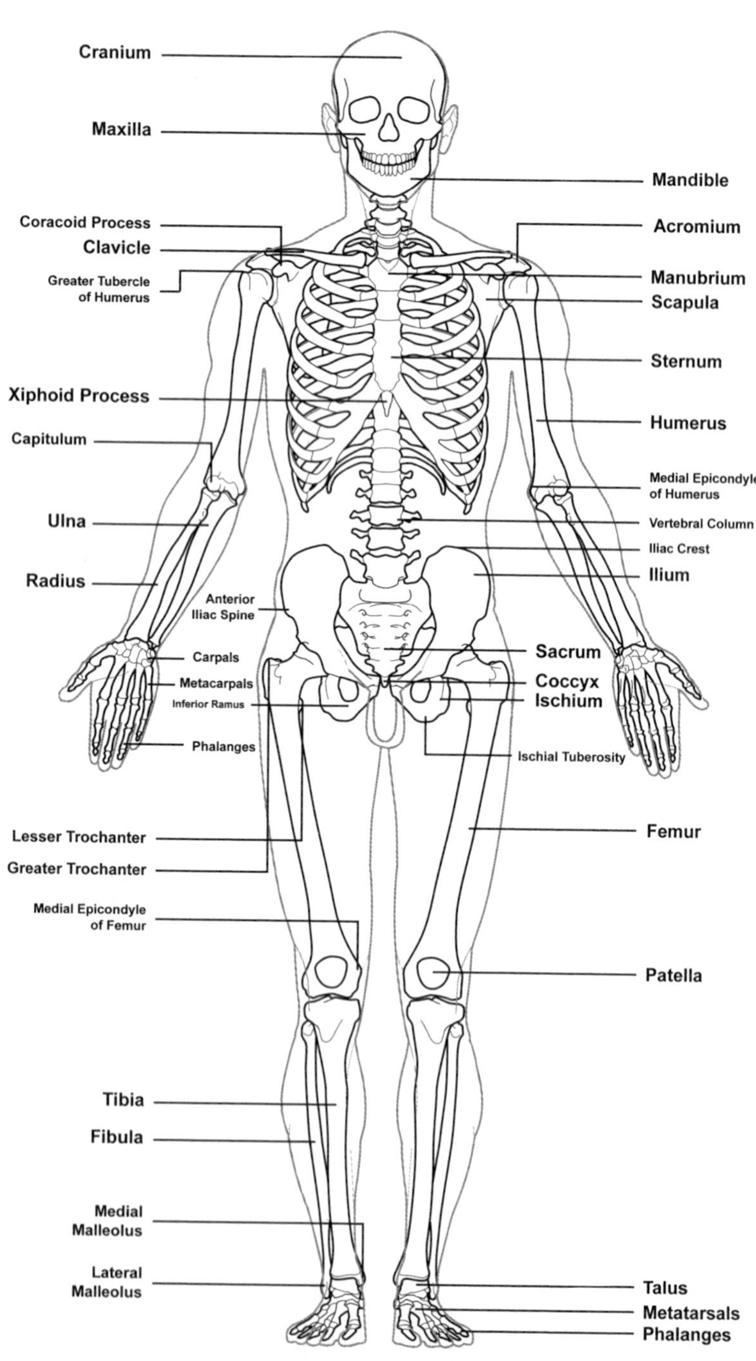
Cranium
Maxilla
Mandible
Coracoid Process
Clavicle
Greater Tubercle of Humerus
Acromium
Manubrium
Scapula
Sternum
Xiphoid Process
Humerus
Capitulum
Medial Epicondyle of Humerus
Ulna
Vertebral Column
Iliac Crest
Radius
Ilium
Anterior Iliac Spine
Carpals
Sacrum
Metacarpals
Coccyx
Inferior Ramus
Ischium
Phalanges
Ischial Tuberosity
Lesser Trochanter
Femur
Greater Trochanter
Medial Epicondyle of Femur
Patella
Tibia
Fibula
Medial Malleolus
Lateral Malleolus
Talus
Metatarsals
Phalanges

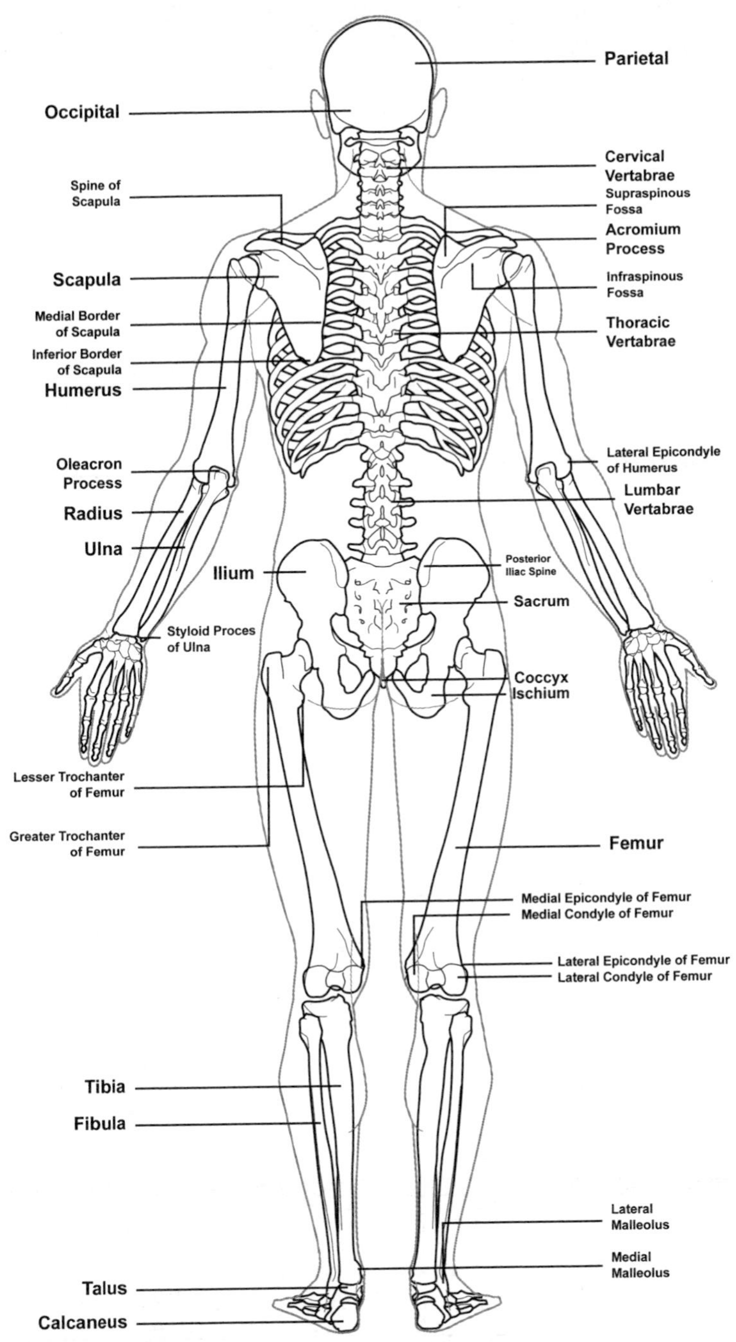
Parietal
Occipital
Cervical Vertabrae
Spine of Scapula
Supraspinous Fossa
Acromium Process
Scapula
Infraspinous Fossa
Medial Border of Scapula
Thoracic Vertabrae
Inferior Border of Scapula
Humerus
Oleacron Process
Lateral Epicondyle of Humerus
Lumbar Vertabrae
Radius
Ulna
Ilium
Posterior Iliac Spine
Sacrum
Styloid Proces of Ulna
Coccyx
Ischium
Lesser Trochanter of Femur
Greater Trochanter of Femur
Femur
Medial Epicondyle of Femur
Medial Condyle of Femur
Lateral Epicondyle of Femur
Lateral Condyle of Femur
Tibia
Fibula
Lateral Malleolus
Medial Malleolus
Talus
Calcaneus

Muscle	Origin	Insertion	Action
Upper Extremities			
Acts on Scapula and Shoulder			
Trapezius	EOP, ligamentum nuchae of cervical spine, C7-T12	Spine of the scapula, acromion, lateral 1/3 of clavicle	Adducts, rotates, elevates, and depresses scapula
Upper	Occiput and ligamentum nuchae of cervical spine	Lateral 1/3 of clavicle and acromion	Elevates and helps upward rotation of scapula, extends neck
Middle	Spinous process of C7-T5	Spine of the scapula	Retracts scapula medially
Lower	Spinous process of T5-T12	Spine of the scapula	Depresses and helps upward rotation of scapula
Rhomboid			
Major	Spinous process of T2-T5	Medial border of the scapula inferior to spine	Retracts and rotates scapula downward. Fixes scapula to thoracic wall
Minor	Ligamentum nuchae and spinous process of C7-T1	Medial border of the scapula at the root of the spine	(Same as Rhomboid major)
Levator Scapulae	Transverse processes of C1-C4	Superior third of vertebral border of scapula	Elevates the scapula and moves neck laterally. Assists trapezius and rhomboids
Serratus Anterior	Anterior ribs 1-8	Anterior aspect of vertebral border of scapula	Stabilizes, rotates scapula upward and protracts anteriorly toward thoracic wall
Pectoralis Minor	Anterior ribs 3, 4, 5	Coracoid process of scapula	Rotates forward and depresses scapula
Acts on Upper Arm and Shoulder			
Pectoralis Major	Clavicle, sternum, six upper ribs, aponeurosis of external oblique muscle of abdomen	Intertubercular sulcus of the humerus	Both heads; Rotates medially and adducts arm at shoulder and flexes arms
Clavicular	Medial half of clavicle, clavicular head	Lateral ridge of bicipital groove distal to Pectoralis major sterna insertion	Flexes arm at shoulder
Sternal	Sternum, costal cartilage of ribs 1-6	Lateral ridge of bicipital groove proximal to Pectoralis major clavicular insertion	Flexes and extends arm at shoulder
Deltoid	Lateral third of clavicle, acromion, spine of scapula	Deltoid tuberosity of humerus	Abducts, flexes, and extends arm at shoulder
Anterior	Lateral third of clavicle	Deltoid tuberosity of humerus	Flexes and medially rotates arm at shoulder
Middle	Acromion and lateral spine of the scapula	Deltoid tuberosity of humerus	Abducts arm at shoulder
Posterior	Lower lip of the spine of the scapula	Deltoid tuberosity of humerus	Extends and laterally rotates arm at shoulder
Supraspinatus	Supraspinous fossa of scapula	Top of greater tubercle of the humerus	Abducts arm at shoulder, assists deltoid, acts with rotator cuff muscles
Coracobrachialis	Coracoid process of scapula	Middle third of medial surface of humerus	Flexes and adducts the arm at shoulder
Infraspinatus	Infraspinous fossa of scapula	Greater tubercle of humerus	Rotates arm at shoulder laterally, helps hold head in glenoid cavity
Subscapularis	Subscapular fossa of scapula	Lesser tubercle of humerus	Adducts and rotates arm at shoulder medially, helps hold humeral head in glenoid cavity
Teres Minor	Upper axillary border of scapula	Inferior aspect of greater tubercle of humerus	Rotates arm at shoulder laterally, draws humerus toward glenoid fossa of scapula to stabilize shoulder
Teres Major	Lateral border, inferior angle of scapula	Medial ridge of bicipital groove of humerus	Extends arms and medially rotates arm at shoulder
Latissimus Dorsi	Spines of T7-T12 thoracolumbar fascia, iliac crest, lower ribs, inferior angle of scapula	Intertubercular groove of humerus	Extends, adducts, and medially rotates humerus at shoulder
Acts on the Arm and Forearm			
Biceps Brachii	Long head - Supraglenoid tubercle, Short head - apex of coracoid process of scapula	Radial tuberosity of radius and bicipital aponeurosis	Flexes forearm at the elbow and supinates hand
Long Head	Supraglenoid tubercle of scapula	Posterior portion of the tuberosity of the radius	Flexes the elbow and supinates hand
Short Head	Coracoid process of the scapula	Posterior portion of the tuberosity of the radius	Flexes arm and forearm, supinates hand

Muscle	Origin	Insertion	Action
Brachialis	Distal half of anterior surface of the humerus	Ulnar tuberosity and coronoid process	Flexes forearm at the elbow in all directions
Brachioradialis	Proximal two thirds of lateral supracondylar ridge of humerus	Lateral surface of distal end of radius	Flexes forearm at the elbow
Triceps Brachii			Extends the forearm at elbow, main extensor of elbow, steadies head of abducted humerus
Long Head	Infraglenoid tuberosity of the scapula and upper lateral border of the scapula	Posterior olecranon process of ulna	Extends the forearm at elbow
Lateral Head	Proximal portion of posterior humerus, superior to radial groove	Posterior olecranon process of ulna	Extends the forearm at elbow
Medial Head	Inferior to radial groove on humerus	Posterior olecranon process of ulna	Extends the forearm at elbow
Supinator	Lateral epicondyle of humerus, supinator crest of ulna, radial collateral ligament, annular ligament	Lateral, posterior, and anterior surfaces of proximal third of radius	Assists biceps to supinate hand and forearm
Pronator Teres	Medial epicondyle of humerus and coracoid process of ulna	Midlateral surface of radius	Pronates the forearm, flexes the elbow
Anconeus	Lateral epicondyle of humerus	Olecranon process of ulna	Assists triceps in elbow extension, abducts ulna during pronation
Pronator Quadratus	Distal fourth of anterior surface of the ulna	Distal fourth of anterior surface of the radius	Pronates the forearm
Acts on the Wrist and Hand			
Flexor Carpi Radialis	Medial epicondyle of the humerus	Base of the second and third metacarpals	Flexes and abducts hand at wrist
Flexor Carpi Ulnaris	Medial epicondyle of the humerus	Pisiform, hamate and base of fifth metacarpal	Flexes and abducts hand at wrist
Humeral Head	Medial epicondyle of humerus	Pisiform, hamate and base of fifth metacarpal	Flexes and abducts hand at wrist
Ulnar Head	Proximal 2/3 of posterior ulna and olecranon	Common insertion with humeral head	Flexes and abducts hand at wrist
Palmaris Longus	Medial epicondyle of humerus	Distal half of flexor retinaculum and palmar aponeurosis	Flexes wrist joint
Extensor Carpi Radialis Brevis	Lateral epicondyle of humerus	Dorsal surface of base of third metacarpal	Extends and abducts hand at wrist
Extensor Carpi Radialis Longus	Distal third of supracondylar ridge of humerus	Dorsal surface of base of second metacarpal	Extends and abducts hand at wrist
Extensor Carpi Ulnaris	Lateral epicondyle of humerus and by aponeurosis from proximal posterior ulna	Lateral dorsal side of base of fifth metacarpal	Extends and adducts hand at wrist
Acts on the Fingers			
Flexor Digitorum Superficialis			Flexes middle phalanges of digits 2-5 and flexes the wrist
Humeral Head	Medial epicondyle of humerus and ulnar collateral ligament	By four tendons to the sides of the middle phalanges of digits 2-5 on palmar aspect	Flexes middle phalanges of medial four digits
Ulnar Head	Medial side of coronoid process of ulna	By four tendons to the sides of the middle phalanges of digits 2-5 on palmar aspect	Flexes middle phalanges of medial four digits
Radial Head	Superior half of anterior border of radius	By four tendons to the sides of the middle phalanges of digits 2-5 on palmar aspect	Flexes middle phalanges of medial four digits
Flexor Digitorum Profundus	Proximal 3/4 of anterior and medial ulna and interosseus membrane	By tendons to anterior bases of distal phalanges 2-5	Flexes distal phalanges 2-5 and flexes the wrist
Flexor Digiti Minimi	Hamate bone and flexor retinaculum	Base of proximal phalanx of little finger	Flexes metacarpophalangeal (MP) joint of little finger
Extensor Digitorum	Lateral epicondyle of humerus	By four tendons to digits 2-5. To the forsal base of the middle and distal phalanges	Extends medial four digits at the MP and interphalangeal joints
Extensor Indicis	Distal third of posterior ulna and interosseus membrane	Extensor expansion of index finger with Extensor digitorum tendon	Extends the second digit and helps extend hand at wrist
Extensor Digiti Minimi	Lateral epicondyle of humerus	Extensor expansion of little finger with extensor digitorum tendon	Extends the fifth digit at MP and interphalangeal joints
Abductor Digiti Minimi	Tendon of flexor carpi ulnaris and pisiform	Ulnar side of proximal phalanx of little finger	Abducts the little finger at MP joint

Muscle	Origin	Insertion	Action
Opponens Digiti Minimi	Hook of the hamate and flexor retinaculum	Ulnar side of fifth metacarpal	Opposes the fifth metacarpal, brings it into opposition with thumb
Palmar Interossei			Adducts the digits of the hand, flexes digits at MP joint and interphalangeal joints
First	Ulnar side of first metacarpal	Ulnar side of proximal phalanx of first digit	Adducts the digits of the hand, flexes digits at MP joint and interphalangeal joints
Second	Ulnar side of second metacarpal	Ulnar side of proximal phalanx of second digit	Adducts the digits of the hand, flexes digits at MP joint and interphalangeal joints
Third	Radial side of fourth metacarpal	Radial side of proximal phalanx of fourth digit	Adducts the digits of the hand, flexes digits at MP joint and interphalangeal joints
Fourth	Radial side of fifth metacarpal	Radial side of proximal phalanx of fifth digit	Adducts the digits of the hand, flexes digits at MP joint and interphalangeal joints
Dorsal Interossei	Adjacent surfaces of all metacarpal bones	Extensor expansion and proximal bases of digits two, three and four	Abducts the index, middle and ring fingers. Assists lumbrical in MP flexion and extension
Lumbricals	Flexor digitorum tendons at level of metacarpals	Radial side of extensor expansion at proximal phalanx of digits 2, 3, 4 and 5	Flexes MP joints and extends the interphalangeal joints
Acts on the Thumb			
Abductor Pollicis Longus	Middle third of posterior surface of ulna, radius and interosseus	Base of radial side of first metacarpal	Abducts and extends the MP joint of thumb
Abductor Pollicis Brevis	Flexor retinaculum, trapezium and scaphoid	Radial side of proximal phalanx of thumb	Abducts the thumb at MP joint
Adductor Pollicis			
Transverse Head	Anterior surface of third metacarpal	Medial side of the base of the proximal phalanx of the thumb and the ulnar sesamoid	Adducts the thumb toward middle digit
Oblique Head	Capitate bone and base of second and third metacarpals	Medial side of the base of the proximal phalanx of the thumb and the ulnar sesamoid	Adducts the thumb toward middle digit
Flexor Pollicis Longus	Anterior surface of middle radius and adjacent interosseus membrane	Base of palmar surface of distal phalanx of thumb	Flexes distal phalanx of thumb
Flexor Pollicis Brevis	Flexor retinaculum and tubercles of scaphoid and trapezium	Radial side of proximal phalanx of thumb and extensor expansion	Flexes distal phalanx and assists with opposition of thumb
Extensor Pollicis Longus	Posterior surface of middle 1/3 of ulna and interosseous membrane	Base of dorsal surface of distal phalanx of thumb	Extends distal phalanx of thumb and abducts the wrist
Extensor Pollicis Brevis	Posterior surface of radius and interosseus membrane distal to origin of abductor pollicis longus	Base of proximal phalanx of thumb	Extends distal phalanx of thumb and abducts the wrist
Opponens Pollicis	Flexor retinaculum and tubercles of scaphoid and trapezium	Entire radial side of first metacarpal	Opposes the thumb toward center of palm and rotates it medially
Lower Extremities Acts on the Gluteal and Thigh			
Psoas Major	Anterior surfaces of transverse processes of L1-L5 and discs of T12-L-5	Lesser trochanter of the femur	Acts with iliacus to flex hip, flexes vertebral column laterally, balances trunk in sitting position, flexes trunk
Gluteus Maximus	Posterior gluteal line of ilium and adjacent iliac crest, the posterior inferior surface of the sacrum and lateral surface of coccyx	Iliotibial tract of fascia lata and gluteal tuberosity of femur	Extends thigh at the hip and rotates thigh laterally, supports extended knee, raises trunk from flexed position
Gluteus Medius	Iliac crest and external surface of ilium	Lateral and superior surface of greater trochanter of the femur	Abducts and rotates thigh medially at hip, steadies pelvis on leg when opposites leg is raised
Gluteus Minimus	External surface of ilium inferior to gluteus medius muscle and margin of greater sciatic notch. Anterior portion of iliac spine and ASIS	Anterior surface of the greater trochanter of femur	Abducts and rotates thigh medially at hip, steadies pelvis on leg when opposite leg is raised
Iliacus	Superior 2/3 of iliac fossa and iliac crest	With psoas major at lesser trochanter of the femur	(Same as psoas major). Flexes hip and stabilizes hip joint

Muscle	Origin	Insertion	Action
Tensor Fascia Latae	Anterior superior iliac spine, outer lip of anterior iliac crest and fascia lata	Iliotibial tract of fascia lata	Abducts and rotates thigh medially. Maintains extension of knee
Pectineus	Pecten pubis and pectineal surface of the pubis	Pectineal line of femur, inferior to lesser trochanter	Adducts, flexes and rotates thigh at hip. Assists with rotation of thigh medially
Adductor Brevis	Anterior surface of inferior pubic ramus, inferior to origin of adductor longus	Pectineal line and superior part of medial lip of linea aspera of femur	Adducts, flexes and rotates thigh medially
Adductor Longus	Anterior surface of body of pubis, just lateral to pubic symphysis	Middle third of linea aspera of femur, between the medial adductor magnus and brevis insertions and lateral origin of the vastus medialis	Adducts, flexes and rotates thigh medially
Adductor Magnus	Inferior pubic ramus, ischial ramus and ischial tuberosity	Gluteal tuberosity of femur, medial lip of linea aspera, medial supracondylar ridge, and adductor tubercle of femur	Powerful adduction. Anterior fibers flex and rotate medially, posterior fibers extend and rotate laterally
Acts on the Thigh and Rotators			
Sartorius	Anterior superior iliac spine and superior part of notch inferior to it	Superior aspect of the medial surface of the tibial shaft near the tibial tuberosity	Flexes, rotates and abducts thigh laterally at hip joint. Assists with flexion and medal rotation of knee
Gracilis	Inferior 1/2 of symphysis pubis and inferior ramus of pubis	Superior part of medial surface of tibia, just posterior to sartorius	Adducts thigh at hip, flexes and rotates leg at knee, helps medial rotation
Piriformis	Anterior surface of lateral process of sacrum and gluteal surface of ilium at the margin of the greater sciatic notch	Superior edge of greater trochanter of the femur	Rotates thigh laterally at hip, abducts thigh and stabilizes hip joint
Gemellus Superior	Outer surface of ischial spine	Medial surface of the posterior greater trochanter of the femur	Rotates thigh laterally at hip, abducts flexed thigh
Obturator Internus	Internal surface of obturator membrane and posterior bony margins of obturator foramen	Medial surface of greater trochanter of femur, in common with superior and inferior gemelli	Rotates thigh laterally at hip and abducts the thigh when flexed
Gemellus Inferior	Upper border of ischial tuberosity	Medial surface of the posterior greater trochanter of the femur	Rotates thigh laterally at hip, abducts flexed thigh
Obturator Externus	Pubis and ischium around medial side of obturator foramen	The fossa of the greater trochanter of the femur	Rotates thigh laterally at hip and steadies femoral head in acetabulum
Quadratus Femoris	Lateral margin of obturator ring above ischial tuberosity	Quadrate tubercle and adjacent bone of intertrochanteric crest of proximal posterior femur	Rotates thigh laterally at hip and adducts the hip
Acts on the Lower Leg			
Hamstrings			
Biceps Femoris	Ischial tuberosity and sacrotuberous ligament	Head of the fibula and the lateral condyle of the tibia	Both heads; flexes thigh at hip and rotates leg laterally when knee is flexed
Long Head	Ischial tuberosity	Lateral side of head of fibula. Tendon at this site split by fibular collateral ligament of the knee	Extends thigh at hip and rotates leg laterally when knee is flexed
Short Head	Linea aspera and lateral supracondylar line of femur	Lateral side of head of fibula. Tendon at this site split by fibular collateral ligament of the knee	Flexes leg at the knee and rotates leg laterally when knee is flexed
Semitendinous	Ischial tuberosity	Medial surface of superior part of the tibia. Pes anserine	Extends thigh at hip. Flexes and rotates knee medially
Semimembranosus	Ischial tuberosity	Posterior part of medial condyle of the tibia	Extends thigh at hip. Flexes and rotates knee medially
Quadriceps Femoris			
Rectus Femoris	Anterior inferior lilac spine and the groove above the acetabulum	Via quadriceps expansion and patella through patellar ligament to tuberosity of tibia	Extends the leg at the knee joint. Steadies hip joint. Helps iliopsoas flex thigh at hip
Vastus Lateralis	Anterior and inferior border of greater trochanter, proximal 1/2 of lateral linea aspera	Lateral base and border of patella; also forms the lateral patellar retinaculum and lateral side of quadriceps femoris tendon	Extends the leg at the knee joint
Vastus Intermedius	Anterior and lateral surfaces of proximal two-thirds of femur	Lateral border of patella; also forms the deep portion of the quadriceps tendon	Extends the leg at the knee joint
Vastus Medialis	Medial lip of linea aspera and posterior femur	Medial base and border of patella; also forms the medial patellar retinaculum and medial side of quadriceps femoris tendon	Extends the leg at the knee joint
Tensor Fasciae Latae	Anterior superior Iliac spine and anterior iliac crest	Iliotibial tract that attaches to lateral condyle of tibia	Adducts, rotates medially, and flexes thigh at hip joint. Helps keep knee extended

Muscle	Origin	Insertion	Action
Acts on the Foot and Lower Leg			
Gastrocnemius			
Medial Head	Popliteal surface of femur, superior to medial condyle	Middle of posterior surface of the calcaneus via the Achilles tendon	Plantar flexes foot at ankle, assists flexion of leg at the knee joint, raises heel during walking
Lateral Head	Lateral aspect of lateral condyle of femur	Middle of posterior surface of the calcaneus via the Achilles tendon	Plantar flexes foot at ankle, assists flexion of leg at the knee joint, raises heel during walking
Popliteus	Lateral epicondyle of femur and lateral meniscus	Posterior surface of proximal tibia, superior to soleal line	Initiates leg flexion by unlocking the knee
Tibialis Anterior	Lateral condyle and proximal 1/2 of tibia, interosseus membrane, and deep surface of the fascia cruris	Medial and plantar surface of medial cuneiform and base of first metatarsal	Dorsiflexes the ankle and inverts the foot
Peroneus Tertius	Distal 1/3 of anterior fibula and interosseus membrane	Base of fifth metatarsal	Dorsiflexes the ankle, everts the foot
Extensor Digitorum Longus	Lateral condyle of tibia and proximal 3/4 of the anterior interosseous membrane and fibula	By four tendons to the dorsal surfaces of the second and third phalanges of the four lateral toes	Extends lateral four toes and dorsiflexes the foot at ankle
Extensor Hallucis Longus	Anterior surface of the fibula and the adjacent interosseous membrane	Base of distal phalanx of large toe	Extends large toe, dorsiflexes the foot at ankle
Plantaris	Distal lateral supracondylar line of the femur and oblique popliteal ligament	Posterior surface of the calcaneus via the Achilles tendon	Assists gastrocnemius in plantar flexing foot at the ankle or flexion of the knee
Soleus	Head and proximal 1/3 of posterior fibula and middle border and soleal line of tibia	Middle of posterior surface of the calcaneus via the Achilles tendon	Plantar flexes foot at the ankle, stabilizes leg on foot
Flexor Digitorum Longus	Middle 1/3 of posterior surface of tibia	By four tendons to the plantar surface of the distal phalanges of the four lateral toes	Flexes lateral four toes. Assists in plantar flexion and inverts the foot, supports longitudinal arches of foot
Flexor Hallucis Longus	Distal 2/3 of posterior fibula and adjacent interosseus membrane	Base of plantar surface distal phalanx of large toes	Flexes large toe. Assists plantar flexion and inverts the foot
Tibialis Posterior	Middle third of posterior tibia, proximal 2/3 of medial fibula and interosseus membrane	Plantar surfaces of navicular, cuboid, second and third and fourth metatarsals	Inverts the foot. Assists in plantar flexion of ankle
Peroneus Longus	Head and proximal 2/3 of lateral surface of fibula and lateral condyle of tibia	Plantar surface of medial cuneiform and base of first metatarsal	Everts the foot. Assists plantar flexion of ankle
Peroneus Brevis	Distal 2/3 of lateral surface of fibula	Lateral surface of base of fifth metatarsal	Everts the foot. Assists plantar flexion of ankle
Acts on the Abdomen			
Transverse Abdominis	Inguinal ligament, Iliac crest and thoracolumbar fascia and lower six ribs	Abdominal aponeurosis to linea alba and iliac crest	Tenses abdominal wall and compresses contents
Rectus Abdominis	Crest of the pubis and pubic symphysis	Xiphoid process and costal cartilage of ribs 5, 6, 7	Flexes the trunk. Tenses abdominal wall and compresses contents
External Oblique	External surface of eight lower ribs	Abdominal aponeurosis to linea alba and iliac crest	Bilateral - (Same as above). Unilateral - Flexes laterally and rotates to the opposite side
Internal Oblique	Inguinal ligament, Iliac crest and thoracolumbar fascia	Abdominal aponeurosis, linea alba, and costal cartilages of four lower ribs	Bilateral - (Same as above). Unilateral - Flexes laterally and rotates to the same side
Muscles for Respiration			
Diaphragm	The xiphoid process, six lower ribs and costal cartilages, ligaments, bodies and transverse processes of upper lumbar vertebrae	Central tendon of the diaphragm, a strong aponeurosis with no bony attachment.	Main muscle of respiration, contracts during inspiration increasing thoracic volume. Separates abdominal and thoracic cavities
Serratus Posterior Superior	Spinous process of C7-T2, ligamentum nuchae C6-T1 supraspinous ligament	Posterior superior surfaces of ribs 2-5	Raises ribs during deep inspiration
Serratus Posterior Inferior	Spinous process of T11-L3, supraspinous ligament	Inferior borders of ribs 8-12	Retracts ribs outward and downward, opposes diaphragm

Muscle	Origin	Insertion	Action
Intercostals			
External	Inferior margin of the rib above	Superior margin of the rib below. Fibers angle 45% lateral to medial	Pulls ribs together and elevates ribs during respiration
Internal	Inferior margin of the rib above	Superior margin of the rib below. Fibers angle 45% medial to lateral	Pulls ribs together and elevates ribs during respiration
Innermost	Sternum and inferior margin of lower ribs	Inner surface of ventral ribs	Pulls ribs together and elevates ribs during respiration
Acts on the Spine and Back			
Quadratus Lumborum	Posterior iliac crest and iliolumbar ligament	Transverse processes of L1-L4 and inferior border of rib 12	Flexes and extends spine laterally, fixes 12th rib during respiration
Intertransversarii	Transverse processes of cervical, lumbar and T10-T12 vertebra	Transverse process of vertebra directly above origin	Flexes laterally and stabilizes the spine
Rotatores	Transverse process of each vertebra	Lamina of vertebra directly above	Extends, rotates to the opposite side and stabilizes the spine
Multifidus	Transverse processes of C4-L5, PSIS, posterior sacrum, and iliac crest	Spans 2-4 vertebrae. Inserts on spinous process	Extends, rotates to the opposite side and stabilizes the spine
Semispinalis			Extends head, neck and thorax and rotates them to opposite side
Capitis	Transverse processes of C4-T7	Occipital bone between inferior and superior nuchal lines	Unilateral; Rotates to the opposite side. Stabilizes the spine
Cervicis	Transverse processes of T1-T6	Spinous process of C2-C5	Extends, rotates vertebral column
Thoracis	Transverse processes of T6-T12	Spinous process of C6-T8	Extends, rotates vertebral column
Spinalis			Bilateral; Extends the spine. Unilateral; Flexes spine laterally
Capitis	Inseparable from Semispinalis	(Same as semispinalis)	Extends head
Cervicis	Ligamentum nuchae	Spinous process of C2-C4	Extends vertebral column
Thoracis	Spinous process of T10-L2	Spinous process of T4-T8	Stabilizes the spine
Longissimus			Bilateral; Extends the spine. Unilateral; Flexes spine laterally
Capitis	Articular processes of C4-C7, Transverse processes of T1-T4	Posterior surface of mastoid process	Extends and laterally bends vertebral column and head
Cervicis	Transverse processes of T1-T5	Transverse processes of C2-C6	Extends and laterally bends vertebral column and head, stabilizes the spine
Thoracis	Thoracolumbar fascia, transverse processes of lumbar vertebra	Transverse processes of T1-T12 and posterior surface of lower ten ribs	Extends and laterally bends vertebral column and head
Acts on the Neck and Back			
Sternocleidomastoid	Sternal head: Superior aspect of manubrium. Clavicular head: Medial one third of clavicle	Mastoid process and superior nuchal line of occipital bone	Bilateral; Flexes the neck. Unilateral; Rotates the head to opposite side, flexes laterally
Iliocostalis Lumborum	Common origin by broad tendon arising from spinous process of T12-L5, medial lip of iliac crest and medial and lateral crest of the sacrum	Inferior borders of the posterior angle of ribs 7-12	Bilateral; Extends the spine Unilateral; Flexes spine laterally. Stabilizes the spine
Thoracis	Upper borders of posterior angles of ribs 7-12	Transverse process of C7 and angles of ribs 1-6	Keeps thoracic spine erect
Cervicis	Posterior angles of ribs 3-6	Transverse processes of C4-C6	Extends cervical spine
Splenius Capitis	Lower one half of ligamentum nuchae, Spinous process of C7-T4	Mastoid process and lateral 1/3 of occiput	Bilateral; Extends the head Unilateral; Bends laterally, rotates the face to same side
Splenius Cervicis	Spinous process of T3-T6	Transverse processes of C1-C3	Bilateral; Extends the neck Unilateral; Bends laterally, rotates the head to same side
Scalene			
Anterior	Anterior tubercles of transverse processes of C3-C6	Anterior superior aspect of first rib	Bilateral; Raises rib cage in deep inspiration, flexes the neck Unilateral; Flexes neck laterally, rotates neck to opposite side
Medial	Posterior tubercles of transverse processes of C2-C7	Lateral anterior aspect of first rib	Flexes neck laterally, elevates first rib
Posterior	Posterior tubercles of transverse processes C5-C7	Lateral anterior aspect of second rib	Flexes neck laterally, elevates second rib

ANATOMY

Muscle	Origin	Insertion	Action
Rectus Capitis			
Lateralis	Upper surface of transverse process of C1	Jugular process of occipital bone	Flexes head laterally, stabilizes head
Anterior	Anterior surface and transverse process of C1	Base of occipital bone, anterior to occipital condyle	Flexes the neck, rotates to the same side
Posterior Minor	Tubercle of posterior arch of atlas	Median inferior nuchal line	Extends the head and neck
Posterior Major	Spine of axis	Lateral inferior nuchal line	Extends the head, flexes laterally
Obliquus Capitis			
Inferior	Spinous process of C2	Posterior aspect of transverse process of C1	Rotates to the same side
Superior	Superior aspect of transverse process of C1	Between inferior and superior nuchal lines of occiput	Extends the head, rotates to the same side
Longus Capitis	Anterior tubercles of transverse processes of C3-C6	Inferior surface of occiput	Flexes and rotates the head
Longus Colli	Anterior tubercles of C3-5, Anterior vertebral bodies C5-T3	Anterior surface of vertebral bodies of C1, Anterior tubercles of C5-6	Flexes head, flexes laterally and rotates to the same side
Acts on the Hyoid and Neck			
Infrahyoid Muscles			
Sternohyoid	Manubrium of sternum and medial end of clavicle	Inferior body of hyoid bone	Depresses hyoid bone and larynx after swallowing
Sternothyroid	Top of sternum and costal cartilage of 1st rib	Lamina of thyroid cartilage	Depresses larynx after swallowing
Thyrohyoid	Lamina of thyroid cartilage	Inferior body of hyoid bone	Depresses hyoid bone, raises larynx when hyoid bone is fixed
Omohyoid	Superior border of scapula near suprascapular notch	Inferior border of hyoid bone	Depresses, retracts and fixes hyoid bone
Suprahyoid Muscles			
Geniohyoid	Mental spine of mandible	Body of hyoid, superior aspect	Elevates hyoid or depresses mandible
Mylohyoid	Mylohyoid line of mandible	Body of hyoid, superior aspect	Elevates hyoid bone, floor of mouth, and tongue during swallowing and speaking
Stylohyoid	Styloid process of temporal bone	Body of hyoid, superior aspect	Elevates and retracts hyoid bone
Digastric		Intermediate tendon to hyoid bone	Depresses mandible, elevates hyoid bone, steadies it during speaking and swallowing
Anterior Belly	Digastric fossa on deep surface of inferior border of mandible near symphysis	By tendon to body of hyoid, superior aspect	Elevates hyoid or depresses mandible
Posterior Belly	Mastoid notch of temporal bone	By tendon to body of hyoid, superior aspect	Elevates hyoid or depresses mandible
Muscles for Mastication			
Masseter	Lower border and medial surface of zygomatic arch	Lateral surface of ramus of the mandible	Elevates and retracts mandible, closes jaw
Superficial	Aponeurosis from the zygomatic process of the maxilla	Coronoid process and ramus of mandible	Elevates and retracts mandible
Deep	Posterior third of the lower border and from the whole of the medial surface of the zygomatic arch	Coronoid process and ramus of mandible	Elevates and retracts mandible
Buccinator	Ridge of mandible, alveolar process of maxilla, pterygomandibular ligament	Angle of mouth, blending with Orbicularis oris	Holds cheeks near teeth positioning food for chewing, aids chewing
Temporalis	Temporal lines on the parietal bone of the skull	Coronoid process and ramus of mandible	Elevates mandible, closes and retracts jaw
Medial Pterygoid	Medial surface of pterygoid plate of sphenoid	Medial surface of ramus of the mandible	Closes jaw, elevates and protracts mandible, Unilateral; protrudes side of the jaw
Lateral Pterygoid	Lateral surface of pterygoid plate of sphenoid	Anterior surface of condyle of mandible and TMJ capsule	Depresses chin, protracts and depresses mandible to open mouth, Unilateral; moves jaw to opposite side

Muscle	Origin	Insertion	Action
Muscles for Expression			
Platysma	Superficial fascia of upper thorax and anterolateral aspect of neck	Inferior border of mandible and skin over lower face and angle of mouth	Depresses angle of mouth and wrinkles skin of neck
Epicranius			
Occipitalis	Posterior occiput above occipital ridge	Epicranial aponeurosis	Draws epicranius towards posterior
Frontalis	Blended into procerus, corrugator and orbicularis oculi	Epicranial aponeurosis	Raises eyebrow and wrinkles the forehead
Orbicularis Oculi	Medial palpebral ligament to maxilla, nasal bone, nasal part of frontal bone	Fibers surround eye and blend with adjacent muscles	Closes the eye
Nasalis	Maxilla above incisors	Blends into procerus	Compresses nostrils
Corrugator	Medial aspect of supraorbital ridge	Deep surface of skin in middle of supra-orbital arch	Draws eyebrows together
Procerus	Fascia over upper nasal cartilage and lower nasal bone	Deep surface of skin between eyebrows	Draws nose up, causing wrinkles across nose
Dilator Naris	Greater ala cartilage	Point of the nose	Expands opening of nostril
Quadratus Labii Superioris	Lower margin of orbit, frontal process of maxilla	Blends into orbicularis oris on upper lip	Raises upper lip
Zygomaticus			
Minor	Continuous from inferior border of orbicularis oculi	Blends into orbicularis oris on upper lip	Raises upper lip
Major	Anterior surface of zygomatic bone	Blends into orbicularis oris muscle at upper angle of mouth	Draws angle of mouth back and up
Auricularis	Temporal bone	Deep skin around ear	Raises and moves ear
Anterior	Superficial temporal fascia	Cartilage of ear	Draws ear forward
Posterior	Mastoid process	Cartilage of ear	Draws ear backward
Superior	Galea aponeurotica	Cartilage of ear	Raises ear
Orbicularis Oris	From numerous adjacent muscles surrounding mouth	Lips, external skin around mouth and mucous membrane adjacent to the lips inside of mouth	Closes and protrudes lip as if whistling
Risorius	Fascia over masseter	Blends into orbicularis oris and skin at corner of the mouth	Draws angle of mouth backward
Depressor Anguli Oris	Anterior inferior surface of mandible	Blends into orbicularis oris and skin at corner of the mouth	Draws angle of mouth downward
Depressor Labii Inferioris	Anterior inferior surface of mandible	Blends into orbicularis oris and skin on lower lip of the mouth	Depresses lower lip
Mentalis	Mandible below incisors	Deep skin at point of chin	Raises chin and protrudes lower lip as if pouting
Acts on the Eyes			
Levator Palpebrae Superiores	Inferior aspect of lesser wing and anterior optic nerve	Superior tarsal plate and skin of upper eyelid	Elevates and opens upper eyelid
Superior Rectus	Common tendinous ring within the orbit	Anterior superior aspect of eyeball	Elevates, adducts, and rotates eyes medially
Inferior Rectus	Common tendinous ring within the orbit	Anterior inferior aspect of eyeball	Depresses, adducts, and rotates eyes medially
Medial Rectus	Common tendinous ring within the orbit	Anterior medial aspect of eyeball	Rotates eye medially
Lateral Rectus	Common tendinous ring within the orbit	Anterior lateral aspect of eyeball	Rotates eye laterally
Inferior Oblique	Orbital surface of maxilla behind orbital margin	Posterior lateral aspect of eyeball	Elevates and rotates eyes laterally
Superior Oblique	Common tendinous ring within the orbit	Posterior lateral aspect of eyeball	Rotates eye upward and outward

Bodywork as Energy Work

Energy fields and currents exist everywhere in nature. Energy can neither be created nor destroyed, but can be manipulated and transformed. This concept is related to theories of quantum mechanics which states that matter and energy actually fluctuate, meaning that our thoughts can become physical and our bodies energetic. Energy healing means different things to different people. All bodywork practitioners as energy workers, regardless of expertise and training, whether you are Reiki Master or doing massage for the first time. Energy work is a natural part of performing bodywork. Our bodies have electrical charges and chemical impulses that originate from the somatic nervous system. Thoughts and intent are the powerful mechanisms behind the somatic nervous system. How else could you explain the ability of energy to affect clients without touch? Whether we believe in energy work or not, and no matter what you want to call it, we send energy healing to clients from our intention.

As an acupuncture student, I studied traditional Chinese medicine in China, and had seen some remarkable results from acupuncture and qi gong treatments that could not be explained by Western medicine, so I was open to chi, qi, prana, and energy work. I practiced with the intent of moving qi through the needles or placing my hands on a patient at the beginning of the treatment as a form of energy healing. Some patients would describe the feeling as a physical sensation, vibration or heat. While it's not always the same, it's energy moving through the body. In acupuncture school, we learn the fundamentals of qi and energy; when energy is unbalanced, blocked or fixed due to stress or other factors, pain and disease arise. Blockages generally manifest in sequence from the subtle (energetic) to the dense (physical) levels of the field. The practitioner seeks to find the blockages and release energy to normal flow patterns, and to maintain the energy field in an open, flexible condition.

Energy work is the general term for describing all the therapy modalities that are based on energy healing. They are all focused on the belief that the human body contains many levels of energy that, when stimulated through various techniques, will promote overall health and well-being. The idea of energy fields can be traced back to some of the oldest traditional medicine systems. Shamanism, with its connection to the spiritual as a source of healing energy, was the earliest form of energy work in many cultures. Indigenous cultures throughout the Americas, Australia, Polynesia, Africa and the Arctic have practiced the art of setting intent, connecting with healing energy, transmission of that intent into healing of the physical body for thousands of years. The word "shaman" is derived from an indigenous people in Siberia that still practices their healing arts today. Some techniques such as acupressure and shiatsu have roots in ancient traditional medicine while techniques like Reiki to Zero Balancing to Polarity Therapy are more modern approaches to energy medicines. But the underlying principle of these treatments remains the same - the idea of energy flowing in the body.

Energy work can be appropriate when clients are in extreme pain and cannot be touched or they have recently undergone surgery. Energy work can be interactive, when a client and practitioner engage in dialogue during the bodywork session, or non-interactive, when a client relaxes and receives work which balances out his or her energy. Energy work can be integrated into the healthcare plan for clients with cancer, HIV, and emotional challenges, and it is known for relieving emotional tensions which appear in the physical body as pain.

Energy work techniques can be combined with massage treatments, or they may be used as a stand-alone modality, to affect physical, emotional, mental and spiritual imbalances. They can be used as a form of natural healing and guide treatment. Above all, it should be remembered that it is a subjective experience. Many of the changes that take place during a treatment are registered at a subconscious level, so that a practitioner may be more aware of events in the healing process than a client. The client may become aware of these changes hours, days, weeks and even months later, once they process them on a conscious level. Additionally, an interesting aspect of energy work is that the more open a recipient is to the shifts that may occur during treatment, the more possible it is for them to experience benefits. This is because their open attitude causes their energetic system to respond more to treatment. Literally, the more energy flow is occurring in the field of the client, the easier it is for them to heal.

Introduction to Energy Work

Energy work is a general term for a group of healing modalities that focus on creating balance and harmony in the physical body by facilitating balance in the energetic anatomy of the client. The approach in energy work is holistic; the belief is that the physical, emotional, mental and spiritual aspects work synergistically to create a healthy condition. If there are imbalances on one level, they may also appear on another level, so the root of the problem must be addressed in order to fully heal. Typical issues addressed in energy work are traumatic events: emotional wounding, physical disease and spiritual issues.

The energy work therapist recognizes that there is electromagnetic energy flowing around and through the body in very specific currents (meridians and nadis) and vortexes (chakras), as well as through the human energy field (also called the aura). When energy currents, vortexes and fields are disrupted, an imbalance occurs in the energy system. If allowed to persist long enough, energetic imbalances can create pain and even disease in the physical body. The paradigm is that once the root of a problem is fully addressed, health returns.

Thank you to Ariel F. Hubbard, of the California Academy for the Healing Arts for her contribution on energy work chapter.
www.cahaschool.com

There are many different healing modalities in energy work, such as Reiki, Sound Healing, HighSelf Resonance Therapy, Light Work, Zero Balancing, Polarity Therapy, Shamanism and Crystal Healing. However, all of these modalities, despite using different treatment protocols, contain similar general approaches:

Approach	Protocol
Preparing the practitioner and the client for the session	The practitioner may use various energy work techniques to enhance, clear and balance their own energy flow prior to working; they may also prepare the space in which they are working for the client; they may also ask the client for their intent for healing
Creating rapport with and assessing the client	This gives the therapist the information they need to develop a plan of care and generate confidence in the client. This may be accomplished through a client intake form, interview, scanning of the client's energy system, intuitive reading of the client's energy system, or a combination of techniques
Determining energetic stagnation, deficiency or energetic excess and selecting tools to facilitate wellness	This may be accomplished through various protocols used to read a client's energetic flow, such as by scanning with hands; client interview, clairvoyant/clairsentient/clairaudient reading of the client's energy system and selecting the best method to correct imbalances
Making corrections in the client's energy system (with their permission)	Some energy work approaches use hands-on techniques, such as Reiki Hand Placements, laying on of hands, crystal layouts or shamanic ritual to encourage energy flow, remove stagnation, correct deficiencies and remove excess energy.
Closing the treatment	Once the appropriate corrections have been made, the facilitator uses a variety of techniques, such as grounding or sealing the Auric Field to close the session.

Techniques

Energy work, like massage, is a multifaceted collection of techniques and approaches, usually limited only by the creativity of the practitioner. The therapist usually practices more than one style of energy work so that they have multiple tools available for their client. A few examples include:

Technique	Practice
Energy work through touch	• Reiki practitioners use Reiki hand positions to transmit Reiki to the client (they may also send Reiki long-distance) • Shamans may also touch their clients to transmit healing energy, ground energy or remove spirits from the client • Psychic surgeons palpate and remove cysts and other diseased tissue through physical touch
Energy work through transmission of energy	• Sound, Crystal, Shamanic, Psychic, Faith, Qi Gong, Pranic, Reiki and other healers may transmit healing energy to a client through the client's energy system. This may occur through the auric field, the chakras, the meridians or nadis, or even through prayer, chanting, or hypnotic suggestion
Energy work through counseling	• Many energy workers use psychic ability to "read" the conditions in a client's life and to give suggestions to assist the client to choose a healthy lifestyle. Some give counseling for the present time; others read potential outcomes for the future to assist clients to make beneficial decisions
Energy work through emotional release work	• Gestalt Therapy, Rebirthing, Constellation Healing Work, Reiki, Hypnotherapy, High-Self Resonance Therapy and a variety of other energy work modalities work with emotional release and healing as a part of restoring energetic balance and harmony

Energetic Anatomy Structures

The Chakra System: The word "chakra" means "wheel" in Sanskrit and refers to this energy vortex's ability to spin energy into and out of the body. Chakras are located all over the body at intersections of energy flow through nadis. There are many minor chakras, and several major chakras. Minor chakras lie in the hands, feet, ears, eyes and other organs of the body. Major chakras lie on the Sushumna (also called the Central Channel).

Nadis: Nadis are energetic and physical tubes that transmit bodily fluids and energy throughout the body. The most important three are the Sushumna (the central channel), Ida (the feminine), and Pingala (the masculine). The main chakras in the body connect into the central channel. Some examples are nerves, meridians, intestines and blood vessels.

ENERGY

Chakra System 1

Chakras are energy centers along the spine located at major branchings of the human nervous system, beginning at the base of the spinal column and moving upward to the top of the skull. It is believed to be a center of activity that receives, assimilates, and expresses life force energy. There is a belief that when there are imbalances in certain chakras centers, unusual physical manifestations of illness can arise. Some practitioners focus on areas of blockages in order to rebalance the chakras incorporating ayurvedic medicine, massage and manual therapy into their treatment.

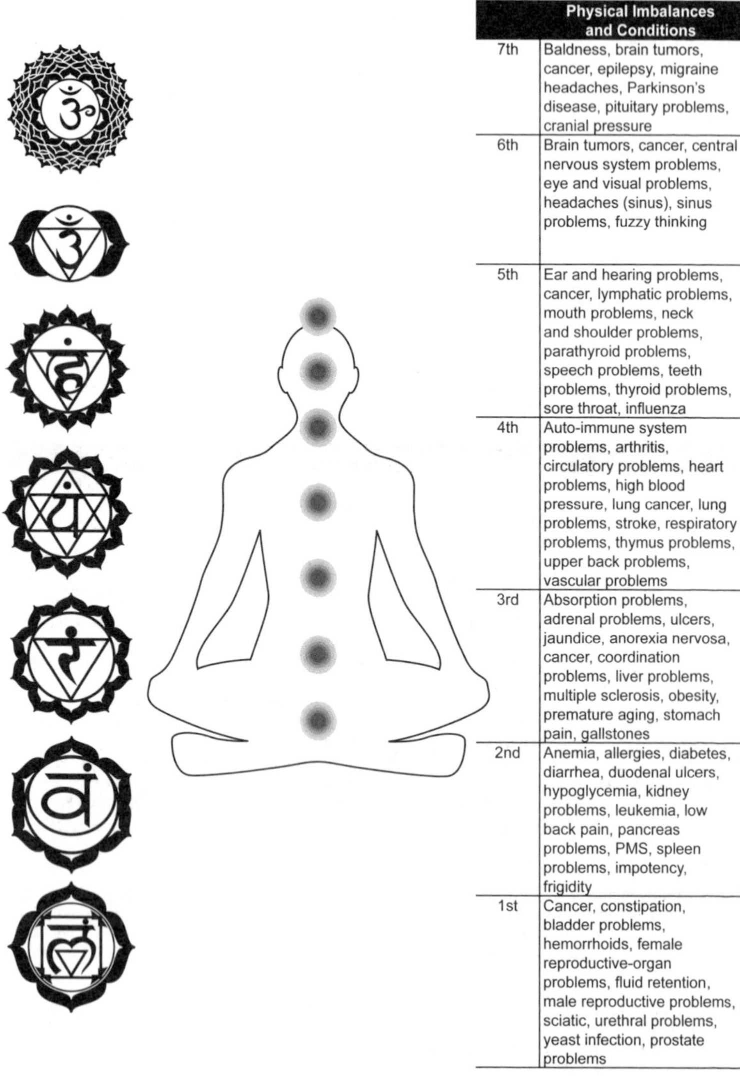

	Physical Imbalances and Conditions
7th	Baldness, brain tumors, cancer, epilepsy, migraine headaches, Parkinson's disease, pituitary problems, cranial pressure
6th	Brain tumors, cancer, central nervous system problems, eye and visual problems, headaches (sinus), sinus problems, fuzzy thinking
5th	Ear and hearing problems, cancer, lymphatic problems, mouth problems, neck and shoulder problems, parathyroid problems, speech problems, teeth problems, thyroid problems, sore throat, influenza
4th	Auto-immune system problems, arthritis, circulatory problems, heart problems, high blood pressure, lung cancer, lung problems, stroke, respiratory problems, thymus problems, upper back problems, vascular problems
3rd	Absorption problems, adrenal problems, ulcers, jaundice, anorexia nervosa, cancer, coordination problems, liver problems, multiple sclerosis, obesity, premature aging, stomach pain, gallstones
2nd	Anemia, allergies, diabetes, diarrhea, duodenal ulcers, hypoglycemia, kidney problems, leukemia, low back pain, pancreas problems, PMS, spleen problems, impotency, frigidity
1st	Cancer, constipation, bladder problems, hemorrhoids, female reproductive-organ problems, fluid retention, male reproductive problems, sciatic, urethral problems, yeast infection, prostate problems

Note: Chakra System 1, This chart is based on the traditional Indian system of 7 chakras.

Human Energy Anatomy System 2

Auric Layers

Etheric Layer - (Closest to the body) Reveals the Condition of the Physical Body

Emotional Layer - Reveals the Condition of the Emotions

Mental Layer - Reveals the Condition of the Mind

Astral Layer - Reveals the Condition of the Self

Etheric Template - Reveals Alignment with Divine Will

Celestial Body - Reveals Alignment with Divine Love

Ketheric Template - Reveals Alignment with Divine Consciousness

Chakras Above the Body

Universal - Ultimate Divine Connection

Galactic - Connection with our Galaxy

Solar System - Connection with our Solar System

Upper Earth - Portal of Incarnation onto the Earth Plane

Transpersonal Point - Portal of Incarnation into the Human Body

Body

Crown Chakra / Sahasrara - Unity with Divine Consciousness

Third Eye / Ajna - Spiritual Vision

Zeal Point - Spiritual Enthusiasm

Throat / Vishuddhi - Self-Expression, Receiving, Relationship and Work

Thymus - Life Purpose

Heart / Anahata - Unconditional Love

Diaphragm - Deeply-Held Emotions

Solar Plexus / Manipura - Personal Power

Sacral / Swadhisthana - Creativity, Sexuality

Root / Muladhara - Physical Vitality and Enthusiasm for Life

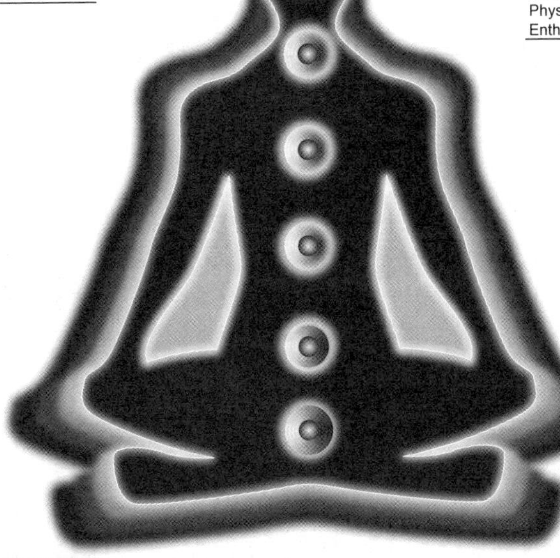

Hara Line

Upper Dan Tien - Connection with the Divine

Middle Dan Tien - Connection with Your Life Purpose

Lower Dan Tien - Connection with Your Personal Power

Below the Body

Knees - Grounding

Feet - Grounding

Earth - Connection with the Earth

Note: Human Energy Anatomy System 2, This system includes chakras from the traditional system as well as including new chakras that have been more recently discovered. The names of the auric field layers are based on Barbara Brennan's teaching tradition. The names of the Dan Tians are based on Chinese and Japanese teachings.

Source: from The *Human Energy Anatomy System* Chart: (Adapted) with permission from Ariel F. Hubbard

Chakra & Location	Acupressure Points	Psychic Abilities	Spiritual Symbology	Psychological Correlations	Physical Imbalances & Conditions	Psychological Imbalances & Conditions
7th **Crown Chakra** (Crown of head)	Du-16, Du-17, Du-18, Du-19, Du-20, Du-21	• To be open • To know • Intuition • Precognition • Connection with infinite intelligence	The state of the one's relationship to the Divine. Trusting the Divine	• Pineal gland • Old mammalian brain • Greater right-hemisphere correlation	Baldness, brain tumors, cancer, epilepsy, migraine headaches, Parkinson's disease, pituitary problems, cranial pressure	• Excessive gullibility • Memory disorders • Multiple personalities • Nightmares • Split personality
6th **Third Eye** (Center of forehead)	Sj-4, Du-17, Du-18, Du-19, Du-24, Du-25, E-Yintang, Ub-2	• Clairvoyance • Psychic reading • To have vision or insight • Photographic memory • Telekinesis	The ability to see events from a spiritual perspective	• Pituitary glands • Neo-mammalian brain • Greater left-brain hemisphere correlation	Brain tumors, cancer, central nervous system problems, eye and visual problems, headaches (sinus), sinus problems, fuzzy thinking	• Extreme confusion • Inability to focus • Intelligence deficiencies • Living in a fantasy world • Paranoia • Psychotic behavior • Schizophrenia
5th **Throat Chakra** (Expression) (Center of the throat)	St-9, Ub-10, Ren-22, Ren-23	• Communication center • Telepathy • Clairaudience • Inner voice • Tone healing	The ability to speak one's truth and the state of one's feelings regarding their job (posterior throat)	• Thyroid • Parathyroid • Lymphatic system • Brain stem	Ear and hearing problems, cancer, lymphatic problems, mouth problems, neck and shoulder problems, parathyroid problems, speech problems, teeth problems, thyroid problems, sore throat, influenza	• Inability to express oneself in words • Logorrhea (nonstop verbal chatter) • Poor auditory memory • Stuttering
4th **Heart Chakra** (Center of the chest)	Ren-17, Ren-18, Du-10, Du-11, Du-12	• To be in affinity with • To be at one with • To connect with • Compassion • Unconditional love	The state of unconditional love and emotional openness	• Thymus gland • Heart • Vascular system • Lungs • Respiratory system	Auto-immune system problems, arthritis, circulatory problems, heart problems, high blood pressure, lung cancer, lung problems, stroke, respiratory problems, thymus problems, upper back problems, vascular problems	• At war with oneself • Feelings of alienation • Inability to bond with another • Self-destructive tendencies • Suicide
3rd **Solar Plexus** Personality Chakra (Above the navel)	K-17, K-18, K-19, Ren-10, Ren-11, Ren-12, Ren-13	• Astral projection • To be empowered • To manifest • To be in control of yourself • Psychic healing	The state of one's thoughts and ego; also the development of one's personal power	• Adrenal glands • Solar plexus (neural center) • Autonomic control center	Absorption problems, adrenal problems, ulcers, jaundice, anorexia nervosa, cancer, coordination problems, liver problems, multiple sclerosis, obesity, premature aging, stomach pain, gallstones	• Addictive personality • Catatonic schizophrenia • Compulsive behavior • Excessive anger or fear • Manic-depressive behavior • Obsessive behavior • Sleep problems
2nd **Feeling Center** Sexual Chakra (Center of the abdomen)	K-11, K-12, K-13, Ren-3, Ren-4, Ren-5, Ren-6, Ren-7, Du-3, Du-4, Du-5, Ub-23, Ub-24, Ub-46, Ub-47, Gb-25	• Clairsentience • Emotional feelings • Balance of male and female energies	The state of close personal relationships (anterior) and one's relationship to oneself. Also sexuality, money and creativity	• Insulin-producing glands in the pancreas and spleen	Anemia, allergies, diabetes, diarrhea, duodenal ulcers, hypoglycemia, kidney problems, leukemia, low back pain, pancreas problems, PMS, spleen problems, impotency, frigidity	• Chameleon personality • Depression • Hysteria • Unable to be sexually intimate
1st **Root Chakra** (Base of the spine)	Du-1, Du-2, Du-3, Ren-1, Ren-2, Ren-3, Sp-12, Sp-13, St-29, St-30, Liv-12	• Grounding • Realizing • Letting go • Surviving	Vital enthusiasm for life, the state of the physical body	• Ovaries • Testes • Placenta	Cancer, constipation, bladder problems, hemorrhoids, female reproductive-organ problems, fluid retention, male reproductive problems, sciatic, urethral problems, yeast infection, prostate issues	• Accident prone • Being in survival • Dependent personality • Identity crisis • Weak ego structure

The Central Channel: The Central Channel, or the Sushumna, is the most important nadi in the body. It connects the energies of the Cosmic Universe, with the energies of the earth through our bodies. This connects us with the male and female energies and grounds those energies through our physical bodies. The chakras connect to the Central Channel through "seals." They open out the front *and* the back of the body (except the Crown Chakra, which points upward, and the Root Chakra, which points downward). The Ida is the main feminine nadi, and the Pingala is the main masculine body. These two nadis either parallel or spiral around the Central Channel (different teachings give them different placements).

The Hara Line: The Hara Line is a Nadi that connects the Center of the Earth, the Lower Dan Tien, the Middle Dan Tien and the Upper Dan Tien with the Universe. The Hara Line lies parallel, yet deep to the Central Channel. The Lower Dan Tien indicates the state of our personal power. The Middle Dan Tien indicates the life direction, and the Upper Dan Tien indicates the state of our divine connection.

The Auric Field: The Auric Field is a field of energy around the physical body. The Auric Field is a repository of thoughts, feelings, beliefs, and experiences as a human being. It can indicate karma as well as the history of life experiences. It is divided into layers, each of which has a different structure and purpose.

Ability to Read Energy

When energy workers read the energetic system to gain information or to facilitate healing, they are reading information that is continuously changing. The condition of these layers may change moment to moment, depending on a client's thoughts, feelings, reactions to events, karma, physical condition and belief systems. A client's thoughts and beliefs can influence their energetic and physical state. When energy workers are reading their energetic anatomy to gain information about them, the energy workers' clear-mindedness and impartiality will enhance their ability to read this information accurately.

Not all energy workers see energetic anatomy structures. Some may hear, sense, or even know the state of a client's energetic anatomy intuitively.

Physiologic Effects. The practitioner may also notice changes while working, including:

- **Increased blood, lymphatic, and qi circulation:** You may notice a change in a client's complexion. Be aware of changes in breathing patterns, shifts in lymphatic distribution or an opening of meridians, chakras, or acupressure points.
- **Increased heart rate, pulse, respiration, and perspiration:** Clients and practitioners both may feel increased heart rate and pulse, usually signaled by increased body temperature.
- **Improved immunological function:** Energy work, like massage, improves immune function, especially with consistent treatments.
- **Altered mood:** Clients frequently experience mood elevation, calming from stress, a feeling of being centered or a sense of mental and spiritual clarity.
- **Improved organ function:** Many clients report enhanced digestive, urinary, integumentary and other organ system functions after energy work treatments (often evidenced by accelerated elimination, increased appetite, perspiration and other effects)
- **Altered brain chemistry:** Clients with depression and other conditions affected by brain chemistry have reported altered moods, increased clarity, reduced stress and anxiety. Energy work is not a replacement for medication, but it may enhance its effects.

How Practitioners Learn Energy Work Modalities

Many call the process of learning and developing their skill in energy work a "journey." Developing proficiency in energy work requires dedication - not only to learning the modality, but also to self-development, communication skills and healing oneself.

In order to become an energy worker, practitioners need to develop sensitivity to energy flow, the ability to read energy, and the ability to manage their own energy flow. They also undergo their personal healing process, where they address and heal internal issues.

Practitioners should learn to develop an awareness of what is occurring in their own energy system and how to manage that flow. Self-management is key so that the practitioner is energetically clear and balanced. Many people do sense energy from others; however, in order to receive accurate information, reading energy flows must be clear, present and grounded. If they allow their own emotions, thoughts or beliefs to intervene, their information about other people may not be accurate, and accuracy is vital to providing beneficial treatments.

ENERGY WORK

Energy workers learn the modality of choice and understand its theory and practical applications. They work with this modality until they achieve proficiency. Some modalities, such as Reiki, are easy to learn and apply, but fully understanding their true impact may take years. Other modalities, such as Polarity Theory, are much more complex, and require consistent dedication in order to master.

Developing proficient client communication skills also requires years of practice, as well as the confidence to explain the more esoteric aspects of energy work. Energy work, itself, by its very nature, may seem mysterious and complicated to those who have not yet had experience with it. Therefore, a practitioner must be clear when communicating with people new to energy work. Developing the ability to speak with people in terms that they understand when discussing energy work requires the ability to listen and to understand people from their own perspective.

There are several qualities that are essential to energy work:

- Having faith in the healing process. When there is faith that, under the right circumstances, energy work may make a difference for the appropriate clients, powerful healing occurs.
- Having humility to be sourced by a Universal Energy. This is the energy that flows through to bring healing to the client.
- Self-esteem is key in this work, since energy workers, like practitioners of other healing professions, must have trust in themselves and their work in order to gain the trust of their clients.
- Developing trust in intuition is also necessary, since energy workers use their intuition consistently while reading energy flow and providing treatments and information to clients.
- Recognizing an appropriate course of treatment for a client. An energy worker understands what they can contribute to a client, the amount of treatment necessary to achieve their objective and the proper time to close treatment.
- Referring to other practitioners when appropriate. Energy work may not be the correct modality for everyone.

Finally, energy work is an excellent adjunct to massage, acupuncture, chiropractic or even allopathic treatments for a variety of conditions and disorders. Energy work may help clients address issues they may not have been able to access through other modalities.

In closing, when person is "called" to the energy work journey, they may feel an intuition to study a particular modality, read a particular book, or hear a talk on the subject. When this occurs, they should follow their intuition, because that is the part of their consciousness that is "in tune" with the Divine consciousness. They are receiving an invitation to make a powerful contribution to others.

Recommended reading and resources on energy work:

Ariel F. Hubbard, *Come From the Heart: A Practical Guidebook to Healing with Divine Energy, Part One* and *Part Two*, California Academy for the Healing Arts, Costa Mesa, CA 2000. www.cahaschool.com

Robert O Becker & Gary Selden, *The Body Electric, Electromagnetism and the Foundation of Life*, Quill, William Morrow, New York, 1985.

Barbara Brennan, *Hands of Light* and *Light Emerging, The Journey of Personal Healing*, Bantam Books, New York, 1991 and 1993.

Donna Eden, *Energy Medicine*, Tarcher/Putnam, New York, 1999.

Mantak Chia, *Awaken Healing Energy Through the Tao*, Aurora Press, 1983.

Michael Gerber, *Vibrational Medicine for the 21st Century: A Complete Guide to Healing with Energy and Vibrational Medicine*, Eagle Brook/Harper Collins, New York, 2000.

Diane Goldner, *Infinite Grace: Where the Worlds of Science and Spiritual Healing Meet*, Hampton Roads Publishing Co., Inc., Charlottesville, VA, 1999.

Fritz Pearls, *Bodymind,* Harper and Row Publishers, New York, 1986.

Sanaya Roman & Duane Packer, *Personal Power through Awareness*, H.J. Kramer, Inc., Tiburon, CA 1986.

Franklyn Sills, *The Polarity Process, Energy As A Healing Art*, Element Inc., Rockport, MA, 1989.

Twelve Benefits of Qi Gong

1. **Well-being and improved health.** Qi gong emphasizes the whole-body, whole-system health. While it is true that qi gong will often cure specific ills, this is not the primary reason for practice. It is not only a matter of adding years to your life, but life to your years.

2. **Clear and tranquil mind.** When the mind is at peace, the whole universe seems at peace. World peace begins with you; it is your responsibility to find a peaceful heart and mind. Then you can heal and transform others just through your presence. If you have a tranquil mind, you will make better decisions and have the skill to know when act and when to be still.

3. **Deeper, more restorative sleep.** Qi gong will help you find the deep relaxation and mental quiet necessary for sleep.

4. **Increased energy, including sexual vitality and fertility.** Qi gong people have more energy; it can "reverse aging and restore youthfulness."

5. **Comfortable warmth.** Qi gong is great for cold hands and feet. Circulation improves, and the body generates more internal warmth when it is cold.

6. **Clear skin**. The skin, like the intestines, is an organ of elimination. According to Chinese medicine, as your qi gong improves, your body eliminates toxins, and the skin becomes clear.

7. **Happy attitude**. There is an old Tibetan saying, "You can tell a Yogi by his or her laugh." Correct and moderate qi gong practice usually creates an optimistic and joyous disposition.

8. **More efficient metabolism.** Digestion improves, and hair and nails grow more quickly.

9. **Greater physiological control.** This means that aspects of the body that were imbalanced or out of control begin to normalize, for example, breathing rate, heart rate, blood pressure, hormone levels, and states of chronic inflammation or depletion.

10. **Bright eyes.** The qi gong master's eyes are said to glow in the dark, like a cat's. The eyes also appear bright because the spirit and soul are luminous and the heart is open.

11. **Intuition and creativity.** Intuition and creativity generate each other and come from the same source, an awakened brain and being, an ability to think with the gut, to feel with the mind.

12. **Spiritual effects.** Advancement in qi gong is often accompanied by a variety of spiritual experiences. For example, synchronicity, meaningful coincidences, become more common. When the qi is abundant, clear, and flowing, the senses perceive and are permeated by a sweetness. "

Recommended reading and resources on Qi Gong:

Master Hong Liu, *The Healing Art of Qi Gong, Ancient Wisdom from a Modern Master,* Warner Books, New York, NY, 1997.

Ken Cohen, T*he Essential Qi Gong Training Course: 100 Days to Increase Energy, Physical Health & Spiritual Well-Being,* Sounds True, Boulder, CO, 2005.

Charles McGee, Effie Chow, *Miracle Healing from China...Qi Gong*, Medipress, Coeur d' Alene, ID, 1996.

The above Twelve Benefits of Qi gong are abridged with permission from pages 17-18 of Ken Cohen's *The Essential Qi Gong Training Guide* (workbook accompanying *The Essential Qi Gong Training Course: 100 Days to Increase Energy, Physical Health, and Spiritual Well-Being*. Boulder, CO, Sounds True; 2005)

Propellar Turns - Warm-up

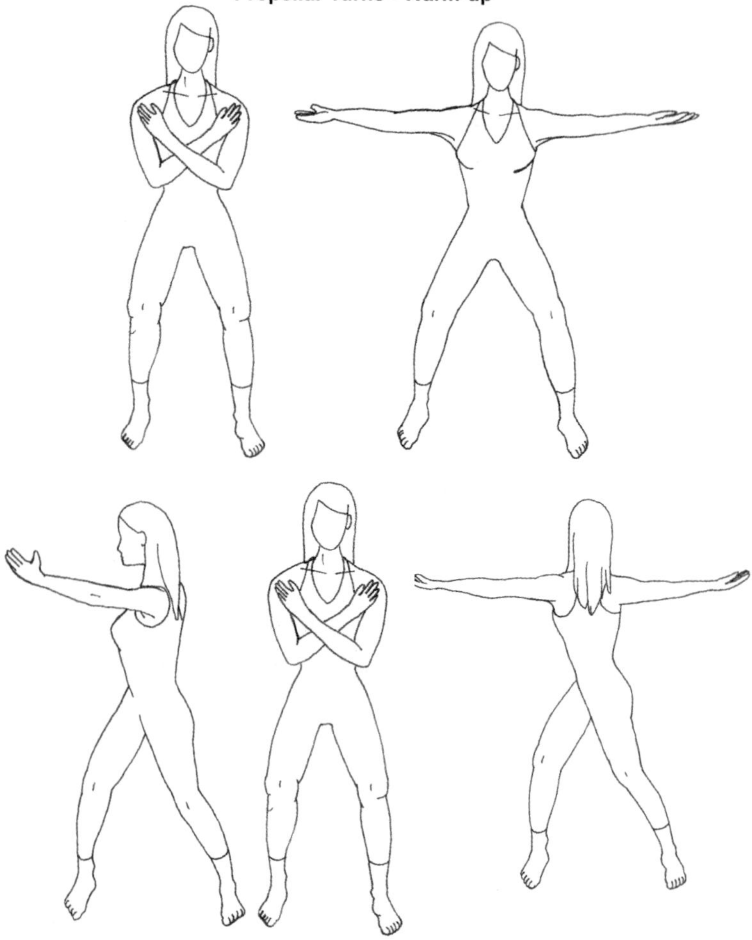

Warm-up - Propeller Turns	Benefits
1. Stand straight with your feet shoulder-width apart, arms stretched out to the side with palms facing up. 2. Keeping your feet firmly planted on the ground, rotate your upper body to the side, stretching your spinal column. Turn as far as possible to a comfortable position, and then hold for a count of ten. 3. Rotate back very slowly, and repeat the opposite direction.	The "propeller turns" is a great warm-up exercise that increases flexibility of the waist and hips, tightens the abdominal muscles, strengthens the shoulders and arms, and increases stamina.

Hip Rotation - Warm-up

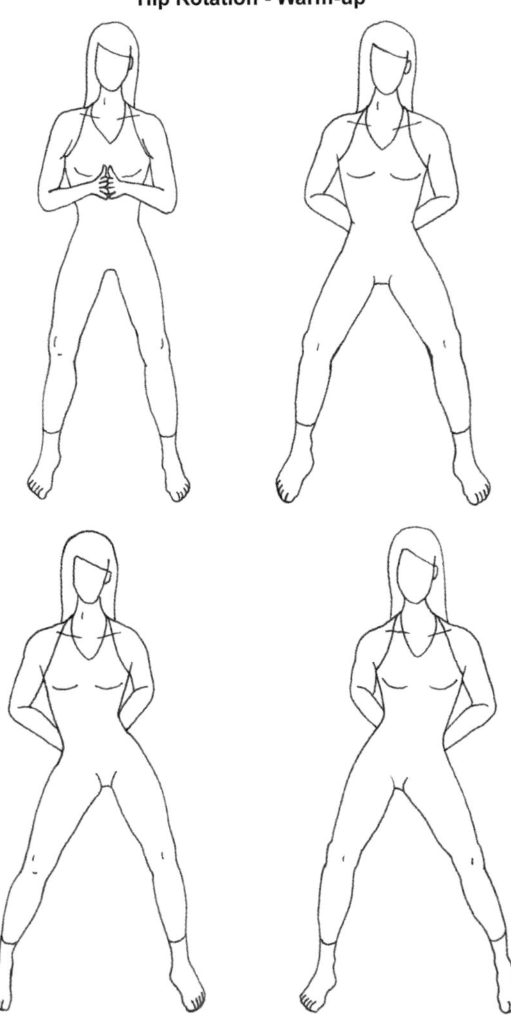

Warm-up - Hip Rotation	Benefits
1. Stand straight with your feet shoulder-width apart. Place your hands on the back of your hips with your fingertips pointing down. 2. Rotate your hips clockwise by moving to one side and then forward to the opposite side in a swirling motion. 3. Repeat for ten rotations, and then reverse the direction to move counter-clockwise.	The "hip rotation" is a great warm-up exercise that lubricates hips and knee joints, loosens low back, and strengthens the thigh, leg and lower body. It can also prevent osteoporosis and improve digestion, elimination, and sexual energy and function.

Propellar Turns - Warm-up

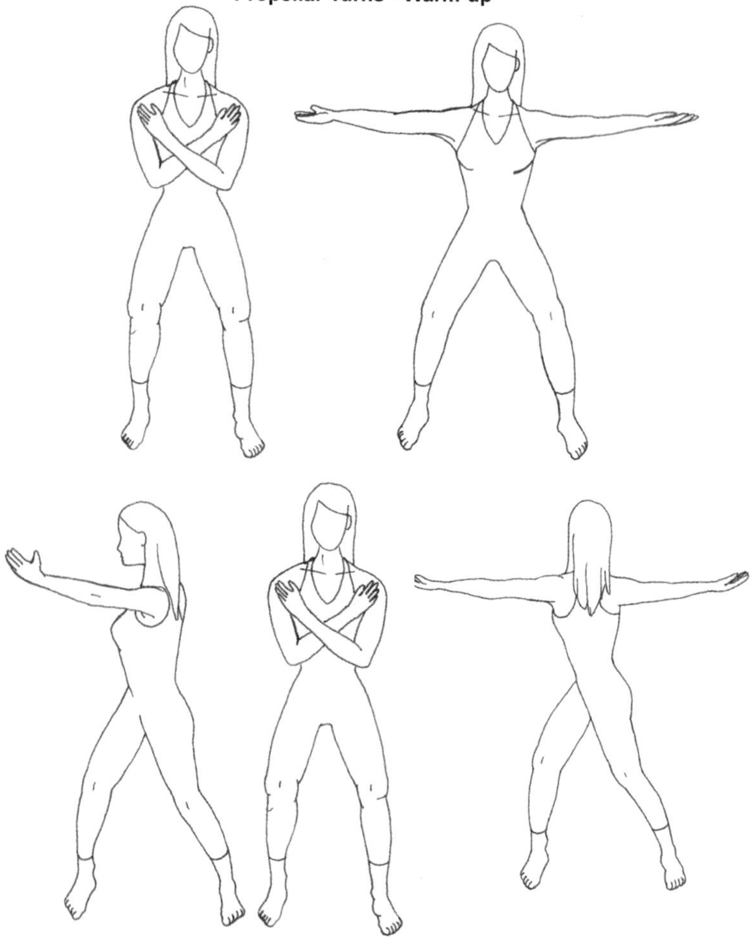

Warm-up - Propeller Turns	Benefits
1. Stand straight with your feet shoulder-width apart, arms stretched out to the side with palms facing up. 2. Keeping your feet firmly planted on the ground, rotate your upper body to the side, stretching your spinal column. Turn as far as possible to a comfortable position, and then hold for a count of ten. 3. Rotate back very slowly, and repeat the opposite direction.	The "propeller turns" is a great warm-up exercise that increases flexibility of the waist and hips, tightens the abdominal muscles, strengthens the shoulders and arms, and increases stamina.

Hip Rotation - Warm-up

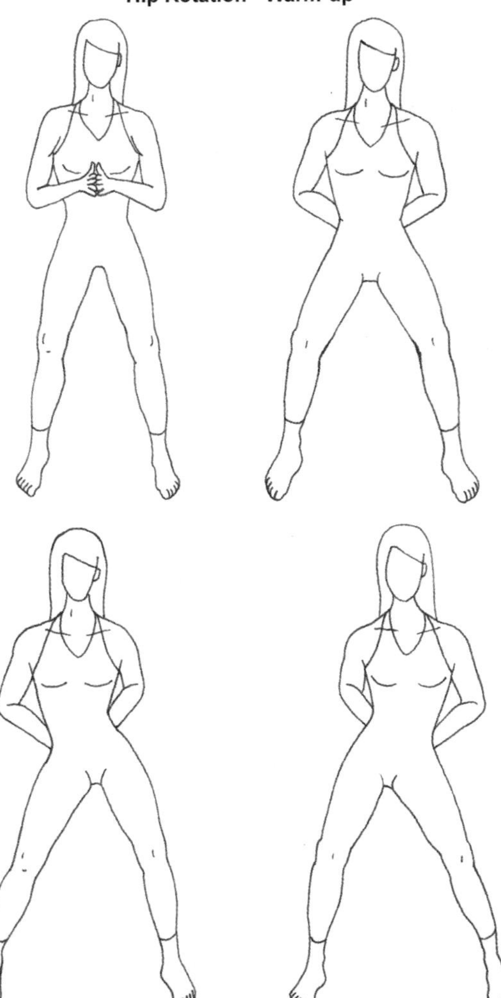

Warm-up - Hip Rotation	Benefits
1. Stand straight with your feet shoulder-width apart. Place your hands on the back of your hips with your fingertips pointing down. 2. Rotate your hips clockwise by moving to one side and then forward to the opposite side in a swirling motion. 3. Repeat for ten rotations, and then reverse the direction to move counter-clockwise.	The "hip rotation" is a great warm-up exercise that lubricates hips and knee joints, loosens low back, and strengthens the thigh, leg and lower body. It can also prevent osteoporosis and improve digestion, elimination, and sexual energy and function.

Side Bends - Warm-up

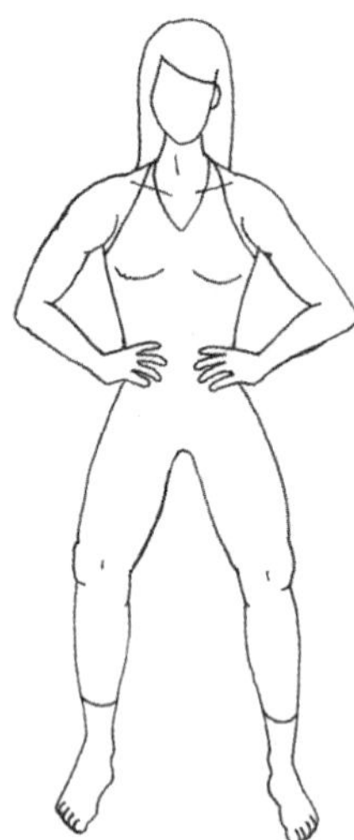

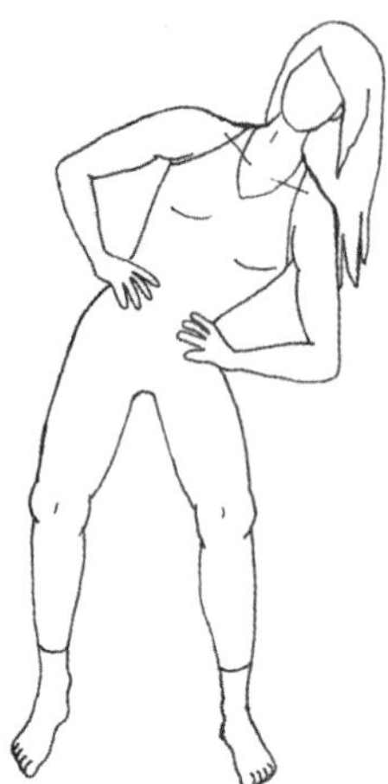

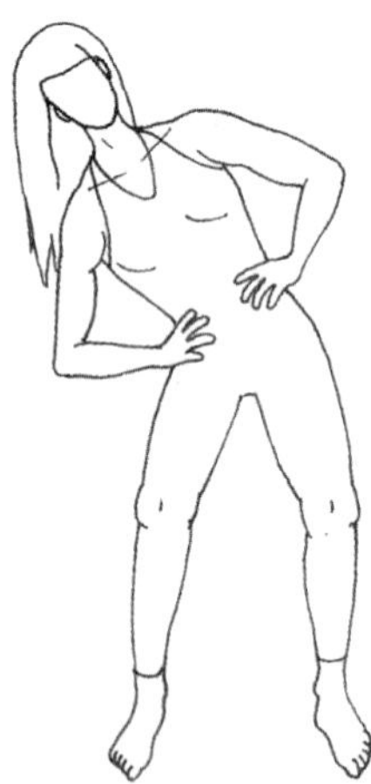

Warm-up - Side Bends	Benefits
1. Stand straight with your feet shoulder-width apart. Inhale and bend to one side. 2. As you exhale, slowly return to the starting position and hold. 3. Repeat the opposite side while bending.	The "side bends" exercise is a great warm-up exercise that increases flexibility of the spine, strengthens low back, hips, and thighs, loosens the body and joints, and assists in relaxation.

Knee Rotation - Warm-up

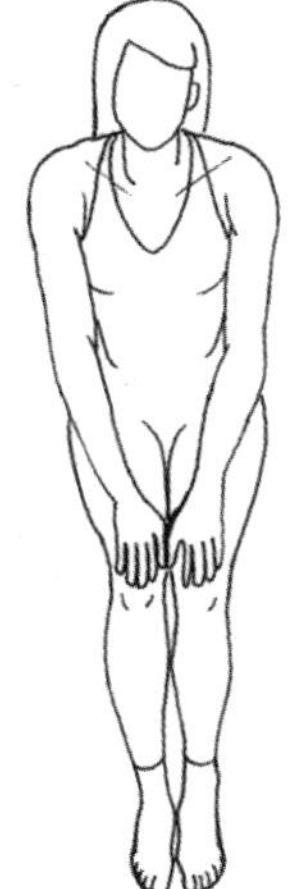

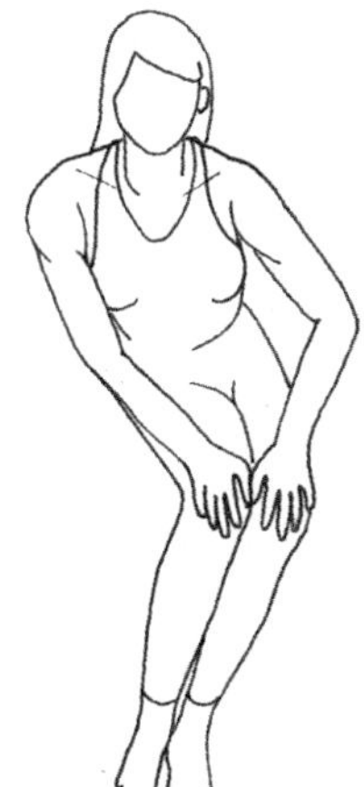

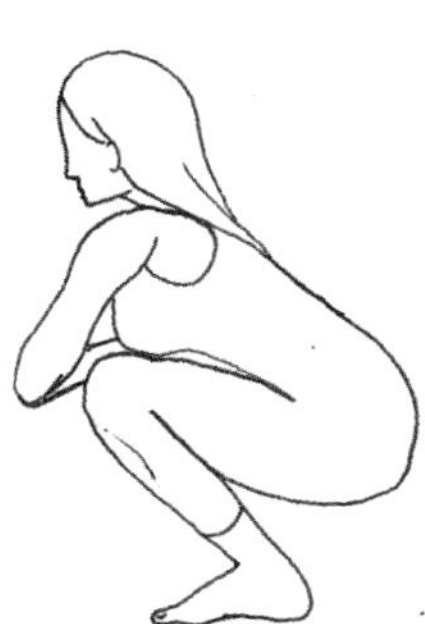

Warm-up - Knee Rotation	Benefits
1. Stand straight with your feet and knees together. Bend at the waist and place your hands over your kneecaps. 2. Slowly move your knees to one side and rotate them downward by bending your knees. Do not lift your heels off the ground. While you move, maintain a comfortable position as you stretch your Achiles tendon at the back of the heel. 3. Rotate your knees in the opposite direction as you come back up.	The "knee rotation" exercise is a great warm-up that increases flexibility of the knees, ankles, and hips while it strengthens thigh and leg muscles.

Reaching for Happiness - Posture

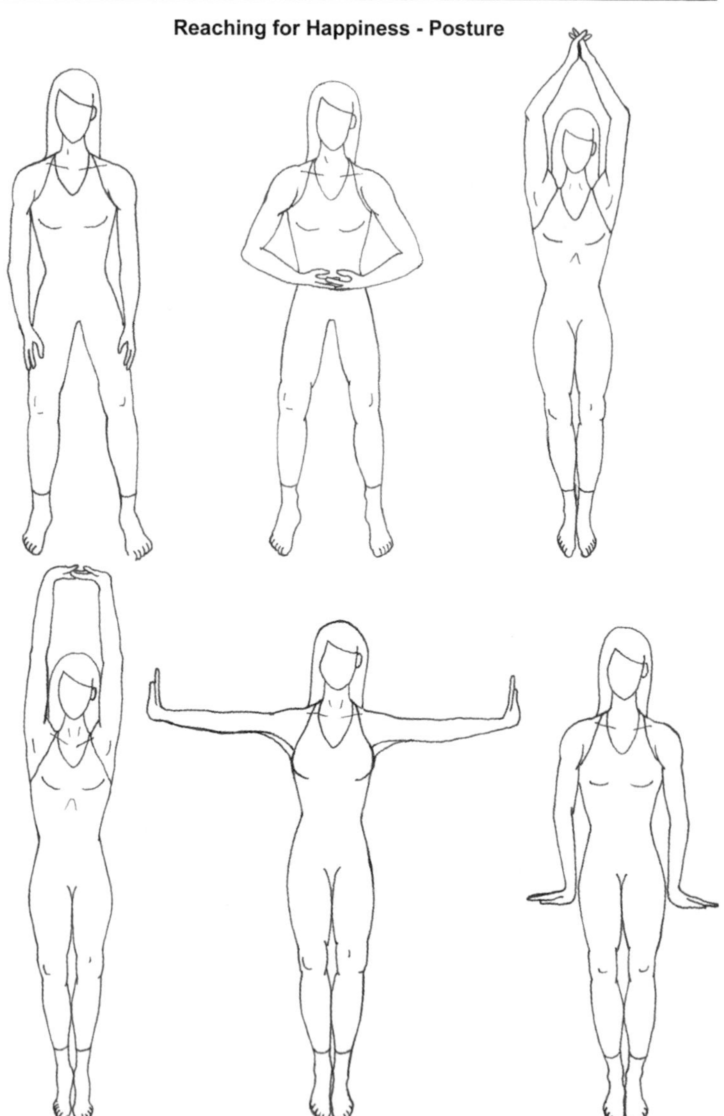

Posture - Reaching for Happiness with Both Hands	Benefits
1. Let your arms hang loosely at your sides as you stand with your feet shoulder-width apart. Slowly raise your hands in front of your body with palms facing upward while inhaling. 2. When your hands are above your head, twist the palms to face the sky and press upward gently, interlacing the fingers. 3. Look up at your fingers and lift your heels so you are standing on the balls of your feet. 4. As you exhale, separate your fingers and lower your arms slowly to the side until your hands rest in the starting position.	The "reach for happiness" exercise benefits the Heart, Lungs, and Spine. It also addresses digestive problems, increases circulation to heart and abdominal area, increases lung capacity, increases oxygen flow to the brain, and loosens the shoulder muscles and tendons.

Drawing the Bow - Posture

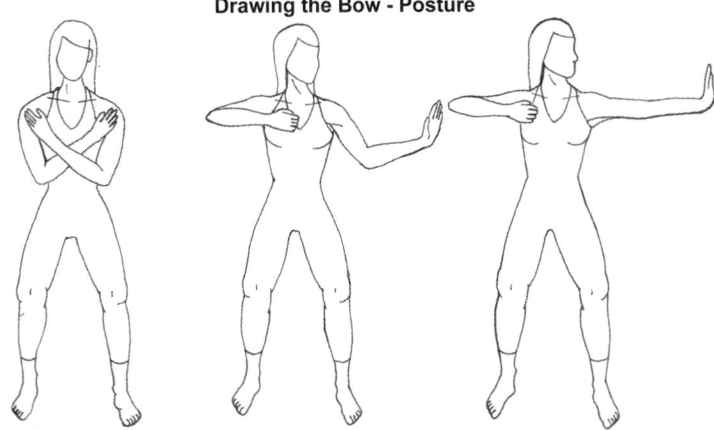

Posture - Drawing the Bow and Letting the Arrow Fly	Benefits
1. Spread your feet so they are two shoulder-widths apart and facing forward. Bend your knees and assume the "horse stance" position. 2. Cross your arms in front of your throat, palms facing you, left arm in front. Slowly extend your left arm and then sweep it out to the side, index finger and thumb forming an "L" shape and the other fingers bent. 3. While the left arm is moving, make a fist with your right hand. Draw back your right elbow and focus your gaze on your left hand, as if you are shooting a bow. 4. Bend your knees deeper in the horse-stance position, as you gaze through the "L" shape of the extended hand. 5. Slowly bring your arms back to the neutral position crossed in front of your throat, right hand in front. 6. Repeat in the opposite direction. Keep your weight centered at all times.	The "drawing the bow" exercise benefits the Heart and Lungs, improves circulation in the neck area, and prevents structural and functional disorders associated with poor posture. It is an ideal exercise for people who have respiratory problems.

Energy Jump - Posture

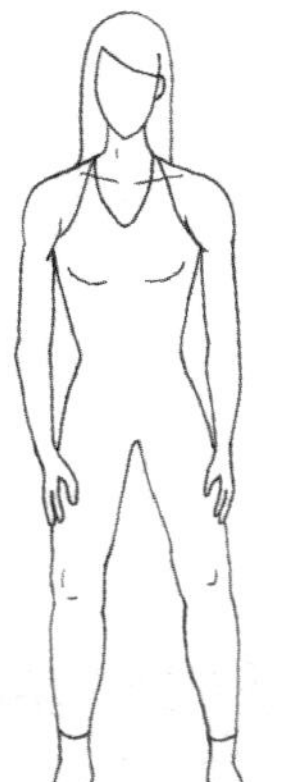

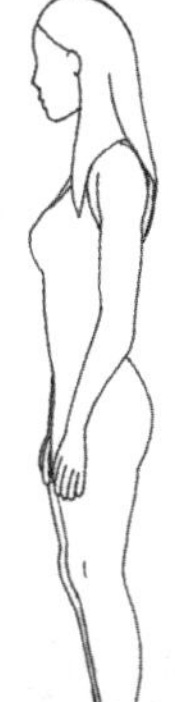

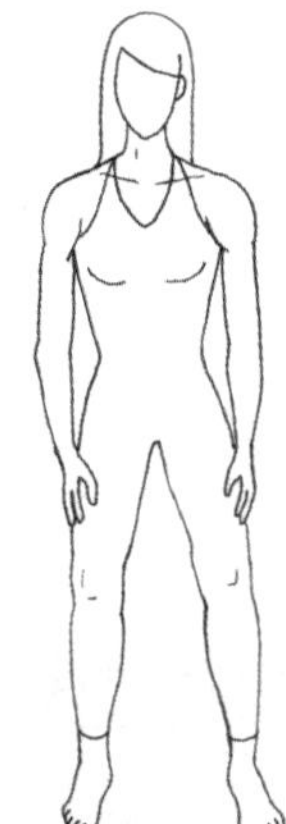

Posture - Energy Jump	Benefits
1. Stand with your feet shoulder-width apart, knees bent. Lift your heels, raise your body and inhale. 2. Exhale and drop your heels suddenly. Your body should feel a little jolt. If the sensation of this exercise is too strong, lower the heels more gently. 3. The head should be kept erect to prevent shock to the cervical vertebrae.	The "energy jump" exercise benefits the circulation of energy in all meridians, stimulates and energizes nervous system, skeletal system and blood circulation, stimulates growth of bone marrow, and balances internal organs.

Separating Heaven and Earth - Posture

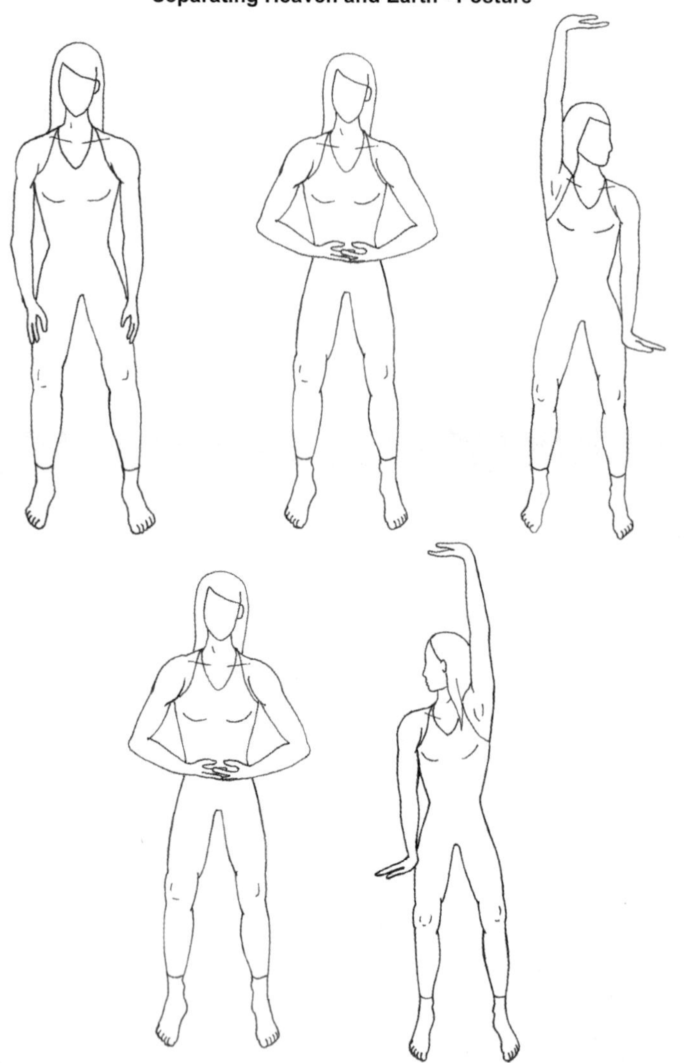

Posture - Separating Heaven and Earth	Benefits
1. Stand with your feet shoulder width apart, arms relaxed at your side. 2. Turn your palms to face forward, and then lift your hands to the stomach, fingertips touching, while inhaling. 3. Separate your hands, slowly reaching your left hand up while slowly pushing your right hand down while exhaling. 4. Slowly return your hands to meet in front of your body at the level of the stomach. 5. Once your hands meet, reverse the direction, reaching your left hand down and your right hand up. 6. Slowly return your hands to meet in front of your body at the level of the stomach.	The "separating heaven and earth" exercise benefits the Stomach, Spleen, Liver, Gallbladder, and improves digestion.

Twist and Release - Posture

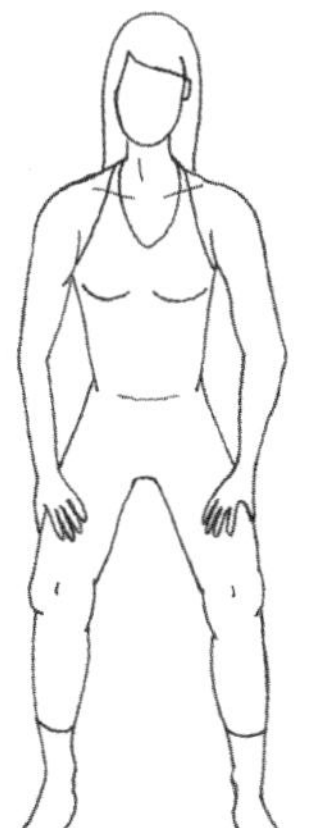
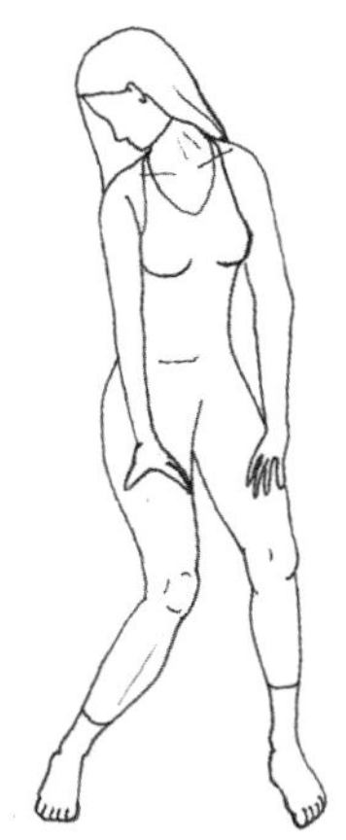
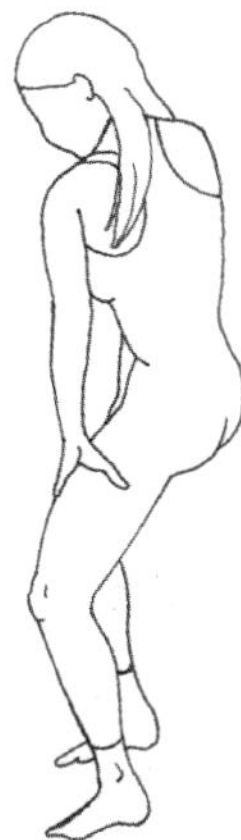

Posture - Twist and Release	Benefits
1. Stand with your feet parallel and two shoulder-widths apart. Bend forward at the waist and let your arms hang down loosely or placed on the thighs. There are two movements to this posture and both should be done in a relaxed state. 2. Raise your left shoulder while lowering your right and let your right hand drag on the ground. Repeat on the opposite side. 3. The second is to turn your hips while moving your left arm and shoulder inward. Repeat on the opposite side.	The "twist and release" exercise benefits the Liver and the circulation of qi through all meridians. It increases circulation and breathing capacity, releases tension, lowers blood pressure, calms the Heart, and releases anger.

Look Back and Letting Go - Posture

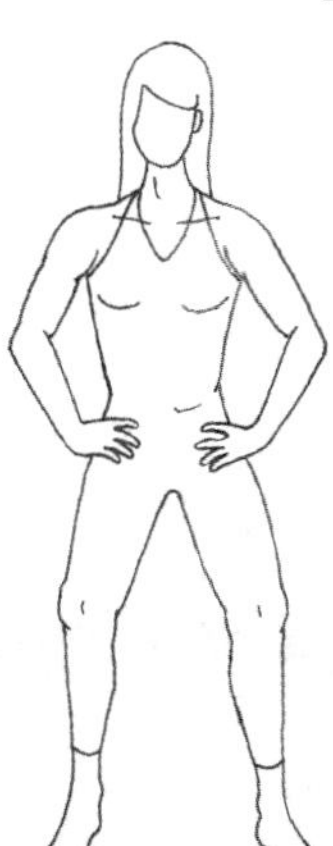
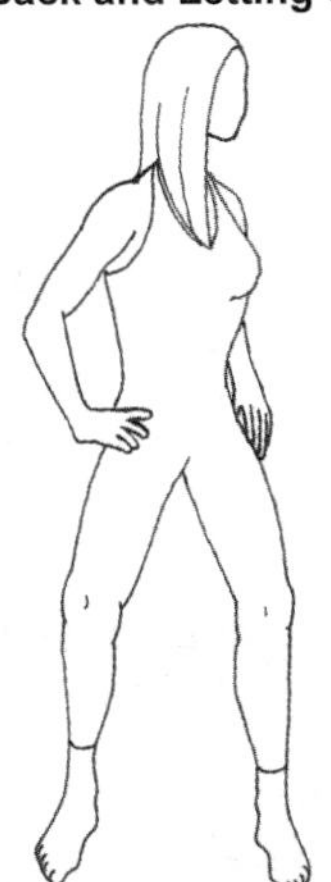
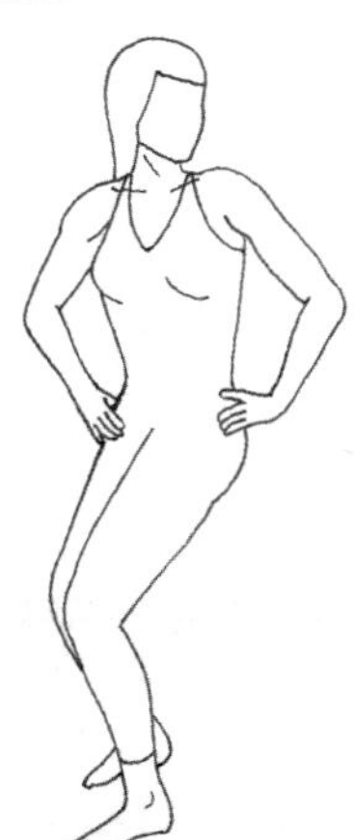

Posture - Looking Back and Letting Go	Benefits
1. Stand with your feet shoulder-width apart. Look straight in front of you, eyes relaxed. Place your hands on your waist, hooking your thumbs behind your back to make a *V* and with your palms facing down. 2. As you exhale, bend your knees slightly to distribute your weight firmly. 3. As you inhale, turn your upper body to left, and look over your left shoulder. Hold the position for a few seconds. 4. As you exhale, return your body to the center position. 5. Repeat the movement on the opposite side.	The "look back and let go" exercise benefits the flow of energy in all the primary meridians. It benefits the central nervous system, lowers stress and emotional turmoil, prevents high blood pressure, and stimulates internal organs by improving circulation. This exercise also stimulates circulation in the body, head, neck, and eyes.

Touching Toes then Bend Backwards - Posture

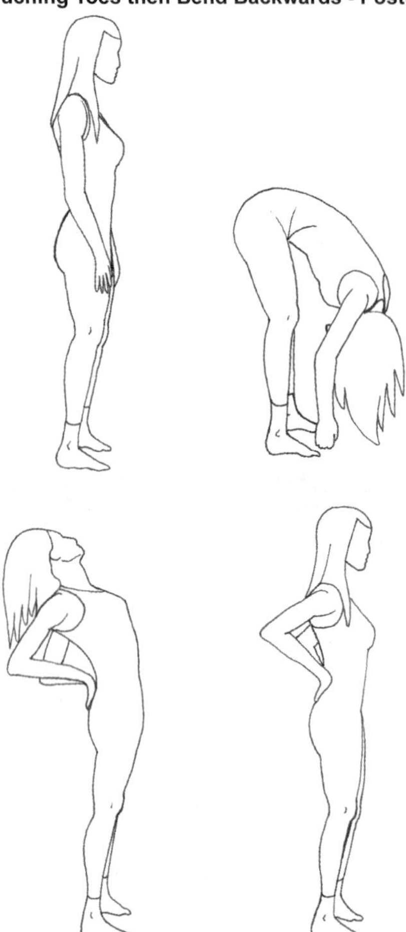

Posture - Touching Toes then Bending Backwards	Benefits
1. Stand with knees bent and feet shoulder-width apart. 2. As you inhale, bend at the waist and let your hands hang at your side. You should be looking between your legs, allowing your head to hang in a relaxed position. 3. As you exhale, slowly lift your torso back to the starting position, placing your palms on your mid-back. 4. As you inhale again, lengthen your spine and lean back as far as comfortably possible. 5. Exhale and return to the starting position, letting your arms hang comfortably at your sides.	The "bending backwards for health" exercise benefits the Kidneys, adrenals, urinary system, prostate and reproductive organs. It stimulates circulation in the lower abdomen, strengthens the nervous system, adjusts overall body metabolism, increases blood flow to the brain, and nurtures personal Qi.

Punching with Angry Eyes - Posture

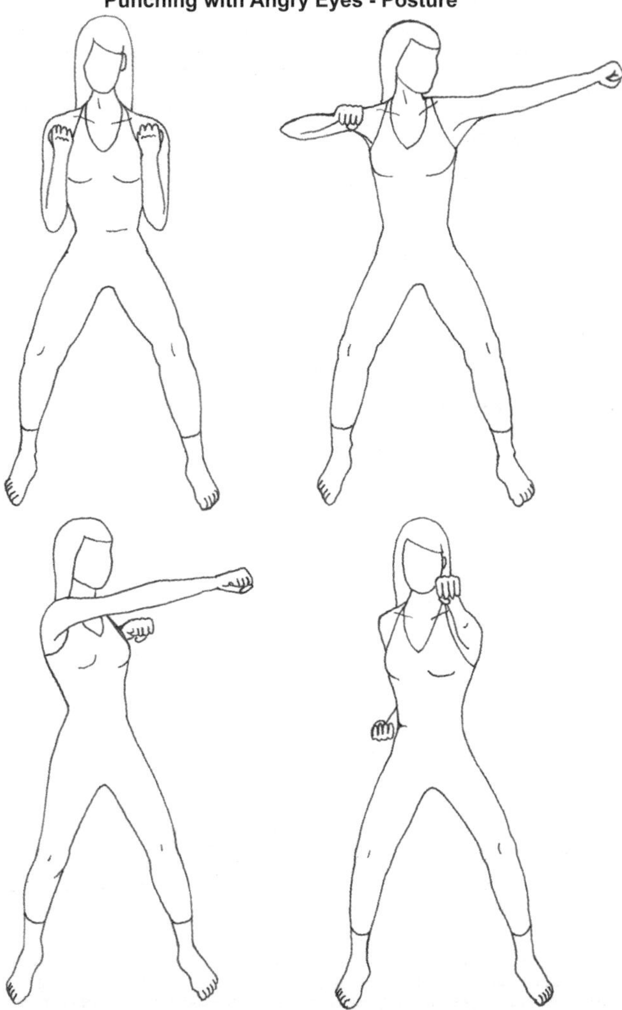

Posture - Punching with Angry Eyes	Benefits
1. Stand with your feet parallel and two shoulder-widths apart. Bend your knees and clench your hands into loose fists. Hold your hands next to your waist, knuckles down. 2. Inhale deeply. While exhaling, slowly extend the right arm, punching directly in front of your throat, focusing your eyes on a point 20 to 30 feet ahead. As you extend your arm, twist the fist so that the knuckles face upward. 3. Clench your teeth and keep your eyes wide as you release your punch. 4. Withdraw the hand while twisting it back and to rest at the side of the waist, knuckles facing up, and relax the face. 5. Repeat the exercise using the opposite arm. Grip the ground firmly with your feet during this posture. Keep your stomach muscles engaged so that your buttocks do not stick out behind you.	The "energy punch with angry eyes" is an exercise that harmonizes a client's emotions. It also benefits the Lungs, central nervous system, skeletal and muscular systems, adjusts breathing to increase vitality, and promotes qi and blood circulation.

Health Benefits of Regular Exercise

Regular exercise and stretching provides enormous health benefits. Regular exercise, combined with massage and good diet, is essential to balancing organ disharmonies associated with neuromuscular pain, tightness, and tension. A daily exercise routine with stretching can help reduce heart disease, cancer, type-2 diabetes and many other diseases and metabolic conditions. Regular fitness exercise is also highly beneficial for weight reduction and weight maintenance and may improve brain chemistry to reduce depression.

The Health Benefits of Exercise

- Improves your chances of living longer
- Improves quality of life
- Reduces the risk of heart disease
- Helps lower high blood pressure and high cholesterol
- Helps protect you from developing certain cancers
- Helps prevent or control type-2 diabetes
- Reduces the risk of arthritis and alleviates associated symptoms
- Helps prevent osteoporosis
- Improves mobility and strength in later life
- Alleviates symptoms of depression and anxiety
- Benefits weight reduction and weight management

The Health Benefits of Stretching

- Increases flexibility and daily performance of muscles
- Improves range of motion of your joint for better balance
- Improves circulation and increases blood flow to your muscles
- Promotes better posture and minimizes aches and pains
- Relieves stress associated with tense muscles
- Prevents injury

For the greatest overall health benefits, experts recommend that you do 20 to 30 minutes of aerobic activity three or more times a week and some type of muscle-strengthening activity and stretching at least twice a week. However, if you are unable to do this level of activity, you can gain substantial health benefits by accumulating 30 minutes or more of moderate-intensity physical activity a day, at least five times a week. For people in their thirties and beyond, many of whom have pain in targeted areas, it may still be a very good idea to do static stretching exercise in conjunction with their treatment.

If you have been inactive for a while, you may want to start with less strenuous activities such as walking or swimming at a comfortable pace. Beginning at a slow pace will allow you to become physically fit without straining your body. Once you are in better shape, you can gradually do more strenuous activity.

The following section provides exercise programs to target areas of the neck, shoulder, back, wrist, knee, ankle, elbow and upper body. As a general rule: when you're stretching or exercising, focus on big muscle groups first - hamstrings, calves, and quads, which support the surrounding structures and then move to smaller groups later. Stretching for longer periods of time is preferable over more repeitions. Stretch muscles and joints that you routinely use at work or play. Warm your body up first. Stretching muscles when they're cold increases your risk of injury, including pulled muscles. Warm up by walking while gently pumping your arms, or do a favorite exercise at low intensity for five minutes. Better yet, try qi gong and warming-up exercises so your muscles are more receptive to stretching.

If you plan to stretch only after your work out, increase the intensity of the activity more slowly than you would if you had stretched your muscles before exercising. (You can download full pdf versions of exercises that target specific areas at www.acupuncturedeskreference.com. Use caution when recommending exercise programs to your clients.)

General rule and caution: You can exercise anytime, anywhere in your home, at work or when you're traveling. If you have a chronic condition or an injury, however, you may need to alter your approach to exercise. For example, if you have a strained muscle, exercise may cause further harm. Discuss with your physician, physical therapist and exercise consultant the best approach to strengthening your body. Each exercise program will depend on your client. We have provided an average based on recommendations for a normal able-bodied person. Please adjust your recommendations according to your client's needs, especially if there is an injury.

Exercise and Fitness Consultant: Martina Sturm, LAc, gofitnessgo@mac.com
Sources: Brian Sharkey, *Fitness and Health, 6th Edition*, Human Kinetics, Champaign, IL, 2007.
Bob Anderson, *Stretching*, Shelter Publications, Bolinas, CA, 2000.
Michael Reed Galch, *Acu-Yoga: Self Help Techniques to Relieve Tension*, Japan Publications, Tokyo, 1981.

Lung Balancing - Exercise

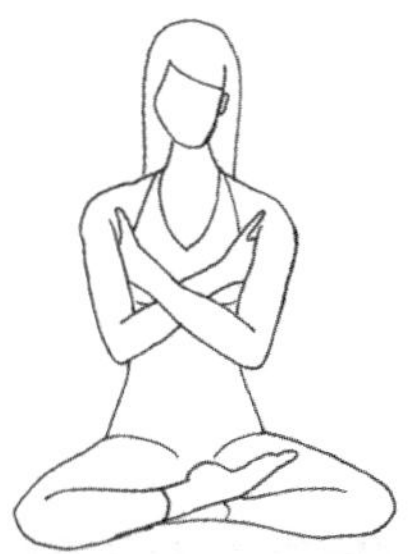

Exercise - Lung Meridian Balancing	Benefits
1. Sit in a comfortable position. Interlace your hands at the center of the chest, and stretch your thumbs out so that you can press them into the muscles on your upper chest. 2. Close your eyes and begin long, deep breathing, allowing the diaphragm to open and ribs to expand. Be sure to inhale completely. 3. Hold the breath at the top of the inhalation for a few seconds. Then exhale slowly, releasing the breath gently for one full minute. 4. Imagine a circuit of electricity or energy circulating through your mind and body as you allow your breath to be full and deep. This is only a breathing exercise, but it takes concentration and discipline.	

Large Intestine Balancing - Exercise

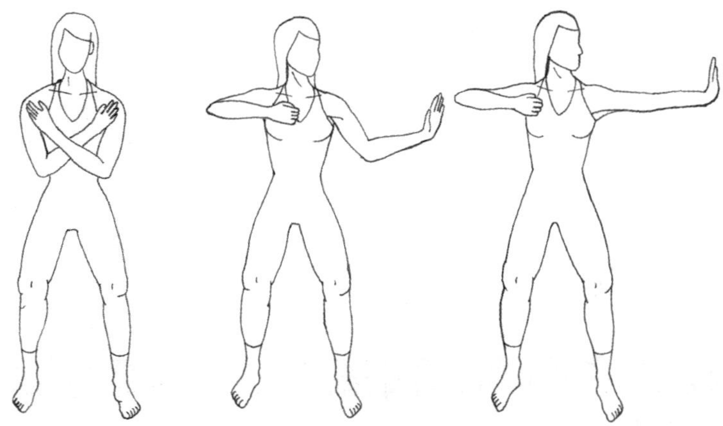

Exercise – Large Intestine Meridian Balancing (See Drawing the Bow)	Benefits

Elimination Large Intestine - Exercise

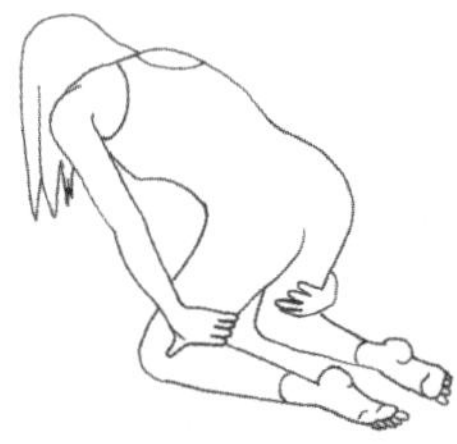
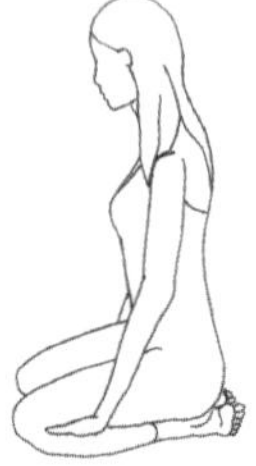

Exercise – Elimination Balancing	Benefits
1. Sit on your heels with your legs folded under you in a kneeling position. Rock forward with your palms facing up, spreading your index fingers and thumbs apart underneath your knees. 2. Lower your body down slowly, stretching the webbing between the thumbs and index fingers apart to press LI-4. 3. Stimulate this point further by rocking back and forth as if you are on a rocking horse.	The "elimination balancing" exercise is used to treat constipation, front headaches, insomnia, nervous depression, pains, and toothaches. Ideally suited for problems association with poor bowel elimination.

Stomach Balancing - Exercise

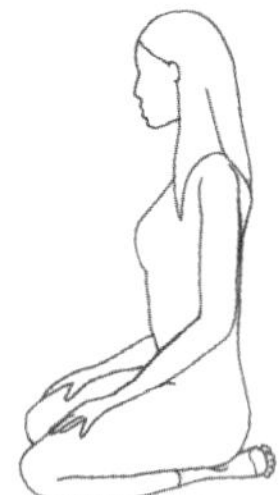
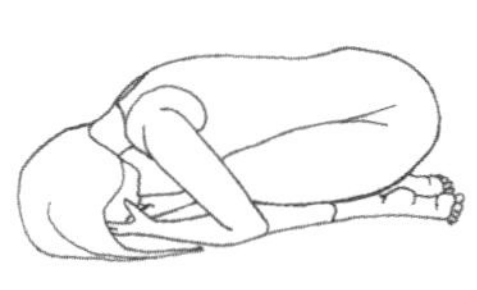
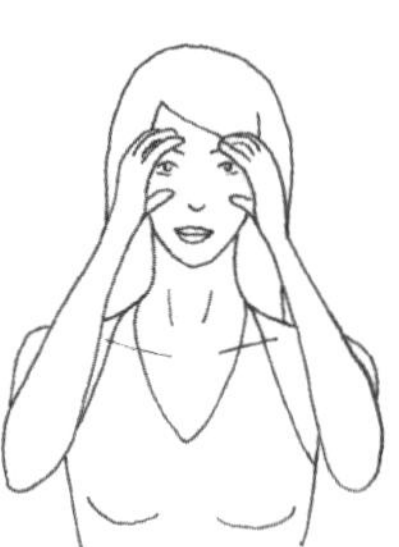

Exercise – Stomach Balancing	Benefits
1. Sit on your heels in a kneeling position and take a deep breath with your spine straight. 2. As you exhale, slowly lower your chest to your knees. Let your body compress the breath outward naturally. 3. Use your thumbs to press on St-3, as you exhale and bend over. Palpate for other tender points on the cheekbone. 4. Inhale as you slowly sit up and return to the starting position. 5. Repeat the first three steps for one to two minutes, inhaling up and exhaling down.	

Spleen Balancing - Exercise

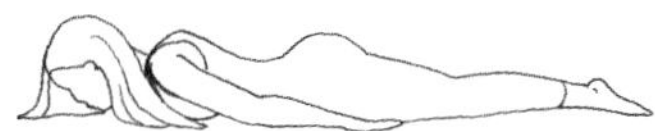
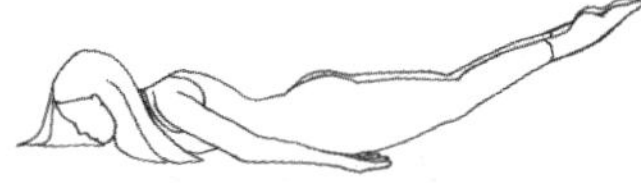

Exercise – Spleen Balancing	Benefits
Locust Pose 1. Lie flat on your stomach, placing your arms underneath your body. Make fists with your hands and place them underneath your groin. 2. Bring your forehead or chin to the floor, whichever is most comfortable. 3. Bring your feet together. Inhale and raise your feet up with the thighs off the ground. This puts pressure on Spleen and Stomach points in the groin area where these two meridians intersect. 4. Breathe deeply, and keep your legs elevated as long as possible. 5. Lower your legs, and rest for at least 30 seconds. After 30 seconds, inhale deeply and stretch your torso up. Hold the breath for 10 seconds.	The "locust pose" exercise strengthens the muscles of the upper legs and lower back, stimulates the stomach and intestines, strengthens the urinary bladder, and stretches the spine

Heart Balancing - Exercise

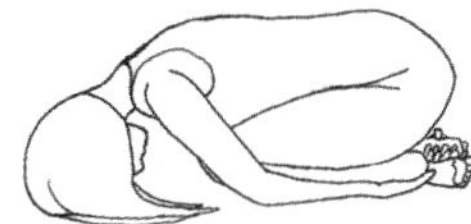

Exercise – Heart Balancing	Benefits
1. Sit on your heels in a kneeling position. Bend forward, allowing your head to rest on your knees, or in front of your knees with your forehead resting on the floor. 2. Place your hands underneath your feet so that the palms are facing upwards, while interlacing your little fingers between your large and second toes. 3. Move your hips back and forth for one minute.	

Small Intestine Balancing - Exercise

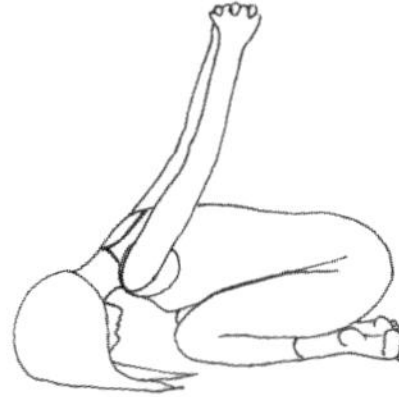

Exercise – Small Intestine Balancing	Benefits
1. Sit on your heels in a kneeling position. Place forehead on the floor. Interlace your fingers and hands behind your back, palms facing each other. 2. Inhale and stretch your arms upwards holding them up for 30 seconds. Breathe deeply through the nose. 3. After 30 seconds, inhale and stretch the arms up further, then exhale and let the arms relax down by your sides.	

Urinary Bladder Balancing - Exercise

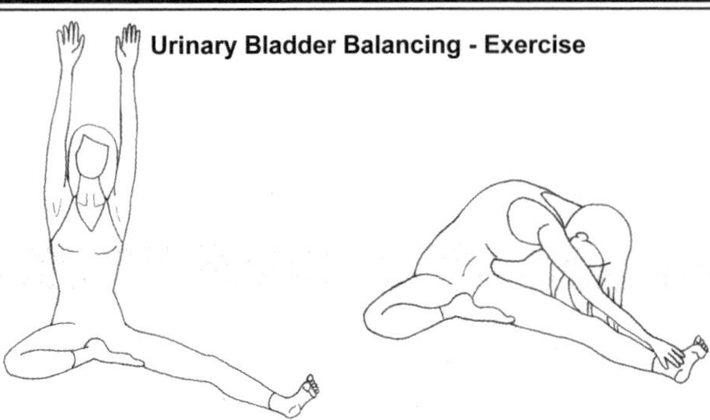

EXERCISE

Exercise – Urinary Bladder Balancing	Benefits
1. Sit on the floor with your legs stretched out in front of you. Bend one knee, bringing your foot into the groin area. Keep the other leg stretched out in front of you. 2. Inhale and stretch up to the sky. Exhale and stretch down toward the extended leg keeping your shoulders relaxed. Pull your chin in slightly so your spine is aligned. Exhale down over your straight leg, using your arm muscles to pull yourself further, bringing your forehead toward the knee. 3. Continue to stretch for about one minute, and then release, switch to the other leg and repeat. 4. Finish by stretching both legs out straight out in front of you.	
1. Sit with your back straight and legs stretched out in front of you. Rotate your ankles and wrists a few times. 2. Grab hold of your ankles, or calves, wherever you can reach without straining and without bending your knees. Straighten the spine and take a deep breath. The backs of the knees remain flat against the floor. 3. Inhale as you stretch up, and exhale bending forward, pulling yourself down with your arms. 4. Continue for one minute, establishing your own full breathing pace.	

Kidney Balancing - Exercise

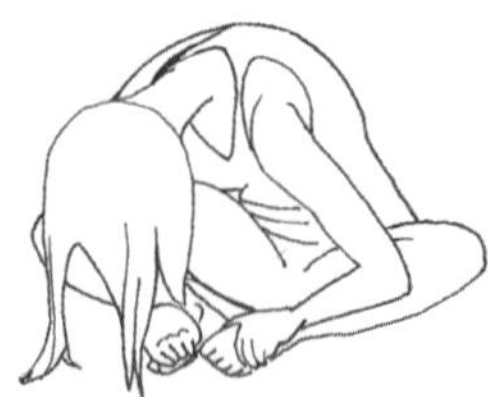

Exercise – Kidney Balancing	Benefits
1. Sit on the floor, bend your knees and bring the bottoms of your feet together. 2. Hold your feet, using your thumbs to press K-2 on both feet. 3. Pull your feet close to the genital area, your heels touching your body. 4. Inhale and straighten your spine, bringing your forehead down toward your toes. Repeat the exercise as needed.	

Pericardium Balancing - Exercise

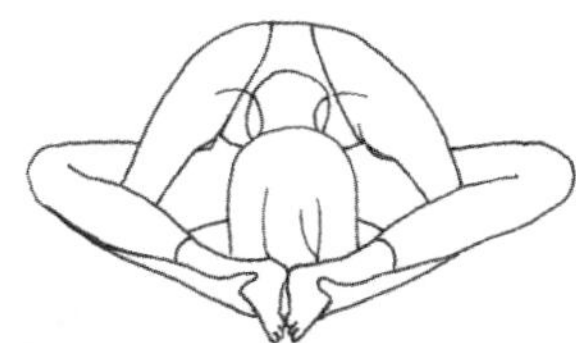

Exercise – Pericardium Balancing	Benefits
1. Sit on the floor with the soles of your feet together. 2. Lean forward, placing your wrists under your feet palms facing up. The outside of the ankle bones should be used to press Pc-7 in the center of the wrist fold. 3. Allow your body to relax forward. Breathe deeply in this position for 30 seconds. 4. Slide your hands two inches to apply pressure on Pc-6. Let your body relax forward for another 30 seconds.	

San Jiao Balancing - Exercise

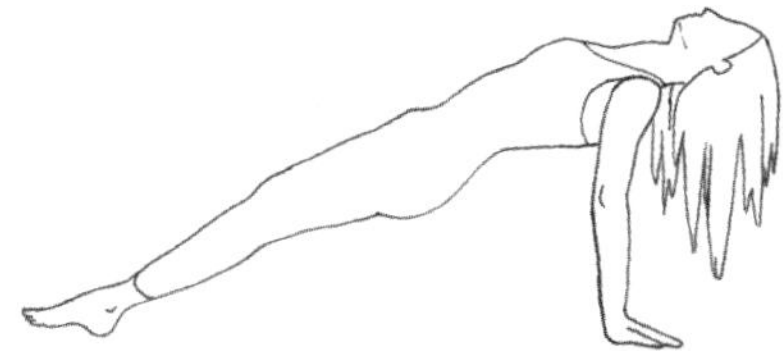

Exercise – San Jiao Balancing	Benefits
Platform Pose 1. Sit on the floor with your legs stretched straight out in front of you. Put your hands on the floor behind you with the fingers pointing away from your body. 2. Arch the pelvis so that your body forms a straight line between toes and shoulders. 3. Begin long deep breathing or the "breaths of fire" for one minute.	

Gallbladder Balancing - Exercise

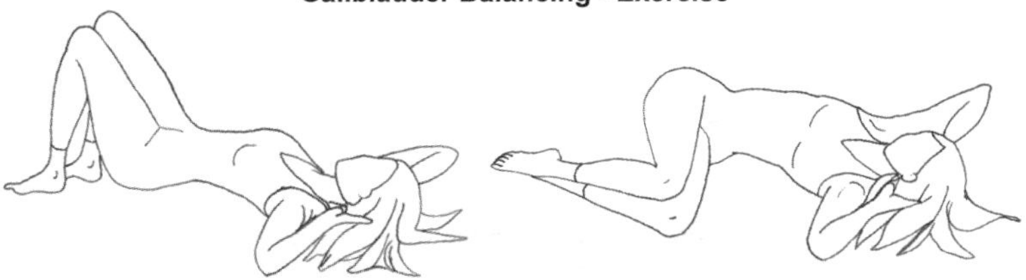

Exercise – Gallbladder Balancing	Benefits
1. Lie on your back, bending your knees, and bringing your feet up toward your buttocks. Grab hold of your ankles, keeping your feet on the floor. 2. Inhale, arching the pelvis up, and exhale, bringing it back down. 3. After a minute, inhale and stretch up to the maximum. Tighten your buttocks muscles. Contract them, squeeze more, and relax the body down as you exhale. 4. Lie flat on your back with your eyes closed and relax completely.	

Liver Balancing - Exercise

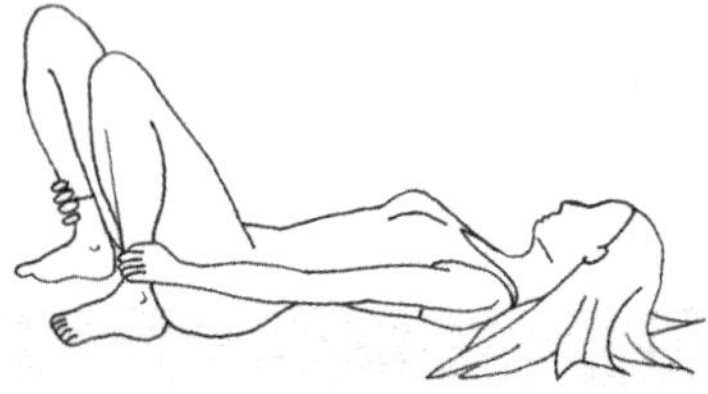
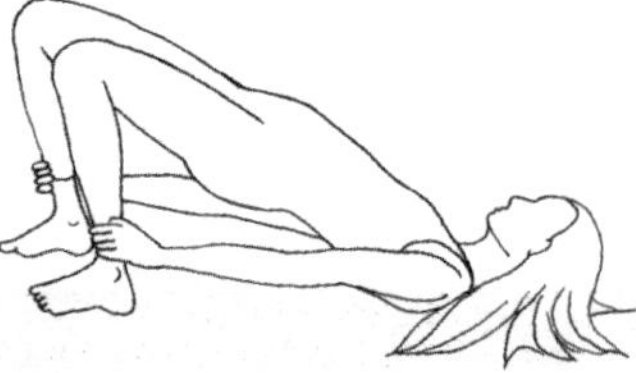

Exercise – Liver Balancing	Benefits
1. Lie on your back, bending your knees, and bringing your feet up towards your buttocks. Grab hold of your ankles, keeping your feet on the floor. 2. Inhale, arching the pelvis up, and exhale, bringing it back down. 3. After a minute, inhale and stretch up to the maximum. Tighten your buttocks muscles. Contract them, squeeze more, and relax the body down as you exhale. 4. Lie flat on your back with your eyes closed and relax completely.	

Yin Balancing - Exercise

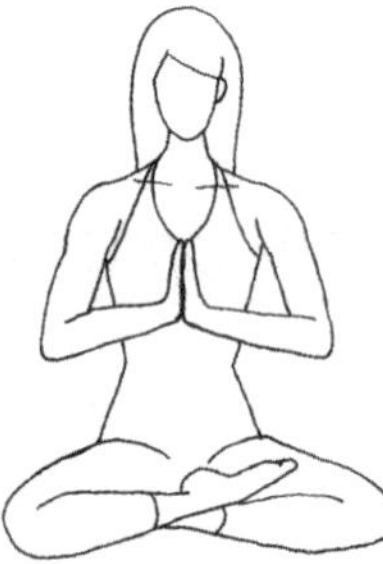

Exercise – Yin Balancing	Benefits
Prayer pose 1. Sit on the floor with the soles of your feet together, palms placed on the center of the chest at Ren-17. 2. Close your eyes and breathe deeply. Inhale and exhale to calm the nervous system. 3. Allow the energy to circulate through your body while sitting and meditating for one minute.	The "prayer pose" exercise is an excellent way to induce a meditative state of awareness and balance the yin meridian.

All Eight Channels Balancing - Exercise

Exercise – All Eight Channel Balancing (See Locust Pose or Spleen Balancing)	Benefits

All Channels Balancing - Exercise

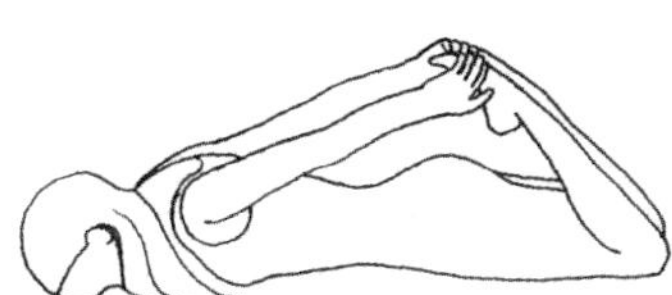

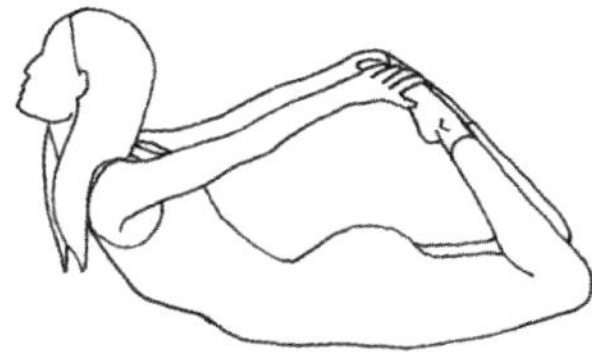

Exercise – All Channels Balancing	Benefits
Bow Pose 1. Lie on your stomach, with your arms on your sides. Bend your knees and bring your feet towards your buttocks. 2. Inhale and grab hold of the tops of your feet by bending your legs and reaching your arms back. Let your weight rest on your stomach and not on your pelvis. Bring your fingers over the arches to hold Sp-4. 3. Arch yourself back like a bow. Begin rocking as you inhale back and exhale coming forward. Breathe through your nose. Continue rocking back and forth for 15 seconds. 4. Come out of the pose slowly and lie flat on your stomach. Relax for three minutes with your hands by your sides. Breathe through your nose into and out of the lower abdomen, during the relaxation period.	The "bow pose" exercise is good for the entire length of the spine, building both strength and flexibility in the back. It also relieves constipation and improves digestive functions.

Du and Ren Balancing - Exercise

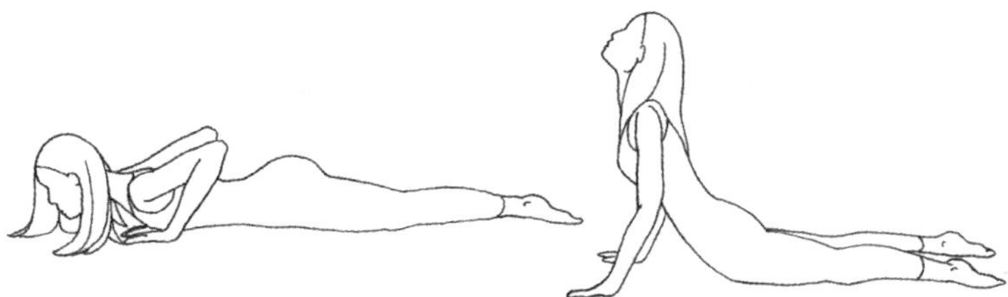

Exercise – Du and Ren Balancing	Benefits
Cobra Pose 1. Lie on your stomach with your chin on the ground, bringing your hands underneath your shoulders with the palms pressing down. Your fingers should point forward and your toes should point behind you. 2. Make sure your hands are close to your body beside your rib cage. 3. As you inhale, raise your head all the way up and back, gently pushing off your hands. Keep your pelvis on the ground. 3. Begin breathing into your abdomen. 4. After a minute or two in this position, exhale completely and squeeze your buttocks muscles, stretch back, and press your navel toward the ground. This will put pressure on Du-4. 5. Inhale slowly and deeply through the nostrils. Exhale slowly coming down by bending your arms. 6. Bring your hands to your sides, and let your head rest on its side.	The "crobra pose" exercise is great for the health and flexibility of your back and spine, stretching the chest and shoulders, excellent for regulating your digestive system and tonifying the Du and Ren meridians.

Chong Mai and Dai Mai Balancing - Exercise

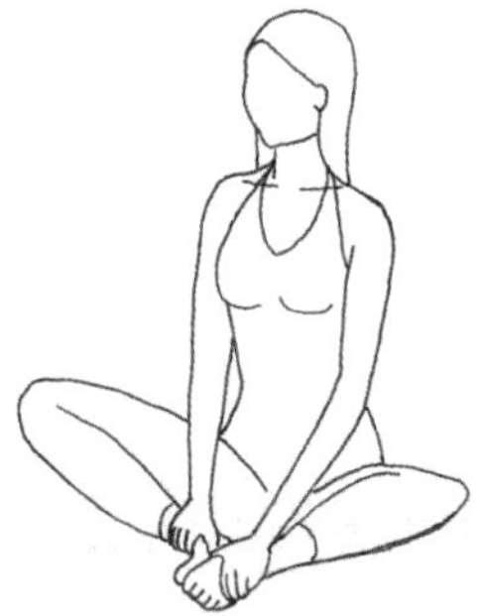

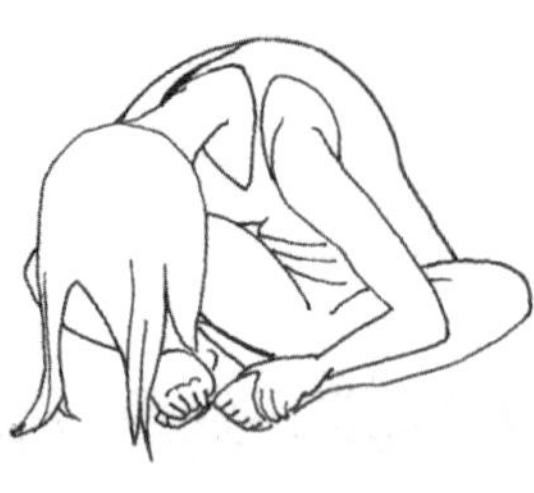

Exercise – Chong Mai and Dai Mai Balancing	Benefits
Butterfly pose 1. Sit with your legs straight out in front of you. Bend both knees and bring your feet together. 2. Use your thumbs to hold Sp-4 and press your fingers on Gb-41. 3. Inhale as you lengthen your spine, drawing your belly button towards your spine and your chest up and out. 4. Exhale and bend forward, drawing your torso and head towards your legs. Continue this for 60 seconds or you can keep this down for an extended stretch. 5. Then inhale, and lift your body back to the original position.	The "butterfly pose" exercise lengthens and strengthens the spine, increases blood flow to the Large and Small Intestines, lengthens muscles around the inner thighs and hips, and increases mobility of the shoulder joints.

Yin Qiao and Yang Qiao Balancing - Exercise

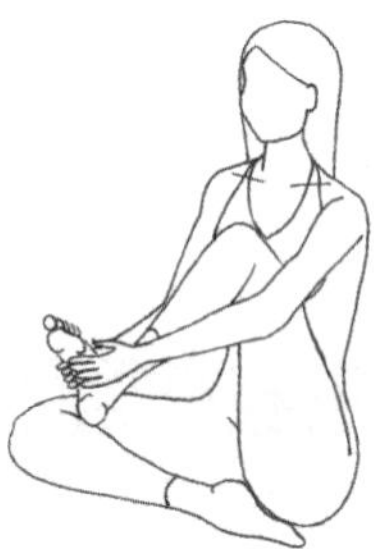

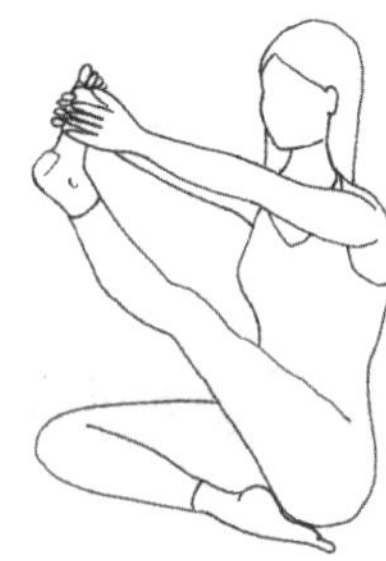

Exercise – Yin Qiao and Yang Qiao Balancing	Benefits
Extended Pose 1. Remain in a seated position on the floor. Bend your left leg and grasp hold of the bottom of the left foot at K-1. 2. As you inhale, stretch this leg out in front of you at a 45-degree angle from the ground and exhale as you bring the leg down to the floor. 3. After a minute, switch legs and equally stretch out the right leg.	The "extended pose" exercise distributes energy to all parts of the body and highly beneficial for nervous and muscular skeletal systems and Kidney. It is beneficial for low back pain and reproductive problems associated with yang qiao mai and yin qiao mai.

Yin Wei and Yang Wei Balancing - Exercise

Cross Heart Pose

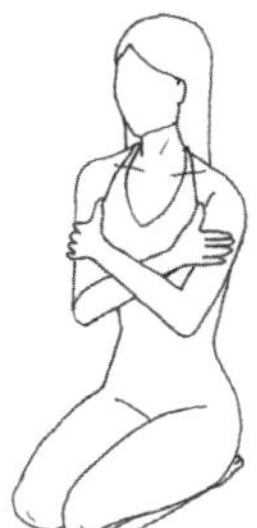

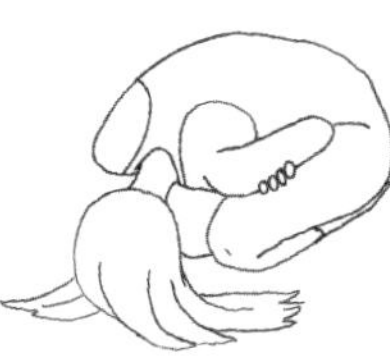

Exercise – Yin Wei and Yang Wei Balancing	Benefits
Cross my Heart pose 1. Sit on your heels in a kneeling position. 2. Cross your arms at your heart's center holding the upper arms. 3. Inhale as you lengthen your spine, sitting comfortably and upright. 4. Exhale as you bend forward, drawing your head forward towards the ground. 5. Remain in this position for a minute as you visualize energy moving up and down the front of your body as you breathe.	The "cross the heart pose" exercise circulates the qi to body's vital centers and chakras. It restores the body's vital energy and calms the mind.

Mind Clearing Pose

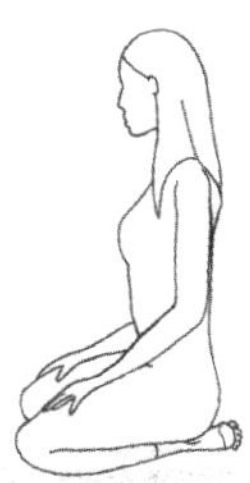

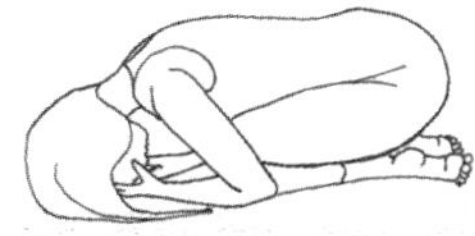

Mind-Clearing Pose 1. Sit in a comfortable cross-legged position on the floor. 2. Slowly lower your head forward, supporting it by gently placing your fingers on the forehead of Gb-14. 3. Use your thumbs to press on the jaw muscles of St-6. 4. Relax forward, breathing into the abdomen for about one minute.	The "mind-clearing pose" is good for clearing the mind and cultivating focus and attention. It opens the yin wei mai and yang wei mai meridians.

Yin Qiao and Yang Qiao Balancing - Exercise

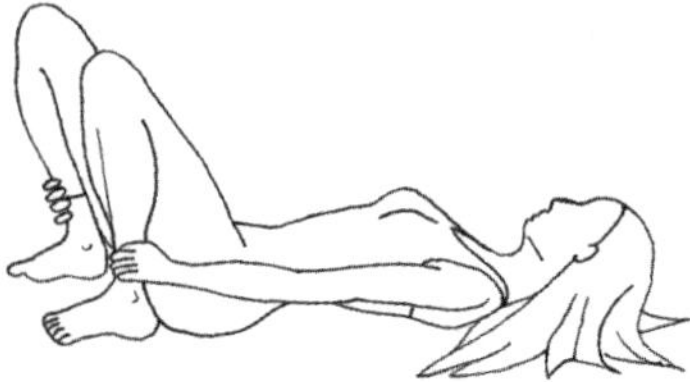
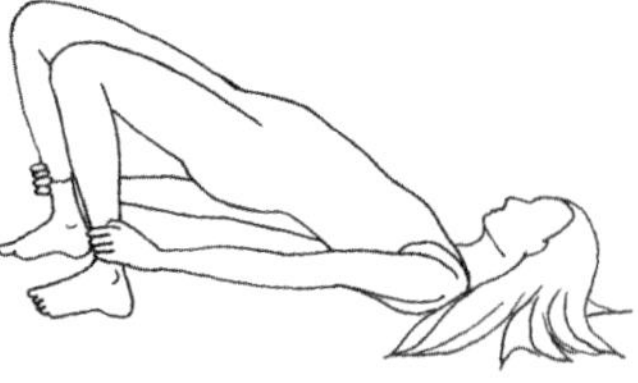

Exercise – Yin Qiao and Yang Qiao Balancing	Benefits
Under Bridge Pose 1. Lie on your back, bend your knees, and bring the soles of the feet parallel on the floor close to your buttocks. 2. Grasp hold of your ankles and lift the hips towards the ceiling and hold this pose for 30 seconds. 3. Breathe deeply as you press the shoulder blades firmly into the back. Draw the chest toward the chin, but do not move the chin toward the chest. 4. To exit the position, exhale and move the shoulder out from underneath as you slowly lower the spine starting from the upper back down through to the hips. 5. Relax quietly for a few minutes with your eyes closed.	The "under bridge pose" exercise strengthens back muscles, buttocks, and hamstrings. It calms the brain and central nervous system, and helps alleviate stress and mild depression. This pose is beneficial for lung and thyroid function, and helps relieve the symptoms of menopause.

Yin Wei and Yang Wei Balancing - Exercise

Plow Pose

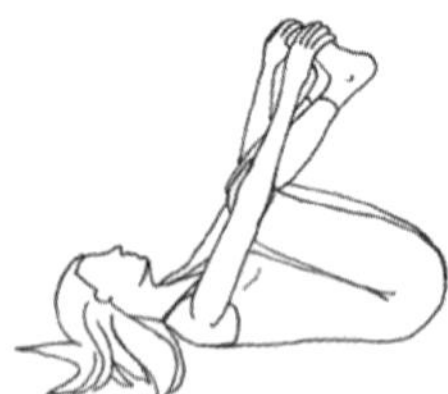
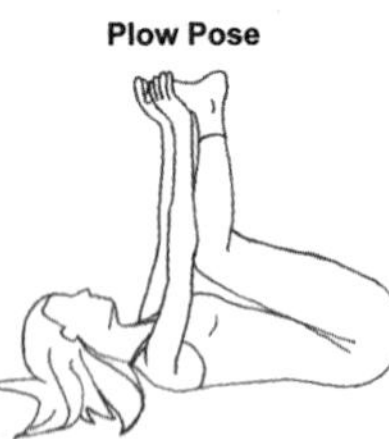
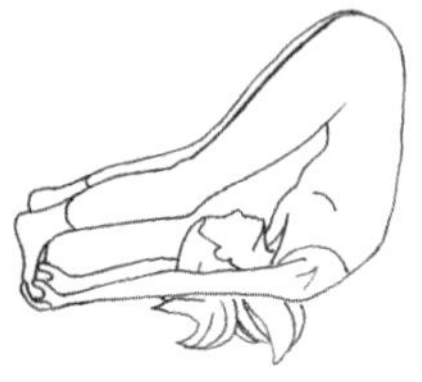

Exercise – Yin Wei and Yang Wei Balancing	Benefits
Plow Pose 1. Lie flat on your back, ankles together and hands at your sides. 2. Inhale deeply through the nostrils and raise the legs straight up, perpendicular to the floor. 3. Exhale and raise the legs over the head, bending at the waist. Interlace your fingers and toes, and lift the back and buttocks until the toes touch the floor directly in back of the head. 4. Breathe slowly through the nostrils and hold the posture for 30 seconds. 5. Slowly reverse the pose, unfolding one vertebra at a time. Keep the legs straight and feet together.	The "plow pose" exercise is good for stretching the shoulders and improving the flexibility of the spine. It calms the brain and nervous system and helps relieve stress and fatigue.

BACK EXERCISES

These movements are intended to stretch out and develop the strength in your back. Prior to engaging in any exercise, read all the directions. During the exercise, inhale and exhale naturally and perform it with fluid movements. If you experience pain at any time, discontinue the exercise. If the pain continues, contact your healthcare provider.

HAMSTRING STRETCH

1. Lying on your back, keep both your knees somewhat bent. Lift your left leg as far off the floor as you can without discomfort. Wrap a towel around the back of your left knee or calf.
2. Grab both ends of the towel and, keeping your leg rather straight, gradually pull it in the direction of your chest. Be aware of the stretch in the back of the leg. Hold for 15-30 seconds. Return to the initial position.
3. Do 3-5 repetitions, switching sides, 1-3 times a day.

CAUTION

- A pillow can be used to prevent your neck from arching.
- Maintain the supporting leg in a bent position and your foot flat on the floor.

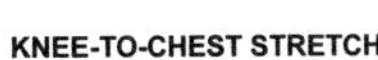

KNEE-TO-CHEST STRETCH

1. Lying on your back with knees bent, keep your feet on the floor.
2. Clutch the back of your right thigh. Gradually pull your knee to your chest. Experience this stretch in your buttock. Make sure you keep your left foot on the floor. Hold for 15-30 seconds. Go back to beginning position.
3. Do 3-5 repetitions, switching legs, 1-3 times a day.

CAUTION

- You can use a little pillow to prevent your neck from arching.

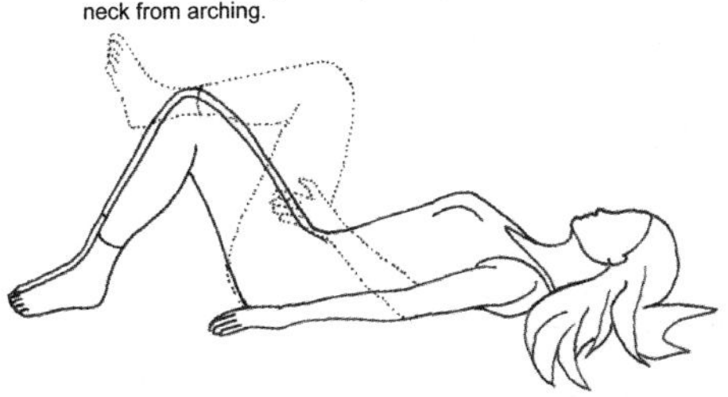

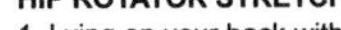

HIP ROTATOR STRETCH

1. Lying on your back with knees bent, rest your left ankle on your right knee.
2. Wrap a towel behind the right thigh. Clutch both ends of towel. Slowly pull the right knee toward the chest. You should feel the stretch in the left buttock. Hold for 15-30 seconds.
3. Do 3-5 repetitions, switching sides,1-3 times a day.

CAUTION

- You can use a pillow to prevent neck from arching.
- Keep the back and hips flat on the floor.

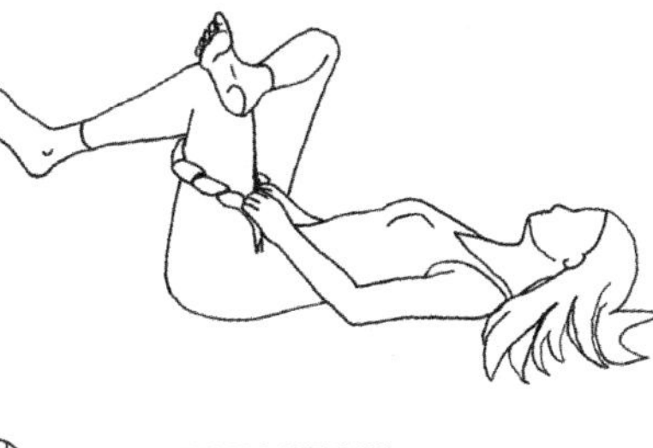

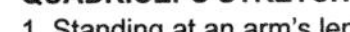

QUADRICEPS STRETCH

1. Standing at an arm's length from the wall, look straight ahead.
2. Placing the left hand against wall, grasp right ankle with right hand. Slowly pull straight up.
3. When a stretch is felt in your right thigh, hold for 15-30 seconds.
4. Do 3-5 repetitions, switching legs, 1-3 times a day.

CAUTION

- Don't arch the back.
- Don't twist the back to reach leg.

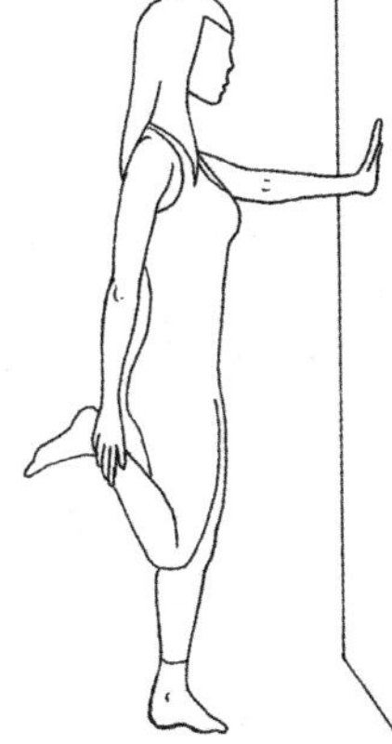

Please use caution. This information is not intended as a substitute for professional health care. Follow your health care provider's instructions. Downloadable exercise forms are available at www.acupuncturedeskreference.com for clinical usage. Permission to use granted.

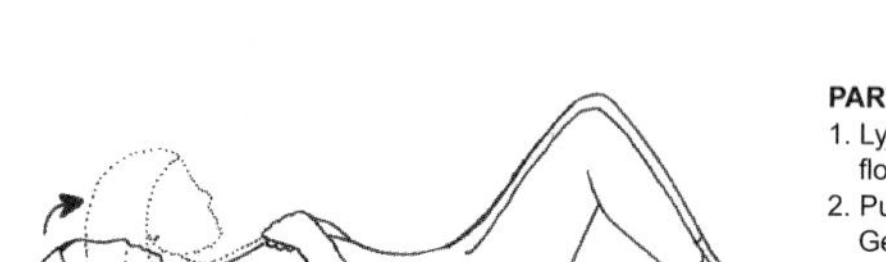

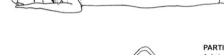

PRONE PRESS-UP

1. Lying on stomach with feet slightly apart, rest forehead on floor. Relax stomach, back and muscles in legs.
2. Press yourself up onto forearms, keeping the neck straight. Quit when you feel light pressure in the lower back. Hold for 5-10 seconds. Then gradually return to lying position.
3. Do 5-10 repetitions 1-3 sets a day.

CAUTION

- Keep stomach and hips on floor.
- Keep chin tucked in but don't arch the neck.

PARTIAL CURL-UP

1. Lying on back with bent knees and feet flat on floor, cross hands on chest.
2. Pull in to constrict the muscles in stomach. Gently raise shoulder blades until they begin to leave the floor. Hold for 3-5 seconds, breathing as you normally would. Gradually lower yourself back to floor.
3. Do 8-15 repetitions 1-3 sets a day.

CAUTION

- Do not pull up with your neck.
- Keep your arms relaxed.

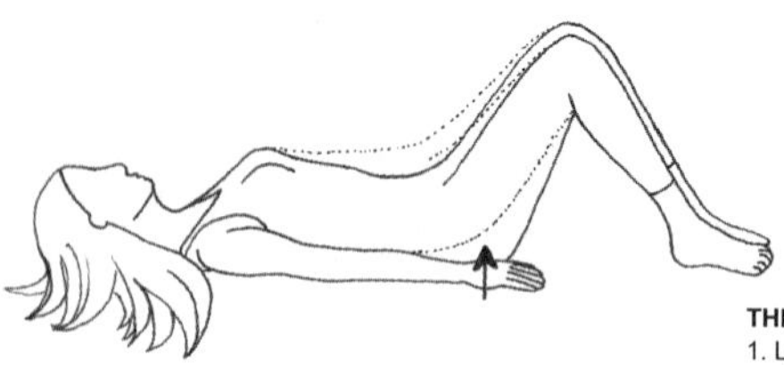

THE BRIDGE

1. Lying on floor with back flat and knees bent, keep feet and palms flat on floor.
2. Draw in and squeeze the stomach muscles. Constrict your buttocks and gently lift hips from floor. Hoist the hips just high enough to make your lower back straight. Hold for 5-10 seconds.
3. Do 8-15 repetitions 1-3 sets a day.

CAUTION

- You can use a pillow to ensure that your neck doesn't arch.
- Don't arch the back.

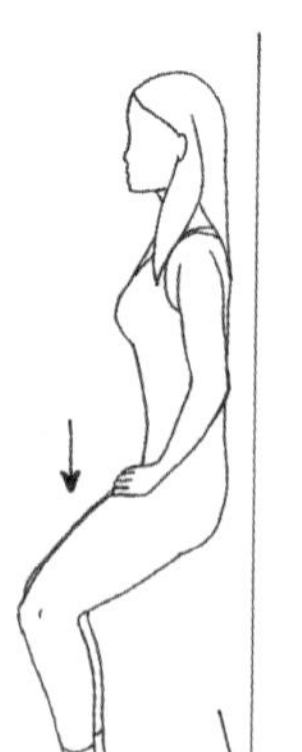

WALL SLIDE

1. Stand with back and head against wall. Looking straight ahead, keep feet shoulder-width apart and at least 12 inches away from wall. Relax shoulders and squeeze muscles in stomach.
2. Gradually slide directly down until there is a stretch in the front of the thighs. Hold for 5-20 seconds, then slowly slide back upward.
3. Do 8-15 repetitions 1-3 sets a day.

CAUTION

- Don't let your buttocks descend below the knees.
- Gaze straight ahead and breathe in a normal fashion.

NECK EXERCISES

These exercises are intended to stretch and reinforce your neck. Before you start the exercise, read all the directions. While you're doing the exercise, breathe as you normally would and move smoothly. If you experience pain, discontinue the exercise. If the pain continues, let your healthcare provider know.

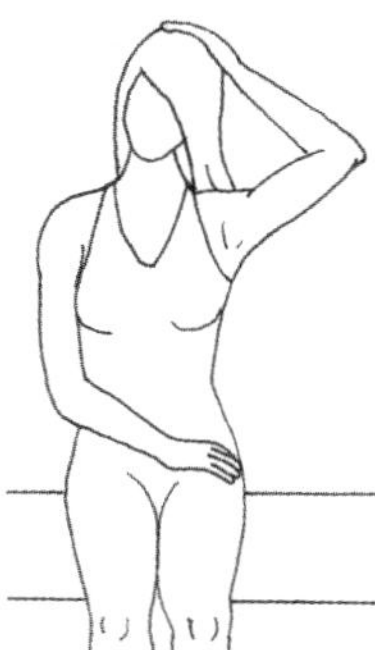

TENSION RELEASE

1. Sit straight in a chair. While tucking your chin in somewhat, tilt head to the left.
2. Putting left hand on upper right side of head, carefully pull head to the left. Hold for 10-20 seconds, then return to initial position.
3. Do 5-10 repetitions on each side 1-3 sets a day.

CAUTION

- Avoid overstretching.
- Quit if you experience any pain or tingling sensation.

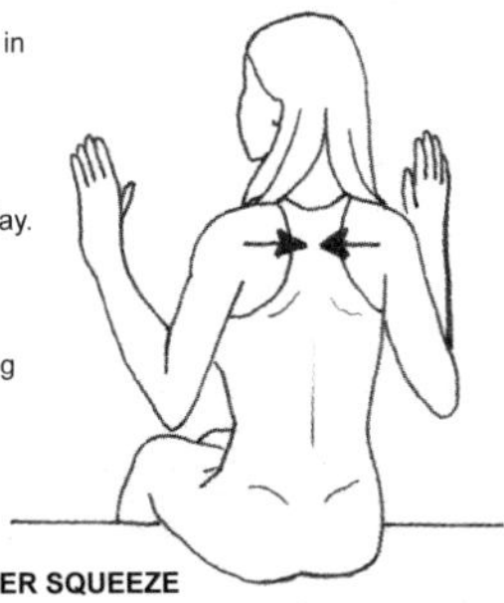

SHOULDER SQUEEZE

1. Bend the elbows and point the fingers toward the ceiling. Lift elbows out away from your sides until the wrists are at shoulder height.
2. Maintaining your fingers in an upward-pointing position, press the elbows back to squeeze the shoulder blades toward each other. Hold for 5-10 seconds. Gradually go back to the beginning position.
3. Do 5-10 repetitions 1-3 sets a day.

CAUTION

- Don't arch the back.
- Don't draw the shoulders up.

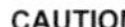

ACTIVE NECK ROTATION

1. Lying on the back with knees bent and feet flat on floor, look straight ahead. If you experience discomfort, put a neck roll or a rolled-up towel beneath the neck.
2. Rotate head gradually from side to side, while keeping the chin level.
3. Do 8-15 repetitions on each side, returning the head to beginning position between each turn 1-3 sets a day.

CAUTION

- Don't force any movement.
- Go just as far as possible with comfort.

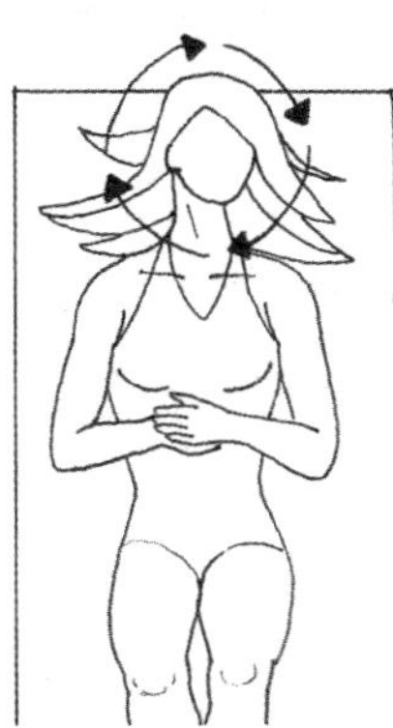

FACE CLOCK

1. Lying on back with knees bent and feet flat on floor, look straight ahead.
2. Visualize your head touching the face of a clock. Little by little, trace the outside edge of the clock with your nose. First go in a clockwise direction, then go counterclockwise.
3. Do 5-10 repetitions in each direction 1-3 sets a day.

CAUTION

- Don't stay in one stance for too long. Keep the head moving to prevent constricting your muscles.

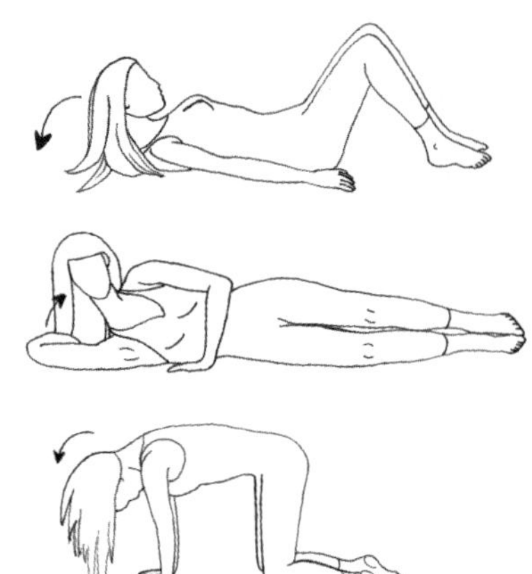

HEAD LIFTS

1. Lying on your back with knees bent and feet flat on the floor, tuck in the chin and raise the head toward the chest, keeping shoulders on the floor. Hold for 5-10 seconds. Repeat 10-15 times. Do 1-3 sets a day.

2. Lying on the right side, with the head relaxing on the right arm, lift the head bit by bit toward the left shoulder. Hold for 5-10 seconds. Repeat 10-15 times on each side. Do 1-3 sets a day.

3. On your hands and knees, and keeping your back straight, slowly release the head toward the chest. Tuck in your chin, and raise the head until the neck is level with the back. Hold for 5-10 seconds doing 10-15 repetitions 1-3 sets a day.

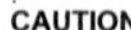

CAUTION

- To protect the knees, kneel on carpet or a pad.

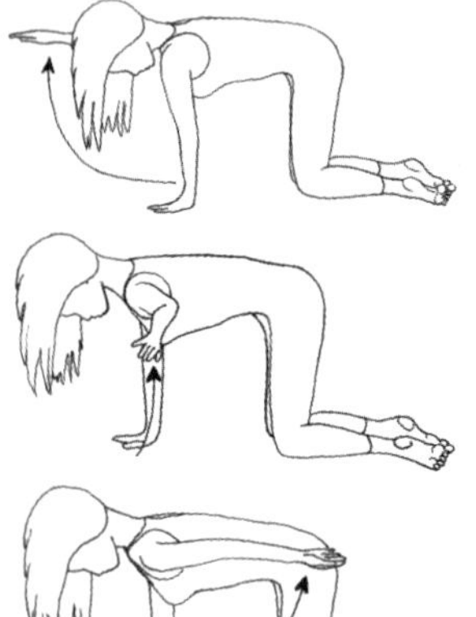

REACH AND HOLD

1. On your hands and knees, with knees apart under your hips, tighten the stomach muscles. Keeping the head and neck straight, lift an arm straight ahead. Hold for 5-10 seconds. Repeat 8-12 times with each arm.

2. Raise one arm to the side. Hold for 5-10 seconds. Repeat 8-12 times with each arm.

3. Raise one arm to the back with the palm facing up. Hold for 5-10 seconds. Do 8-12 repetitions with each arm 1-3 sets a day.

CAUTION

- Avoid arching your back or neck.
- To protect your knees, kneel on carpet or a pad.

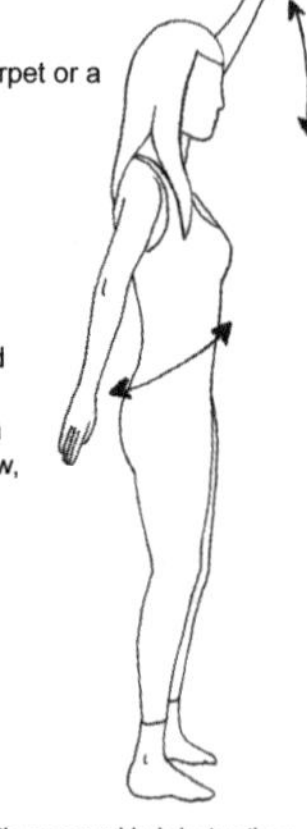

ARM LIFT

1. Standing with back straight, keep your head and neck straight as well.
2. Keeping the arms straight, raise and lower them in front of you, alternating left and right. Use slow, smooth arc motions.
3. Do 8-15 repetitions 1-3 sets a day.

CAUTION

- Avoid locking the knees.
- Don't arch the back.

ELBOW EXERCISES

These exercises stretch and strengthen your elbows. Prior to starting the exercise, read all the directions. While exercising, breathe as you would normally and utilize fluid motions. If you experience pain, stop the exercise. If pain continues, let your healthcare provider know.

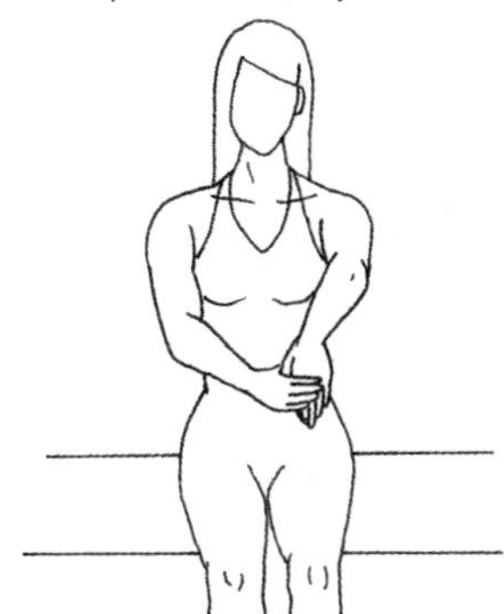

WRIST FLEXION

1. Hold your hand in front of yourself with palm facing downward and the elbow bent.
2. Grab the back of that hand with other hand. Pull back so the fingers point downward as you straighten the arm. The stretch will be felt in the forearm and wrist. Hold for 10-20 seconds. Relax.
3. Do 3-5 repetitions with each hand 3 sets 1-3 times a day.

CAUTION

- Quit immediately if you feel pain.
- Keep the arms in front of your body.

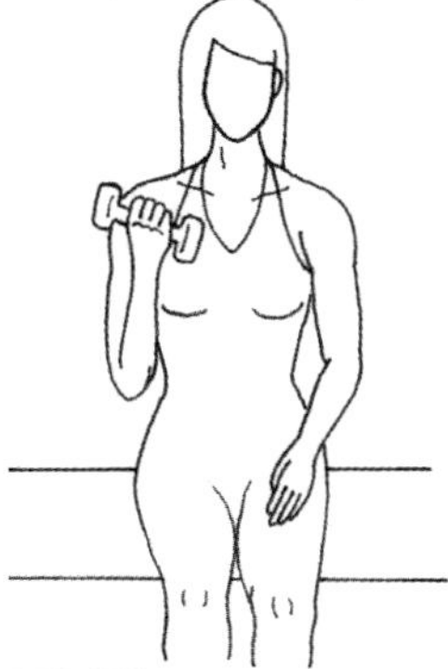

BICEPS CURL

1. Sitting straight, grasp a 5-20 pound weight.
2. Keeping the elbow close to the body and the wrist straightened, bend the arm, moving the hand up to the shoulder, then lower gradually.
3. Do 8-15 repetitions with each arm 3 sets 1-3 times a day.

CAUTION

- Keep the wrist straight.
- Maintain alignment in the head, neck, and back.

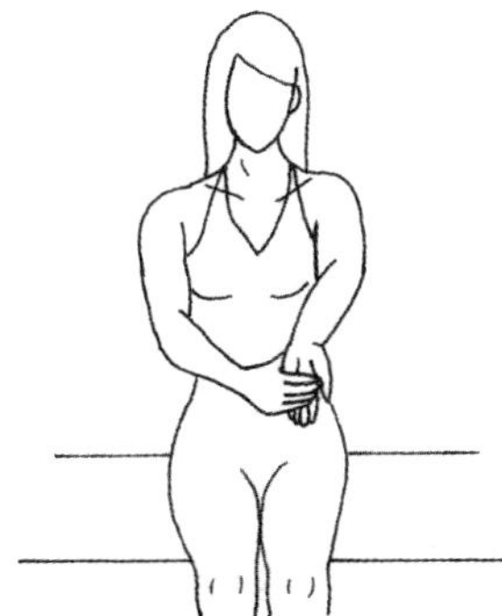

WRIST EXTENSION

1. Holding the hand palm up in front of yourself with the fingers extended and the elbow bent, grasp palm of that hand with the other hand. Pull back so the fingers point down as you straighten the arm. Feel the stretch in the forearm and wrist. Hold for 10-20 seconds. Then relax.
2. Do 3-5 repetitions with each hand 3 sets 1-3 times a day.

CAUTION

- Quit immediately if you experience pain.
- Keep the arms in front of your body.

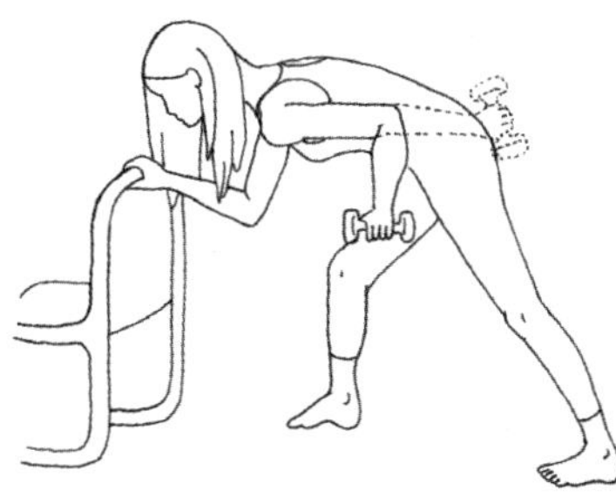

TRICEPS EXTENSION

1. While holding onto the back of a chair with one hand, hold a 5-15 pound weight in your other hand. Bend your elbow so your forearm is perpendicular to floor. Bend forward from waist, with back flat.
2. Gently straighten the elbow, extending the arm up and back.
3. Do 8-15 repetitions with each arm 3 sets 1-3 times a day.

CAUTION

- Keep the elbow close to the body.
- Use smooth, gradual movements and avoid swinging the arm.
- Be sure to keep the head, neck, and back aligned.

Please use caution. This information is not intended as a substitute for professional health care. Follow your health care provider's instructions. Downloadable exercise forms are available at www.acupuncturedeskreference.com for clinical usage. Permission to use granted.

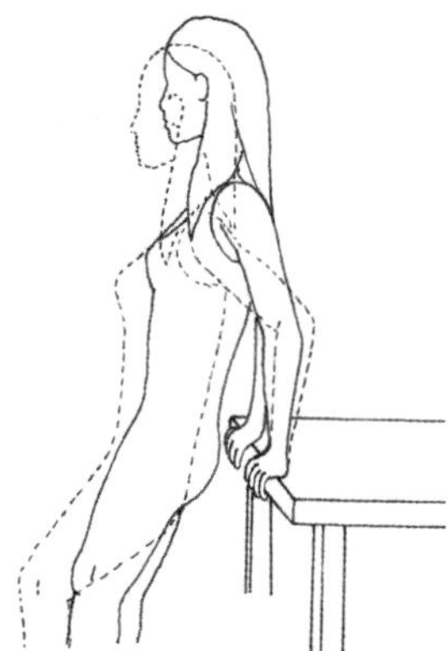

FOREARM ROLL

1. Sit down while clutching a hammer or a 1-5 pound weight in your hand. Place the wrist, palm down, over the end of the knee.
2. Keeping the forearm against the thigh, rotate the hand until the palm is up. Hold for 5 seconds. Then return to beginning position.
3. Do 5-8 repetitions with each arm 2-3 sets 1-3 times a day.

CAUTION

- Quit immediately if you experience pain.
- Avoid lifting the elbow or forearm off the thigh.

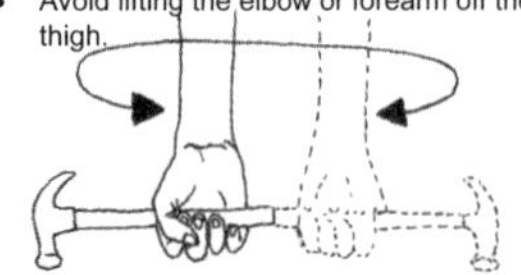

TABLE DIP

1. Stand with your back to a sturdy table or the back of a sofa. Grab the edge of it using both hands and fingers facing out. Keep the elbows straight, without them being locked. Place your feet two to three feet in front of you with legs straight.
2. Keep legs straight as you slowly lower your body until the elbows are bent at a right angle and you experience a pull in the triceps muscles. Go back to beginning position.
3. Do 8-15 repetitions 3 sets 1-3 times a day.

CAUTION

- Don't dip beyond a right angle.
- Wear proper shoes to avoid slipping.

WAND ROLL-UP

1. Tie a three- to four-foot rope to a 1-5 pound weight. Tie other end of rope to the middle of a broom handle or other rounded pole.
2. Standing with feet shoulder-width apart, grasp pole with hands shoulder-width apart, palms facing downward. Extend arms in front of yourself at shoulder height. Use your wrists to roll the rope around the pole, thus lifting the weight up. Reverse to gradually roll the weight back down.
3. Do 3-5 repetitions 3 sets 1-3 times a day.

CAUTION

- Keep the elbows and back straight.
- Use gradual movements.

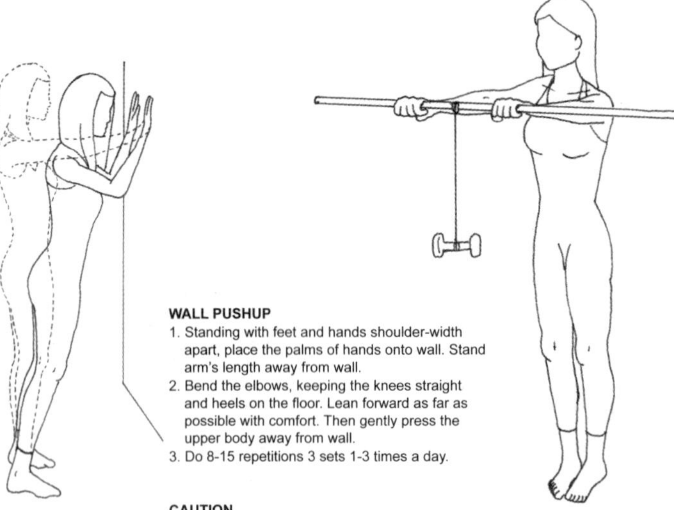

WALL PUSHUP

1. Standing with feet and hands shoulder-width apart, place the palms of hands onto wall. Stand arm's length away from wall.
2. Bend the elbows, keeping the knees straight and heels on the floor. Lean forward as far as possible with comfort. Then gently press the upper body away from wall.
3. Do 8-15 repetitions 3 sets 1-3 times a day.

CAUTION

- Wear proper shoes that will keep you from slipping.
- Don't arch the back.

ADVANCED BACK EXERCISES

These exercises stretch and strengthen your back. Prior to starting the exercise, read all the directions. While exercising, breathe as you would normally and utilize fluid motions. If you experience pain, stop the exercise. If pain continues, let your healthcare provider know.

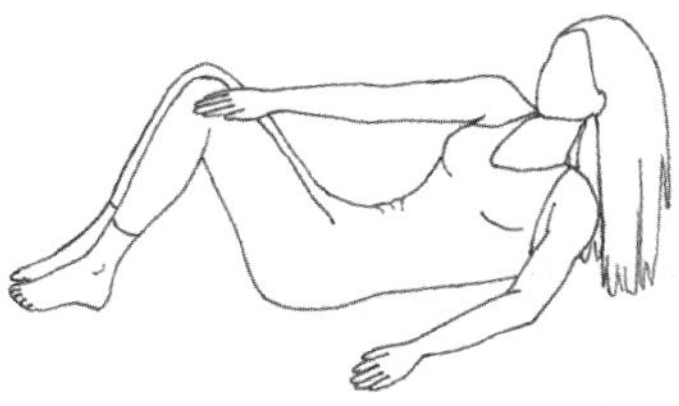

DIAGONAL CRUNCH

1. Lying flat on the floor, rest the left arm on the floor for balance. Put the right arm on the left thigh. Then tilt the pelvis to flatten the back.
2. Keep back flat. Raise the head and shoulders from floor while reaching right arm past the left knee. Hold for 2-5 seconds. Gradually lower the head and shoulders back to floor.
3. Do 8-15 repetitions on each side 3 sets 1-3 times a day.

CAUTION

- Keep lower back pressed to floor while raising head and shoulders.
- Keep head aligned with shoulders.

SEATED TRUNK ROTATION

1. Sitting straight with legs shoulder-width apart and feet flat on floor, cross arms on chest.
2. Keeping the head, neck, and trunk aligned, turn as far as possible to one side. Look over the shoulder. Hold for 5-10 seconds, and then gradually go back to beginning position. Do again with opposite side.
3. Do 8-15 repetitions 3 sets 1-3 times a day.

CAUTION

- Keep the back straight, with head, neck and trunk in a straight line.
- Don't turn too far.

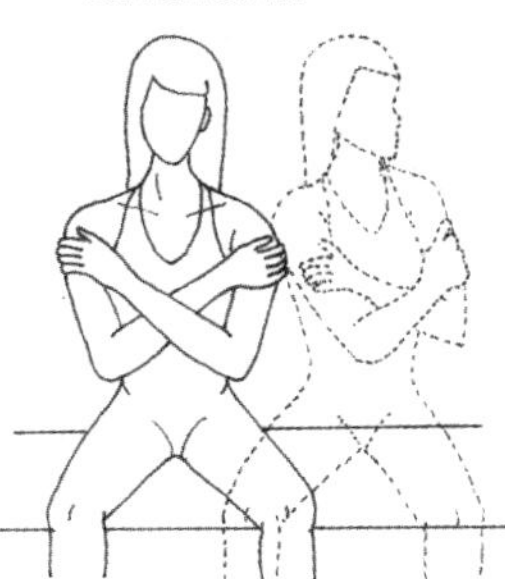

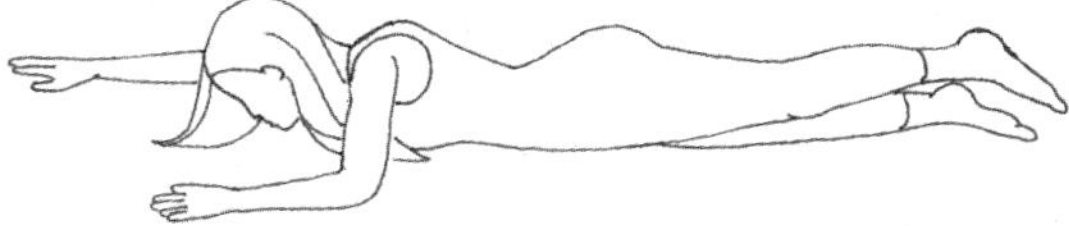

SWIMMING

1. Lying on your stomach with forehead resting on a rolled towel and a pillow under the hips, straighten your legs and put your arms out in front of you.
2. Keep the knees and elbows straight as you raise the left leg and right arm three to six inches from floor. Hold 2-5 seconds, then lower. Lift the right leg and left arm. Hold 2-5 seconds, then lower.
3. Do 8-15 repetitions 3 sets 1-3 times a day.

CAUTION

- Avoid arching the back.

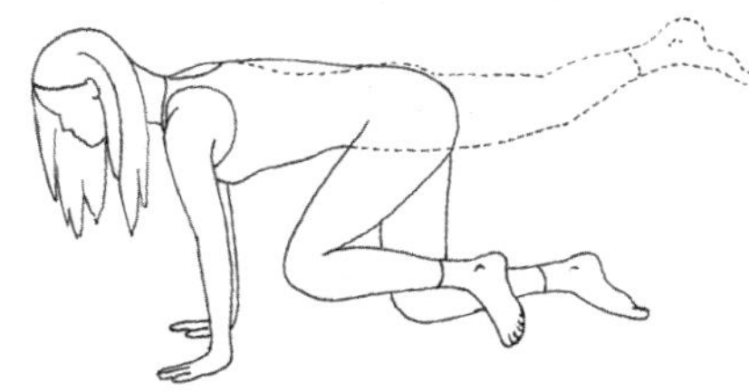

DONKEY KICK

1. Start out on hands and knees. Keep head and neck aligned and back flat.
2. Pull one knee in toward the chest, then push that leg straight back. Hold 2-5 seconds, the return to starting position.
3. Do 8-15 repetitions with each leg 3 sets 1-3 times a day

CAUTION

- While straightening the leg, don't arch the back or overextend the neck.
- Use fluid movements and do not jerk.

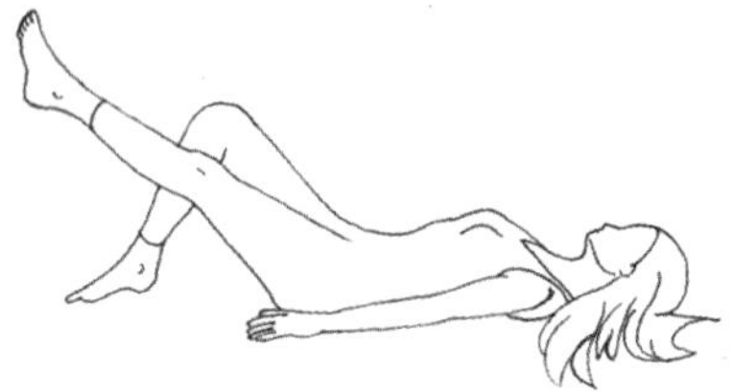

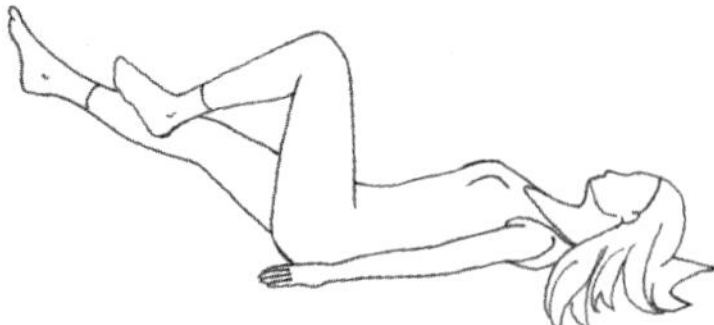

BRIDGE WITH LEG LIFT

1. Lying on floor with one leg straight and one bent, place hands and palms flat on the floor.
2. Raise the buttocks two to three inches while lifting the straight leg. Lower the buttocks, only touching them lightly onto the floor. Then repeat.
3. Do 8-15 repetitions with each leg 3 sets 1-3 times a day.

CAUTION

- Avoid arching the back.
- Keep the head and neck straight.

LEG PRESS

1. Lying with the lower back pressed flat to floor, bend your knees at a right angle, hips parallel to floor.
2. Lift both feet off floor. Keep the stomach tight and back flat as you push the heel of one leg out at a 45-degree angle. Hold for 2-5 seconds. As you slowly return that leg to the beginning position, push out with the heel of the opposite leg. Continue by alternating legs.
3. Do 8-15 repetitions 3 sets 1-3 times a day.

CAUTION

- Avoid arching the back.

WALL SQUAT

1. Stand with back against wall. Position feet shoulder-width apart and at least 24 inches out in front of you with legs straight.
2. Grasp a 5-20 pound weight in each hand with arms straight and palms toward your body. Bend the knees until you feel tightness in the thighs. Hold for 5-10 seconds. Return to beginning position.
3. Do 5-10 repetitions 3 sets 1-3 times a day.

CAUTION

- Consult your healthcare provider before doing this exercise if you have any knee problems.
- Don't allow your bent knees to extend past your toes.

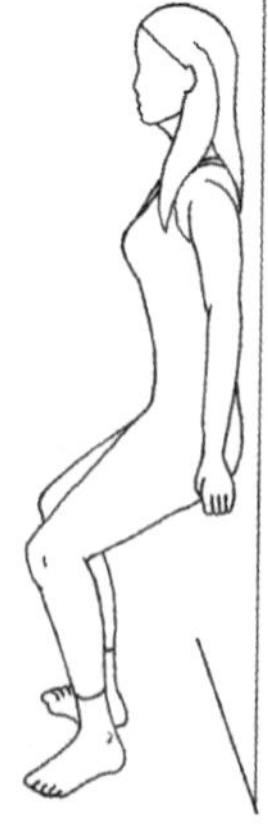

SIDE LUNGE

1. Stand with feet shoulder-width apart and hands on hips as you bend your knees slightly.
2. Holding your stomach muscles tight, take a big step (about 45 degrees) to the side with one leg. Bend front leg as you keep your back leg straight. Return to the beginning position.
3. Do 8-15 repetitions with each leg 3 sets 1-3 times a day.

CAUTION

- Don't allow the bent knee to extend past the toe.
- Keep head level.

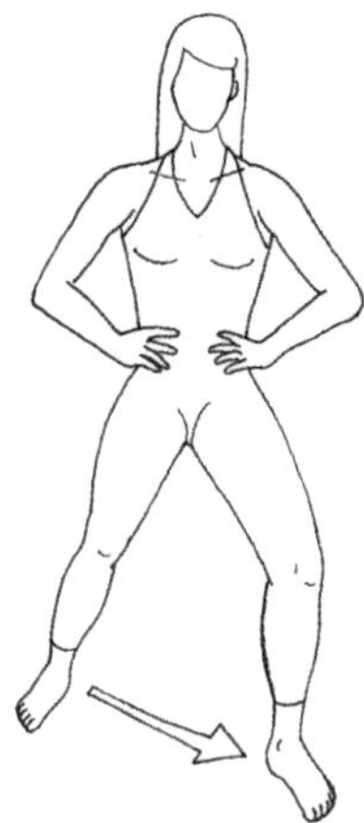

SHOULDER EXERCISES

These exercises are intended to stretch and reinforce the shoulders. Prior to starting the exercise, read all the directions. While exercising, breathe as you would normally and utilize fluid motions. If you experience pain, stop the exercise. If pain continues, let your healthcare provider know.

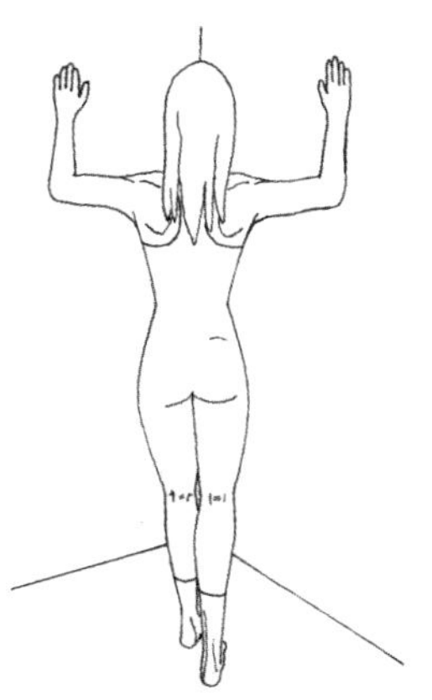

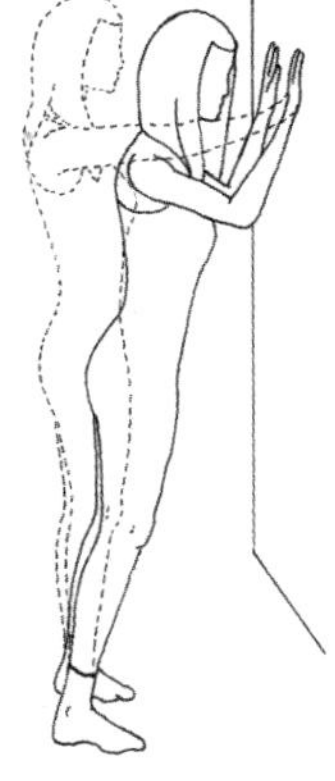

WALL PUSH-UP

1. With your feet and hands shoulder-width apart, put the palms of your hands on a wall and stand about an arm's length away from it.
2. Keeping the knees straight and heels on floor, bend the elbows and lean forward as far as you can comfortably. Then push away from wall.
3. Do 10-15 repetitions 1-3 sets a day.

CAUTION

- Wear shoes that will prevent you from slipping.

CORNER STRETCH

1. Standing facing a corner, with one of your feet slightly in front of the other and elbows at shoulder level, place your forearms onto each wall.
2. Lean into corner until you experience a stretch across the chest. Hold for 15-30 seconds. Go back to initial position.
3. Do 3-5 repetitions 1-3 sets a day.

CAUTION

- Keep the ears, shoulders, and hips aligned.

BROOM STRETCH

1. Lay the palm of your left/right hand over the end of a stick (or a broom or cane). Grab farther down the stick with the other hand, with the palm down.
2. Push the end of stick up to your left/right side as far as you can without any discomfort. Hold for 5-10 seconds. Return to the beginning position.
3. Do 3-5 repetitions 1-3 sets a day.

CAUTION

- Stand straight as you do exercise.
- Don't force the stretch.

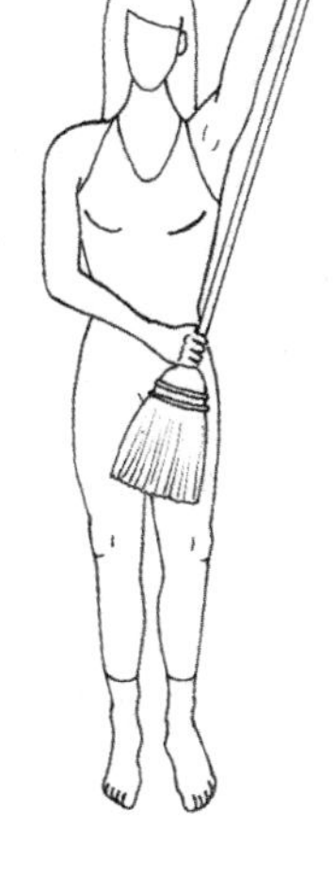

PENDULUM EXERCISE

1. Step forward with the left/right foot and grab the back of a chair with the hand on that same side. Allow the other arm to hang.
2. Swing the free arm backward and forward a few times, then in circles that start out small and steadily get bigger.
3. Continue the circles for 30-60 seconds. Switch directions. Relax.
4. Do 3-8 repetitions 1-3 sets a day.

CAUTION

- Keep the shoulders relaxed.
- Keep the back straight.

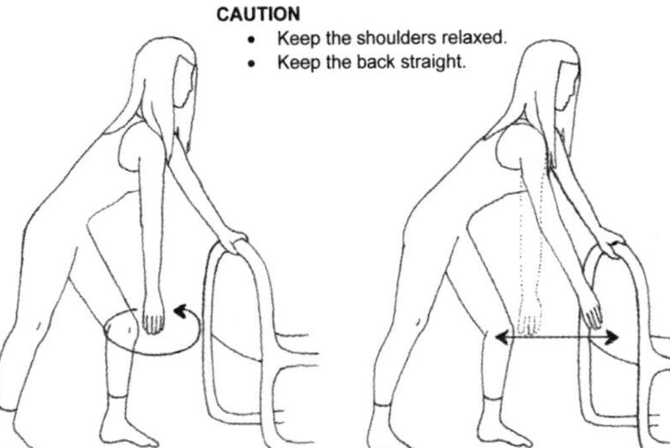

Please use caution. This information is not intended as a substitute for professional health care. Follow your health care provider's instructions. Downloadable exercise forms are available at www.acupuncturedeskreference.com for clinical usage. Permission to use granted.

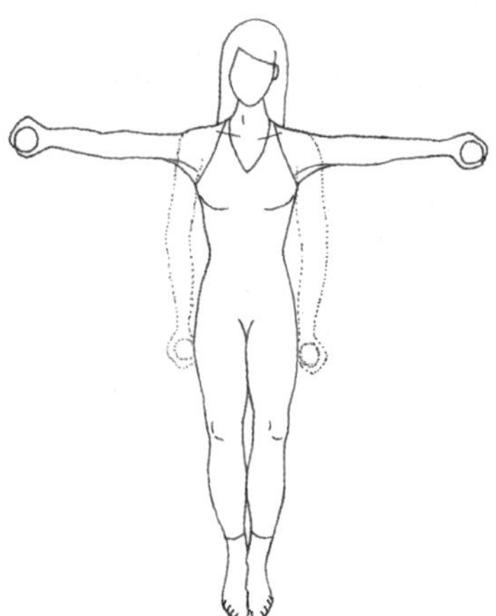

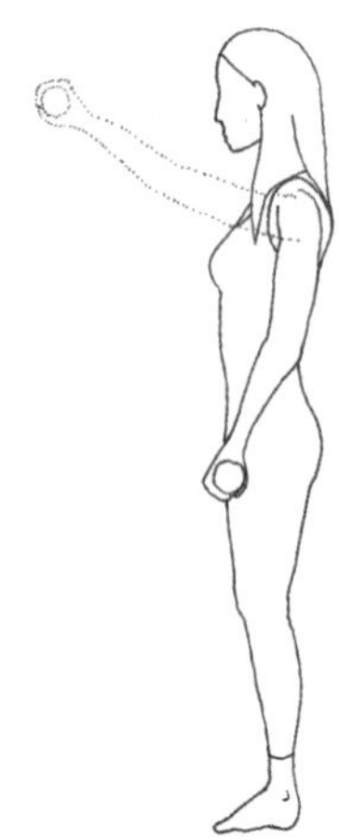

SIDE RAISE

1. Hold a 3-10 pound weight in each hand and stand with arms at your sides, palms facing your body.
2. Keeping your elbows straight, gradually raise your arms no more than shoulder level.
3. Gradually drop your arms to initial position.
4. Do 8-15 repetitions 1-3 sets a day.

CAUTION

- Keep neck and shoulders relaxed.

FRONT RAISE

1. Stand with your palms back and hands at sides. Grab a 3-10 pound weight or in your left/right hand.
2. Lift the arm in front of your body as high as you can comfortably, keeping both your back and elbow straight. Resume

the beginning position.

3. Do 8-15 repetitions 1-3 sets a day.

CAUTION

- Keep the hand in front of the body.
- Keep the back straight and shoulders relaxed.

EXTERNAL ROTATION

1. Lie on your left/right side with head supported with a pillow or your arm.
2. Put a small, rolled-up towel beneath your top elbow. Clutch a 1-8 pound weight with the top hand and bend that arm to a 90-degree angle, relaxing the forearm against the stomach.
3. Leaving the elbow against the towel, gradually lift weight until the forearm is a little higher than the elbow. Come back slowly to beginning position.
4. Do 8-15 repetitions 1-3 sets a day.

CAUTION

- Keep elbow against towel

INTERNAL ROTATION

1. With your knees bent, lie on your back on a firm surface. Grasp a 1-8 pound weight in your left/right hand. Bend that arm to 90-degree angle, resting the elbow and forearm, with palm up, on a pillow.
2. With your elbow next to your side, lift your hand and forearm toward stomach.
3. Gradually return your forearm to the pillow.
4. Do 8-15 repetitions 1-3 sets a day.

CAUTION

- Stabilize head with pillow.

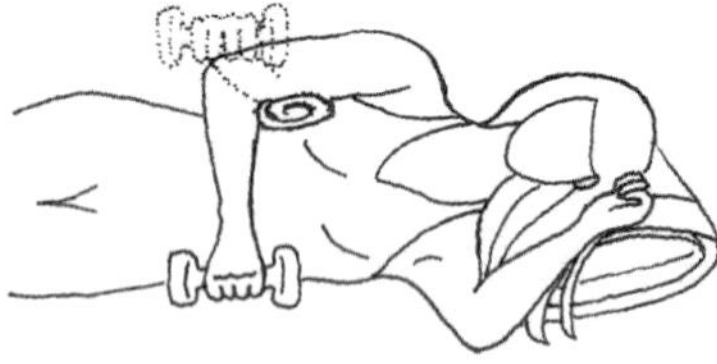

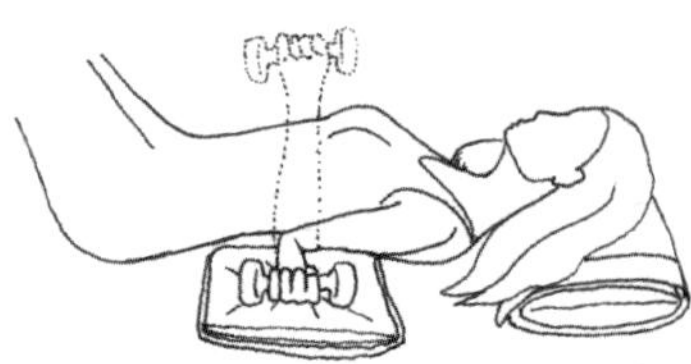

KNEE EXERCISES

These exercises are intended to stretch and strengthen the knees. Prior to starting the exercise, read all the directions. While exercising, breathe as you would normally and utilize fluid motions. If you experience pain, stop the exercise. If pain continues, let your healthcare provider know.

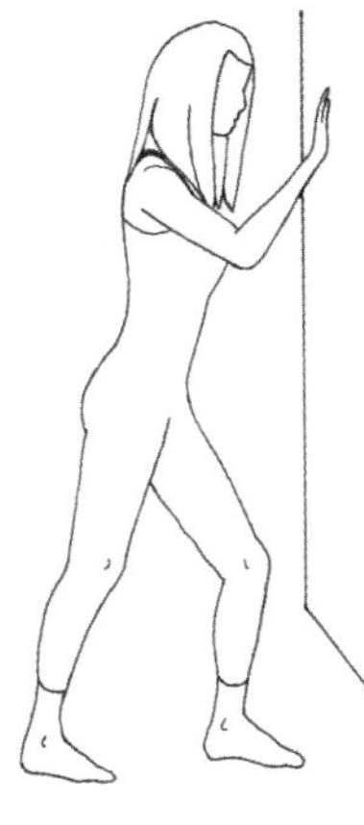

CALF STRETCH

1. Stand with arms supported against wall, with both your feet pointing straight ahead. Put your left/ right foot several inches behind the other.
2. Bend the front leg. Both heels should remain on floor and the back leg should be straight. There should be a slight pull in the calf. Hold for 15-30 seconds. Bend the back leg and hold for 15-30 seconds.
3. Do 3-5 repetitions 1-3 sets a day.

CAUTION

- Don't lift the back heel.
- Don't arch the back.

QUADRICEPS STRETCH

1. Stand at arm's length from a wall, looking straight ahead.
2. Put your left/right hand against wall. With the other hand, grab the ankle of the foot on the same side. Carefully pull heel to the buttocks.
3. When there is a mild stretch in your thigh, hold for 15-30 seconds.
4. Do 3-5 repetitions 1-3 sets a day.

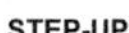

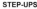

CAUTION

- Don't arch the back or bend forward.
- Don't twist the back to reach leg.

STEP-UPS

1. Stand with the left/right foot on a 3 to 5-inch support (such as a wood block) and other foot flat on the floor.
2. Transfer weight onto foot that's on the block, while straightening that knee and lifting the other foot off floor. Then smoothly lower the foot until just the heel touches the floor.
3. Do 8-15 repetitions 1-3 sets a day.

CAUTION

- Don't lock the knees.
- Keep your body weight on foot on the block but don't push off from floor.

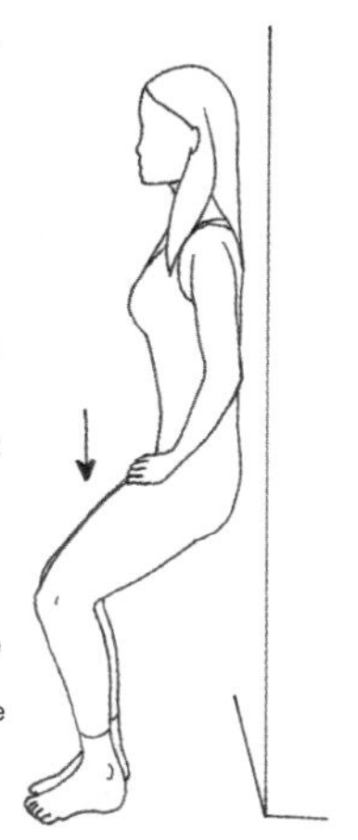

Wall Slide

1. Standing with the back and head against a wall, look straight ahead. Keeping feet shoulder-width apart and at least 12 inches from the wall, relax shoulders and tighten the muscles in stomach.
2. Gradually slide directly down until a stretch is felt in front of thighs. Hold for 5-10 seconds. Slide back up slowly.
3. Do 8-12 repetitions 1-3 sets a day.

CAUTION

- Don't allow the knees to go forward past the toes.
- Don't allow the buttocks to go lower than the knees.

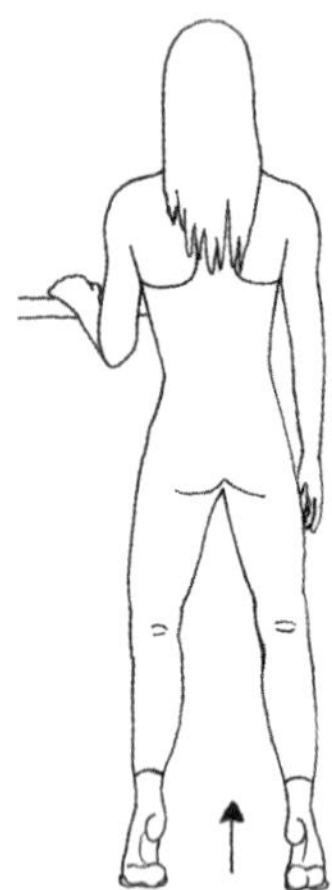

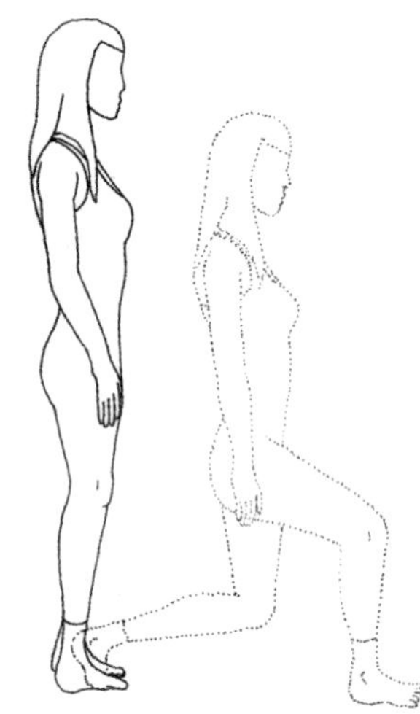

CALF RAISES

1. Start by standing with both feet flat on the floor, shoulder-width apart. If support is necessary, balance yourself with your hand on a wall or table.
2. Lift both heels so you're standing on toes. Hold for 5-10 seconds. Gradually lower heels to the floor.
3. Do 8-12 repetitions 1-3 sets a day. As your strength increases, stand on one foot at a time, and lift that heel off the floor.

CAUTION

- Don't lock the knees.
- Don't arch the back.

LEG LUNGE

1. Stand with feet shoulder-width apart.
2. With the left/right foot, step out and sink your body into a position that's comfortable. Keeping the back straight and feet pointing straight ahead, the heel of the other foot lifts off the floor as you step. Smoothly go back to the starting position.
3. Do 8-12 repetitions 1-3 sets a day.

CAUTION

- Don't allow the forward knee to go past the toes.
- Don't lunge so far that the rear knee touches the floor.

QUAD SET

1. Sit down on floor, one leg straight and the other bent.
2. Flex foot of straight leg by pointing toes toward you. Push back of knee into floor while you tighten muscles on the top of your thigh, holding for 5-10 seconds.
3. Do 8-12 repetitions 1-3 sets a day.

CAUTION

- Don't arch the back.
- Don't hunch the shoulders.

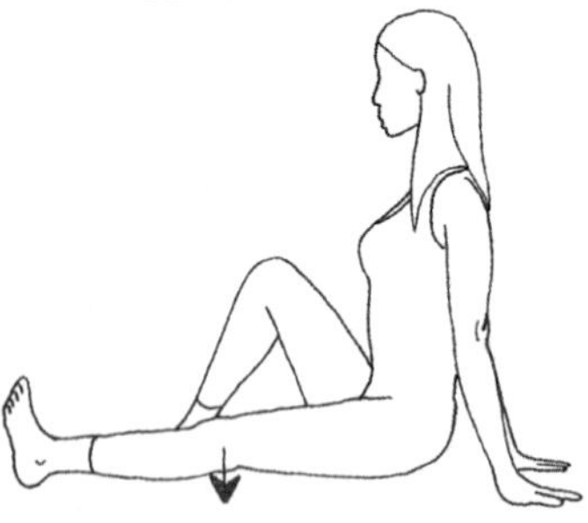

LEG RAISE

1. Sit on floor with the left/right leg straight and the other leg bent.
2. Squeeze the thigh muscles on top of the leg that is straight. You should experience the muscles contracting. Lift that leg up 6 to 8 inches. Then lower it gradually to the floor. Then relax.
3. Do 8-12 repetitions 1-3 sets a day.

CAUTION

- Don't arch the back.
- Don't hunch the shoulders.

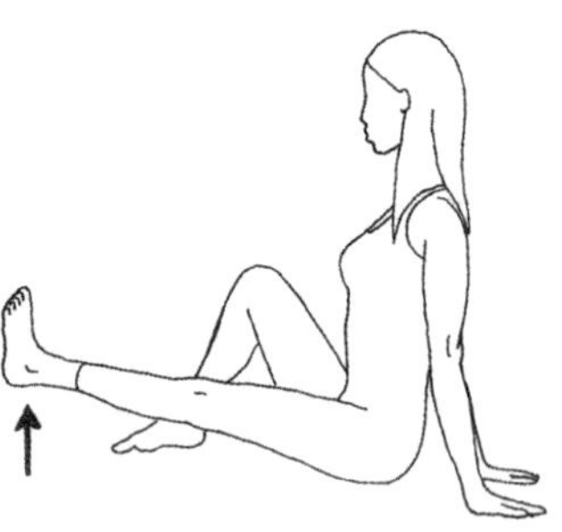

HAND AND WRIST EXERCISES

These movements are intended to stretch out and develop strength in your hands and wrists. Prior to engaging in any exercise, read all the directions. During the exercise, inhale and exhale naturally and perform it with fluid movements. If you experience pain at any time, discontinue the exercise. If the pain continues, contact your healthcare provider.

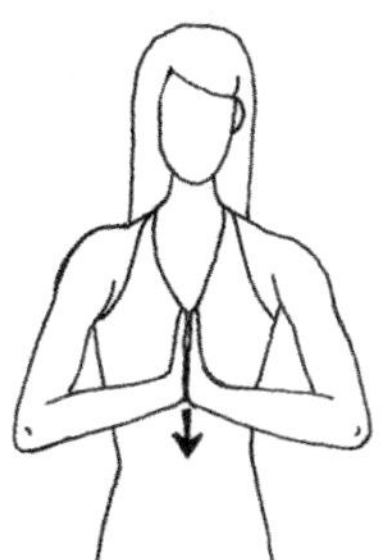

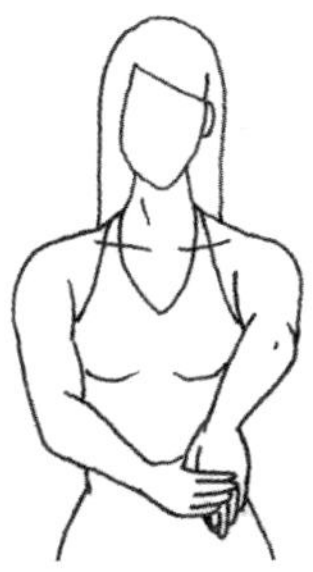

PRAYER STRETCH

1. Sitting or standing with elbows out, put palms together at chest level.
2. Pressing your palms to each other and slowly lowering your wrists until you feel a stretch, hold for 10-15 seconds. Then relax.
3. Do 3-5 repetitions 1-3 sets a day.

CAUTION

- Keep arms close to body.

WRIST FLEXION

1. With palm down and elbow ben, hold your left/ right hand in front of you.
2. Grab back of that hand with other hand. Pull back so that fingers point to floor as you straighten arm. Experience stretch in forearm and wrist. Hold for 10-15 seconds. Relax.
3. Do 3-5 repetitions 1-3 sets a day.

CAUTION

- Keep arms in front of body.

PINCHING

1. Carefully but firmly press left/right thumb to each of the fingertips on the same hand.
2. Then press thumb to middle section of each finger, then to lower part of each finger.
3. Do 10-15 repetitions 1-3 sets a day.

CAUTION

- Be sure wrist is straight.

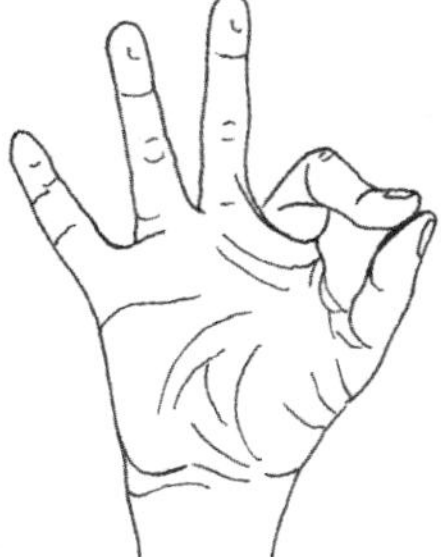

FINGER GRIP AND RELEASE

1. Using left/right hand, form a tight fist. (Or clutch sponge or flexible ball.) Hold 3-5 seconds. Relax.
2. Spread fingers apart as far as possible. Hold for 3-5 seconds. Relax.
3. Do 10-15 repetitions 1-3 sets a day.

CAUTION

- Be sure wrist is straight.

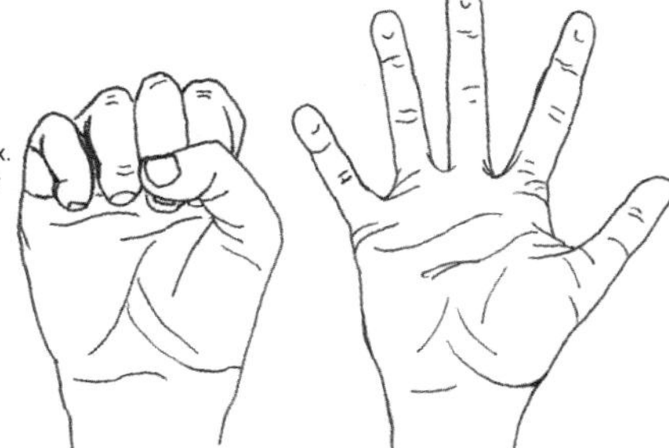

Please use caution. This information is not intended as a substitute for professional health care. Follow your health care provider's instructions. Downloadable exercise forms are available at www.acupuncturedeskreference.com for clinical usage. Permission to use granted.

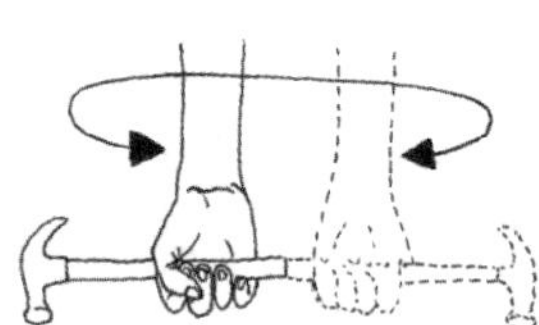

FOREARM ROLL
1. Clutch hammer or hand weight with lef/right hand. Place the wrist, with palm facing down, over the end of knee.
2. With forearm against thigh, rotate hand until palm is up. Hold for 5-10 seconds, then return to beginning position.
3. Do 8-15 repetitions 1-3 sets a day.

CAUTION
- Avoid lifting forearm or elbow off thigh.

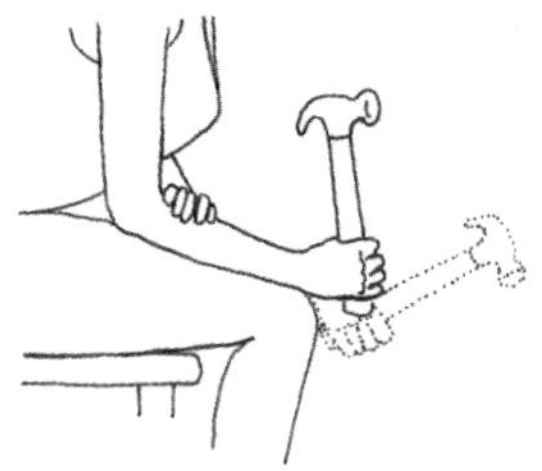

HAMMER EXERCISE
1. While clutching a hammer in left/right hand as if ready to pound a nail, sit. Rest the same forearm on thigh.
2. Keeping forearm and elbow on thigh, raise hammer as high as possible, then lower hammer as quickly as possible.
3. Do 8-15 epetitions 1-3 sets a day.

CAUTION
- Use slow, steady movement.

WRIST CURLS
1. Sit comfortably grasping a 5-10 pound weight or soup can in your left/right hand. Place your wrist, palm up, over the end of your knee.
2. With forearm and elbow against the thigh, curl the weight and lower to starting position.
3. Do 8-15 repetitions 1-3 sets a day.

CAUTION
- Be sure back is straight.

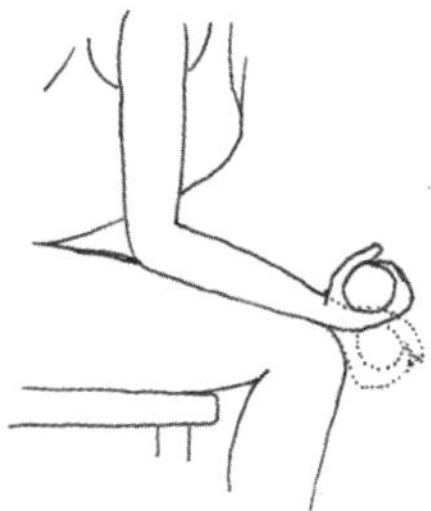

WRIST REVERSE CURLS
1. Sit comfortably grasping a 5-10 pound weight or soup can in your left/right hand. Place your wrist, palm down, over the end of your knee.
2. With forearm and elbow against the thigh, curl the weight and lower to starting position.
3. Do 8-15 repetitions 1-3 sets a day.

CAUTION
- Be sure back is straight.

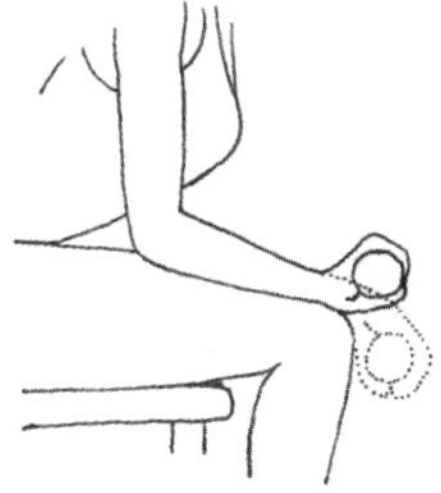

UPPER BODY EXERCISES

These movements are intended to stretch out and develop strength in your upper body. Prior to engaging in any exercise, read all the directions. During the exercise, inhale and exhale naturally and perform it with fluid movements. If you experience pain at any time, discontinue the exercise. If the pain continues, contact your healthcare provider.

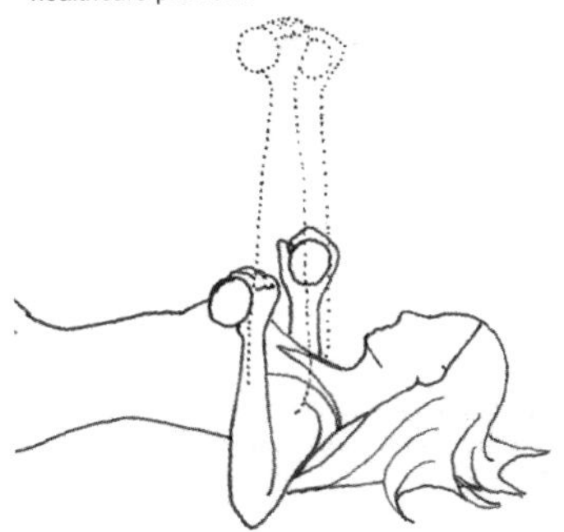

CHEST PRESS

1. Holding a 8-20 lb. weight in each hand, lie on your back on flat bench with your knees bent. Hold arms straight up, positioning weights aligned with chest.
2. Lower arms down and out until elbows are bent at a right angle. Go back to beginning position.
3. Do 10-15 repetitions 1-3 sets a day.

CAUTION

- Avoid arching the back.
- Be sure knees are bent.

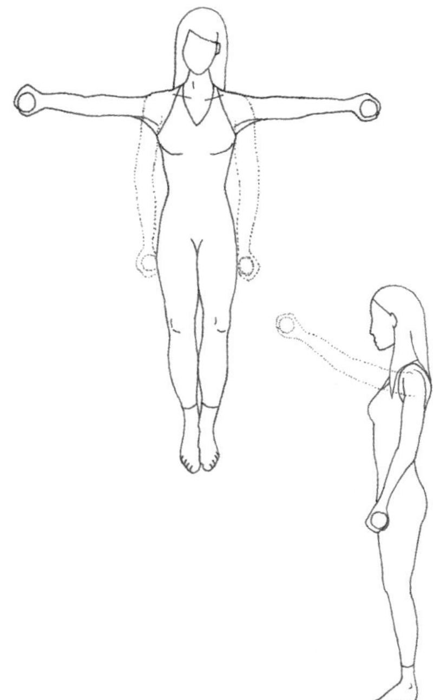

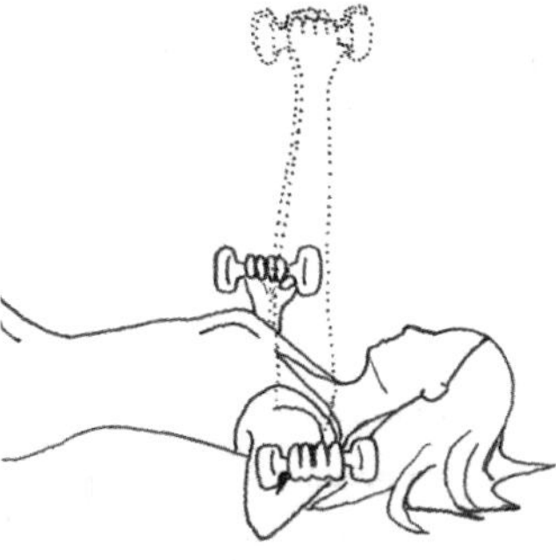

CHEST FLY

1. Lying face up on a flat bench or on floor with knees bent, hold a 5-15 lb. weight in each hand. Extend arms out to sides, keeping elbows somewhat bent and palms facing upward.
2. Keep elbows bent and raise arms upward until the weights touch each other. Go back to beginning position.
3. Do 10-15 repetitions 1-3 sets a day.

CAUTION

- Move slowly, using controlled motions
- Be sure knees are bent.

STANDING SIDE RAISE

1. Stand up straight while holding a 5-10 lb. weight in each hand, with arms at sides and feet shoulder-width apart.
2. Gently extend arms up and out until weights are at shoulder height. Slowly return to starting position.
3. Do 10-15 repetitions 1-3 sets a day.

CAUTION

- Avoid swinging weights. Instead, use slow, controlled movements.
- Avoid lifting weights above shoulder height.

STANDING FRONT RAISE

1. Standing with legs shoulder-width apart, hold a 5-10 lb. weight in each hand, palms facing body. Extend arms straight down until weights touch the thighs.
2. Lift one arm up to shoulder or eye level. Hold for one second, then lower arm. As arm lowers, raise opposite arm to shoulder or eye level.
3. Do 10-15 repetitions 1-3 sets a day.

CAUTION

- Avoid swinging weights. Instead, use slow, controlled movements.

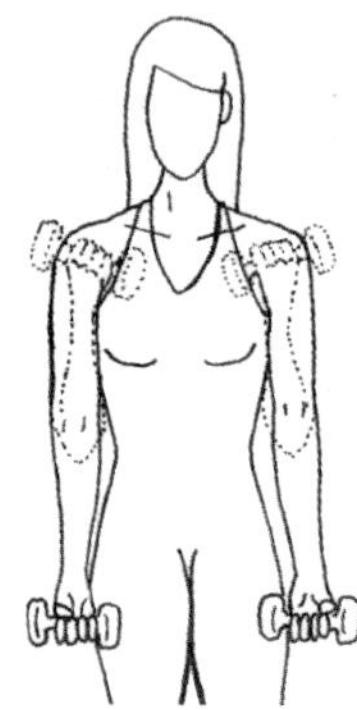

BICEPS CURL

1. Hold a 5-20 lb. weight in each hand, with palms away from the body.
2. Tucking arms near sides of body, bend left elbow and raise weight to left shoulder. Lowering that weight, bend right elbow and raise weight to right shoulder. Continue exercise by alternating arms.
3. Do 10-15 repetitions 1-3 sets a day.

CAUTION

- Keep arms near body during exercise.
- Be sure wrists are straight.

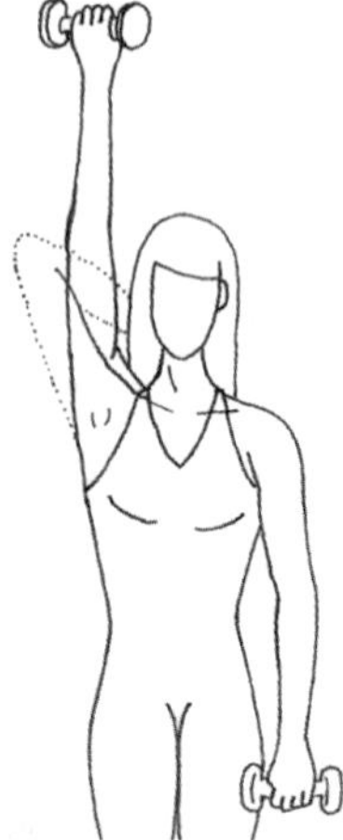

TRICEPS PRESS

1. Grasp a 5-15 pound weight in each hand. Raise one arm overhead. Hold that arm close to your ear. Bend your elbow and lower the weight behind your head, as far as you can.
2. Slowly straighten your elbow, extending your arm upward. Return to starting position.
3. Repeat 10-15 times with each arm, 1-3 sets a day.

CAUTION

- Keep head still and neck straight.
- Keep arm close to ear.
- Avoid arching the back.

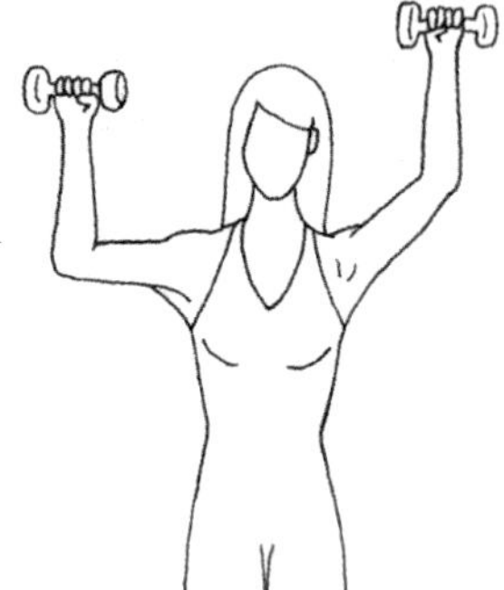

SHOULDER PRESS

1. Holding a 5-15 lb. weight in each hand, keep elbows at shoulder level, with palms facing forward.
2. Lift one arm upward until it is almost straight. Hold for one second, then lower weight, extending the other arm upward.
3. Repeat 10-15 times with each arm, 1-3 sets a day.

CAUTION

- If shoulder problems exist, consult healthcare provider before performing this exercise.
- If it is difficult keeping correct form, use a weight that's lighter.

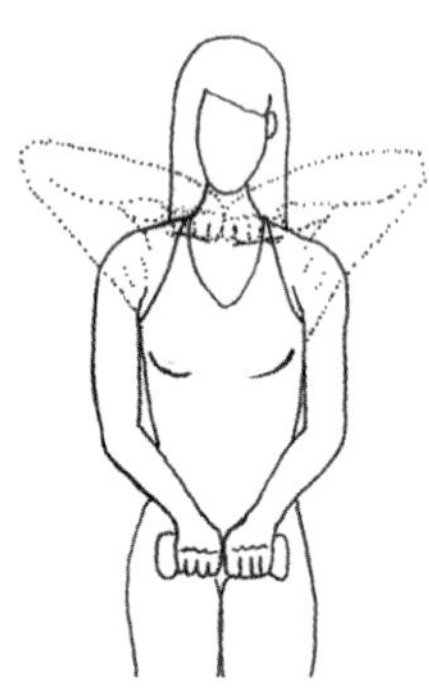

UPRIGHT ROW

1. Standing with feet shoulder-width apart, clutch a 5-20 lb. weight in front of yourself with both hands, palms facing downward, and elbows straight.
2. Keeping the weight close to body, raise it along the midline of body to collarbone. Elbows should extend out to the sides. Return to beginning position.
3. Do 10-15 repetitions, 1-3 sets a day.

CAUTION

- If shoulder problems exist, consult healthcare provider prior to performing exercise.
- Keep head and body still while doing exercise. Just arms should be moving.

ANKLE AND FOOT EXERCISES

The following exercises are intended to stretch and strengthen the feet and ankles. Prior to starting the exercise, read all the directions. While exercising, breathe as you would normally and utilize fluid motions. If you experience pain, stop the exercise. If pain continues, let your healthcare provider know.

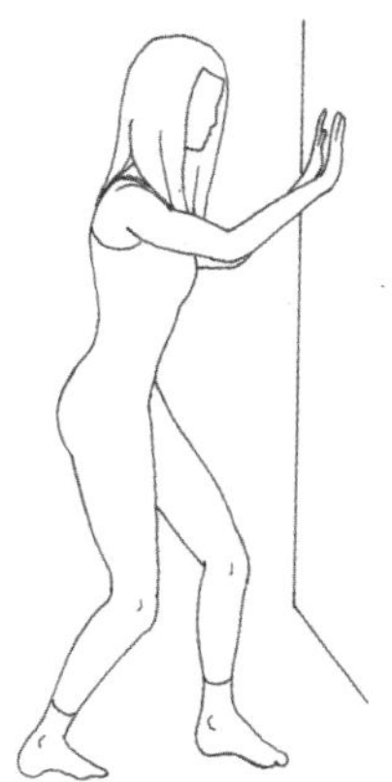

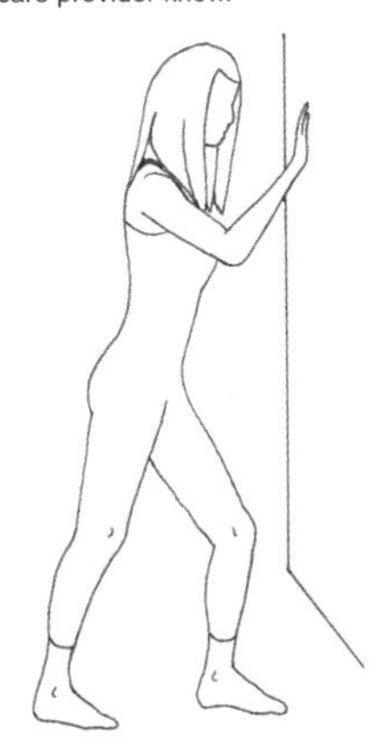

BENT-KNEE CALF STRETCH

1. Stand arm's length away from wall. Put palms of hands on wall. Step forward approximately 12 inches with your left/right foot.
2. With toes pointed forward and both heels on floor, bend both knees and lean forward. Hold for 15-30 seconds. Then relax.
3. Do 3-5 repetitions 1-3 sets a day.

CAUTION

- Don't arch your back.
- Don't hunch your shoulders.

STRAIGHT-KNEE CALF STRETCH

1. Stand arm's length away from wall. Place palms of hands onto wall. Step forward approximately 12 inches with your left/right foot.
2. Lean toward wall, keeping toes pointed forward and both heels on the floor. Bend the forward leg, keeping the back leg straight. Hold for 15-30 seconds. Then relax.
3. Do 3-5 repetitions 1-3 sets a day.

CAUTION

- Don't arch the back.
- Don't hunch the shoulders.

ANKLE CIRCLES

1. Sit on the floor with legs straight.
2. Rest your left/right calf on a rolled-up towel, using the foot to draw circles in both directions or write the letters of the alphabet in the air.
3. Continue for 30-60 seconds 1-3 times a day.

CAUTION

- If your ankle is swollen, make sure it is elevated above your hip.

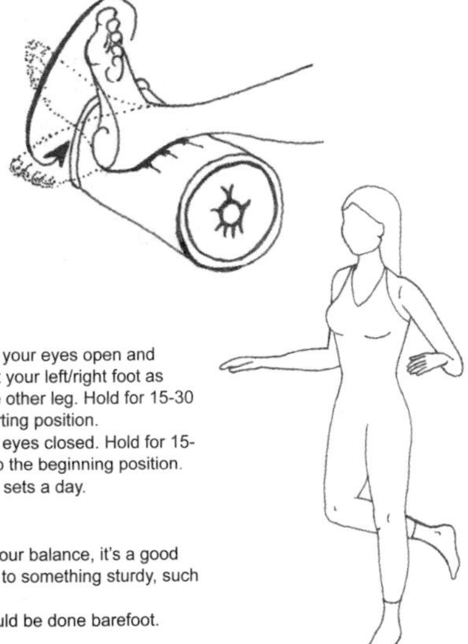

BALANCING EXERCISE

1. Stand up straight. With your eyes open and arms out to the side, lift your left/right foot as you're balancing on the other leg. Hold for 15-30 seconds. Return to starting position.
2. Do first step again with eyes closed. Hold for 15-30 seconds. Go back to the beginning position.
3. Do 5-10 repetitions 1-3 sets a day.

CAUTION

- In case you lose your balance, it's a good idea to stand next to something sturdy, such as a wall or table.
- This exercise should be done barefoot.

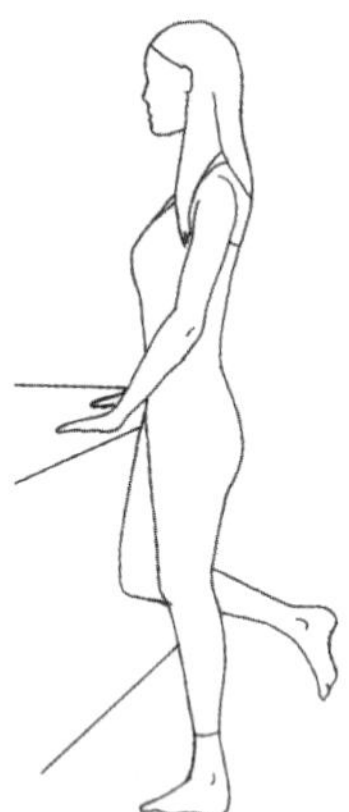

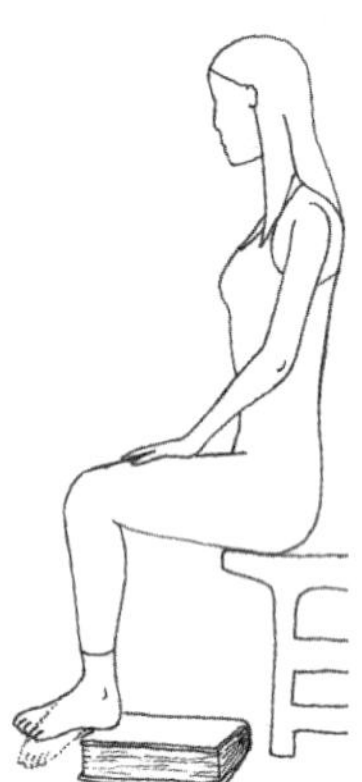

STANDING CALF RAISE

1. Stand up while using a sturdy table for balance only. Raise the left/right foot so that you're standing on the other foot.
2. Rise up on your toes, then lower yourself back onto your heel.
3. Do 8-15 repetitions 1-3 sets a day.

CAUTION

- Be sure to keep back straight.
- Don't lean on the table.

REVERSE CALF RAISE

1. Take off shoes and socks and sit down with your left/right heel on the edge of a block of wood.
2. While keeping your heel on the wood, lift the front of foot as far as possible, then lower it back down.
3. Do 8-15 repetitions 1-3 sets a day.

CAUTION

- A book or block that is thicker than 3 inches should be used for this exercise.

ISOMETRIC ANKLE EXERCISE

1. Start by sitting down in a chair next to something sturdy to help maintain balance.
2. With heel on floor, push the outside of foot against the hard surface. Hold for 5-10 seconds. Repeat 8-15 times.
3. With heel on floor, push the inside of foot against the hard surface. Hold for 5-10 seconds. Repeat 8-15 times.
4. Do 1-3 sets a day.

CAUTION

- Don't push with the rest of the leg, only with your foot.

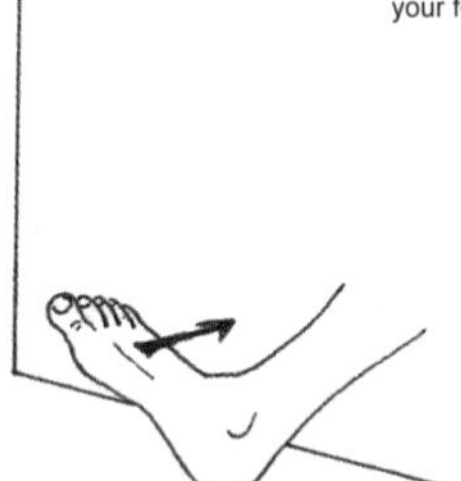

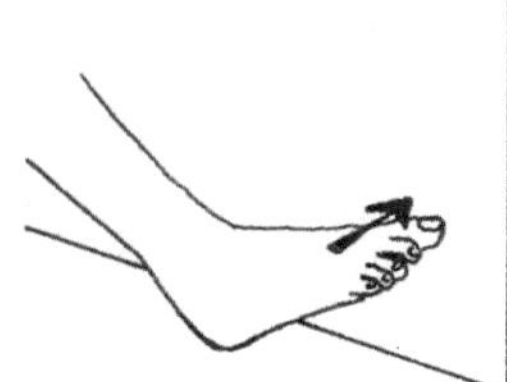

Abdominal obstruction	Tofu
Abdominal pain	Buckwheat, fennel seed, ginger, fresh green onion - white part only, hawthorn fruit, rosin, mutton or goat meat, sorghum, brown sugar, wild cabbage
Abdominal pain with chills	Grapefruit, lychee, black pepper, red or green pepper (chili pepper, cayenne pepper)
Acute gastroenteritis	Tea
Aging	Common button mushroom, royal jelly, walnut
Alcoholism	Freshwater clam
Alcoholism, chronic	Yam bean
Altitude sickness	Fenugreek seed
Anemia	Corn silk, longan
Angina pectoris	Bee venom, hawthorn fruit
Appendicitis	Purslane
Arrhythmia	Chicken egg yolk
Arsenic poisoning	Eggplant, radish leaf
Arteriosclerosis	Tea, tofu, eggplant, wheat bran, yam
Arthritis	Bee venom, loquat root, red vine spinach, royal jelly, sunflower disc or receptacle, vinegar
Asthma	Bamboo liquid oil, black sesame seed, cinnamon bark, cuttlebone, squash, grapefruit peel
Asthma, bronchial	Castor bean, pork testes, bee venom
Bleeding	Black fungus, day lily, white fungus, lotus rhizome, radish, shepherd's purse, water spinach
Bleeding after childbirth	Lotus rhizome
Bleeding gums	White sugar
Blocked urination	Prickly ash
Blood in stools	Black sesame seed, kumquat cake, lychee, longan, mung bean sprouts, chestnut, eggplant, kohlrabi, leaf or brown mustard
Blood in urine	Celery, lettuce towel gourd
	Food cure for blood in urine with diminished urination: Cut up 50g celery into small pieces. Place celery, 25g broad beans, and 100g rice in a saucepan and cover with water to about an inch above. Boil until soft. Eat at mealtime.
Blurred vision	Liver (beef, chicken, pork), matrimony vine leaf
Breast cancer	Crab, squash calyx
Breast lump	Cucumber, green onion (fibrous root), squash calyx
Bronchitis	Chicken, jellyfish, pork gallbladder, tangerine peel, water chestnut
Bronchitis, chronic	Fungus, white fungus, yam
	Food cure for bronchitis: Rinse 100g dried jellyfish. Place jellyfish and 100g fresh chestnuts in a saucepan and cover with water to about an inch above. Boil until soft. Eat at mealtime, once a day, until the symptoms disappear.
Burn	Cucumber, mung bean, mung bean powder, pork skin, watermelon
Cancer	Apricot, button mushroom, carrot, Chinese gooseberry, eggplant leaf, garlic, lily bulb leaf, ling, mulberry root bark, snail (river snail), wild cabbage
Canker, mouth	Watermelon
Cardiovascular diseases	Chinese chive
Cervical cancer	Shiitake mushroom, walnut twig (young branches)
Chicken pox	Potato
Childbirth, difficult	Pork
Cirrhosis	Azuki bean
Colon cancer	Chinese chive
Common cold	Coriander (Chinese parsley), duck egg, honeysuckle stem leaf, pine leaf, green onion - white part
	Food cure for the common cold: Combine 6 green onions, white part only, 50g maltose (or brown sugar if not available), and 2 cups (500mL) water. Bring to a boil for a few seconds. Discard the onions. Add an egg white into the soup and stir. Divide into three doses to drink morning, afternoon, and evening.
Concussion	Peanut plant
Conjunctivitis	Peanut oil, pork gallbladder
Constipation	Bamboo shoot, black sesame seed, carrots, green onion - white part, loquat leaf, potato, red vine spinach, small white cabbage, sweet potato, water spinach
	Food cure for constipation: Cut 250g carrots into cubes. Boil in water until soft. Eat at mealtime.
Constipation in the elderly	Walnut
Constipation with dry stools	Amaranth, banana, beef, black sesame seed, carrot, fungus, white fungus, honey, longevity fruit, mulberry, peach, pine-nut kernel, pork, spinach
	Food cure for constipation with dry stools: Boil 100g spinach in water until soft. Drain. Pour 1 teaspoon sesame oil over the spinach. Eat at mealtime.
Corns	Yellow soybean sprout
Coronary heart disease	Tofu, black fungus, chrysanthemum, hawthorn fruit
	Food cure for coronary heart disease: Immerse 6g black fungus in water for 20 minutes. Cut up 50g lean pork. Combine the pork and the black fungus with 30g cornstarch and add to 2 cups (500mL) water. Boil to make soup. Eat the soup at mealtime, once a day.
	Food cure for coronary heart disease with hypertension: Place 50g cornstarch, 10g rice, and 10g of tofu in a saucepan. Cover with water to about an inch above. Boil to make soup. Eat at mealtime, once a day.
Cough	Betel pepper, citron, crown daisy, goose meat, mandarin orange, olive, peanut, pear, squash
Cough, chronic	Chicken, lily bulb leaf
Cough (dry cough)	Apple, autumn bottle gourd, banana, fungus, white fungus, honey, peanut, pine-nut kernel, pork, sand pear, sugar cane
Cough due to weak lungs	Plum (prunes)
Cough with chills	Leaf or brown mustard

FOOD

Cough with copious phlegm	Apricot, bamboo shoot, chicken egg, ginkgo (cooked), grapefruit, towel gourd, water chestnut
Coughing up blood	Duck, loquat, persimmon
Cystitis	Magnolia vine fruit - Chinese, red vine spinach
Decreased vision	Matrimony vine leaf
Dehydration	Coconut meat
Depression	Red date, wheat
Dermatitis	Chicken egg, pork gallbladder, rice bran oil, safflower, tea, walnut, walnut twig (young branches)
Diabetes	Bottle gourd, black fungus, corn (sweet or Indian), eggplant, hyacinth bean, kiwi fruit, mulberry, palm seed, pear, pork pancreas, radish, sand pear, sheep or goat's pancreas, spinach, squash, sweet potato vine leaves, tangerine, orange, water spinach, wheat bran, wintermelon, yam
	Food cure for diabetes: Cut 150g squash and 100g yam into small pieces. Place in a saucepan and cover with water to about an inch above. Eat the soup at mealtime.
Diarrhea	Black pepper, brown sugar, buckwheat sprout, chestnut, chicken, garlic, grapefruit leaf, hyacinth bean, onion, papaya, purslane, rabbit liver, red bayberries, tangerine, orange, watermelon, yam
	Food cure for diarrhea: Place 30g hyacinth beans and 100g rice in a saucepan. Cover with water to about an inch above. Eat at mealtime.
Diarrhea, chronic	Apple, carrot, fig, gorgan fruit, guava, lychee, lotus rhizome, plum (prunes), pomegranate (sweet fruit), sword bean, wheat
	Food cure for chronic diarrhea: Peel 2 apples. Remove the seeds. Cut up and place in a saucepan. Cover with water to about an inch above. Boil until soft. Drink the liquid like tea.
Diarrhea, with indigestion	Pineapple
Diarrhea in infant	Tea
Digestive tract disorders	Black fungus
Diminished urination	Amaranth, asparagus, barley, bottle gourd, cantaloupe, carp, celery, Chinese cabbage, crown daisy, cucumber, grapes, green onion - white part, hami melon, kidney bean, lettuce, mandarin orange, mango, mulberry, red vine spinach, star fruit, string bean, wintermelon
Diphtheria	Pork gallbladder, walnut
Dizziness	Corn silk
Dog bite	Apricot seed (bitter)
Dry eyes	Liver (pork)
Dry throat	Apricot
Dysentery	Amaranth, bitter gourd (balsam pear), cantaloupe, chicken gallbladder, Chinese toon leaf, chrysanthemum, cucumber vine (stem), date tree bark, fig, garlic, ginger - fresh, grape, guava, hawthorn fruit, honeysuckle, hyacinth bean flower, lotus root, magnolia vine fruit - Chinese, olive, papaya, plum (prunes), pomegranate (sweet fruit and peel), purslane, radish leaf, red vine spinach, scallion bulb, smoked prunes, tea, tomato, towel gourd, walnut leaf
Earache (Otitis media)	Pork gallbladder
Eczema	Broad bean shell, chicken egg yolk, clam - freshwater, coconut shell, mung bean powder, olive, potato, soybean - black
Edema	Areca nuts, autumn bottle gourd, beef, bottle gourd, carp (common and gold), chicken, corn (Indian corn, maize), day lily, duck, grapes, kidney bean, kohlrabi, mulberry, radish leaf, shepherd's purse, sorghum root, wintermelon
	Food cure for edema: Cut 50g wintermelon into cubes. Place melon and 50g kidney beans in a saucepan. Cover with water to about an inch above. Boil until soft. Eat at mealtime.
Edema during pregnancy	Carp
Encephalitis	Banana rhizome, buffalo's horn, pine leaf
Enteritis	Chicken egg, Chinese toon leaf, date tree bark, ginkgo (cooked), kumquat, pork gallbladder, purslane, tea
Epilepsy	Castor bean root, green turtle, olive
Fatigue	Beef, goose meat, honey
Fatigue, chronic	Matrimony vine fruit, mutton
Food poisoning	Ginger - fresh
Forgetfulness	Longan
Fracture	Chicken egg shell inner membrane, mung bean powder
Frostbite	Cherry, cherry juice, chili rhizome, rosin, tangerine, orange peel
Fungus infections	Bee secretion
Gallstone	Radish
Gastroduodenal ulcer	Barley, green peel of unripe walnut, honey, potato, royal jelly
Gastric ulcer	Wild cabbage
Gastritis	Papaya, rice (polished)
Genital itch	Apricot seed (bitter), chicken egg yolk
Glaucoma	Areca nuts
Goiter	Kelp, laver
	Food cure for goiter: Place 50g kelp and 50g laver in a saucepan. Cover with water to about an inch above. Boil until soft. Eat at mealtime.
Headache	Buckwheat, carp, radish
Headache with the common cold	Green onion - white part
Heart disease	Ginkgo leaf, hawthorn fruit, loquat seed, pineapple, tea plant root
Hemophilia	Lotus rhizome, peanut
Hemorrhoid	Black fungus, clam - freshwater, chicken egg, eggplant, fig, leaf or brown mustard, pork, pork gallbladder, spinach, walnut leaf, water spinach, fig leaf
Hepatitis	Button mushroom, cotton root, garlic, glutinous rice stalk, honeysuckle stem leaf, loach, loquat root, magnolia vine fruit - Chinese, malt, muskmelon calyx receptacle, pork gallbladder, red and black date, rice straw, royal jelly, tea
Hernia	Green onion - white part/outer skin, pork
Herpes	Purslane, water spinach

FOOD

Hiccups	Brown sugar, Chinese chive seeds, duck egg, ginger - fresh, persimmon calyx receptacle, rice (polished), sword bean and seed
	Food cure for hiccups: Grind 10 dried lychee nuts (shells removed) into a fine powder. Mix the powder in 1 cup (250mL) water with 2 tablespoons of brown sugar. Drink it as a tea.
Hiccups triggered by cold	Lychee
High cholesterol	Celery, corn (Indian corn, maize), cucumber, garlic, kiwi fruit, onion, shiitake mushroom, sunflower seed, tofu
Hookworm	Purslane
Hot sensations	Pear
Hyperglycemia	Black sesame seed, water spinach
Hypersensitive teeth	Tea
Hypertension	Apple, betel pepper, black sesame seed, broad bean flower, carrot, celery, chrysanthemum, corn (Indian corn, maize), cucumber vine (stem), eggplant, garlic, hawthorn fruit, jellyfish, matrimony vine root bark, onion, peanut, peanut plant, peony root bark, persimmon, persimmon calyx receptacle, royal jelly, sand pear, seaweed, spinach, sunflower sic or receptacle, sunflower leaf, tofu, tomato, watermelon
	Food cure for hypertension with high cholesterol: Crush 250g fresh celery to make celery juice. Drink in 1 day.
	Food cure for hypertension with heart disease: Immerse 50g hawthorn fruit in water for 15 minutes. Remove the fruit from the water and squeeze to obtain juice. Boil the juice over low heat to increase its concentration. Mix it with 50g rice to make soup. Drink the soup at mealtime.
Hyperthyroidism	Persimmon
	Food cure for hyperthyroidism: Crush 1kg unripe persimmons. Fry until soft. Add 3 teaspoons honey and continue to fry until very sticky. Take 1 teaspoon 3 times a day.
Hypothyroidism	Kelp, laver
Hysteria	Wheat
Impotence	Chinese chive, lobster, mutton, walnut
Indigestion	Apricot seed (bitter), chicken egg yolk, coriander - Chinese parsley, corncob, grapefruit, hawthorn fruit, lemon, papaya, pomegranate leaf, prickly ash, sorghum, tea, water chestnut
Indigestion in children	Coconut meat
Induced labor	Asparagus (lucid asparagus), sweet potato vine leaves
Infertility	Ginger - fresh
Inflammatory disease	Chili pepper (cayenne pepper)
Influenza	Garlic
Injury	Chili pepper (cayenne pepper), glutinous rice stalk, safflower
Lactation problems	Carp, button mushroom, day lily, fig, lettuce, papaya, towel gourd
Insomnia	Lotus (fruit, seed, root), grapes, lily bulb leaf, longan, peanut plant
	Food cure for insomnia: Place 15 longan nuts, 7 red dates, and 50g rice in a saucepan. Cover with water to about an inch above. Boil until soft and eat.

Intestinal obstruction	Brown sugar, ginger - fresh, green onion - white part, peanut oil, prickly ash, radish, rapeseed (canola) oil, soybean oil, tea oil
Intestinal parasites	Areca nuts
Intoxication	Apple, grapefruit, ling, mandarin orange, peanut, sand pear, tea, tea melon
Itch	Mung bean powder
Jaundice	Autumn bottle gourd, brown sugar, citron leaf, corn male flower, crab, eggplant, hawthorn fruit, jackfruit, kiwi fruit
	Food cure for jaundice: Cut 50g eggplant into cubes. Place eggplant, 100g rice and 5 pieces ginger into saucepan. Cover with water to about an inch above. Boil until soft. Eat at mealtime.
Kidney disease	Hami melon, watermelon
Laryngitis	Watermelon
Lead poisoning	Mung bean, water chestnut
Leukemia	Hairtail
Loss of voice	Fig, longevity fruit, loquat, mango, radish
Malaria	Areca nuts, black pepper, chicken egg
Malnutrition	Squash
Mastitis	Chicken egg yolk, eggplant, grapevine leaf, green onion - white part, honeycomb - wax cells, kumquat seed, pomegranate peel, sunflower disc or receptacle, tangerine, orange peel, seed
Mastitis, acute	Antler (deer horn)
Measles	Shepherd's purse, towel gourd
Measles, early stage	Cherry
Measles, delayed eruption	Bamboo shoot, coriander - Chinese parsley, shiitake mushroom, sugar cane
Meningitis	Garlic
Menorrhagia	Sorghum root
Menstrual cramps	Hawthorn fruit, lychee seed
Menstruation, irregular	Brown sugar, ginger - fresh, safflower
Migraine	Muskmelon calyx receptacle, radish
Miscarriage	Azuki bean sprout
Motion sickness	Mango
Mumps	Black pepper, mung bean, potato
Nervousness	Longan, wheat
Neurosis	Red date
Night blindness	Alfalfa root, carrot, liver (beef, chicken, pork), matrimony vine leaf, spinach
Night sweats	Duck, grapes, oyster shell, peach, rock sugar
	Food cure for night sweats: Peel and cut up 10g yam. Place yam, 50g rock sugar and 50g rice in a saucepan. Cover with water to about an inch above. Eat at mealtime.
Nipple, sore	Clove
Nosebleed	Chestnut, Chinese chive, green onion leaf, radish, spinach, vinegar
Numbness	Black fungus

FOOD

Numbness of four limbs	Cherry
Obesity	Wintermelon, yam
	Food cure for obesity: Boil 250g wintermelon in 3 cups (750mL) water until soft. Eat the soup as a daily tonic.
Osteoporosis	Chestnut
Pain in the arm	Carp (gold carp)
Pain in the leg	Chili pepper (cayenne pepper)
Pain in penis	Sunflower root
Pain in the testes	Kumquat seed
Pain in the tongue	Bee venom
Palpitations	Grapes, longan
	Food cure for palpitations: Place 50g longan nuts, 10g lotus fruit and seed, and 50g rice in a saucepan. Cover with water to about an inch above. Boil the three ingredients until soft. Eat at mealtime.
Penis swelling	Green onion leaf
Peptic ulcer	Banana, wild cabbage
Periodontal disease	Bee secretion
Perspiration	Radish
Pink eye (conjunctivitis)	Chicken egg, cucumber, shepherd's purse
Pneumonia	Garlic, honeysuckle (dried), jackfruit
	Food cure for pneumonia: Prepare an infusion of 30g dried honeysuckle and 6g peppermints to make tea. Drink the tea at mealtime.
Poor appetite	Black pepper, cantaloupe, honey, kiwi fruit, onion, shiitake mushroom, tangerine, orange, tomato
Poor memory	Tofu
Postnatal anemia	Liver, chicken
Postnatal spasm	Black fungus
Pregnancy, bleeding during	Chinese chive
Premature ejaculation	Lotus (fruit, seed, root)
Psoriasis	Chicken egg, smoked prunes, walnut
Pulmonary tuberculosis	Ginkgo (cooked), mutton
Rheumatoid arthritis	Bee venom, chili pepper (cayenne pepper), royal jelly
Rhinitis	Aloe vera, garlic, magnolia flower bud, peony root bark, sesame oil, sword bean seed
Ringing in the ears	Day lily
Scarlet fever	Burdock, garlic
Scrotum swelling	Lychee seed
Seminal emission	Duck, gorgan fruit, string bean, yam
Sinusitis	Peanut
Skin disease	Castor bean

Skin inflammation	Green onion - white part
Sore throat	Chicken egg, cucumber, fig, longevity fruit, olive, radish, star fruit
Stomach cancer	Chinese chive, shiitake mushroom, sunflower stem and pith, walnut twig (young branches), wild cabbage
Stomachache	Green peel of unripe walnut, longan, papaya, potato, sorghum leaf, root
Stomachache with chills	Garlic, ginger - fresh, grapefruit, lychee
Sunstroke	Bitter gourd (balsam pear), hyacinth bean
Swallowing difficulty	Chinese chive
Swollen scrotum	Garlic
Swollen testes	Kelp
Tetanus	Green onion - white part, mulberry branch juices
Thirst	Apple, apricot, bitter gourd (balsam pear), kiwi fruit, lemon, loquat, mandarin orange, olive, pear, pineapple, plum (prunes), pomegranate (sweet fruit), red bayberries, sand pear, star fruit, tomato
Thrush	Sesame oil
Thyroid cyst	Seaweed
Toothache	Olive, prickly ash, star fruit, wax cells of honeycomb
Tuberculosis	Chicken egg yolk, garlic, ginkgo (fresh or cooked), honeysuckle, rabbit, radish, seaweed, sheep or goat's gallbladder
Tumors	Asparagus (lucid asparagus), sunflower disc or receptacle, kidney bean, sword bean seed
Tympanic membrane perforation	Ginger - dried
Ulcer	Chicken egg shell inner membrane, clam shell powder, cuttlebone, ginger - fresh, mung bean, onion, peanut oil, potato, safflower, soybean - yellow
Urinary infection	Watermelon
Urination difficulty	Arrowhead, autumn bottle gourd, garlic, kohlrabi, pear, white cabbage, wheat
Urination, frequent	Gorgan fruit, lotus (fruit, seed, root), mutton
Vaginal bleeding	Asparagus (lucid asparagus), cuttlefish ink sac, persimmon cake, sunflower disc or receptacle
Vaginal bleeding and discharge	Chicken
Vaginal bleeding during pregnancy	Liver, chicken
Vaginal discharge	Cuttlefish, ginkgo (cooked)
Vaginitis	Chinese toon leaf
Vertigo	Celery, day lily, liver - beef, mulberry, shepherd's purse
Vomiting	Ginger - fresh, loquat, lotus sprout, mango, red bayberries, sugar cane, sword bean and seed, tangerine, orange
	Food cure for vomiting: Cut up fresh ginger into five pieces. Boil in water. Drink like tea.
Wart	Yellow soybean sprout
Whooping cough	Aloe vera, asparagus, chestnut, chicken egg yolk, purslane, celery, chicken egg, chicken gallbladder, cow's gallbladder, garlic, longevity fruit, pork gallbladder, sweet orange peel, tofu

Source: Henry Lu, *Traditional Chinese Medicine, How to Maintain Your Health and Treat Illness*, Basic Health Publications, 2005

Alfalfa sprouts	Vitamin A, C, B, E and K, calcium, silicon	The nervous system, bones and skin.
Apples	Carotenes, pectin, vitamin C, potassium, ellagic acid	The immune system, digestion, heart and circulation. Especially good for constipation, diarrhea and lowering of cholesterol.
Apricots	Beta-carotene, potassium, iron, soluble fiber	Skin and respiratory problems, protects against cancer. Dried apricots relieve constipation and high blood pressure.
Artichokes (Jerusalem and globe)	Inulin, phosphorus, iron	Digestion, as they stimulate liver and gallbladder function. Useful for gout, arthritis and rheumatism.
Asparagus	Vitamin C, riboflavin, folic acid, asparagines, potassium, phosphorus	Gentle diuretic treatment, hence it is excellent for cystitis and fluid retention. Good for rheumatism and arthritis, but not for gout.
Avocado	Potassium, vitamins E and A, essential fatty acids	Heart, circulation and skin. Relieves symptoms of PMS, and protects against cancer.
Bananas	Potassium, fiber, energy, magnesium, vitamin A, folic acid	Preventing cramps. Excellent for digestion, chronic fatigue syndrome and glandular fever.
Basil	Volatile oils: linalool, limonene, estragole	Stimulating the digestion and as a calming, stress-fighting herb.
Beans, dried	Protein, carbohydrates, fiber, B vitamins, minerals, folic acid, selenium, iron, zinc. Choose chickpeas for calcium, soy beans for cancer- and osteoporosis- fighting genistein	Maintaining a healthy heart and circulatory system, also fighting high blood pressure and lowering cholesterol. Offers excellent protection against cancer and regulates bowel function.
Beans, green	Vitamins A and C, potassium, folic acid	Skin, hair and digestive problems.
Beetroot	Vitamins B6 and C, beta-carotene, potassium, folic acid, iron, calcium	Anemia, chronic fatigue and convalescence.
Blackberries	Vitamins E and C, potassium, fiber, cancer-fighting phytochemicals	Heart, circulation and skin. Also good protection against cancer.
Blackcurrants	Vitamin C, carotenoids, anti-inflammatory and cancer-fighting phytochemicals	The immune system. Also protects against colds, flu and some cancers. Good for lowering blood pressure and reducing stress.
Blueberries	Vitamin C, carotenoids, antibacterial and cancer-fighting phytochemicals	See Blackberries.
Brazil nuts	Protein, selenium, vitamin E, B vitamins	One of the richest sources of selenium (five provide a day's dose), an essential mineral that protects against heart disease, breast cancer and prostate cancer.
Bread	Fiber, iron, B vitamins, vitamin E, protein	Everyone – except those with wheat intolerance. Especially valuable for combating stress, physically active people, and the prevention of constipation, Diverticulitis and piles.
Broccoli	Vitamins A and C, folic acid, riboflavin, potassium, iron, cancer-fighting phytochemicals	Anemia, chronic fatigue, before and during pregnancy, skin problems and protection against cancer.
Brussels	Especially rich in cancer-fighting phytochemicals, vitamin C and beta-carotene	Protection against cancer, skin problems.
Cabbage family	Vitamins A, C, E, folic acid, potassium, cancer-fighting phytochemicals	Protection against cancer, stomach ulcers, chest infections, skin problems, anemia.
Carrots	Vitamin A, carotenoids, folic acid, potassium, magnesium	Eyesight, circulation, and protection against heart disease and cancer. Also good for the skin and all mucous membranes.
Cauliflower	Vitamin C, folic acid, sulphur	Protection against cancer, natural immunity and skin problems.
Celeriac	Vitamin C, folic acid, potassium, fiber	Pre-pregnancy and pregnancy, constipation and lowering cholesterol levels.
Celery	Beta-carotene, potassium, vitamin C, coumarins, flavonoids, fiber	Fluid retention, constipation, rheumatism, gout, arthritis and stress.
Chard (Swiss)	Vitamins A and C, iron, calcium, phosphorus, carotenes, cancer-fighting phytochemicals	Protection against eye diseases such as macular degeneration. Also protection against cancer and good for anemia.
Cheese	Protein, calcium and vitamin B12. Also a valuable source of zinc, essential for normal growth, reproduction (especially sperm production) and immunity	Bones, teeth, and prevention/treatment of osteoporosis. Excellent pre-conceptual, pregnancy and breastfeeding food (avoid unpasteurized ones).
Cherries	Vitamin C, potassium, magnesium, flavonoids, cancer-fighting phytochemicals	Natural resistance, arthritis and rheumatism, protection against cancer. Especially good for gout.

Chestnuts	Fiber, vitamins E and B6, potassium	Energy. They are also easily digestible and make excellent gluten-free flour for those with wheat allergies.
Chicory	Folic acid, potassium, iron, vitamins C and A (the latter only if unblanched), liver-stimulating terpenoids	Before and during pregnancy. Has excellent detoxifying and cleansing properties and is mildly diuretic and liver stimulating.
Chilies	Vitamin C, carotenoids, capsaicin	Circulation, especially helpful for chilblains, sinus, digestion, chest problems. Fights stomach bugs.
Coriander	Flavonoids, coumarins, linalool	Digestion. Relieves gas, bloating, irritable bowel syndrome, stress.
Courgettes and other curcubits	Beta-carotene, vitamin C, folic acid, potassium	Skin problems, natural resistance and promotes weight loss.
Cranberries	Vitamin C, cancer-fighting phytochemicals, specific urinary antibacterial	Treatment/prevention of cystitis. Powerful cancer-fighter and immune system booster.
Cucumber	Tiny amounts of beta-carotene in the skin, also a little silica, potassium, and folic acid	Skin and eyes. The juice is useful for relieving fevers.
Dandelion leaves	Beta-carotene, other carotenoids, iron, diuretic, liver-stimulating phytochemicals	Fluid retention, bloating, liver problems, PMS.
Dates	Iron, potassium, folic acid, fiber, fruit, sugar	Anemia, fatigue, constipation, pregnancy. An excellent and easily digested energy source before and during sports.
Eggs	Protein, vitamin B12, iron, lecithin. Also a good source of zinc and vitamins A, D and E	Protection against cancer and heart disease, cholesterol stories are untrue. Also helps relieve anemia, rheumatoid arthritis, osteoarthritis and supports the male sexual function.
Fennel	Low in vitamins, but rich in volatile oils, including fenchone, anethole and anisic acid – all liver and digestive stimulants	Digestive problems, flatulence, and fluid retention.
Figs	Beta-carotene, iron, potassium, fiber ficin (a digestive aid), cancer-fighting phytochemicals	Energy, constipation, digestive problems, anemia and protection against cancer.
Fish	Protein, vitamin B, minerals – especially iron, zinc and iodine. Oily fish has the added bonus of vitamin D and essential fatty acids	Oily fish: joint diseases, brain development, pregnancy, and all inflammatory diseases. White fish: heart protection. Shellfish: male sexual function, heart protection.
Garlic	Antibacterial and anti-fungal sulphur compounds, cancer-fighting and heart-protective phytochemicals	Preventing heart disease, lowering cholesterol levels, and high blood pressure. Useful as an anti-fungal and antibacterial agent, and helps relieve sinus and chest infections.
Ginger	Circulatory-stimulating zingiberene and gingerol	Morning sickness in pregnancy, travel sickness, post-operative sickness, circulation, fevers and coughs.
Grapes	Vitamin C, natural sugars, powerful antioxidant flavonoids	Convalescence, anemia, fatigue, cancer protection and weight gain, especially after illness.
Grapefruit	Vitamin C, beta-carotene, potassium, bioflavonoids – especially naringin, which thins the blood and lowers cholesterol	Natural resistance, circulatory problems, sore throats and bleeding gums.
Kale	Beta-carotene, vitamin C, phosphorus, sulphur, iron, potassium, calcium, folic acid, cancer-fighting phytochemicals	Protection against cancer, provides a boost to immunity. Good for skin and eyes thanks to high content of beta-carotene.
Kiwi fruit	Vitamin C, beta-carotene, potassium, bioflavonoids, fiber	The immune system, skin, constipation and digestive problems.
Kohlrabi	Vitamin C, folic acid, potassium, cancer-fighting phytochemicals	Protection against cancer, immune fighter, and skin problems.
Lamb's lettuce	Vitamins A, C and B6, folic acid, iron, potassium, zinc. Contains calming phytochemicals	Anemia, stress and anxiety. Great before/ during pregnancy, and when breastfeeding.
Leeks	Vitamins A and C, folic acid, potassium, diuretic, anti-arthritic, anti-inflammatory, cancer-fighting phytochemicals	Chest and voice problems, especially sore throat. Helps reduce high blood pressure and cholesterol, and is particularly good for gout and arthritis.
Lemons	Vitamin C, bioflavonoids, potassium, limonene	This powerful immune booster is also good for digestive problems. Particularly beneficial for mouth ulcers and gum disease.
Lettuce	Vitamins A and C, folic acid, potassium, calcium, phosphorus, sleep- inducing phytochemicals	Insomnia, stress and bronchitis.

FOOD

Lime	Vitamin C, bioflavonoids, potassium, limonene	Immune fighter, terrific for the relief of coughs, colds and flu. Also highly cancer-fighting.
Mango	Vitamin C, beta-carotene, potassium, flavonoids, other antioxidants	Convalescence, skin problems, protection against cancer and a boost to the immune system.
Meats	Protein, iron, B vitamins, other minerals	Anemia, stress, and all-round nutrition, as meat contains a broad spread of essential nutrients.
Melon	Vitamins A, C, potassium, folic acid, some B vitamins	Mild constipation, gout, arthritis and urinary problems.
Milk	Calcium, riboflavin, zinc, protein	Growth, strong bones, and convalescence.
Mint	Antispasmodic volatile oils, menthol, flavonoids	Indigestion, irritable bowel syndrome, gastritis, bloating and flatulence.
Mushrooms	Some protein, vitamins B12 and E, zinc	Important nutrient for vegetarians and vegans. Valuable for depression, anxiety and fatigue.
Nuts and seeds	Protein, unsaturated fats, minerals (especially zinc and selenium), fiber, energy	Diabetes, male sexual function, fertility, constipation and varicose veins. Also cancer-fighting.
Oats	Calcium, potassium, magnesium, B-complex vitamins, some vitamin E	Reducing blood cholesterol, stress, digestion. Specifically protective against bowel cancer, heart disease and high blood pressure.
Olives	Protective antioxidants, vitamin E and monounsaturated oil	Skin, heart and circulation.
Onions	Vitamin C, sulphur-based phytochemicals similar to garlic	Reducing cholesterol, preventing blood clots, bronchitis, asthma, chest infections, gout, arthritis and chilblains.
Oranges (mandarins, satsumas, tangerines)	Vitamins C and B6, bioflavonoids, potassium, limonene, thiamine, folic acid, calcium, iron	Fighting infection and improving resistance, fighting heart disease and high blood pressure.
Pak choi	Vitamin C, beta-carotene, folic acid, B vitamins, cancer-fighting phytochemicals	Cancer protection, boosting immunity, anemia, pregnancy and skin problems.
Parsley	Vitamins A and C, iron, calcium, potassium	A strong diuretic and anti-inflammatory, relieves fluid retention, PMS, gout, rheumatoid and osteoarthritis. Also useful against anemia.
Parsnip	Vitamin E, folic acid, potassium, B vitamins, inulin	Fatigue, constipation, good for pregnancy and diabetes.
Pawpaw	Vitamin C, beta-carotene, flavonoids, magnesium, the digestive enzyme papain	Digestive problems, skin, improved immunity. Also for convalescence, particularly after gastric illness as they are extremely easy to digest.
Peaches	Beta-carotene, flavonoids, vitamin C, potassium	Good for pregnancy, people on low-salt diets, reducing cholesterol. Also good as a gentle laxative.
Pears	Soluble fiber, vitamin C	Energy, lowering cholesterol, convalescence and constipation.
Peas	Thiamine (B1), folic acid, beta-carotene, vitamin C, protein	Protein, stress, tension and all digestive problems.
Peppers	Vitamin C, beta-carotene, folic acid, potassium, phytochemicals that prevent blood clots, strokes and heart disease	All skin problems, mucus membranes, night and color vision. Also a good booster for the immune system.
Pineapple	Vitamin C, but most valuable for enzymes, especially bromelain	Angina, arthritis, constipation, fevers, sore throats and all soft tissue injuries.
Plums	Beta-carotene, vitamins C and E, malic acid	Heart, circulation, fluid retention and digestion.
Potatoes	Rich in vitamin C, fiber, B vitamins, contains some minerals	Anemia, digestive problems, fatigue, growth and natural resistance.
Poultry	Protein, vitamin B12, iron, zinc	Convalescence, anemia, natural resistance, PMS, good for pregnancy and growth.
Prunes	Beta-carotene, niacin, vitamin B6, potassium, iron, fiber, phytochemicals	High blood pressure, fatigue, exhaustion and constipation. Also contains high concentrations of cancer-fighting phytochemicals.
Pumpkin	Vitamins A, C, potassium, folic acid, some B vitamins	Protection against cancer, respiratory problems and skin disorders.
Radishes	Vitamin C, iron, magnesium, sulphur, potassium, phytochemicals	Protection against cancer, liver and gallbladder problems, indigestion and respiratory problems.
Raspberries	Vitamin C, soluble fiber, calcium, potassium, iron, magnesium	Immune system, protection against cancer and mouth ulcers.
Rhubarb	Calcium, potassium, manganese, some vitamin A and C	Relieving constipation.
Rice, brown	Protein, B vitamins	Good for people with diarrhea and celiac disease as it contains no gluten. Excellent source of energy.

FOOD

Spinach	Chlorophyll, folic acid, beta-carotene, lutein, iron, cancer-fighting phytochemicals	Skin, protection against cancer, prevention of vision loss in old age. Also good before and during pregnancy.
Spring greens	Vitamin C, beta-carotene, carotenoids, iron, cancer-fighting phytochemicals	Protection against cancer, skin problems and anemia.
Strawberries	Vitamins C and E, beta-carotene, anti-arthritic phytochemicals, soluble fiber	Protection against cancer, gout, arthritis, kidney problems and anemia.
Swede	Vitamin C, useful amounts of vitamin A, trace minerals	Protection against cancer, skin problems and an ideal weaning food for babies.
Sweet corn	Fiber, protein, some vitamins A and E, some B vitamins, folic acid	Energy and fiber.
Sweet potato	Vitamins C and E, beta-carotene and other carotenoids, protein, cancer-fighting phytochemicals	Eye problems, night vision and all skin problems. Also a powerful cancer-fighting food.
Tea	Vitamins E and K, protective phenolic compounds. Also trace minerals, tannin and powerful protective antioxidants	Mild stimulant for fatigue and exhaustion. Also cancer-fighting and heart protective.
Tofu and other soy products	Protein and enormous quantities of cancer-fighting genistein	Protection against cancer – especially breast and prostate. Good for vegetarians and diabetics. Good replacement for those with milk intolerance.
Tomatoes	Vitamins C and E, potassium, beta-carotene, lycopene	Protection against cancer, skin problems, fertility and heart protection.
Watercress	Vitamins C and E, beta-carotene, antibacterial mustard oils, phenethyl isothiocyanate, iron	Essential protection against lung cancer. Food poisoning, anemia, skin and underactive thyroid.
Wheat, wholegrain	B-complex vitamins, vitamin E, fiber, zinc, magnesium and (if North American or Canadian) selenium	A vital source of energy and essential nutrients.
Wine	Excellent source of heart-protective substances	The heart (in modest doses), improves circulation and helps mild depression.
Yogurt	Calcium, riboflavin, zinc, protein, beneficial bacteria	Diarrhea, natural resistance, prevention and treatment of osteoporosis, thrush and cystitis.

Meridian Clock balance with diet

There are two major cycles at work in our bodies: The meridian clock and the pH (acid/alkaline balance). See the following pages for acid/akaline balance. The meridian/organ clock provides us with bioenergetic insights; the pH cycles are the basis of our biochemical life processes. If we work in accord with these natural cycles, nature rewards us with better health and longevity. If, in contrast, we fight or live in conflict with our natural cycles, then dispassionate nature allows only the survival of the fittest. The time of day that you eat a certain food is often of greater importance than what the food is. Poor foods eaten at the "right" time do less damage than good foods eaten at the "wrong" time. Basically, there is a time to eat, a time to live, and a time to sleep. All eating causes the body to work and adapt. This activity occurs best at certain times of the circadian rhythms.

Times	Channels	Functions
5-7AM	Large Intestine	Drinking water triggers bowel evacuation, making room for the new day's nutritional intake. Removes toxins from cleansing during the night.
7-9AM	Stomach	Stomach energies are the highest so eat the most important meal of the day here to optimize digestion/assimilation.
9-11AM	Spleen	The stomach passes its contents on. Enzymes from the pancreas continue the digestive process. Carbohydrate energy made available during this time.
11AM-1PM	Heart	Food materials enter the blood stream. The heart pumps nutrients throughout the system and takes its lipid requirements.
1-3PM	Small Intestine	Foods requiring longer digestion times complete their digestion/ assimilation.
3-5PM	Urinary Bladder	Metabolic wastes from morning's nutritional intake clear, making room for the kidney's filtration to come.
5-7PM	Kidney	Filters blood (decides what to keep, what to throw away), maintains proper chemical balance of blood based on nutritional intake of day. Blood to deliver useable nutrients to all tissues.
7-9PM	Pericardium	Circulation nutrients are carried to groups of cells (capillaries) and to each cell (lymphatic).
9-11PM	San Jiao	The endocrine system adjusts the homeostasis of the body based on electrolyte and enzyme replenishment.
11PM-1AM	Gall Bladder	Initial cleansing of all tissues, processes cholesterol, enhances brain function.
1-3AM	Liver	Cleansing of blood. Processing of wastes.
3-5AM	Lung	Respiration, Oxygenation, Expulsion of waste gasses.

The Chinese Acupuncture "meridian clock" is an example of a 24-hour cycle that portrays the body's complete functions as well as its relationship with diet. The clock delineates which meridian system is activated and dominant at a given time and help us make better decisions about when it is generally best to eat, exercise and sleep.

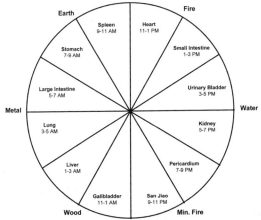

FOOD

Vitamin	Major Functions	Reported Usage	Deficiency Signs and Symptoms	Toxicity Signs and Symptoms	Top Food Sources	Therapeutic Research
Vitamin A (retinol) RDA 5000 IU RDA males 1000 IU RDA females 800 IU	Strengthens mucus membranes, the immune system immune response; required for normal vision, healthy epithelial membranes and skin; high doses have been used for acne and to prevent immune compromise during radiation and chemotherapy	Acne, AIDS, cancer prevention, circulation, colds/flu, Chrohn's disease, eczema, glaucoma, hemorrhoids, measles, menorrhagia, PMS, psoriasis, rosacea, sore throat, ulcerative colitis, UTI	Poor night vision, Bitot's spots, eye problems, fatigue, anemia, poor growth, frequent infections, impaired wound healing, follicular hyperkeratosis (rough, dry, scaly skin), brittle nails, loss of appetite, kidney stones, reduced sweat glands, birth defects; deficiencies may result from low dietary intake, malabsorption or depletion caused by infection	Vomiting, headaches, malaise, loss of appetite/weight, difficult sleep, birth defects, abortion, rough skin, hair loss, bone/joint pain, eye irritation, blurred vision, constipation	Retinol form: Liver, beef, egg yolks, butter, cream, cod liver oil, cheese	Vitamin A plays a major role in wound and bone fracture healing. Has cancer prevention effects 15,000 IU. Can improve menstrual pain. Topical and oral application can improve skin and scalp conditions.
Beta carotene No RDA	Converted to vitamin A by the liver; diabetics have a decreased ability to make this conversion; although not technically a vitamin, it is the only source of vitamin A in many multi formulas	Asthma, cancer prevention, immune support	Low dietary levels are associated with higher rates of several types of cancer	Orange skin (palms, soles, nasolabial folds) are seen with high levels of ingestion but pose no health risks; large supplemental amounts in heavy smokers can increase lung cancer rates	Carotenoid form: carrot, sweet potatoes, red peppers, yams, mangos, apricots, spinach, dark greens vegetables, most orange and yellow fruits	It also acts as an antioxidant and an immune system booster. Ingestion of large dosages can result in orange coloring of the skin.
Vitamin D (cholecalciferol) RDA 400 IU RDA 70+ is 600 IU	Supports bone and tooth formation and muscle function; aids in calcium, phosphorus, and magnesium absorption, thus, critical for healthy bones; supports healthy functioning of the thyroid glands; inhibits proliferation of several types of cancer; may slow the progression of multiple sclerosis	Chrohn's disease, epilepsy, hearing loss, osteoporosis, psoriasis, rickets, scleroderma	(Rickets in children, i.e. bent and bowed legs), late teeth development, osteoporosis, osteomalacia, osteopenia, impaired immune response, muscle weakness around hip/pelvis.	Most toxic; weakness, tiredness, excessive thirst, loss of appetite, nausea, vomiting, headache, constipation, mental retardation, hypercalcuria (which can lead to decreased kidney function and calcium deposits), liver damage, high cholesterol and blood pressure, fetal abnormalities, slow growth	Fortified milk products, liver, seafood, salmon, sunflower seeds, cod liver oil, eggs, mushrooms, herring	Treatment of bone disorders can slow or prevent bone loss with calcium. Can decrease hyperproliferation of skin cells in psoriasis. Stimulates white blood cells and increases resistance to infection. May reduce the risk of colorectal and breast cancer. 4000-5000 IU provides protection for multiple sclerosis and autoimmune conditions.

Vitamin	Major Functions	Reported Usage	Deficiency Signs and Symptoms	Toxicity Signs and Symptoms	Top Food Sources	Therapeutic Research
Vitamin E (tocopherols) "d" natural form "dl" synthetic form RDA males 15mg RDA females 12mg for d alpha tocopherol	Helps the formation of red blood cells, neurological and lung tissue; slows the aging of cells; helps maintain normal enzyme function, aids in tissue healing	Acne, Alzheimer's disease, atherosclerosis, BPH, cataracts, cancer, diabetes, heart attacks, increase immune function, lupus, osteoarthritis, peptic ulcer, peripheral circulation, PMS, rheumatoid arthritis, sunburn	Rare: peripheral neuropathy, fluid in arms and legs, increased RBC fragility (hemolytic anemia), ataxia, muscle weakness	Generally safe; can cause stomach upset, fatigue, muscle weakness, breast tenderness, emotional problems; may increase blood pressure in hypertensives; may augment anticoagulant activity in persons with clotting disorders; women with heart disease on hormone-replacement therapy should avoid high doses.	Wheat germ, vegetable oil, nuts, seeds, cabbage, liver, wheat flour	Cardiovascular diseases 300-1600 IU for 3 months. Enhances immunity, age-related eye disease; may help reduce nocturnal leg cramps and PMS. May slow progression of Parkinson's & Alzheimer's disease. May be beneficial for osteoarthritis and rheumatoid arthritis. May decrease oxidative damage and enhance use of insulin in diabetics. Use with caution in individuals with history of bleeding.
Vitamin K (phylloquinone) RDA males 80 mcg females 65 mcg	Critical for blood clotting; activates proteins essential for bone mineralization and calcium binding.	Blood clotting, osteoporosis	Easy bruising, GI bleeding, nose bleeds, heavy periods	Natural forms are safe; persons on warfarin or other anti-coagulants should avoid supplements	Green, leafy vegetables, Brussels sprouts, broccoli, cabbage, spinach, cauliflower, liver, oats, cheddar cheese	Counteracts anticoagulant overdoses. May help optimize bone mineralization and remodeling. Deficiency may be dietary, malabsorption, or loss of storage sites (liver disease).
Vitamin B1 (thiamin) RDA males 1.5 mg RDA females 1.2 mg	Energy production from carbohydrates; required for healthy nervous tissue and brain cells	Alcoholism, Alzheimer's' disease, anemia, CHF, diabetes, fibromyalgia, insomnia, psychiatric patients	Fatigue, weakness, depression, neuropathy, loss of appetite, depression, nervous system problems, severe deficiency is seen in beriberi, muscle weakness, decreased reflex activity, edema, heart enlargement	Non-toxic	Brewer's yeast, wheat germ, whole grains, nuts, beans, oats, bran, pork, sunflower seeds, lean beef or pork, soybeans, peanuts	Used to treat chronic alcoholics. May ease chronic pain, trigeminal neuralgia, diabetic neuropathy in many nervous system disorders. May improve outcome of myocardial infarction.
Vitamin B2 (riboflavin) RDA males 1.8 mg RDA females 1.2 mg	Energy production from carbohydrates, fats, and proteins; antioxidant effects by regeneration of glutathione; supports the production of adrenal hormones; helps the body utilize other vitamins	Cataracts, depression, migraines	Usually not seen alone; cheilosis (chapped, swollen, fissured lips), angular stomatitis (sores at the corner of the mouth), glossitis (swollen, fissured, sore tongue), photophobia, seborrheic dermatitis (crusty, scaly skin) especially around nasolabial folds, scrotum, and labia	Non-toxic; high doses over long periods may cause diarrhea; harmless coloring of urine (orange/ yellow) appears a few hours following ingestion	Liver, lean beef or pork, chicken, spinach, brewer's yeast, almonds, wild rice, mushrooms, egg yolks	Substantial intake may reduce the risk of developing cataracts. Maintains healthy skin and may help prevent stomatitis and cheilosis. May help fatigue and depression if symptoms are due to riboflavin deficiency.

Vitamin	Major Functions	Reported Usage	Deficiency Signs and Symptoms	Toxicity Signs and Symptoms	Top Food Sources	Therapeutic Research
Vitamin B3 Niacin, niacinamide (nicotinic acid and nicotinamide) RDA 20 mg	Involved with over 200 reactions in the body; supports healthy function of the nervous and digestive systems; involved in the production of sex hormones; helps maintain healthy skin	Acne, cataracts, circulation, diabetes, high cholesterol, glucose intolerance, heart attack prevention, osteoarthritis, Raynaud's disease, rheumatoid arthritis, schizophrenia	Dermatitis, diarrhea, inflamed tongue and mouth, psychiatric changes; pellagra includes the above symptoms with irreversible dementia and is seen with acute deficiency	Burning flush on hands and face, hypersensitivity which may be accompanied with upset stomach, cramps, nausea, vomiting, itching, dizziness, palpitations, and sweating; severe toxicity from time release forms can cause liver damage, elevated blood glucose, peptic ulcers, rash on large areas, gouty arthritis	Lean beef, white meat, tuna, salmon, milk, eggs, legumes, chicken, rice bran, wheat bran, peanuts, rabbit, peanut butter	May help prevent headaches associated with PMS and migraines. Niacin may be beneficial for osteoarthritis especially involving the knee. May lower LDL and serum triglycerides and increase HDL levels.
Vitamin B5 (pantothenic acid, pantothenate) RDA 7 mg	A component of coenzyme A, it is used for energy production from carbohydrates, proteins, and fats; it is also involved in the synthesis of acetyl choline, adrenal hormones, heme, and cholesterol; supports the sinuses; supports normal growth and development	Adrenal support, allergies, arthritis, constipation, hyperlipidemia, surgery and wound healing	Symptoms are rare. Nausea, numbness and tingling of the hands and feet, muscle cramps of the arms and legs, sleep disturbances, headache, GI disturbances, fatigue, depression, irritability	Non-toxic; megadoses may cause diarrhea	Lobster, beef, pork, chicken, fish, nuts, mushrooms, eggs, corn, peas, soybeans, sunflower seeds	May decrease morning stiffness in both RA & OA sufferers. Improves wound healing after trauma or surgery. B5 supports adrenal function. May decrease serum cholesterol and triglycerides.
Vitamin B6 (pyridoxine, pyridoxal) RDA 2 mg	Protein and amino acid metabolism; it is involved in over 100 enzyme reactions; involved in the production of red blood cells and antibodies; helps maintain healthy skin	Arthritis, asthma, autism, cardiovascular disease, carpal tunnel syndrome, depression, diabetes, epilepsy, kidney stones, MSG, nausea and vomiting, PMS	Symptoms are rare. Cheilosis, glossitis, stomach irritability, depression, anemia	Non-toxic; high dosage (2,000 to 6,000 mg) can cause peripheral neuropathy, insomnia	Lean beef and pork, fish, beans, walnuts, eggs, bananas, sunflower seeds	May help a variety of conditions including carpal tunnel syndrome, anemia, arthritis, epilepsy, depression, osteoporosis, PMS, and kidney stones.
Vitamin B9 (folic acid (folate, folacin) RDA 400 mcg RDA pregnancy 600 mcg	Purine and pyrimidine synthesis, heme production converts homocysteine to methionine and helps in the formation of tyrosine, serine, and glutamic acid; deficiency while pregnant can cause neural tube defects	Alcoholism, anemia, atherosclerosis, cancer prevention, coronary heart disease, Chrohn's disease, dementia, depression, osteoporosis, pregnancy and lactation, ulcer	Megaloblastic anemia can cause fatigue, weakness, headache, sleeping difficulty, irritability, depression, restless leg syndrome, facial color loss; anemia is similar to that of vitamin B12 deficiency and include increased MCV, MCH, and MCHC	Safe unless there is a B12 deficiency; high doses will correct the hematological symptom complex, thus masking inadequate B12 which will result in neurological damage	Black-eyed peas, wheat germ, bran, beans, green, leafy vegetables, nuts	May reduce premature birth defects, cleft lip and neural tube defects. Diabetics may improve circulation and visual acuity in elderly diabetics.

Vitamin	Major Functions	Reported Usage	Deficiency Signs and Symptoms	Toxicity Signs and Symptoms	Top Food Sources	Therapeutic Research
Vitamin B12 (cobalamins, cyanocobalamin) RDA 2 mcg	Red blood cell production; healthy myelin; DNA and RNA synthesis; converts homocysteine to methionine; helps the body use folic acid; supports healthy function of the nervous system	AIDS, atherosclerosis, bronchial asthma, depression, diabetes, male infertility, memory loss, multiple sclerosis, pernicious anemia	Pernicious anemia, loss of reflexes and nerve sensation, tingling hands and feet, fatigue, shortness of breath, pallor; neuropathy, especially over age 60; hematological signs are very similar to folic acid; age-related loss of hearing, memory, and concentration; loss of bladder, bowel control; impotence, glossitis, weight loss, insomnia	Non-toxic; GI upset, urticaria, rash, and pruritus have been reported; megadoses can lead to kidney stones and gout	Most animal products; meats, fish, shellfish, dairy, clams, oysters, egg yolks, sardines, liver	May decrease dementia. May inhibit HIV replication. May decrease pain and symptoms of trigeminal neuralgia and accelerate healing time in nerve injuries.
Biotin RDA 300 mcg	Energy production, fatty acid synthesis, healthy hair and nails, sweat glands, nerves and bone marrow	Diabetes, brittle nails, diabetic peripheral neuropathy, dermatitis	Dermatitis around orifices (mouth, nose, ears, eyes, perianal), hair loss, depression, gray skin	Non-toxic	Soy, liver, organ meats, oatmeal, egg yolk, soy, mushrooms, bananas, peanuts, brewer's yeast, egg yolk, peanuts, walnuts	May be supportive for people with diabetes by lowering blood glucose levels and by preventing diabetic neuropathy.
Vitamin C (ascorbic acid, ascorbyl palmitate, ascorbate) RDA males 90 mg RDA females 75 mg	Most important water-soluble antioxidant in the body; reduces several species of free radicals; regenerates vitamin E; involved in the formation of collagen formation, which is important for healthy intervertebral discs, teeth, bones, gums, ligaments and blood vessels; involved in the synthesis of the neurotransmitters and adrenal gland hormones; plays an important role in immune response to infection and support wound healing	AIDS, allergies, asthma, atherosclerosis, cancer, cervical dysplasia, Chrohn's disease, common cold, diabetes, gingivitis, immunity Parkinson's disease, peptic ulcer, wound healing	Fatigue, shortness of breath, bleeding gums, easy bruising, slow wound healing, frequent infections; severe deficiency is seen in scurvy which has the above symptoms along with weakness, inability to stand, pain, shrunken black tendons, depression, anemia, hemorrhage, purple spots on skin, loose teeth	Rare; high amounts can cause diarrhea, nausea, bloating	Rose hips, red peppers, broccoli, citrus fruit, guavas, greens (kale, collard, parsley, turnip, mustard), spinach, kiwis, strawberries, black currants	May act as an anti-inflammatory, and helps the body fight inflammatory diseases, including arthritis, fibromyalgia, chronic fatigue and angina. May reduce the toxicity and improve effectiveness of chemotherapy and radiation of cancer patients

Vitamin	Major Functions	Reported Usage	Deficiency Signs and Symptoms	Toxicity Signs and Symptoms	Top Food Sources	Therapeutic Research
Calcium RDA 1000 mg RDA 50+ and pregnancy 1200 mg	Calcium is crucial to building and maintaining strong bones, teeth, and connective tissue; it is helpful for muscle contraction, nerve impulse stimulation, blood clotting, enzyme activation, ion transport in cell membranes, cardiac rhythm, hormone secretion; helps regulate insulin secretion	Blood pressure regulation, cancer prevention, hypertension, kidney stones, osteoporosis, poison ivy, PMS, pregnancy	Nocturnal cramps; chronic deficiency results in rickets, osteomalacia, osteopenia, osteoporosis. Excess dietary fiber, fat, vitamin A, caffeine along with high stress and low activity reduces the absorption and/or increases the excretion of calcium. Epidemiological association between low intake and obesity	Non-toxic; constipation, may reduce absorption of biphosphate drugs; kidney stones may develop in severe cases	Cheese (except cottage cheese), milk, yogurt, bran, carob, almonds, sesame seeds, tofu, sardines	May help with osteoporosis; suggested dose is 1000 mg and 1500 mg for postmenopausal women. Reduces hypertension in some patients and may reduce risk of colon cancer. Can reduce irritability and depression for PMS sufferers.
Magnesium RDA males 350 mg RDA females 280 mg	Reputed to be the “antistress” mineral and part of enzymatic reactions including muscle contractions, nerve impulse relaxation, cardiac rhythm, ATP phosphate transfer, vascular tone, glycolysis, protein and fatty acid synthesis; essential for healthy teeth and bones; decreases platelet stickiness, helps thin the blood, blocks calcium uptake, and relaxes blood vessels	ADD, PMS, asthma, cardiovascular disease, circulation, CHF, diabetes, dysmenorrhea, epilepsy, fatigue, fibromyalgia, gallbladder, heart disease, hypertension, insomnia, kidney stones, migraine headaches, multiple sclerosis, muscle cramps, osteoporosis	Muscle spasticity, cramping, fasciculations, tremors, twitches, weakness, arrhythmias; cerebral vasospasm, confusion, irritability, insomnia, decreased appetite, osteoporosis	Rare toxicity; diarrhea, nausea, abdominal cramping, reduced heart and breathing rate; persons with renal failure should avoid large doses	Whole grains, molasses, fish, nuts, green, leafy vegetables, soybeans, shellfish, almonds, cocoa, most processed foods are low in magnesium	The adequate intake of magnesium may help to control blood pressure, kidney stone prevention, muscle cramps, migraine headaches, asthma and PMS. Dosages over 1000 mg can cause diarrhea, drowsiness, weakness and lethargy.
Phosphorus RDA adults 800 mg RDA teens 1250 mg	Components of bone, teeth, and energy molecules, ATP, ADP, AMP, and creatine phosphate; required for phospholipid synthesis; regulates extracellular pH; plays a role in cell growth and repair; supports kidney function	No reported use	Rare; loss of appetite, weight, and strength, and bone demineralization	Diarrhea, hypocalcemia, vomiting, nausea, abdominal pain	Found in almost all foods, fish, pumpkin seeds, dairy, almonds, soft drinks, fast food, grains, beef, chicken, beans	May increase endurance performance in athletes and increase libido.

Vitamin	Major Functions	Reported Usage	Deficiency Signs and Symptoms	Toxicity Signs and Symptoms	Top Food Sources	Therapeutic Research
Sodium DV 2000 mg EMR 500 mg	Involved in muscle contraction, nerve function, carbohydrate absorption, and fluid balance as the principle extracellular ion; supports blood and lymph system	No reported use	Most often seen in athletes during competition in the heat; symptoms include muscle cramps, dehydration, heat exhaustion, and heat stroke caused by excessive loss of sweat w/insufficient replacement	Hypertension, water retention, bloating and increase in urinary calcium excretion	Processed foods including canned, frozen, fast, chips, cheeses; sauces, condiments, and restaurant foods	We consume most of our sodium through normal table salt. Most often excess sodium can be a factor in high blood pressure.
Potassium DV 3500 mg EMR 2000 mg	Muscle contraction, nerve transmission and steady function of the nervous system; supports the heart, muscles, kidneys and blood; important for fluid balance and acid-base balance	Cardiac arrhythmias, CHF, hypertension, kidney stones	Rapid and/or irregular heart beat, abnormal EKG	Muscle pain and weakness; hyperkalemia which may lead to life-threatening cardiac dysfunction	Almost all fruits and vegetables, beef	May help a variety of conditions including lowering blood pressure, constipation, cardiac arrhythmias, and exercise.
Iron RDA males 10 mg RDA females 15 mg RDA 50+ 10 mg RDA pregnancy 30 mg	A component of both hemoglobin and myoglobin, it is involved in oxygen transportation; required for collagen synthesis, and immune function; helps build resistance to disease; necessary for energy production	Anemia, menorrhagia, pregnancy, restless leg syndrome	Microcytic anemia, fatigue, shortness of breath, pallor, angular stomatitis, decreased cold tolerance (esp. hands and feet), restless leg Syndrome	One percent of people of European descent have hemochromatosis, a genetic error that causes excessive iron absorption which can lead to liver disease and coma; vomiting, cramps, diarrhea, weak pulse, exhaustion; frequent cause of poisoning in children who mistakenly take their parent's supplements	Red meat, oysters, beans, raisins, egg yolks, molasses, sunflower seeds	Mainly used to prevent iron deficiency anemia.
Zinc RDA males 15 mg RDA females 12 mg	Involved in over 100 enzymatic reactions; important for growth, development, wound healing, and immune response; has antioxidant activity, sperm production, normal fetal growth; needed for proper functioning of insulin and Vitamin A transport	Acne, athletes foot, BPH, common cold, Chrohn's disease, diabetes, diaper rash, immune function, osteoporosis, skin conditions, ulcers, wound healing	Poor wound healing, frequent infections, decreased libido, stunted growth in children, white spots on nails, multiple dermatological problems (eczema, acne, skin ulcer, rashes, seborrhea)	Diarrhea, delayed growth development, vomiting, GI pain, kidney failure, poor coordination	Red meat, lamb, crab, seafoods, nuts, seeds, beans, oysters, egg yolks, dark meat, poultry	May help a variety of conditions including acne, wound healing, male infertility, diabetes, gastric ulcers.

Vitamin	Major Functions	Reported Usage	Deficiency Signs and Symptoms	Toxicity Signs and Symptoms	Top Food Sources	Therapeutic Research
Selenium RDA males 70 mcg RDA females 55 mcg	A component of glutathione peroxidase, a powerful antioxidant; required for thyroid hormone conversion (T_4 to T_3); works synergistically with vitamin E; detoxification of heavy metal; has antiviral activity, increase T lymphocytes and enhance natural killer cell activity	Acne, AIDS, atherosclerosis, cancer prevention, cataracts, chemotherapy, circulation, eczema, epilepsy, hemorrhoids, herpes simplex virus, hypothyroidism, ulcerative colitis	Low dietary levels are associated with increased risk of heart disease and several types of cancer including prostate and colorectal	Tooth decay, nerve problems; doses over 1000 mcg may in time cause brittle hair, brittle nails with white horizontal streaks, skin rash, and garlic breath	Wheat (germ, bran, and unprocessed flour), butter, organ meats, scallops, lobster, shrimp, crab	May help a variety of conditions including cancer prevention, RA, hypothyroidism, heavy metal accumulation in the body, and act as an immune stimulant.
Copper ESSADI 1.5-3.0 mg	A component of enzymes required for collagen cross linking, melanin, hemoglobin, phospholipids, and norepinephrine synthesis; has antioxidant activity; plays a role in mental and emotional processes	Anemia, osteoporosis, rheumatoid arthritis	Elevated cholesterol, triglyceride, and glucose levels; depigmentation of skin and hair; anemia and osteoporosis	Nausea, vomiting, muscle aches, diarrhea, GI pain; persons with liver and kidney disease should use with extreme caution; Wilson's disease is a genetic disorder which results in excessive copper accumulation	Oysters, soy lecithin, potatoes w/skin, beans, almonds, walnuts, sunflower seeds, brazil nuts, pecans, split peas	May help reduce symptoms of RA and certain types of anemia. Use in Wilson's disease is contraindicated.
Chromium ESSADI 50-200 mcg	Helps control blood glucose by activating insulin membrane receptors enabling insulin to promote glucose, amino acid, and triglyceride uptake by cells; influences the metabolism of carbohydrates and fats	Atherosclerosis, diabetes, glaucoma, hypothyroidism, PMS, weight loss	Glucose intolerance, hypoglycemia, craving for simple carbohydrates, fatigue, and irritability	Rare toxicity; disturbances in fat, sugar and protein metabolism; there have been a few reports where the picolinate form was taken in large amounts by people who developed renal failure, however, there was no proof chromium picolinate was the cause	Oysters, brewer's yeast, beef, whole wheat, chili, potatoes, wheat bran, wheat germ	May help improve glucose tolerance, reduce serum cholesterol and increase lean body masses during weight training.
Iodine RDA 150 mcg	Synthesis of thyroid hormones are involved in basal metabolic rate, heart rate, endocrine secretion, respiration, digestion, carbohydrate and fat metabolism	Fibrocystic breast disease, goiter prevention, hypothyroidism	Causes reduced levels of T_3 and T_4 which cause increases in thyroid stimulating hormone (TSH); this results in goiter, hypothyroidism, and myxedema	Metallic taste, paresthesias, arrhythmias, rashes, acne, hyperthyroidism, cretinism, nervousness and anxiety	Iodized salt, kelp, seafood, seaweed or sea plants, milk	Mainly used to prevent or reduce iodine deficiency and hypothyroid deficiency.
Manganese ESSADI 2-5 mg	Participates in formation connective tissue, fats, cholesterol, bones, blood clotting factors, proteins and glucose transport; functions as antioxidant cofactor for enzymes	Diabetes, epilepsy, osteoporosis	Poor growth of hair and nails, both demineralization which may lead to fracture and osteoporosis	Psychiatric and nerve disorders; persons with liver failure may accumulate high levels in the basal ganglia which leads to Parkinson-like symptoms	Whole grains, nuts, especially pecans, brazil, and almonds; fruits, barley, rye, buckwheat, wheat, and split peas	May help a variety of conditions including osteoarthritis, diabetes, and schizophrenia.

Vitamin	Major Functions	Reported Usage	Deficiency Signs and Symptoms	Toxicity Signs and Symptoms	Top Food Sources	Therapeutic Research
Boron No established value	Appears to influence intracellular and extracellular calcium transport; helps the kidney in the synthesis of the active form of vitamin D; helps regulatory effect on the production of estrogens and testosterone	Osteoarthritis, osteoporosis, rheumatoid arthritis	Increased urinary losses of calcium and magnesium, bone demineralization, osteoarthritis	Huge doses (100 mg plus) may cause nausea, diarrhea, abdominal pain, appetite and weight loss	Most fruits and vegetables	May help levels of estrogen and testosterone in the body and this has belief that boron can enhance lean muscle mass for bodybuilding purposes and can also be used to treat menopausal symptoms by raising estrogen levels.
Molybdenum RDA 75 mcg	Component of enzymes used to detoxify alcohol, sulfites, and uric acid	No reported use	Headache, tachycardia (caused by sulfate buildup)	Gout-like symptoms	Meats, lentils, peas, brown rice, whole grains	Too much molybdenum is not a good thing, and can cause painfully swollen joints and deplete the body of copper.

Source: *Natural Medicines Comprehensive Database, 4th Edition,* Therapeutic Research Faculty; *Vitamins Herb, Minerals & Supplments, The Complete Guide,* H.Winter Griffith, Da Capo Press; Doug Andersen, Andersen Chiropractic at www.andersenchiro.com

Condition	Supplements / Vitamins	Nutrition
Acne	1. Multivitamins and minerals daily. 2. Vitamin C, 500 to 1,000 mg tid is essential for healthy collagen. 3. Vitamin E, 200 to 400 IU daily enhances healing. 4. Chromium, 400 to 600 mcg daily aids in reducing infections of the skin. 5. Zinc, 45 to 60 mg daily is important for healthy skin. 6. Selenium, 100 to 200 mcg daily encourages tissue elasticity and is a powerful antioxidant. 7. Vitamin B6 is helpful for premenstrual acne. Take 50 mg B-Complex before and during premenstrual flare-ups. 8. Homeopathic silica reduces pus formation. 9. Vitex and saw palmetto alleviates hormone-related acne. 10. Kombucha tea, which has antibacterial and immune-boosting properties, has been found by many people to be beneficial for acne.	1. Make sure the diet contains an adequate amount of fruits, vegetables, whole grains, and dietary fiber. 2. Other foods: squash, cucumbers, watermelon, winter melon, celery, carrots, cabbage, beet tops, dandelions, aloe vera, mulberry leaves, carrot tops, lettuce, potatoes, cherries, papayas, pears, persimmons, raspberries, buckwheat, alfalfa sprouts, millet, brown rice, mung beans, and plenty of water. 3. Increase intake of raw foods especially foods that contain oxalic acid, including almonds, beets, cashews, and Swiss chard. 4. Avoid high fat foods, junk foods, fried foods, processed foods, saturated fats, refined carbohydrates, sugar, caffeine, chocolate, citrus fruits, oily foods, spicy foods, alcohol, smoking, ice cream, soft drinks, and emotional stress.
Allergy	1. Multivitamins and minerals daily. 2. Nutrients that give immune systems an extra boost include: Vitamin A, C, E, B-complex, zinc, quercetin, pycnogenol, EFAs and gamma linolenic acid. 3. Vitamin A, 10,000 IU daily is a great immune supporter. 4. Vitamin C, 1,000 mg tid detoxifies, strengthens the immune system, and reduces histamine levels in the blood. 5. Vitamin D, 600 IU daily. 6. Quercitin, 1,000 mg tid. 7. Take EFAs, which include 1 to 2 tablespoons of flaxseed oil or 3 grams of fish oil daily. 8. Coenzyme Q10, 100 mg daily improves cellular oxygenation. 9. L-Tyrosine, 500 mg daily has an important function in protein synthesis. 10. MSM, 1,000 mg tid improves allergies, asthma, headache and skin problems.	1. Make sure the diet contains an adequate amount of vitamin A and C. Vitamin A is essential for healthy mucus lining of the respiratory tract. Vitamin C is well recognized for its effect to prevent and treat infection. 2. Reduce or eliminate intake of dairy products, as they increase mucus production. 3. Drink plenty of distilled water throughout the day to help drainage.
Alopecia	1. Cysteine, 2,000 mg daily. 2. Vitamin B-complex, 150 mg daily with niacin, 50 mg daily. 3. Zinc, 75 mg daily prevents hair loss. 4. EFAs, in the form of flaxseed oil, fish oil, and evening primrose oil are rich in fatty acids and are essential for healthy hair. 5. Natural silica is the building block that boosts hair growth. 6. MSM, 700 mg daily is a vital substance to the life of hair and skin. 7. L-Cysteine and L-methionine improve quality, texture, and growth of hair. 8. Kelp 500 mg daily, supplies needed minerals for proper hair growth. 9. Consider Aangamik DMG from Food Science Labs or Ultra Hair Plus from Nature's Plus for good circulation to the scalp.	1. Biotin, found in green peas, oats, soybeans, sunflower seeds, and walnuts, is essential for healthy hair and skin. Kelp and seaweed are also excellent choices to include in the daily diet. 2. Protein is the essential make-up of hair. Therefore, the intake of food high in protein such as milk, fish, eggs, and beans is recommended. 3. Foods that are high in collagen will improve the elasticity and shine of hair, such as wild yams, taro, lotus root, and tendons. 4. Intake of vitamins A and B are also recommended, as they can improve circulation to the scalp and promote hair growth. 5. Increase intake of water, vegetables, fruits, seeds, and nuts for patients with dry skin.
Alzheimer's	1. Multivitamins and minerals daily. 2. Vitamin C, 500 to 1,000 mg tid. 3. Vitamin E, 400 to 800 IU daily is a beneficial antioxidant. 4. EFAs, Flaxseed oil, 1 tablespoon daily. 5. Thiamin, 3 to 8 grams daily. 6. Phosphatidylserine, 100 mg tid. 7. Methylcobalamin (active vitamin B12), 1,000 mcg bid. 8. Melatonin, one to three time-release tablets before sleep. 9. SAMe, 400 to 1,600 mg daily. 10. CoQ10, 50 mg daily augments the supply of oxygen to the brain. 11. DHEA supplementation during the later years can aid mental abilities and alleviate stress. 12. Huperzine A, 200 mcg bid, slows disease progression, improves memory, and inhibits destruction of acetylcholine.	1. Consume adequate amounts of vegetables for vitamins A, B1, B2, C, and E. 2. Encourage a diet with a diverse source of all nutrients, including raw fruits, vegetables, whole grains, nuts, and seeds. B vitamins are important to maintain nerve health. 3. Small frequent meals are recommended, instead of a few large meals. Weight loss is recommended if obese. 4. Avoid fried foods, smoked or barbecued foods, meat, alcohol, hot sauces, spicy foods, fatty foods, rich foods, salty foods, coffee, caffeine, sweet foods, and sugar. 5. Encourage more white meat and less red meat.
Amenorrhea		1. Adequate intake of calcium is important to prevent menstrual cramps. Calcium level in the body is decreased about 10 days before a period. 2. Increase the intake of vegetable oil and fish. They are rich resources of prostaglandin, which relieves cramping and pain associated with painful menstruation. 3. Soy products are also beneficial as they help to regulate hormone imbalance. 4. Increase the intake of foods that are warm in nature, such as onions, garlic, mutton, chili, or chives.
Angina	1. L-carnitine, 1,000 to 3,000 mg daily helps improve functioning of the heart. 2. Vitamin E, 200 to 800 IU daily is a powerful antioxidant and reduces clotting. 3. Selenium, 200 mcg daily keeps tissue elastic. 4. Multivitamins and minerals daily that include vitamins A, C, and E. 5. EFAs, in the form of fish oils help reduce chest pain. 6. Melatonin, 500 to 3,000 mcg prevents free-radical damage. 7. CoQ10, 90 to 180 mg daily prevents heart disease. 8. Magnesium, 500 to 1,000 mg daily helps reverse heart disease.	1. Increase the intake of fresh fruits and vegetables, including broccoli, Brussels sprouts, carrots, pumpkin, and cantaloupe. 2. Avoid MSG, meat, fat, aged foods, alcohol, diet soft drinks, preservatives, sugar substitutes, meat tenderizers, and soy sauce. 3. Garlic is effective to lower blood pressure, lower bad LDL, and increase good HDL.

Condition	Supplements / Vitamins	Nutrition
Ankle Pain		1. Glucosamine sulfate and chondroitin sulfate are well recognized for their nutritional support, as they are important for the formation of bones, tendons, ligaments, and cartilage. 2. Sulfur helps the absorption of calcium. Consume foods high in sulfur such as asparagus, eggs, fresh garlic, and onions. 3. Sea cucumber is very beneficial for synovial joints and joint fluids. 4. Fresh pineapples are recommended as they contain bromelain, an enzyme that is excellent in reducing inflammation. 5. Avoid spicy foods, caffeine, citrus fruits, sugar, milk, dairy products, and red meat.
Anxiety	1. EFAs, flaxseed oil, 1 tablespoon daily. 2. Calcium, 500 to 1,000 mg daily. 3. Magnesium, 250 to 500 mg daily. 4. Niacin, 250 to 500 mg daily. 5. Zinc, 15 mg bid. 6. Consider Liquid kyolic with B12 from Wakunaga. 7. Consider Floradix Iron. 8. 5-HTP, 50 to 100 mg tid, but do not take with any pharmaceutical antidepressant or anti-anxiety medication. 9. B-complex, 50 mg bid. 10. GABA, 500 mg tid between meals, has a calming effect.	1. A diet high in calcium, magnesium, phosphorus, potassium, and vitamins B and E is recommended. These nutrients are easily depleted by stress. 2. Encourage the consumption of fruits and vegetables such as apricots, wintermelon, asparagus, avocados, bananas and broccoli in addition to brown rice, dried fruit, figs, salmon, garlic, green leafy vegetables, soy products, and yogurt. 3. Avoid caffeine (coffee, tea, soda, chocolate), tobacco, alcohol, and sugar whenever possible.
Arthritis	1. Bioflavonoids, 500 mg daily. 2. Chondroitin sulfate, 1,000 to 2,000 mg daily, holds cartilage together, prevents damage, and stimulates repair. 3. Digestive enzymes. 4. Glucosamine sulfate, 700 to 1,000 mg daily repairs joint cartilage and tissue damage, reduces symptoms of osteoarthritis. 5. Omega-3 fatty acids (fish oil capsules), 50 mg tid. 6. MSM, 500 to 1,000 mg tid reduces inflammation. 7. Sea cucumber. 8. Silica. 9. Vitamin E, 400 to 800 IU daily reduces symptoms. 10. NSAIDs.	1. Consume more foods containing iron, such as broccoli, Brussels sprouts, cauliflower, fish, lima beans, and peas. 2. Eat more sulfur-containing foods, such as asparagus, eggs, garlic, and onions. 3. Eat fresh pineapple, which contains bromelain, an enzyme that reduces inflammation. 4. Avoid nightshade vegetables, greasy foods, and NSAIDs. 5. Avoid iron supplements because they are suspected of being involved in pain, swelling, and joint destruction. 6. Avoid all forms of hydrogenated oils, which include peanut butter, cooking oils, snack chips, margarine, and processed foods.
Asthma	1. Multivitamins and minerals daily. 2. Vitamin C, 10 to 30 mg for every two pounds of body weight, daily. 3. Vitamin E, 200 to 400 IU daily. 4. EFAs, Flaxseed oil, 1 tablespoon daily. 5. Magnesium, 200 to 400 mg tid prevents bronchial spasm attacks. 6. Adrenal cortex extract, 250 mg tid. 7. Asthma-X5, 500 to 1,000 mg tid, from Olympian Labs is an herbal combination for chronic sufferers of asthma. 8. B6, 50 to 200 mg daily decreases frequency of attacks. 9. Quercetin, 500 to 1,000 mg tid acts as an antihistamine.	
Back pain	1. Multivitamins and minerals daily. 2. Calcium, 1,500 to 2,000 mg daily. 3. DLPA (dl-phenylalanine), 375 mg capsule prn 4/24 for discomfort. 4. Glucosamine sulfate, 700 to 1,200 mg daily. 5. Chondroitin sulfate, 1,200 mg daily. 6. Magnesium, 700 to 1,000 mg daily. 7. Zinc, 50 mg daily. 8. Consider Arth-X from Trace Minerals Research containing herbs, sea minerals, calcium and other nutrients for bones and joints. 9. Consider horsetail, alfalfa, burdock, oat straw, slippery elm, white willow bark in capsules or extract, tea form to reduce inflammation. 10. MSM, 3,000 to 8,000 mg daily in divided dosages for inflammation. 11. Bromelain, 500 mg tid between meals. 12. Consider bovine cartilage and shark cartilage as added support for back pain.	1. Eat a diet with a wide variety of raw vegetables and fruits, and whole-grain cereals to ensure a complete supply of nutrients for the bones, nerves, and muscles. 2. Adequate intake of calcium is essential for the repair and rebuilding of bones, tendons, cartilage, and connective tissues. 3. Fresh pineapples are recommended for reducing inflammation. 4. To relieve cramps and spasms, eat plenty of fruits and vegetables, especially those high in potassium, such as bananas and oranges. 5. Avoid red meat and seafood as they contain high levels of uric acid, which strain the kidneys. 6. Avoid cold beverages, ice cream, caffeine, sugar, tomatoes, milk, and dairy products.
Bronchitis	1. Selenium, 200 mcg daily. 2. Vitamin C, 500 to 1,000 mg daily neutralizes free-radicals and aids mucus lining. 3. Goldenseal root extract and bromelain at a dosage of 400 mg of each, tid on an empty stomach decrease bronchial secretions. 4. Vitamin E, 400 to 800 IU daily protects lung tissue and increases oxygen supply. 5. Vitamin A, 25,000 IU daily protects lung tissue. 6. Carnitine, 2,000 mg bid eases breathing during exercises. 7. EFAs, in the form of flaxseed oil and fish oil daily are helpful anti-inflammatory. 8. Magnesium, 300 to 500 mg daily strengthens muscles and relaxes the bronchi. 9. Colloidal silver is a natural antibiotic that destroys bacteria, viruses, and fungi and promotes healing.	1. Always drink plenty of water, juice, soup, and tea as they can help flush out the body and prevent dehydration. 2. Vitamin C is well recognized for its effect to prevent and treat common colds and influenza. Foods high in vitamin C, such as oranges, are strongly recommended. 3. Vitamin A, a vital nutrient for the mucus membranes throughout the respiratory system, should also be consumed in adequate quantity. Foods rich in vitamin A include raw fruits and vegetables, such as carrots. 4. To avoid infection, a diet high in garlic and onions is recommended as these two foods contain a natural antibiotic effect.
Bursitis	1. Calcium, 400 mg tid, and magnesium 200 mg tid are essential to help relax muscles. 2. Manganese, first 2 weeks, 50 to 200 mg daily in divided dosages; thereafter, 15 to 30 mg daily. 3. Quercitin, 1,000 mcg tid with extra bromelain, 1,500 mg daily. 4. DLPA, mg as needed. 5. Probiotics can help improve digestive function and eliminate bacterial buildups. 6. Omega 3 flax oil, 1 teaspoon tid. 7. Chondroitin sulfate, 500 mg bid. 8. Inositol, 500 mg tid. 9. Proteolytic enzymes work to decrease inflammation and help relieve pain.	1. Eat organically grown foods with no chemical treatments or additives, including vegetarian and alkaline foods like celery, avocados, pineapple, potatoes, wheat germ sweet fruits, sprouts, leafy green vegetables, brewers yeast, oats and sea greens. 2. Eat foods high in magnesium like green and yellow vegetables, broccoli, and cauliflower. 3. Avoid acid-forming foods, such as caffeine, salts, refined foods, red meats and nightshade plants like tomatoes, potatoes and eggplant. 4. Consider carrot or beet juice twice a week to cleanse sediment residues.

Condition	Supplements / Vitamins	Nutrition
Cancer Pain	1. Multivitamins and minerals daily. 2. Vitamin C, 3,000 to 12,000 mg daily in divided dosages protects the immune system. 3. Vitamin E, 400 to 800 IU daily. 4. EFAs, Flaxseed oil, 1 to 2 tablespoons daily. 5. Carotene complex, 50,000 to 100,000 IU daily. 6. Thymus extract, 750 mg crude polypeptide fraction once or bid. 7. Coenzyme Q10, 150 to 300 mg daily during chemotherapy and for 6 months after the last chemotherapy treatment.	1. Consider a raw diet, or whenever possible, eat organically grown food. 2. Foods that are helpful to strengthen the body and fight infection include garlic, citrus fruits, and green vegetables. 3. Limit the intake of sweet foods and refined white sugar because they impair the body's ability to kill bacteria. 4. Eat more fiber, including whole grain, oats and brown rice. 5. Eat lean protein from beans, eggs, tofu, poultry or fish to help keep up your strength and energy. 6. Fermented soy products such as tofu, tempeh, and miso appear to have anticancer properties.
Carpal Tunnel	1. Multivitamins and minerals daily. 2. Vitamin C, 500 to 1,000 mg tid. 3. Vitamin E, 200 to 400 IU daily. 4. EFAs, flaxseed oil, 1 to 2 tablespoons daily. 5. Vitamin B6, 50 to 100 mg daily relieves symptoms, followed by Vitamin B complex to enhance effectiveness of B6. 6. St. John's Wort and Skullcap relieve muscle spasms and pain. 7. Bromelain, take 500 mg tid between meals, has natural anti-inflammatory effect. 8. Calcium and magnesium help reduce muscle tightness and nerve irritation.	1. Deficiency of B6 may be the cause of CTS, so consume plenty of beans, brewer's yeast, and wheat germ. Green leafy vegetables are good sources. 2. Food for SJ and PC related channel problems include: Olives, rye, lima beans, rice bran, bananas, sprouts, watercress, and apples. 3. Drink plenty of water. 4. Reduce intake of salty foods, oranges, tomatoes and wheat which have been shown to exacerbate problems.
Chronic Fatigue	1. Multivitamins and minerals daily. 2. Vitamin C with bioflavonoids, 500 to 1,000 mg tid, plus an additional 3,000 to 8,000 mg has a powerful antiviral effect and increases the energy level. 3. Vitamin E, 200 to 400 IU daily is a powerful free-radical scavenger that protects cells and enhances immune function to fight viruses. 4. EFAs, Flaxseed oil, 1 tablespoon daily. 5. Thymus extract, 750 mg once or bid. 6. Magnesium, 250 mg tid, which is critical for energy production. 7. Vitamin B-complex, 50 mg bid increases energy. 8. CoQ10, 100 mg tid enhances the effectiveness of the immune system. 9. Probiotics can help improve digestive function and eliminate bacterial buildup. 10. Consider proteolytic enzymes or Infla-Zyme Forte from American Biologics or Wobenzyme N from Marlyn Nutraceuticals to reduce inflammation and improve absorption.	1. Increase the consumption of foods rich in Zinc, Vitamins C, and B-complex including: Fresh fruits, vegetables, grains, seeds, and nuts. 2. Eat more fish, fish oils, onions, garlic, olives, olive oil, herbs, beans, spices, soy products, tofu, yogurt, and fiber. 3. Foods with antioxidant effects such as vitamin A, C, and E are beneficial as they neutralize the free-radicals and minimize damage to cells. 4. Sea vegetables, such as kelp and seaweeds, replenish the body with minerals like magnesium, potassium, calcium, iodine, and iron. 5. Ensure adequate intake of vitamin B complex to process and utilize energy. 6. Eat frequent, small meals and drink more liquids. 7. Avoid the use of stimulants, such as coffee, caffeine, and high-sugar products. 8. Avoid meat, processed foods, junk food, alcohol, greasy food, and dairy products.
Common Cold	1. Selenium, 100 to 200 mcg daily. 2. Vitamin C, 500 to 1,000 mg every hour with a glass of water boosts the immune system function. 3. Thymus extract, 750 mg once or bid. 4. Vitamin A, 5,000 to 10,000 IU daily, helps heal the inflamed mucus membranes and strengthens the immune system. 5. Vitamin E, 400 to 500 IU daily. 6. Zinc lozenges, 15 to 25 mg every 2 hours for 4 days. 7. Consider echinacea and goldenseal as they build immune system and fights microbes. 8. Zinc lozenges enhance and stimulate immune function to fight the virus.	1. For treatment of the common cold or influenza, always drink plenty of water, juice, soup, and tea as they can help flush out the body and prevent dehydration. 2. Vitamin C is well recognized for its effect to prevent and treat common colds and influenza. Foods high in vitamin C, such as oranges, are strongly recommended. 3. Vitamin A foods, a vital nutrient for the mucus membranes throughout the respiratory system, should also be consumed in adequate quantity. 4. To avoid infection, a diet high in garlic and onions is recommended as these two foods contain a natural antibiotic effect. 5. Phlegm-producing foods such as sweets, dairy products, and heavy or greasy foods are not recommended.
Constipation	1. Magnesium, 250 to 500 mg daily helps muscle contraction. 2. Probiotics can help improve digestive function and eliminate bacterial buildup. 3. Vitamin C, 500 to 1,000 mg daily encourages regular bowel movements. 4. Dietary fiber, 1 to 3 grams bid. 5. EFAs, flaxseed oil, 1 to 2 tablespoons daily are needed for proper digestion and stool formation. 6. Pysillium, 1 teaspoon or 5 grams of psyillium husks bid. 7. Consider Triphala from Planetary Formulas aids in the formation of odor-free, firm, and healthy stools. 8. Kombucha tea which has detoxifying and immune-boosting properties may be beneficial for relieving constipation and other digestive disorders. 9. Garlic destroys harmful bacteria in the colon.	1. Eat plenty of foods with high-fiber, such as fresh fruits, green leafy vegetables, cabbage, peas, sweet potatoes, and whole grains. Follow a low-fat diet. 2. Drink plenty of water, at least 8 glasses daily. 3. Avoid fried foods, fatty foods, and spicy foods that may irritate the mucus membranes of the intestines. 4. Prunes or prune juice are very effective to regulate bowels and relieve dry stool or constipation. 5. A combination of wild honey with fresh grapefruit will also relieve dry stool or constipation. 6. Black sesame with wild honey or flaxseed oil is a helpful combination to soften stool and facilitate bowel movements.
Depression	1. Multivitamins and minerals daily. 2. Vitamin C, 500 to 1,000 mg tid. 3. Vitamin E, 200 to 400 IU daily. 4. EFAs, flaxseed oil, 1 tablespoon daily. 5. SAMe, 200 mg bid for the first two days, 400 mg bid for three to nine days, 400 mg tid on days ten through twenty, full dosage of 400 mg qid after twenty days if needed. SAMe raises dopamine and serotonin levels and improves binding of neurotransmitters to reception sites. 6. Folic acid and vitamin B12, 1,000 mcg of each daily. 7. 5-HTP, 100 to 200 mg daily at bedtime acts as a mild anti-depressant.	1. Eat plenty of fresh fruits, leafy green vegetables, and whole grains. 2. Avoid greasy and fried foods. A diet high in saturated fat may cause sluggishness, fatigue and slow thinking. 3. Depression may be due in part to nutritional deficiency. Foods such as white bread, flour, saturated animal fats, hydrogenated vegetable oils, sweets, soft drinks, and canned goods deprive the body of vitamin B and increase the probability of depression. 4. Avoid a diet too low in complex carbohydrates as it may cause serotonin depletion and depression. 5. Stay away from wheat products, sugar, alcohol, caffeine, dairy products, and processed foods.

Condition	Supplements / Vitamins	Nutrition
Diabetes	1. Multivitamins and minerals daily. 2. Vitamin C, 500 to 1,000 mg tid improves glucose tolerance reducing insulin needs, fights infections, and strengthens blood vessels. 3. Vitamin E, 400 to 800 IU daily improves glucose tolerance. 4. EFAs, Flaxseed oil, 1 tablespoon daily. Do not take excessive EFAs, fish oil capsules or supplements that contain large amounts of PABA. 5. Chromium picolinate, 400 to 600 mcg daily, improves insulin's efficiency, which lowers blood-sugar levels. 6. Magnesium, 250 mg bid to tid may improve insulin production. 7. Methylcobalamin (active vitamin B12), 1,000 mcg daily. 8. Alpha-lipoic acid, 150 mg daily improves diabetic neuropathy and reduces pain.	1. Eat a high-complex-carbohydrate, low-fat, high-fiber diet focused on whole, unprocessed foods, whole grains, legumes, vegetables, fruits, nuts, and seeds. 2. Get protein from vegetable sources, such as grains and legumes, fish and low-fat dairy products. 3. Eliminate alcohol, caffeine, and sugar. Avoid the consumption of simple sugars, which have an adverse effect on glucose tolerance. 4. Supplement your diet with spirulina which helps stabilize blood-sugar levels. 5. Other foods that help normalize blood-sugar include berries, brewer's yeast, dairy products (especially cheese), egg yolks, fish, garlic, kelp, sauerkraut, soybeans, and vegetables.
Diarrhea	1. Probiotics can help improve digestive function and eliminate bacterial buildup. 2. Calcium, 500 to 1,000 mg daily. 3. Digestive enzyme, 1 to 3 capsules with each meal. 4. Kelp, 150 mcg daily replaces minerals lost through diarrhea. 5. Potassium, 100 mg tid. 6. Colostrum has been shown to reduce acute and chronic diarrhea. 7. Activated charcoal, four to six 250 mg capsules every 2 hours until symptom relief helps remove toxins from the body. 8. Kombucha tea, which has detoxifying and immune-boosting properties, may be beneficial for diarrhea and other digestive disorders.	1. Patients with diarrhea should keep taking in plenty of pure water and appropriate foods to prevent dehydration and malnutrition. Eat oat bran, rice bran, raw foods, yogurt, and soured products daily. A high-fiber diet is important. 2. During the recovery phase of diarrhea, eat foods that are easy to digest early in the meal, such as soup, yogurt, toast, and porridge, and cooked fruits and vegetables. 3. Avoid foods that may trigger diarrhea or are hard to digest, such as sorbitol, dairy products, spicy food, alcohol, and caffeine. 4. Avoid eating raw, cold or unsanitary food and beverages.
Dysmenorrhea		1. Foods and fruits that are cold or sour in nature should be avoided one week prior to or during menstruation. Cold and sour foods create more stagnation, and may worsen the pain. 2. Decrease the consumption of salt, red meats, processed foods, junk foods, and foods with high sodium content. Caffeine should be avoided as it acts as a stimulant to excite the central nervous system and as a diuretic. 3. Increase the consumption of whole-grain foods, and broiled chicken, turkey, and fish. 4. Menstrual cramps due to calcium deficiency should be treated calcium-rich foods, such as green vegetables, legumes, and seaweeds.
Edema	1. Free-form amino acid complex daily. 2. Calcium, 1,500 mg daily and magnesium, 1,000 mg daily to replace minerals lost with correction of edema. 3. Consider SP-6 Cornsilk Blend from Solaray that aids the body in expelling excess fluids. 4. Kelp 1,000 to 1,500 mg daily supplies needed minerals and improves thyroid function. 5. Bromelain aids digestion and metabolism. 6. Vitamin E, 400 IU daily aids circulation.	1. A high-fiber diet is important, eat plenty of apples, beets, garlic, grapes, and onions. 2. Avoid drinking ice-cold beverages, or eating cold or raw foods that are cold in nature such as watermelon, salads, tomatoes and cucumbers. 3. Avoid eating fried, greasy or food high in fat content. 4. Reduce the intake of dairy and sugar. 5. A low-sodium diet is recommended, as sodium may cause fluid retention. 6. Consume an adequate amount of vitamin B complex, which helps to reduce water retention.
Elbow Pain		1. Eat plenty of whole grains, seafood, dark-green vegetables, and nuts. These foods are rich in Vitamin B complex and magnesium, which are essential for nerve health and relaxation of tense muscles, respectively. 2. Adequate intake of minerals, such as calcium and potassium, are essential for pain management. A deficiency of these minerals will lead to spasms, cramps, and tense muscles.
Endo-metriosis	1. Multivitamins and minerals daily. 2. B-complex vitamins, 50 mg bid, are involved in estrogen metabolism. 3. Vitamin E, 400 IU bid. 4. EFAs, flaxseed oil, 1 to 2 tablespoons or fish oil, 3,000 to 5,000 daily. 5. Vitex, 160 to 250 mg daily, balances estrogen and progesterone ratio. 6. Natural progesterone, apply 20 mg to your skin bid from days 6 to 26 of your cycle, and stopping during the week of your menstrual flow. Use under the care of your health care professional. 7. Beta-carotene, 150,000 to 200,000 IU decreases related cramping, fluid retention and fatigue. 8. Calcium, 1,000 to 1,500 mg daily helps to maintain muscle tone and lower chance of cramping.	1. Foods and fruits that are cold or sour in nature should be avoided, especially one week prior to or during menstruation. Cold and sour foods create more stagnation, and may worsen the pain. 2. Decrease the consumption of salt, red meats, processed foods, junk foods, and foods with high sodium content. Caffeine should be avoided as it acts as a stimulant to excite the central nervous system and as a diuretic to deplete many important nutrients. 3. Increase the consumption of whole-grain foods, and broiled chicken, turkey, and fish.
Energy / Fatigue	1. Multivitamins and minerals daily. 2. Vitamin C, 500 to 1,000 mg tid, plus an additional 3,000 to 8,000 mg. 3. Vitamin E, 200 to 400 IU daily. 4. EFAs, Flaxseed oil, 1 tablespoon daily. 5. Thymus extract, 750 mg once or bid. 5. Magnesium, 250 mg tid, which is critical for energy production. 6. Vitamin B-complex, 50 mg bid. Brewer's yeast is a good source of B vitamins. 7. CoQ10, 100 mg tid. 8. DHEA, 25 to 50 mg daily. 9. Pregnenolone, 10 mg daily. 10. Selenium, 100 to 200 mcg daily. 11. Glutamate, 400 mg with each meal helps stabilize blood-sugar levels. 12. Royal jelly increases energy levels. 13. Shiitake or reishi mushrooms help build immunity and boost energy levels.	1. Increase the consumption of fresh fruits, vegetables, grains, seeds, and nuts. 2. Eat more fish and fish oils, onions, garlic, olives, olive oil, herbs, spices, soy products, tofu, yogurt, and fiber. 3. Foods with antioxidant effects such as vitamin A, C, and E are beneficial as they neutralize the free-radicals and minimize damage to cells. 4. Sea vegetables, such as kelp and seaweeds, replenish the body with minerals like magnesium, potassium, calcium, iodine, and iron. 5. Ensure adequate intake of vitamin B complex to process and utilize energy. 6. Eat frequent, small meals and drink more liquids. 7. Avoid the use of stimulants, such as coffee, caffeine, and high-sugar products.

Condition	Supplements / Vitamins	Nutrition
Fever	1. Vitamin C, 500 to 1,000 mg qid, supports immune system. Reduce the dosage if diarrhea occurs. 2. Echinacea, 500 mg qid. 3. Yarrow, 300 mg capsule form or 2 ml tincture qid or until fever breaks.	1. Eat lightly, steamed vegetables, soups, broths, and herbal tea which will let your body focus on healing. 2. Stay hydrated and drink plenty of clean water. 3. Increase consumption of ginger, onions, and garlic. 4. Avoid sugar and be cautious about fruit juices, especially orange juices that contain more sugar than vitamin C. 5. Avoid milk and dairy products while you're sick as they tend to suppress immunity.
Fibromyalgia	1. Coenzyme Q10, 60 mg tid, improves oxygenation of tissues. 2. Arginine, 1,500 mg bid. 3. EFAs, evening primrose oil capsules, 500 to 1,000 mg daily helps to reduce pain and fatigue. 4. Vitamin E, 400 to 500 IU daily protect the body's cells and enhance immune function. 5. Consider chlorophyll tablets form or in "green drinks" such as Kyo-Green from Wakunaga of America to cleanse the bloodstream. 6. Consider Spiratein from Nature's Plus which is a good protein drink. 7. Magnesium, 250 mg tid relaxes muscles. 8. 5-HTP, 50 to 100 mg tid, which reduces pain, improves sleep and mood. 9. SAMe, 400 mg bid, improves detoxification and helps with cartilage formation. 10. Multivitamins and minerals daily. 11. Vanadyl sulfate protects the muscles and reduces overall body fatigue.	1. Eat a well balanced diet of 50 percent raw foods and fresh live juices. 2. Increase the consumption of fresh fruits, vegetables, grains, seeds, soy products, skinless turkey or chicken, deep-water fish, and nuts. 3. Eat more fish and fish oils, onions, garlic, olives, olive oil, herbs, spices, soy products, tofu, yogurt, and fiber. 4. Sea vegetables, such as kelp and seaweeds, replenish the body with minerals like magnesium, potassium, calcium, iodine, and iron. 5. Eat four to five small meals daily and drink plenty of liquids to help flush out toxins. 6. Limit the consumption of green peppers, eggplant, tomatoes and white potatoes, as these foods contain solanin, which interfere with enzymes in the muscle and may cause pain and discomfort.
Flu	1. Selenium, 100 to 200 mcg daily. 2. Vitamin C, 500 to 1,000 mg every hour with a glass of water boosts the immune system function. 3. Thymus extract, 750 mg once or bid. 4. Vitamin A, 5,000 to 10,000 IU daily, helps heal the inflamed mucus membranes and strengthens the immune system. 5. Vitamin E, 400 to 500 IU daily. 6. Zinc lozenges, 15 to 25 mg every 2 hours for 4 days. 7. Consider echinacea and goldenseal as they build immune system and fights microbes. 8. Zinc lozenges enhance and stimulate immune function to fight the virus.	1. For treatment of the common cold or influenza, always drink plenty of water, juice, soup, and tea as they can help flush out the body and prevent dehydration. 2. Vitamin C is well recognized for its effect to prevent and treat common colds and influenza. Foods high in vitamin C, such as oranges, are strongly recommended. 3. Vitamin A, a vital nutrient for the mucus membranes throughout the respiratory system, should also be consumed in adequate quantity. Foods rich in vitamin A include raw fruits and vegetables, such as carrots.
Focus	1. Choline, 500 to 100 mg daily. 2. DMAE, 75 mg bid boosts neurotransmitters, elevates mood, and increases energy. 3. Folic acid, 400 to 800 mg daily. 4. L-Carnitine. 50 to 500 mg daily. 5. Pantothenic acid, 30 to 100 mg daily. 6. High potency multivitamins and minerals that include: Vitamin B, B12, and Zinc for daily nutrients and enhanced memory function.	1. Make sure the diet contains an adequate amount of lecithin, which is essential for transmission of nerve impulses that control memory. Good sources of lecithin include flax seed oil, walnut oil, sesame oil, egg yolk, soybean, and raw wheat germ. 2. The B vitamins are also important for energy and proper brain function. 3. Avoid smoking and drinking alcohol.
Fungal Infection	1. Berberine, has an anti-fungal function. Goldenseal, a berberine-containing herb, works against fungi, including candida. 2. Korlorex from Nature's Sources is an herbal product that has been shown to be effective in treating ringworm and tinea fungi infections. 3. Pau d' arco, 3 cups daily has strong anti-fungal properties. 4. Tea tree oil is a natural anti-fungal treatment for external use.	1. Eat a raw diet. Eat plenty of fresh vegetables and moderate amounts of broiled fish and skinless chicken. 2. Do not eat foods containing sugar or refined carbohydrates, soda drinks, grains, processed foods, greasy and fried foods. 3. Probiotics can help improve digestive function and eliminate bacterial buildup.
Goiter		1. Recommended foods high in iodine, silicon, and phosphorus: Kelp, dulse, swiss chard, turnip greens, egg yolks, wheat germ, cod roe, lecithin, sesame seed butter, seed, nuts, and raw goat milk.
Gout	1. Vitamin C, 500 to 1,000 mg tid increases excretion of uric acid and reduces the levels in the blood. 2. Vitamin E, 200 to 400 IU daily. 3. Flaxseed oil, 1 tablespoon daily. 4. EFAs are beneficial for gout, as they are needed to repair tissues and healing of joint disorders. 5. Vitamin B6, 50 mg daily helps distribute water in the body to keep tissues hydrated. 6. Magnesium, 400 mg daily. 7. AE Mulsion Forte from Biotics SE aids in reducing uric acid in the blood and is a potent antioxidant. 8. Kelp, 1,000 to 1,500 mg daily contains complete protein and vital minerals to reduce serum uric acid.	1. Low purine diet is highly recommended. 2. Since gout attack is caused by excessive deposit of uric acid in the joints, increased intake of food rich in uric acid will increase the risk of gout attacks. Purine-rich food should be avoided, including meat, soup (bone broth), gravies, meat extracts, seafood, anchovies, fish, herring sardine, mussels, shellfish, internal organ meats (liver and kidneys), alcoholic beverages, spinach, asparagus, mushrooms, and cauliflower. 3. Increase intake of cherries, blueberries and strawberries, all of which are excellent in neutralizing uric acid.
Hair Loss	1. Cysteine, 2,000 mg daily. 2. Vitamin B-complex, 150 mg daily with niacin, 50 mg daily. 3. Zinc, 75 mg daily prevents hair loss. 4. EFAs, in the form of flaxseed oil, fish oil, and evening primrose oil which are rich in fatty acids are essential for healthy hair. 5. Natural silica is the building block that boosts hair growth.	1. Biotin, found in green peas, oats, soybeans, sunflower seeds, and walnuts, is essential for healthy hair and skin. Kelp and seaweed are also excellent choices to include in the daily diet. 2. Protein is the essential make-up of hair. Therefore, the intake of food high in protein such as milk, fish, eggs, and beans are recommended. 3. Foods that are high in collagen will improve the elasticity and shine of hair, such as wild yams, taro, lotus root, and tendons.

Condition	Supplements / Vitamins	Nutrition
Headache	1. Calcium, 500 to 1,000 mg daily. 2. Magnesium, 250 to 500 mg daily may relieve and reduce migraines in young women and individuals with low tissue or low magnesium levels. 3. Pantothenic acid, 30 to 100 mg daily. 4. Vitamin C, 500 to 1,000 mg daily. 5. Vitamin E, 500 IU daily can help stabilize estrogen levels and prevent migraines. 6. Vitamin D, 400 IU daily. 7. SAMe may relieve symptoms. 8. Vitamin B6, 50 mg daily helps stabilize the brain's serotonin levels. 9. Riboflavin, 400 mg daily can reduce menstrual related migraines.	1. Encourage the patient to consume an adequate amount of fruits, vegetables, grains, raw nuts, and seeds. 2. Drink plenty of water throughout the day to avoid dehydration. 3. Caffeine withdrawal is one of the most common causes of headache. 4. Avoid intake of ice drinks or cold food, as they constrict vessels, channels and collaterals. 5. Avoid foods containing tyramine and MSG, which can trigger headaches, such as alcohol, chocolate, bananas, citrus fruits, avocados, smoked fish, aged cheese, figs, fermented foods, sour cream, lima beans, yeast, red wine, and potatoes.
Hemorrhoids	1. Vitamin E oil or cream to apply to hemorrhoids. 2. Rutin, 50 mg tid reduces swelling, bleeding, and itching. 3. Probiotics can help improve digestive function and eliminate bacterial buildup. 4. Water-soluble fiber, 1 to 2 grams tid. 5. Bromelain, 1,500 mg daily is an effective anti-inflammatory. 6 Vitamin K, 100 mcg bid helps rebuild the colon and rectum. 7. Consider Aerobic Bulk Cleanse (ABC) from Aerobic Life keeps the colon clean, relieving pressure on the rectum. 8. Consider Key-E Suppositories from Carlson Labs which are good for relief of itching and pain.	1. Increase fluids and high-fiber to protect against hemorrhoids, increase cellulose and hemi-cellulose foods in diet. 2. Recommend cooling foods, lubricating foods, and Qi-tonifying foods: Cranberries, black fungus, water chestnut, buckwheat, tangerines, figs, plums, fish, prunes, guavas, bamboo shoots, mung beans, winter melon, black sesame seeds, persimmons, bananas, squash, cucumbers, and tofu.
Herpes (Genital)	1. Vitamin E, 200 to 400 IU daily. 2. EFAs, Flaxseed oil, 1 tablespoon daily. 3. Thymus extract, 750 mg once or bid. 5. Lysine, 500 mg qid or before eating reduces symptoms and recurrence, especially during first 72 hours of the outbreak. 6. Zinc, 15 mg bid internally or zinc sulfate applied topically prevents viral replication. 7. Vitamin C and bioflavonoids, 600 mg tid at first sign of appearance, reduces blister formation and symptoms. 8. Vitamin A, 25,000 IU tid. 9. B-complex, 50 mg bid. 11. Selenium, 200 mcg daily. 12. MSM, 500 mg tid proven relief from herpes outbreak.	1. Consume a diet that focuses on whole, unprocessed foods, whole grains, legumes, vegetables, and fruits. 2. Consume foods that naturally contain lysine including yogurt, cheese, fish, potatoes, eggs, and brewer's yeast since it has been shown to reduce outbreak. 3. Avoid high arginine-containing foods, chocolate, peanuts, almonds, other nuts, and seeds. 4. Eliminate alcohol, caffeine, and sugar.
Herpes (Oral)	1. Lysine, 500 to 1,000 mg daily inhibits herpes virus growth. 2. Consider Oxy C-2 Gel from American Biologics applied topically which is a useful antiviral, antifungal, and bactericide. 3. Vitamin A, 50,000 IU daily prevents spreading of infection. 4. Vitamin B complex, 50 mg tid combats the virus and helps to keep it from spreading. 5. Vitamin C, 5,000 to 10,000 mg daily prevents sores and inhibits the growth of the virus. 6. Vitamin E, 600 IU daily assists in healing sores. 7. Maitake, shiitake, and reishi mushrooms that have immune-boosting and antiviral properties.	1. Patients with oral herpes should avoid heat, UV rays, over-exertion, stress, spicy or greasy foods, seafood, or anything that may trigger an attack. 2. Conversely, they are advised to eat plenty of vegetables or fruits that are cold in nature (cucumbers, pears, watermelon, tomatoes and yogurt). 3. Replacement of their toothbrush is also recommended as some herpes virus may linger on the bristles.
Herpes Zoster	1. Try using essential oils that include bergamot, calophyllum, eucalyptus, geranium, goldenseal, and lemon oil. 2. DMSO has been used with success to relieve the pain of shingles and promote healing of lesions. 3. French Green Clay and tea tree oil can be used topically to dry blisters. 4. Activated charcoal made into a paste with cornstarch or grounded flaxseed can dry healing blisters. 5. Hydrogen peroxide applied topically can speed up shingle healing. 6. Multivitamins and minerals daily. 7. Vitamin C, 1,000 mg tid supports the immune system. 8. Lysine, 1,000 mg daily can help decrease the recurrence of outbreaks.	1. There are many nutrients that are essential for preventing, fighting, and healing of shingles. Some examples include garlic, L-lysine, calcium, magnesium, and vitamins A, B, C, and E. 2. The following foods are also beneficial: Brewer's yeast, brown rice, garlic, raw fruits and vegetables, whole grains, and foods rich in vitamins. 3. Avoid foods that are spicy, fried or greasy. Refrain from foods that are high in L-carnitine, such as peanuts, chocolate, and corn. Shellfish and seafood are also contraindicated. 4. Avoid alcohol and tobacco products.
Hyper-tension	1. Vitamin E, 400 to 800 IU daily. 2. EFAs, Flaxseed oil, 1 tablespoon daily. 3. Magnesium, 800 to 1,200 mg daily. 4. Coenzyme Q10, 150 to 300 mg daily.	1. Eliminate salt from the diet in cases of hypertension. Avoid MSG, baking soda, meat, fat, aged foods, alcohol, diet soft drinks, preservatives, sugar substitutes, meat tenderizers, and soy sauce. Increase the intake of fresh fruits and vegetables. 2. Aspartame should also be avoided, since a high level may increase blood pressure. 3. Increase the intake of fresh, raw vegetables and fruits to control blood pressure. Nuts and seeds should be consumed daily for a source of protein. 4. Garlic is effective to lower blood pressure and thin the blood.
Hyper-thyroidism	1. EFAs help your immune system function properly and provide effective anti-inflammatory. 2. Bromelain, 250 to 500 mg tid reduces swelling. 3. Vitamin C, 250 to 500 mg bid supports immune function and decreases inflammation. 4. Calcium, 1,000 mg daily and magnesium, 200 to 600 daily are cofactors for many metabolic processes. 5. Vitamin E, 400 IU bid can help protect the heart. 6. CoQ10, 50 mg bid can help protect the heart.	1. Consume plenty of the following foods: Broccoli, Brussels sprouts, cabbage, cauliflower, kale, mustard greens, peaches, pears, soybeans, spinach, and turnips. These foods may help to suppress thyroid hormone production. 2. Short-term consumption of foods rich in iodine will provide temporary relief of hyperthyroidism due to a negative feedback mechanism. Foods rich in iodine include sea salt, iodized salt, kelp, and sargassum.

Condition	Supplements / Vitamins	Nutrition
Hypo-thyroidism	1. Iodine, 150 mcg daily. 2. Tyrosine, 500 mg daily is an important amino acid that helps stimulate thyroid function. 3. Vitamin B complex, 25 to 50 mg daily is necessary for regulation of the endocrine system. 4. Thyroid glandular extract, 60 mg daily. 5. Consider ginseng to reduce fatigue and restore energy. 6. Consider natural progesterone. 7. Selenium, 200 to 600 mcg daily assists in the removal of toxins from the body. 8. CoQ10, 100 mg daily is an effective antioxidant and prevents thyroid destruction.	1. Add to your diet rich sources of natural iodine, including seafood, sea vegetables, kelp, dulse, hijiki, and kombu. 2. Avoid eating raw foods, and foods that contribute to sluggish thyroid action, among them cabbage, Brussels sprouts, and broccoli. 3. Avoid tap water because it contains fluorine and chlorine, two chemicals that inhibit the ability to absorb iodine.
Impotence	1. Vitamin C, 500 to 1,000 mg tid. 2. Vitamin E, 400 to 800 IU daily. 3. EFAs, Flaxseed oil, 1 tablespoon daily. 4. Zinc, 30 to 45 mg daily. 5. Arginine, 1,500 mg, bid and 3,000 mg about an hour prior to having sex. 6. DHEA, 50 mg daily for men 40+. 7. Selenium, 100 to 200 mcg daily.	1. Eliminate alcohol from the diet as it decreases the body's ability to produce testosterone. 2. Intake of vitamin E should be increased. Foods high in vitamin E include wheat germ oil, almonds, sunflower seeds or oil, peanuts, soybeans, whole wheat products and asparagus. Kiwi and fresh oysters can also be taken together as an aphrodisiac. 3. Shellfish, oysters, shrimp, cashews, beef and mushrooms are all foods that either contain high protein or zinc that may increase libido. 4. Increase the consumption of niacin foods (eggs, peanut butter, avocado, and fish) and vitamin E (raw wheat germ and vegetable oil) for circulatory problems.
Incontinence	1. Kidney Bladder Formula from Nature's Way and SP-6 Cornsilk Blend from Soloray are herbal formulas that have a diuretic effect and reduce spasms. Take 2 capsules twice daily.	1. Avoid caffeine, alcohol, carbonated beverages, coffee, chocolate, refined and processed foods, and simple sugars. Caffeine acts as an irritant to the bladder and as a diuretic.
Indigestion	1. Probiotics can help improve digestive function and eliminate bacterial buildup.	
Infertility	1. High potency multivitamin and mineral supplement. 2. Vitamin C, 500 to 1,000 mg tid. 3. Vitamin E, 400 to 800 IU daily may improve sperm's impregnating ability. 4. EFAs, Flaxseed oil, 1 tablespoon daily. 5. Beta-carotene, 100,000 to 200,000 IU daily. 6. Folic acid, 400 mcg daily helps normalize blood chemistry. 7. Zinc, 30 to 60 mg daily helps with impotence in men. 8. Panax-ginseng tid. 9. Ginseng-root, 1,500 to 2,000 mg tid. 10. Iron, 35 mg daily helps normalize blood chemistry.	1. Foods that are cold (sushi, uncooked vegetables, salad, tomatoes, watermelon, cucumbers, winter melon, strawberries, tofu, crabs, bananas, pear, soy milk, kiwi, ice cream, cold beverages) or sour (all citrus) in nature should be avoided one week before and during menstruation. Cold and sour foods create stagnation and cause pain. 2. Eat more nuts and seeds in their diet. 3. Avoid overly spicy and pungent food as they may cause excessive bleeding. 4. Decrease processed food and increase organic food. 5. Avoid alcohol, coffee, and cigarette smoking.
Insomnia	1. Melatonin, 0.1 to 3 mg, 30 to 45 minutes before retiring, particularly for the elderly. 2. Magnesium, 500 mg, 30 to 45 minutes before retiring. 3. Valerian root extract, 300 mg, 30 to 45 minutes before retiring. 4. Niacin, 100 mcg, 30 to 45 minutes before retiring. 5. Vitamin B6, 50 mg daily. 6. 5-HTP, 50 to 200 mg before bed to rebalance serotonin. 7. Calcium, 1,500 to 2,000 mg daily has a calming effect.	1. Increase consumption of foods that contain high levels of trytophan such as turkey, bananas, figs, dates, yogurt, milk, tuna, and whole grain crackers as they help promote sleep. 2. A diet high in calcium, magnesium, phosphorus, potassium, and vitamins B and E is recommended. These vitamins and minerals are easily depleted by stress. 3. Encourage the consumption of fruits and vegetables such as apricots, wintermelon, asparagus, avocados, bananas and broccoli in addition to brown rice, dried fruit, figs, salmon, garlic, green leafy vegetables, soy products, and yogurt. 4. Avoid caffeine (coffee, tea, cola, chocolate), tobacco, alcohol, and sugar whenever possible.
IBS	1. Multivitamins and minerals daily. 2. Consider Probiotics can help improve digestive function and eliminate bacterial buildups. 3. Consider digestive enzymes, gentian root, skullcap, or ginger root with each meal to help with food digestion. 4. Aloe vera juice, ¼ cup bid is soothing and healing to the digestive tract and helps fight intestinal infection. 5. Garlic aids in digestion and destruction of toxins in the colon. 6. EFAs, in primrose oil or flaxseed oil are needed to protect the intestinal lining. 7. Vitamin B12, 200 mcg bid for proper absorption of foods. 8. Vitamin B complex, 50 to 100 mg tid, is needed for proper muscle tone in the gastrointestinal tract.	1. Correct nutrient deficiencies with adequate calories. Consider probiotics or acidophilus before meals to help assimilate nutrients. A high-fiber diet based on vegetables and whole grains is essential. Consider eating raw vegetables and fruits. 2. Be careful with food combinations: Especially avoiding starch, sugar, and protein combinations (for example, cheesecake). 3. Avoid, dairy products, caffeine, saturated fats, fried foods, red meat, alcohol, wheat and eating too many types of foods at one time. Minimize intake of gas producing foods such as beans, legumes, cabbage, broccoli, and cauliflower. 4. Suggest foods with high-complex carbohydrates and a high-fiber diet.
Jaundice	1. Multivitamins and minerals daily. 2. Lipoic acid, 100 mg daily helps to improve liver function. 3. Colostrum, 500 mg qid has been shown to strengthen immune function and improve digestion. 4. Vitamin C and bioflavonoids, 500 mg five to six times daily have anti-inflammatory properties and can reduce duration of jaundice. 5. Vitamin E, 400 IU daily.	1. Eat raw vegetables and fruits for one week, then 75 percent raw, then take fresh lemon enemas daily. 2. Drink the following juices: lemon juice and water, beet and beet greens, black radish extract to cleanse the liver. 3. Do not consume any alcohol. 4. Oregano, celandine, chaparral and dandelion aids cleansing the liver. 5. Silymarin, an active flavonoid is known to repair liver damage.

Condition	Supplements / Vitamins	Nutrition
Knee pain	1. Glucosamine sulfate and chondroitin sulfate are well recognized for their nutritional support, as they are important for the formation of bones, tendons, ligaments, and cartilage. 2. Sulfur helps the absorption of calcium. Adequate intake and absorption of calcium is essential for the repair and the rebuilding of bones, tendons, cartilage, and connective tissues.	1. It is important to consume an adequate amount of various vitamins and minerals in foods, as they are essential to prevent bone loss and promote bone growth. 2. Consume foods high in sulfur such as asparagus, eggs, fresh garlic, and onions. 3. Sea cucumber is very beneficial, as it contains a rich source of compounds that are needed in all connective tissues, especially synovial joints and joint fluids. 4. Consume foods high in histidine such as rice, wheat, and rye. 5. Fresh pineapples are recommended as they contain bromelain, an enzyme that is excellent in reducing inflammation.
Libido	1. Ginseng is a primary tonic for male's sexual virility. 2. Consider Yohimbe caps, 750 to 1,000 mg to stimulate testosterone and revitalize male virility. 3. Royal Jelly, 60,000 to 120,000 mg daily helps boost healthy seminal fluids. 4. Vitamin E, 800 IU helps promote vaginal fluids. 5. Niacin, 100 mg, 30 minutes before sex to enhance sexual flush, mucus membrane tingling and intensity of the orgasm.	Women: 1. Increase soy foods for mild estrogenic effect. 2. Eat food rich in EFAs, such as seafoods, green vegetables, sea greens, whole grains, nuts, legumes, and seeds. 3. Vitamin-E-rich foods include soy foods, wheat germ, seeds, nuts and vegetable oils and beta-carotene foods like apricots, mangos and carrots. 4. Boost adrenal energy with brown rice. 5. Magnesium rich foods, like almonds, avocados, carrots, citrus fruits, lentils, and salmon counteract depression and anxiety.
Masses	1. Multivitamins and minerals daily. 2. Vitamin C, 500 to 1,000 mg tid. 3. Vitamin E, 400 to 800 IU daily. 4. EFAs, Flaxseed oil or evening primrose oil, 1 to 2 tablespoons daily help the body process estrogen. 5. Phosphatidylcholine, 500 mg tid. 6. Pancreatin, 350 to 700 mg tid between meals. 7. Magnesium, 1,000 to 1,500 mg daily aids in the stagnation of the uterus.	1. Eat certified organic foods as much as possible. 2. Base your diet around whole grains, unprocessed foods, vegetables, fruits, fish, sea vegetables, beans, beets, carrots, artichokes, dandelion greens, onions, garlic, and soy products. 3. Increase consumption of soy foods and iodine from seaweeds. 4. Vitamin K will encourage proper blood clotting and reduce excessive flow. 5. Flaxseeds have been shown to help balance estrogen levels.
Memory	1. Choline, 500 to 100 mg daily. 2. DMAE, 75 mg bid boosts neurotransmitters, elevates mood, and increases energy. 3. Folic acid, 400 to 800 mg daily. 4. L-Carnitine. 50 to 500 mg daily. 5. Pantothenic acid, 30 to 100 mg daily. 6. High potency multivitamins and minerals that include: Vitamin B, B12, and Zinc for daily nutrients and enhanced memory function.	1. Make sure the diet contains an adequate amount of lecithin, which is essential for transmission of nerve impulses that control memory. Good sources of lecithin include flaxseed oil, walnut oil, sesame oil, egg yolk, soybean, and raw wheat germ. 2. The B vitamins are also important for energy and proper brain function. 3. Avoid smoking and alcohol.
Menopausal Syndrome	1. Vitamin C, 500 to 1,000 mg tid. 2. Vitamin E, 400 to 1,000 IU daily reduces symptoms, also applied topically for vaginal dryness. 3. EFAs, Flaxseed oil, 1 to 2 tablespoons daily. 4. Hesperidin, 900 mg daily. 5. Gamma-oryzanol, 300 mg daily relieves hot flashes. 6. Boron, 3 mg daily increases estrogen blood levels. 7. Vitamin D, 400 to 600 IU daily. 8. Vitamin B-Complex, 50 to 100 mg helps stabilize estrogen levels.	1. Encourage a diet with a high content of raw foods, fruits and vegetables to stabilize blood-sugar. Wild yam is very helpful to nourish yin and reduce menopause symptoms. 2. Discourage dairy products and red meats, as they promote hot flashes. 3. Avoid alcohol, sugar, spicy foods, and caffeine as they trigger hot flashes and aggravate mood swings. 4. Increase the intake of soy products such as tofu, soymilk, and soy nuts. Soy products regulate the estrogen levels and are beneficial for menopause.
Menorrhagia	1. Vitamin A, 50,000 IU daily normalizes blood loss. 2. Vitamin E, 800 IU daily relieves menstrual symptoms and reduces excessive blood loss. 3. Vitamin C and bioflavonoids protect capillaries from damage. 4. Adding cayenne to any herbal tea can regulate bleeding internally and externally. 5. Drinking diluted lemon juice throughout the menstrual period will help reduce the flow.	1. Increase the intake of vegetable oil and fish oil. 2. Soy products are also beneficial as they help to regulate hormone imbalance. 3. Avoid cold or raw foods as they impair the Spleen function and create more dampness and stagnation.
Menstrual Irregularity	1. Multivitamins and minerals daily. 2. Vitamin C, 500 to 1,000 mg tid. 3. Vitamin E, 400 to 800 IU daily is beneficial for cramps and reduces breast tenderness. 4. EFAs, Flaxseed oil, 1 to 2 tablespoons daily aids in the production of prostaglandin and reduces breast tenderness. 5. Calcium, 500 to 1,000 mg daily prevents mood swings and reduces symptoms. 6. EFA capsules, 250 mg 1 to 3 daily. 7. Iron 10 to 15 mg daily. 8. Magnesium, 250 to 500 mg daily soothes the nervous system and reduces irritability. 9. Zinc, 15 mg bid. 10. Melatonin and Pregnenolone, 100 mg daily, or DHEA 10 mg daily.	1. Adequate intake of calcium is important to prevent menstrual cramps. Calcium level in the body is decreased about 10 days before a period. 2. Increase the intake of vegetable oil and fish. They are rich resources of prostaglandin, which relieves cramping and pain associated with painful menstruation. 3. Soy products are also beneficial as they help to regulate hormone imbalance. 4. Increase the intake of foods that are warm in nature, such as onions, garlic, mutton, chili, or chives. 5. Avoid cold or raw foods as they impair the Spleen function and create more dampness and stagnation.
Muscle Tension	1. Vitamin B6, 25 to 50 mg daily. 2. Vitamin B12, 100 to 1,000 mcg daily. 3. Vitamin C, 500 to 1,000 mg daily.	
Multiple Sclerosis	1. Multivitamins and minerals daily. 2. Vitamin C, 500 to 1,000 mg tid. 3. Vitamin E, 400 to 800 IU daily. 4. EFAs, Flaxseed oil, 1 or 2 tablespoons daily may lessen the harshness and duration of MS attacks. 4. Methylcobalamin (active vitamin B12), 1,000 mcg bid. 5. Pancreatin, 350 to 700 mg tid between meals. 6. Niacin, 200 to 500 mg tid. 7. Vitamin B6, 100 to 500 mg daily. 8. Vitamin B12, 1,000 mg daily. 9. L-cysteine, 500 mg daily. 10. Inositol, 1,000 mg daily. 11. DMG, 100 to 400 mg daily contributes to remyelinization of the sheath protecting the spinal column.	1. Eat organically grown foods with no chemical treatments or additives, including eggs, fruits, gluten-free grains, seeds, and vegetables. 2. Eat plenty of dark leafy greens with a normal allowance of protein. 2. Daily intake of 40 to 50 grams of polyunsaturated oils is recommended. At least 1 teaspoon of cod liver oil daily. 3. Consumption of fish three or more times a week is highly recommended. 4. Take a fiber supplement daily. 5. Avoid alcohol, chocolate, coffee, dairy products, meat, refined foods, sugar, wheat, and processed foods.

Condition	Supplements / Vitamins	Nutrition
Neck Pain	1. Multivitamins and minerals daily. 2. Calcium, 1,500 to 2,000 mg daily. 3. MSM, 500 to 1,000 mg tid. 4. DLPA (dl-phenylalanine), 375 mg capsule prn 4/24 for discomfort. 5. Glucosamine sulfate, 700 to 1,000 mg daily. 6. Magnesium, 700 to 1,000 mg daily. 7. Zinc, 50 mg daily. 8. Bromelain, 400 mg tid, or curcimin, 600 mg tid, and grape seed extract for inflammation. 9. Manganese and free form amino acid complexes are good for ligaments and connective tissues. 10. Consider chondroitin sulfate, bovine cartilage, and shark cartilage.	1. Eat plenty of whole grains, seafood, dark-green vegetables, and nuts. These foods are rich in vitamin B complex and magnesium, which are essential for nerve health and relaxation of tense muscles. 2. Adequate intake of minerals, such as calcium and potassium, are essential for pain management. Deficiency of these minerals will lead to spasms, cramps, and tense muscles.
Nosebleed	1. Multivitamins and minerals daily. 2. Vitamin K, 25 mcg bid helps the blood clot more efficiently. 3. Vitamin C and bioflavonoids, 500 to 1,000 mg qid for two days after a nosebleed.	1. Eat organically grown foods with no chemical treatments or additives, including raw and cooked foods with good sources of vitamin K. 2. Avoid refined sugars which slow the healing process.
Obesity / Weight Control	1. 5-HTP, 50 to 100 mg, before meals for the first two weeks, then double the dosage if weight loss is less than one pound per week. Higher dosages are associated with nausea; both symptoms will disappear after six weeks. 2. Chromium, 200 to 400 mcg daily helps stabilize blood-sugar levels and reduce cravings for sweets. 3. Coenzyme Q10, 100 to 300 mg daily. 4. Hydrocitrate, 500 mg tid. 5. Colorad from Enhanced fitness, a liquid food supplement designed to help body lose fat without losing lean muscle. 6. L-carnitine, 500 to 1,000 mg daily helps fatty acids inside cells produce energy burning mitochondria. 7. Lecithin, one tablespoon daily at breakfast helps emulsify fat.	1. Increase the daily intake of cholesterol-lowering foods such as apples, bananas, carrots, cold-water fish, dried beans, garlic, grapefruit, olive oil, and fibers such as bran and oat. 2. Advise the patient to consume large quantities of fresh fruits and vegetables. 3. Decrease the intake of food that will raise cholesterol levels, including but not limited to beer, wine, cheese, tobacco products, aged and cured meats, sugar, and greasy or fried foods. 4. Eat small, frequent meals throughout the day instead of a few large ones. Eat slowly and chew thoroughly.
Obsessive-Compulsive	1. Calcium, 600 mg bid helps strengthen the nervous system. 2. Taurine, 500 mg tid assists in improving brain function and reducing anxiety. 3. Magnesium, 300 mg bid helps strengthen the nervous system. 4. St. Johns wort is useful in mild cases of OCD. 4. Oat straw, 500 mg bid aids in the utilization of calcium.	1. Maintaining a stable blood-sugar level is very important. Avoid sugar, caffeine, and stimulants that cause rapid fluctuation in blood-sugar. 2. Consider food allergies as the culprit for symptoms.
Osteo-arthritis	1. Multivitamins and minerals daily. 2. Vitamin C, 500 to 1,000 mg tid. 3. Vitamin E, 400 to 800 IU daily. 4. EFAs, Flaxseed oil, 1 or 2 tablespoons daily. 5. Vitamin A, 5000 IU daily. 6. Vitamin B6, 50 mg daily. 7. Pantothenic acid, 13 mg daily. 8. Zinc, 30 to 45 mg daily. 9. Glucosamine sulfate, 500 mg tid. 10. Boron (as sodium tetrahydraborate), 6 to 9 mg daily. 11. Topically applied capsain preparation can help reduce pain of osteoarthritis.	1. Raw carrot, beet, celery, parsley or alfalfa juices, 1 to 2 glasses daily can reduce arthritic conditions. 2. Consume iron in foods that include broccoli, Brussels sprouts, cauliflower, fish, lima beans, and peas. 3. Eat more sulfur-containing foods, such as asparagus, eggs, garlic, and onions as they help repair bone, cartilage and connective tissue. 4. Eat fresh pineapple, which contains bromelain, an enzyme that reduces inflammation. 5. Avoid nightshade vegetables, greasy foods, and NSAIDs.
Osteo-porosis	1. Multivitamins and minerals daily. 2. Vitamin C, 500 to 1,000 mg tid. 3. Vitamin E, 200 to 400 IU daily. 4. EFAs, Flaxseed oil, 1 or 2 tablespoons daily. 5. Boron (as sodium tetrahydraborate), 6 to 9 mg daily. 6. Vitamin D, 400 IU daily with calcium is necessary for absorption. 7. Magnesium, 400 to 800 mg daily can improve bone density.	1. Consume a sufficient amount of calcium and vitamin D, including broccoli, chestnuts, clams, dark-green vegetables, flounder, salmon, sardines, shrimp and soybeans. Eat whole grain and calcium-rich foods at different times of the day to prevent grains from binding to calcium, impeding its absorption in the body. 2. Consumption of foods rich in plant estrogen is beneficial, including soybeans and yams. 3. Eat sulfur-rich foods, like garlic and onions, to make bones healthy. 4. Avoid soft drinks, alcoholic beverages, smoking, yeast products, sugar and salt.
Pain	1. Calcium and magnesium, 500 mg of each tid can be effective for pain associated with muscle spasms. 2. Glucosamine sulfate, 500 mg tid effective alternative to aspirin and other NSAIDs. 3. Bromelain, 300 to 500 mg tid is a natural enzyme that reduces inflammation.	1. Eat organically grown foods with no chemical treatments or additives, including pineapple, soups made with garlic, onions, green leafy vegetables, ginger root, and turmeric root. 2. Avoid food containing saturated, hydrogenated fats including butter, red meat, shellfish, margarine, shortenings, and all fried foods.
Palpitations	1. B-complex, 50 mg tid calms and stabilizes your system. 2. Vitamin E, 200 to 800 IU daily is a powerful antioxidant and reduces clotting. 3. Selenium, 200 mcg daily keeps tissue elastic. 4. Multivitamins and minerals daily that include vitamin A, C, and E. 5. Pycnogenol, 400 mg daily keeps collagen elastic and softens platelets. 6. Vitamin C with bioflavonoids, 3,000 to 20,000 strengthens arterial walls. 8. Melatonin, 500 to 3,000 mcg prevents free-radical damage. 7. CoQ10, 60 tid prevents heart disease. 8. Magnesium, 500 to 1,000 mg daily helps reverse heart disease. 9. Bromelain, 1,500 mg daily.	1. A diet which is magnesium and potassium rich includes: fresh leafy green vegetables, sea food, and sea greens are essential in heart disease prevention. 2. Avoid MSG, baking soda, meat, fat, aged foods, alcohol, diet soft drinks, preservatives, sugar substitutes, meat tenderizers, and soy sauce since they can aggravate palpitations and arrhythmias. 3. Increase the intake of fresh, raw vegetables, nuts, sunflower, and sesame seeds.
Paralysis	1. Multivitamins and minerals daily. 2. Vitamin C, 500 to 1,000 mg tid. 3. Vitamin E, 400 to 800 IU daily. 4. EFAs, Flaxseed oil, 1 or 2 tablespoons daily may lessen the harshness of paralysis. 5. DMG, 100 to 400 mg daily contributes to remyelinization of the sheath protecting the spinal column. 6. Calcium, 2,000 mg daily. 7. Magnesium, 1,000 mg daily.	1. Eat soured milk products like yogurt and kefir, including beet greens, chard, eggs, green leafy vegetables, raw cheese, and raw milk. 2. Drink fresh "live" juices made from beets, carrots, green beans, green leafy vegetables, peas, red grapes, and seaweed. 3. Avoid dairy products, meat, sugar and white flour products.

Condition	Supplements / Vitamins	Nutrition
Parkinson's Disease	1. Multivitamins and minerals daily. 2. Vitamin C, 500 to 1,000 mg tid. 3. Vitamin E, 400 to 800 IU daily. 4. Ginkgo biloba, 40 to 80 mg tid increases blood flow to the brain. 5. Phosphatidylserine, 100 mg tid helps boost energy level to the brain. 6. Consider Thiodox from Allergy Research, 200 mg which contains the essential glutathione to support the body. 7. Vitamin B thiamin, 3,000 to 8,000 mg daily and tyrosine, 500 to 1,000 mg daily helps boost dopamine levels for the brain. 8. CoQ10, 200 mg daily is crucial for cellular energy. 9. DHEA, 10 mg for women, 25 mg for men daily is a helpful hormone.	1. Eat a diet consisting of raw foods, with seeds, grains, nuts and raw milk. 2. Include diet foods containing amino acid, such as almonds, fish, pecans, sesame seeds, lentils. 3. Reduce intake of animal protein.
Pelvic Inflammatory Disease		1. Natural, plain yogurt with live cultures helps to minimize yeast infections by establishing a normal environment in the genital tract. 2. Eat plenty of fruits and vegetables, which provide the nutrients needed to resist infection and facilitate healing. 3. Regular consumption of unsweetened cranberry juice will help to prevent and treat urinary tract infections.
PMS	1. Multivitamins and minerals daily. 2. Vitamin C, 500 to 1,000 mg tid. 3. Vitamin E, 400 to 800 IU daily is beneficial for cramps and reduces breast tenderness. 4. EFAs, Flaxseed oil, 1 to 2 tablespoons daily aids in the production of prostaglandin and reduces breast tenderness. 5. Calcium, 500 to 1,000 mg daily prevents mood swings and reduces symptoms. 6. EFA capsules, 250 mg 1 to 3 daily. 7. Iron 10 to 15 mg daily. 8. Magnesium, 250 to 500 mg daily soothes the nervous system and reduces irritability. 9. Zinc, 15 mg bid. 10. Melatonin and Pregnenolone, 100 mg daily, or DHEA 10 mg daily.	1. A diet high in calcium, magnesium, phosphorus, potassium, and vitamins B and E is recommended. These nutrients are easily depleted by stress. 2. Encourage the consumption of fruits and vegetables such as apricots, wintermelon, asparagus, avocados, bananas, and broccoli in addition to brown rice, dried fruit, figs, salmon, garlic, green leafy vegetables, soy products, and yogurt. 3. Avoid caffeine (coffee, tea, soda, chocolate), tobacco, alcohol, and sugar. 4. Reduce exposure to environmental estrogens in foods.
Polycystic Ovarian	1. Multivitamins and minerals daily. 2. Vitamin C, 500 to 1,000 mg tid. 3. Vitamin E, 400 to 800 IU daily is an estrogen antagonist. 4. EFAs, Flaxseed oil or evening primrose oil, 1 to 2 tablespoons daily helps the body process estrogen and reduce inflammation. 5. Pancreatin, 350 to 700 mg tid between meals helps with fat metabolism. 6. Magnesium, 1,000 to 1,500 mg daily aids in the stagnation of the uterus. 7. Quercitin and bromelain are effective anti-inflammatory.	1. Eat certified organic foods as much as possible. 2. Base your diet around whole grains, unprocessed foods, vegetables, fruits, fish, sea vegetables, beans, beets, carrots, artichokes, dandelion greens, onions, garlic, and soy products. 3. Increase consumption of soy foods. 4. Flaxseeds have been shown to help balance estrogen levels. 5. Include green drinks to support detoxification. 6. Avoid red meat, dairy products, sugar, caffeine, alcohol, processed foods, fried foods, and refined sugars.
Rheumatoid Arthritis	1. Multivitamins and minerals daily. 2. Vitamin C, 500 to 1,000 mg tid. 3. Vitamin E, 400 to 800 IU daily. 4. EFAs, Flaxseed oil, 1 to 2 tablespoons daily. 5. Pancreatin, 350 to 700 mg tid between meals.	1. Fasting can bring temporary relief to RA. 2. Consume foods high in an iron which include broccoli, Brussels sprouts, cauliflower, fish, lima beans, and peas. 3. Eat more sulfur-containing foods, such as asparagus, eggs, garlic, and onions. 4. Eat fresh pineapple, which contains bromelain, an enzyme that reduces inflammation. 5. Avoid nightshade vegetables, greasy foods, and NSAIDs. 6. Avoid iron supplements because they are suspected of being involved in pain, swelling, and joint destruction.
Sciatica	1. Multivitamins and minerals daily. 2. Quercitin, 1,000 mg daily, bromelain, 1,500 mg daily to relieve nerve inflammation. 3. Niacin, 500 to 1,500 daily to stimulate circulation. 4. MSM, 3,000 to 8,000 mg daily in divided dosages for inflammation. 5. Consider horsetail, alfalfa, burdock, oat straw, slippery elm, white willow bark in capsules, extract, or tea form to reduce inflammation. 6. EFAs, in the form of flaxseed oil, fish oil, and evening primrose oil which are rich in fatty acids nourish the nervous system. 7. Consider bovine cartilage and shark cartilage as added support for back pain with sciatica.	1. Eat a diet with a wide variety of raw vegetables and fruits, and whole grain cereals to ensure a complete supply of nutrients for the bones, nerves, and muscles. 2. Fresh pineapples are recommended as they contain bromelain, an enzyme that is excellent in reducing inflammation. If the consumption of fresh pineapples causes stomach upset, eat it after meals. 3. Avoid red meat and seafood in the diet as they contain high levels of uric acid, which puts added strain on the kidneys. 4. Avoid cold beverages, ice cream, caffeine, sugar, tomatoes, milk, and dairy products.
Sinusitis	1. Vitamin C, 500 to 1,000 mg every waking hour reduces histamine levels. 2. Thymus extract, 750 mg once or bid. 3. Beta-carotene, 50,000 IU tid.	1. Avoid spicy, fried, or greasy foods. 2. Food or beverages that are cool or cold in nature should be consumed. Among these are watermelon, lotus nodes, melon, seaweed, cranberries, celery, cucumber, cactus and winter melon. 3. Drink plenty of water in order to urinate often. 4. Increase supplementation with vitamin C and B complex.
Smoking	1. Consider Smoking withdrawal from Natra-Bio Homeopathic. 2. Glutamine, 1,000 mg daily, Cysteine, 1,000 mg daily, and Vitamin C, 1,000 mg daily for nicotine toxicity. 3. Magnesium, 800 mg daily to calm nerves. 4. Ginseng and licorice help normalize and control cravings. 5. Lycopene, 10 mg daily, germanium, 150 mg daily, CoQ10, 60 mg tid, aid oxygen flow to the brain and protect heart tissue. 6. Beta-carotene, 200,000 IU daily are great antioxidants and lung protectors. 7. Maitake 1,000 to 4,000 mg daily, inhibits carcinogenesis and protects against metastasis through the lungs.	1. Consume more asparagus, broccoli, cauliflower, spinach, sweet potatoes, nuts, seeds, yellow and deep-orange vegetables, pumpkin, squash, yams, apples, cantaloupe, grapes, legumes, and plums. 2. Drink fresh carrot juice daily as a preventative measure against lung cancer. 3. Avoid junk foods, processed refined foods, sugar, white flour or any animal protein, except for broiled fish.

Condition	Supplements / Vitamins	Nutrition
Sore Throat	1. Vitamin C chewable, 500 mg every hour during acute stages. 2. Consider Emergen-C every few hours. 3. Vitamin C, 5,000 mg daily to fight infection. 4. Zinc lozenges or colloidal silver as needed. 5. Lysine, 500 mg daily. 6. Echinacea to flush lymph glands for at least 7 days. 7. Garlic capsules, 8 daily.	1. Avoid spicy, fried, or greasy foods. 2. Food or beverages that are cool or cold in nature should be consumed. Among these are watermelon, lotus nodes, melon, seaweed, cranberries, celery, cucumber, cactus and winter melon. 3. Drink plenty of water in order to urinate often. 4. Increase supplementation with vitamin C and B complex. 5. Lemon juice and honey in hot water with a pinch of cayenne pepper each morning is helpful.
Stress	1. Calcium 500 to 1,000 mg daily. 2. DHEA, 25 to 50 daily. 3. Magnesium, 250 to 500 mg daily is a muscle relaxant. 4. Vitamin B Complex, 25 to 50 mg daily regulates nerves. 5. Siberian ginseng, astragalus, schisandra, and kava are great adaptogens which strengthen resistance to stress. 6. CoQ10, 100 mg qid helps fight fatigue and is a powerful antioxidant. 7. SAMe, 400 mg daily, glutamine, 1,000 mg daily, tyrosine, 500 mg daily and DLPA, 1,000 mg daily are good amino acids that boost your brain energy. 8. Ginseng, gotu kola, and ginkgo biloba provide excellent support to the nerves. 9. Licorice root extract helps support adrenal functions.	1. A diet high in calcium, magnesium, phosphorus, potassium, and vitamins B and E is recommended. These vitamins and minerals are easily depleted by stress. 2. Consider a raw diet. 3. Encourage the consumption of fruits and vegetables such as apricots, wintermelon, asparagus, avocados, bananas, and broccoli in addition to brown rice, dried fruit, figs, salmon, garlic, green leafy vegetables, soy products, and yogurt. 4. Avoid caffeine (coffee, tea, soda, chocolate), tobacco, alcohol, and sugar whenever possible.
Stroke	1. B-complex, 50 mg tid nourishes the brain and reduces homocysteine levels. 2. Beta-carotene has been shown to reduce the risk of ischemic stroke. 3. Vitamin E, 200 to 800 IU daily is a powerful antioxidant and reduces clotting. 4. Selenium, 200 mcg daily keeps tissue elastic. 5. Multivitamins and minerals daily that include vitamin A, C, and E. 6. Pycnogenol, 400 mg daily keeps collagen elastic and softens platelets. 7. Vitamin C with bioflavonoids, 3,000 to 20,000 strengthens arterial walls. 8. Melatonin, 500 to 3,000 mcg prevents free-radical damage.	1. Eliminate salt and fats from the diet and reduce blood pressure. 2. Avoid MSG, baking soda, meat, fat, aged foods, alcohol, diet soft drinks, preservatives, sugar substitutes, meat tenderizers, and soy sauce. 3. Increase the intake of fresh, raw vegetables and fruits to control blood pressure. Nuts and seeds should be consumed daily for a source of protein. 4. Vitamin C and bioflavonoids help to reduce blood pressure by stabilizing the blood vessel walls. 5. Garlic is effective to lower blood pressure and thin the blood.
Tendonitis	1. Vitamin E, 200 to 400 IU daily reduces trauma and torn cartilage. 2. Vitamin C with bioflavonoids tid is important in the production of collagen and helps speed repair of tissue. 3. Manganese, 3 to 5 mg bid. 4. Bromelain, 400 mg tid is a natural anti-inflammatory. 5. Pine bark and grape seed extract, 50 mg tid. 6. Zinc, 15 mg daily supports the immune system. 7. Flaxseed and fish oil rich in omega-3 fatty acid, 1,000 mg bid. 8. Bromelain, 400 mg tid has natural anti-inflammatory properties. 9. Glucosamine sulfate, 1,500 mg daily or Chondroitin sulfate, 1,200 mg daily to reduce trauma. 10. Creatine, 1,000 mg daily for muscles and joint injuries also help speed up recovery time.	1. Eat organically grown foods with no chemical treatments or additives, including fresh vegetables, especially dark-green vegetables, fruits, lean chicken, fish and tofu. 2. Avoid saturated, hydrogenated, processed foods, sugars, red meat, dairy products, caffeine, and alcohol.
Tinnitus	1. Vitamin A, 25,000 IU daily. 2. Vitamin B1, 100 to 500 mg daily. 3. Vitamin B12, 1 to 5 mcg daily in lozenge form. 4. B-complex, 50 mg bid. 5. Vitamin E, 400 to 800 IU daily helps repair nerves. 6. Vitamin D, 500 to 1,000 daily. 7. Magnesium, 500 mg daily. 8. Potassium, 500 mg daily. 9. Silica helps strengthen vascular walls.	1. Encourage a diet with a high content of raw foods, fruits and vegetables to stabilize blood-sugar. 2. Discourage dairy products and red meats, as they promote hot flashes. 3. Avoid spicy or greasy foods, or anything else that may trigger a recurrent bacterial or viral attack.
TMJ	1. Vitamin B complex daily to relieve anxiety and improve sleep. 2. Vitamin C, 2,000 to 5,000 tid.	1. Eat a diet including lightly steamed vegetables, fresh fruit, whole-grain products, and white fish. Eat more sulfur-containing foods, such as asparagus, eggs, garlic and onions. Sulfur is needed for repair and rebuilding of bones, cartilage and connective tissue. 2. Eat fresh pineapple frequently. 3. Avoid high stress foods: all forms of sugar, all junk foods, alcohol, candy, colas, fast foods, and foods containing caffeine.
Toothache	1. Multivitamins and minerals daily. 2. Calcium, 1,000 mg daily. 3. Magnesium, 600 mg daily for healthy teeth. 4. Hydrogen peroxide, 3 percent, floss and swish in your mouth for few seconds helps kill infection in the gum or nerve of a tooth.	1. A diet consisting of lean protein, good concentration of calcium, phosphorous, and vitamin D. 2. Calcium rich foods include: green leafy vegetables, broccoli, cabbage and Brussels sprouts, figs, kelp, oats, prunes, sesame seeds, and tofu. 3. Phosphorous can be obtained from bananas, whole grain breads and cereals, eggs, fish and poultry. Foods rich in calcium include: eggs, dairy products, and saltwater fish.

Condition	Supplements / Vitamins	Nutrition
Ulcer	1. Vitamin C, 500 to 1,000 mg tid. 2. Vitamin E, 200 to 400 IU daily. 3. EFAs, Flaxseed oil, 1 tablespoon daily. 4. Vitamin A, 20,000 IU daily heals mucosal tissue of the stomach. 5. Zinc, 25 to 30 mg daily speeds the healing process. 6. Chewing tablets containing a special licorice extract, DGL (for deglycyrrhizinated licorice), 380 to 760 mg twenty minutes before meals is very effective in healing ulcers. In fact, clinical studies have shown DGL is more effective than standard anti-ulcer drugs. 7. Fish oil and corn oil can keep ulcers from coming back.	1. Increase the intake of papayas and pineapples as they contain bromelain, a digestive enzyme that helps with indigestion. 2. Acidophilus is also helpful for digestion. 3. For ulcers, intake of vitamin K, found in green leafy vegetables, should be increased as it helps with the healing process. 4. Avoid lentils, peanuts and soybeans because they contain enzyme inhibitors. 5. Avoid fried, spicy or greasy foods, refined sugar, tea, coffee, caffeine, salt, chocolate, strong spices, and carbonated drinks.
UTI	1. Consider Probiotics which can help improve digestive function and eliminate bacterial buildup. 2. Drink unsweetened cranberry juice (16 ounces daily) or take a cranberry extract to acidify the urine and inhibit bacterial growth. 3. Vitamin C, 2,000 to 6,000 mg daily expels infectious bacteria and is an effective preventative agent. 4. Zinc, 50 mg daily assists in WBC production and eliminates bacteria. 5. Vitamin A prevents irritation and improves function of WBC. 6. Colloidal silver is a natural antibiotic. 7. Calcium, 1,500 mg daily and magnesium 750 to 1,000 mg daily reduces bladder irritability.	1. Natural, plain yogurt with live cultures helps to minimize yeast infections by establishing a normal environment in the genital tract. 2. Eat plenty of fruits and vegetables, which provide the nutrients needed to resist infection and facilitate healing. 3. Regular consumption of unsweetened cranberry juice will help to prevent and treat urinary tract infection. 4. Drink watermelon and pear juice tid. 5. Drink carrot and celery juice tid. 6. Drink cornsilk tea freely. 7. Eat squash soup for at least seven days. 8. Eat steamed lotus root and water chestnuts bid.
Varicose Veins	1. Multivitamins and minerals daily. 2. Vitamin C, 500 to 1,000 mg tid strengthen vein walls. 3. Vitamin E, 200 to 400 IU daily. 4. EFAs, Flaxseed oil, 1 tablespoon daily. 5. PCO extracts or flavonoids are excellent at strengthening vein walls. 6. Aorta glycosaminoglycans, 50 mg bid. 7. DMSO has been used to relieve the swelling and pain of severe varicose veins. 8. Bromelain, 1,500 mg daily, quercitin, 1,000 mg daily boost flavonoids for vein tone and reduce inflammation.	1. Eat a diet that is low in fat and refined carbohydrates and includes plenty of fish and fresh fruits and vegetables. 2. Eat as many blackberries and cherries as you wish. 3. Include garlic, onion, and pineapple in your diet. 4. Avoid animal protein, processed and refined foods, sugar, junk foods, tobacco, alcohol, and salt.
Warts Common	1. Adequate vitamin C intake is more important in managing effective immunity against the viruses that cause warts. 2. High potency multivitamin and mineral supplements. 3. Zinc, 75 mg daily, increases immunity against viruses. 4. N-acetyl cysteine, 2,000 mg daily helps boost immune response. 5. Vitamin E, 800 IU daily or apply the oil on the surrounding skin. 6. Vitamin A 100,000 IU daily for one month, then 50,000 IU daily for second month, then reduce to 25,000 IU daily for third month or until warts disappear.	1. Increase the amount of sulfur-containing amino acids in your diet by eating more asparagus, citrus fruits, eggs, onions, and garlic.
Weakened immune system	1. High potency multivitamin and mineral supplements. 2. Vitamin A, 10,000 IU daily. 3. Vitamin C with flavonoids, 5,000 to 20,000 mg daily. 4. Vitamin E, 400 IU daily. 5. Zinc, 50 to 80 mg daily. 6. Coenzyme Q10, 60 mg tid. 7. DHEA, 25 to 50 mg daily. 8. Pregnenolone, 10 mg daily. 9. Selenium, 100 to 200 mcg daily.	1. Begin diet of fresh fruits, vegetables, seeds, grains, and other foods that are high in fiber. 2. Include in your diet: chlorella, garlic, and pearl barley. 3. Consume green drinks daily. 4. Avoid animal products, processed foods, alcohol, smoking, and soda. 5. Follow a fasting program, consider the use of spirulina, especially after fasting.

BOTANICALS

Herbs	Uses	Information	Daily Dose	Cautions
Agar	int: constipation, GI complaints	acts similar to cellulose, absorbing water in intestines	*1 to 2 teaspoons of powder, always with liquid*	none known
Agrimony leaf	int: mild diarrhea, pharyngeal inflammation; ext: mild inflammation of skin	contains tannins and flavonoids: acts as an astringent	*3 g or equivalent*	none known
Aletris	int: dysmenorrhea, amenorrhea, anorexia	may have estrogenic effect, no conclusive studies	*1.5 g drug/100 ml water or equivalent*	none known
Alfalfa	int: anorexia, diabetes, hypothyroidism	no conclusive studies of effectiveness	*as directed*	avoid with SLE or other autoimmune diseases
Almond - sweet and bitter	int: (bitter) cough, nausea; ext: (sweet) skin inflammation	contains fatty acids, especially oleic acid, and cyanide-type compounds	*as directed*	overdose with cyanide-type effects; bitter almond to be used only under strict supervision
Aloe	int: constipation; ext: wound healing, psoriasis	FDA-approved as laxative, increases colonic motility	*int: titrate to soft stool; ext: as directed*	int: avoid in obstruction, IBD, appendicitis, pregnancy/ lactation, or in children; may cause abdominal cramping, hypokalemia- especially with diuretics - as well as albuminuria or hematuria; may cause benign red coloration of urine
Alpha-Lipoic Acid	int: diabetic complications, especially neuropathy; liver disease, cataracts, glaucoma, ischemia-reperfusion injury, amanita mushroom poisoning	water- and fat-soluble antioxidant needed in pyruvate DH reaction; may improve glucose utilization in diabetes and prevent free radical damage: can pass through BBB	*no information: capsules available 30 to 100 mg*	allergic skin reactions and hypoglycemia known; no data on pregnancy; effects of long-term use unknown
Alpine Cranberry	int: UTIs and urinary stones, rheumatism	has antiviral and antibacterial properties	*2 g single dose or equivalent*	contraindicated in pregnancy, nursing, children less than 12 years old; drug effective only with alkaline urine; hepatotoxicity due to hydroquinones is possible
American Hellebore	int: HTN	very effective but no longer used due to severe toxicity	*do not use!*	avoid completely, may cause cardiac arrest
Angelica root/fruit/leaf	int: decreased appetite, early satiety	contains coumarin and essential oil; increases gastric juice/bile production	*4.5 g of drug or equivalent*	may increase photosensitivity or cause dermatitis; may be carcinogenic; no interactions known
Anise fruit/ seed	int: dyspepsia; ext: bronchitis	expectorant, mild antibacterial agent	*3 g of drug or equivalent*	occasional allergic reactions- avoid if allergic to anethole; no interactions known
Arnica	ext: traumatic injuries, such as bruises, dislocations	analgesic and antiseptic activity	*infusion: 2 g of herb per 100 ml of water*	may cause allergic reaction; long-term use may cause edema or dermatitis; no interactions known; has been used internally for throat inflammation, but this is not recommended due to toxicity
Artichoke	int: dyspepsia, biliary complaints, anorexia	may increase bile flow, may be protective against hepatotoxins, may have lipid-lowering effects	*6 g drug or equivalent*	may cause allergic reaction; avoid in cholestasis or cholithiasis
Asarum	int: bronchitis, cough, asthma	may be mucolytic, antibacterial, local anesthetic	*as directed- use purified dry extract*	extremely susceptible mouse strain developed hepatoma after administration; avoid in children less than 12 and in pregnancy
Ash leaf/bark	int: URIs, rheumatism, fever	bark and leaf contain coumarin-like compounds; no evidence of effectiveness	*as directed*	none known
Asparagus root	int: inflammation of urinary tract, prevention of nephrolithiasis	may have diuretic effects	*45 to 60 g of rhizome or equivalent*	avoid if known nephrolithiasis; rare allergic skin reactions
Astragalus	int: general immune stimulant, as in HIV and other infections; memory impairment; anorexia	may increase WBCs (especially T cells), inhibit coxsackievirus replication, increase Liver function, and increase fibrinolysis	*capsule as directed*	caution with immunosuppressive therapy or anticoagulants; no definitive studies about pregnancy or lactation
Autumn Crocus	int: acute gout, familial Mediterranean fever	contains colchicine, an antichemotactic, mitosis inhibitor	*initial dose equal to 1 mg colchicine, then 0.5 to 1.5 mg 1 to 2 hrs until pain free*	avoid in pregnancy, may cause diarrhea, leukopenia, or aplastic anemia
Balm	int: depression, anxiety, insomnia, GI distress, neuralgia	acts as mild sedative: may inhibit TSH	*infusion as recommended*	none known
Barberry fruit/root	int: (fruit) UTIs, immune stimulant; (root) indigestion, constipation	may increase bile flow and have pro-peristaltic, antipyretic effects; contains vitamin C	*as directed*	none known
Barley	int: indigestion, diarrhea	contains numerous vitamins; has soothing effect on GI tract	*taken as malt extract*	avoid during pregnancy
Basil herb	int: fever, URIs, indigestion	may have antimicrobial effects	*not recommended*	potential carcinogen; avoid oil and large amounts of herbs

BOTANICAL

Herbs	Uses	Information	Daily Dose	Cautions
Bayberry fruit/bark	int: diarrhea, colitis, bronchitis	may have mineralocorticoid activity; acts as astringent, circulatory stimulant	*not recommended*	potential carcinogen, cannot recommend
Bean pods (without seeds)	int: supportive therapy for inability to urinate, UTIs, urinary stones	may act as weak diuretic	*5 to 15 g of herb or equivalent*	none known
Belladonna	int: liver and gallbladder complaints, GI spasms	contains atropine and related compounds, with anti-ACh effects	*0.05 to 0.1 g herb or equivalent*	avoid with tachy arrhythmias, BPH, narrow-angle glaucoma, acute pulmonary edema, GI obstruction, megacolon; may cause dry mouth, dry skin, tachycardia, tremor, difficult urination
Bellflower	int: bronchitis, sore throat, tonsillitis	contains saponins, which may inhibit gastric acid and act as expectorant	*6 g powder or equivalent*	none known
Betaine	nutrient which lowers level of homocysteine; found in variety of plant and animal foods	works in tandem with B vitamins and folate, so usually taken together	*no RDA: 500 to 1000 mg for general cardiovascular health*	none known
Bilberry fruit/leaf	int: acute diarrhea, pharyngitis, night vision; may lower blood sugar (leaf used for DM)	contains tannins, anthocyanins, and flavonoids	*fruit: 20 to 60 g or equivalent*	may have some anti-platelet effect; caution with ASA, anticoagulants, hypoglycemics
Biotin	needed for nerves, sweat glands, skin; found in dairy products, nuts, seeds, meats, vegetables	produced by intestinal bacteria	*no RDA; adult estimated need: 30 mcg*	none known
Birch leaf	int: inflammation of urinary tract, adjunct to rheumatic complaints	contains flavonoids, acts as a diuretic	*2 to 3 g of herb several times daily*	no side effects known; avoid if edema due to CHF or renal disease
Bishop's Weed fruit	int: angina, paroxysmal tachycardia, asthma, nonspecific chest pain	may increase coronary circulation with positive inotropic effects; may have antispasmodic effect on smooth muscles	*no information*	reversible cholestatic jaundice and photosensitivity are infrequent; chronic use may lead to dizziness, GI complaints, sleep disorders; high doses may reversibly increase LFTs
Bistort	int: diarrhea, mild GI bleed; ext: throat infections	contains tannins and starch	*as directed*	none known
Bitter Orange peel/flower	int: loss of appetite, dyspepsia	contains essential oil, may have spasmolytic effect on GI tract, increase gastric juice production	*peel: 4 to 6 g or equivalent*	may cause photosensitivity and sensitization with erythema and swelling
Black Cohosh root	int: PMS, dysmenorrhea, promotes labor, menopausal symptoms	may have estrogenic and anti-LH effects	*40 mg drug or equivalent*	occasional GI upset; no interactions known; complications of long-term use unknown; avoid in breast cancer; some use instead of HRT
Black Mustard	ext: pneumonia, sinusitis, sciatica	contains glucosinolates which are released by grinding seeds	*as directed*	contraindicated in peptic ulcer diseases or nephrolithiasis; protect eyes and skin from long-term use; coughing and possible asthma attacks may occur from breathing vapors; avoid in children younger than 6
Black Walnut	int: hemorrhoids, liver/ gallbladder problems	may have antimicrobial effects	*capsules: 95 mg to 500 mg to 3.5 g*	none known; treat overdose with charcoal and shock provisions
Blackberry leaf/root	int: nonspecific diarrhea, inflammation of mouth/throat	contains tannins	*leaf: 4.5 mg or equivalent*	none known
Blackthorn berry	int: inflammation of oral mucosa	contains tannins	*2 to 4 g or equivalent*	none known
Bladderwrack	int: thyroid dysfunction, obesity; ext: sprains	contains high amounts of iodine; may have antimicrobial and hypoglycemic effects	*as directed*	may worsen hyperthyroidism with high doses, as iodine content is not regulated; caution with other hypoglycemics
Blessed Thistle	int: decreased appetite, dyspepsia	promotes saliva, gastric juice production	*4 to 6 g or equivalent*	possible allergic reactions; no interactions known
Blue Cohosh	int: amenorrhea, dysmenorrhea, threatened miscarriage, atonic uterus	may have weak estrogenic, spasmolytic effects	*or equivalent*	avoid during first three months of pregnancy due to possible teratogenicity
Bogbean leaf	int: decreased appetite, dyspepsia	promotes saliva, gastric juice production	*1.5 to 3 g or equivalent*	possible allergic reactions; no interactions known
Boldo leaf	int: mild GI spasm, dyspepsia	contains alkaloids, flavonoids; increases bile and gastric juice production	*3 g or equivalent*	avoid with liver disease or gallstones; no side effects known, but avoid distillates or essential oil
Boneset	int: diaphoretic, emetic, mucolytic	may increase sweating	*as directed*	caution advised due to possible toxic alkaloids
Borage seed	int: astringent, anti-inflammatory such as in arthritis	astringent properties: contains gamma-lineolic acid, which reduces inflammation	*as directed*	caution advised due to potentially hepatotoxic alkaloids

BOTANICALS

Herbs	Uses	Information	Daily Dose	Cautions
Bromelain	int: edema, especially post-traumatic, wounds, burns, Peyronie's disease, angina, HIV	may have anti-edema effects in high dosages	*80 to 320 mg of bromelain*	may prolong PT and bleeding time with possible increased bleeding; may raise level of tetracyclines in blood; hypersensitivity reactions known; occasional GI side effects; no pregnancy data
Buchu leaf	int: irritation of urinary tract/prostate, various GI complaints, gout	no studies of drugs available; popular in South Africa today	*as directed*	avoid during pregnancy
Buckthorn bark/berry	int: constipation	increases colonic motility, GI secretion	*20 to 30 mg hydroxyanthracene derivatives daily*	bark must be aged for one year, fresh bark will cause severe vomiting; avoid with intestinal obstruction or chronic inflammation; may cause hypokalemia, GI cramping; use only if fiber/diet ineffective
Bugleweed	int: mild hyperthyroidism with nervous system dysfunction, mastodynia, PMS	inhibits conversion of T4-> T3; may inhibit prolactin	*water-ethanol extracts equivalent of 20 mg of drug*	may rarely cause goiter; avoid with other thyroactive drugs
Burdock root	int: GI complaints; ext: ichthyosis, psoriasis, seborrhea	may have mild antimicrobial effects; no studies available	*capsules 460 to 475 mg or as directed*	small risk of sensitization
Butcher's Broom	int: chronic venous insufficiency, hemorrhoids, leg cramps, itching	may act as diuretic; may increase venous tone	*raw extract-equivalent to 7 to 11 mg total ruscogenin*	rarely nausea; no interactions known
Cabbage	int: gastritis, ulcers, bronchitis, cough	may protect mucous membrane of stomach from gastric HCl	*tablet 500 mg or juice as directed*	none known
Calamus	int: dyspepsia, related GI complaints; ext: rheumatism, gum disease, tonsillitis	may stimulate appetite and digestion	*tea as directed*	avoid long-term use; susceptible rats developed tumors
Calendula flower/herb	int: pharyngitis/mucositis; ext: wound healing	contains glycosides, aglycones, carotenoids; may have anti-s. aureus, anti-HIV activity; may simulate epithelialization	*as directed*	uncommon dermatitis
Californian Poppy	int: depression, anxiety, sleep disorders	may act as sedative, limited clinical data	*as directed*	avoid during pregnancy; often prescribed with other sedatives
Camphor	int: circulatory regulation disorders; ext: muscular rheumatism, bronchitis, cardiac symptoms	acts as bronchial secretagogue, respiratory antispasmodic	*as directed*	avoid on broken skin; may cause contact eczema; no interactions known
Canadian Goldenrod	int: UTIs, stones of urinary tract	may act as diuretic, weakly spasmolytic	*6 to 12 g or equivalent*	avoid if edema due to CHF, renal failure; take with fluids
Capsicum	ext: analgesia, zoster, diabetic neuropathy	FDA-approved as topical analgesic; contains capsaicinoids, which may have anti-inflammatory actions; blocks substance P in nerves	*as directed*	avoid eyes; use only for 2 days and then again after 2 weeks; rare hypersensitivity reactions; do not add heat; may irritate mucous membranes at low doses; long contact with skin may injure nerves; overdose may cause hypothermia
Caraway oil/seed	int: dyspepsia, early satiety, flatulence	acts as antispasmodic, antimicrobial	*3 to 6 drops of standard preparation*	no side effects or interactions known
Cardamom seed	int: dyspepsia, liver/ gallbladder complaints, URIs, pharyngitis, tendency to infection	may be virustatic, may increase biliary motility	*1.5 g of drug or equivalent*	avoid with gallstones
Carrageen (Irish seaweed)	int: cough, URIs	may act as expectorant	*as directed*	none known
Cascara bark	int: laxative, gallstones, liver ailments	FDA-approved as laxative; may increase peristalsis	*20 to 30 mg hydroxyanthracene derivatives daily*	may cause hypokalemia with chronic use; avoid with chronic GI inflammation or obstruction; fresh bark may cause vomiting--use aged bark
Cashew	int: GI ailments; ext: ulcers, warts, corns	may have anti-Gram positive activity	*as directed*	seed cases contain alkyl phenols and may act as strong skin irritants; nuts do not contain them
Castor oil	int: constipation, intestinal inflammation/parasites	ricolinic acid acts as laxative; also may be antimicrobial	*laxative: 5 g bid or 2 g 5x per day*	contraindicated in obstruction, acute inflammation, abdominal pain of unknown origin, pregnancy/nursing; rare skin rashes; chronic use may cause hypokalemia; castor beans highly toxic
Catechu	int: sore throat; ext: skin diseases, oral ulcers, toothache	may act as astringent and antiseptic	*0.3 to 2 g tid or equivalent*	none known
Catnip	int: fever, cramps, anxiety	limited scientific data	*tea as directed*	avoid during pregnancy; smoking drug may cause mind-altering effects

Herbs	Uses	Information	Daily Dose	Cautions
Cat's Claw	int: immune stimulant	contains hirsutine and sterol components, may stimulate IL-1, IL-6; may inhibit platelets, affect serotonin/dopamine, have anti-HTN effects, induce apoptosis in certain cell lines	*as directed*	contraindicated in pregnancy, nursing; avoid if taking immunosuppressants or with autoimmune disease (one report of ARF in patient with SLE); may lower estradiol and progesterone levels
Cat's Foot flower	int: diuretic, diarrhea	may increase bile flow and decrease GI spasms; limited scientific info	*tea as directed*	no information
Celandine	int: biliary spasm, GI distress	mild antispasmodic, papverdine-like action	*2 - 5 g of herb or equivalent*	may cause mild hypotension; no interactions known
Celery	int: anxiety, GI complaints, edema	may have sedative, anticonvulsant, diuretic effects	*as directed*	avoid volatile oil with pyelonephritis
Centaury	int: decreased appetite, dyspepsia	may increase gastric juice production	*6 g of drug or equivalent*	none known
Chamomile flower	int: GI inflammation, spasms; ext: skin inflammation, pharyngitis	antispasmodic, antiflatulent, antibacterial, promotes wound healing	*as directed*	may cause hypersensitivity or anaphylactic reactions; caution if allergic to ragweed, chrysanthemums, or asters
Chaste Tree fruit	int: PMS, dysmenorrhea, menopausal symptoms, mastodynia	may decrease prolactin secretion via dopaminergic action	*30 to 40 mg or equivalent*	may cause itchy rash; no interactions known; avoid during pregnancy
Chestnut	int: URIs, poor circulation	limited scientific info	*infusion as directed*	none known
Chickweed	int: joint stiffness, gout, Tb; ext: eczema, wounds	limited scientific info	*tea or infusion as directed*	none known
Chicory	int: decreased appetite, dyspepsia	may increase bile production	*3 g of herb or equivalent*	avoid in gallstones; may cause allergic reaction
Chinese Cinnamon	int: anorexia, dyspepsia, bronchitis	may be antibacterial, fungistatic, increase GI motility, inhibit ulcers	*2 to 4 g drug or equivalent*	avoid with pregnancy, as is potential abortifacent
Chinese Foxglove root	int: fever, insomnia, restlessness, rheumatism, eczema, kidney/heart disease	may be antibacterial, immunosuppressive, and hepatoprotective	*as directed - decoction in Chinese fashion*	none known
Chinese thoroughwax	int: fever, pain, inflammatory conditions	contains saponins, which may show antihistaminic, antitumor, and immunoregulatory effects	*often mixed with other herbs; use as directed*	avoid during pregnancy; overdose may cause GI complaints
Choline	found in many foods, in lecithin	important for nervous system functioning (converted to ACh)	*no RDA; recommended (adults): approx. 500 mg*	toxicity can cause rare GI side effects; may need to take if on niacin for hypercholesterolemia
Chondroitin	int: osteoarthritis, other degenerative diseases	carbohydrate which draws fluid into tissues, making them spongier; affects collagen and matrix production	*usually combined with glucosamine - as directed*	may affect coagulability of blood; avoid if pregnant/nursing; will only work for some patients
Chromium	trace element: found in meat, seafood, dairy products, eggs, grain, Brewer's yeast	may have hypoglycemic effect in some patients; most Americans do not receive enough	*no RDA; recommended (adults): 50 to 200 mcg*	toxicity rare, but reported to cause skin problems, liver/kidney disease, and even lung cancer; picolinate form has caused chromosomal damage to animals and rare nephrotoxicity, so chloride form may be preferred
Cinchona bark (quinine)	int: decreased appetite, dyspepsia, bloating	related to quinine-like drugs; may increase saliva, gastric juice production	*1 to 3 g herb or equivalent*	avoid if pregnant, allergic to quinine; rare thrombocytopenia; may sensitize to quinine
Cinnamon bark	int: decreased appetite, dyspepsia, bloating, flatulence	antibacterial, fungistatic, increases GI motility	*2 to 4 g bark or equivalent*	avoid in pregnancy; allergic skin reactions relatively common
Clivers	int: urinary tract inflammation, skin ulcers, rashes	limited scientific data	*tea as directed*	none known
Cloves	ext: topical anesthesia, oral/pharyngeal inflammation	antibacterial, antiviral, antifungal	*mouth washes with essential oil*	none known
Cocoa	int: diarrhea, liver/gallbladder dysfunction, UTIs	contains short-chained fatty acids; no therapeutic effect documented	*as directed*	avoid with migraines
Coenzyme Q10	int: cardiac insufficiency, angina, post-cardiac surgery, immunostimulant	important in ATP production as part of electron transport chain; immunostimulant properties (unproven)	*usually bid or tid as directed as supplement to conventional treatment*	none known; take with some fat to improve absorption
Coffee Charcoal	int: nonspecific diarrhea, mild oral/pharyngeal inflammation	acts as absorbent	*9 g or equivalent*	none known, although may influence absorption of other drugs
Cola Nut	int: mental/physical fatigue	contains methylxanthine, caffeine, similar compounds	*2 to 6 g or equivalent*	may cause insomnia, excitability, tachycardia, diuresis; avoid in peptic ulcer disease
Coltsfoot leaf	int: inflammation of oral/pharyngeal mucosa		*4.5 to 6 g of drug or equivalent*	avoid chronic use and in pregnancy or nursing
Comfrey herb/leaf/root	ext: contusions, sprains, dislocations	fosters callus production	*as directed*	avoid in pregnancy; do not apply to open skin or use internally; do not use more than 4-6 weeks (hepatotoxicity)

BOTANICALS

Herbs	Uses	Information	Daily Dose	Cautions
Condurango bark	int: decreased appetite	increases saliva, gastric juice production	*as directed*	none known
Copper	trace mineral; found in shellfish, nuts, other foods	important for Hb, collagen synthesis	*no RDA; recommended (adults): 2 to 3 mg*	avoid large doses while breastfeeding; take with zinc if taking supplement; balance may be affected by other minerals or antacids; high doses may cause GI side effects; dietary intake preferred to supplements
Coriander seed	int: decreased appetite, dyspepsia	limited scientific data	*3 g herb or equivalent*	avoid in gallstones; may cause allergic reaction
Corn Poppy	int: cough, colds, bronchitis, disturbed sleep	contains small amounts of alkaloids	*tea as directed*	reports of children poisoned with fresh foliage
Cornflower	int: dyspepsia, fever, URI	little evidence of effectiveness	*tea as directed*	small risk of sensitization reaction
Couch Grass	int: inflammation of urinary tract, prevention of urinary stones	contains saponins, essential oil (antimicrobial)	*6 to 9 g or equivalent*	avoid if edema due to CHF, renal failure; take with fluids
Cranberry	int: UTIs, urinary tract stones	may prevent E. Coli from adhering to wall of bladder	*juice or capsules bid to qid*	will not help once bacteria have taken hold; use pure juice, not cocktail or tablets; no known side effects/interactions
Creatine	int: muscle exhaustion, promotes muscle strength, CHF	formed naturally in liver; tends to pull water into muscles; more effective in sprint vs. endurance exercise; effect may be increased with insulin	*as directed during loading cycle, then maintenance*	avoid in renal disease; may lead to dehydration; do not use in pregnancy or breastfeeding
Cumin	int: dyspepsia	may have antimicrobial effect, especially vs. aspergillus	*as directed*	may prolong effect of barbiturates; used as abortifacent, so avoid in pregnancy
Cysteine	nonessential amino acid; changed into N-actetylcysteine (NAC); used for respiratory disease/ ARDS, hyperlipidemia, acetaminophen overdose, HIV, general health	NAC is changed to glutathione, a potent antioxidant (see glutathione)	*no RDA: both NAC and l-cysteine are available; doses depend on indication;: start with 500 mg for general health*	avoid high (> 7 mg) doses of NAC; oral NAC may cause GI side effects and may interact with ACE-inhibitors; IV NAC can cause hypotension with nitroglycerin
Daffodil	int: bronchitis, pertussis, asthma	limited scientific data	*as directed*	may rarely cause itchiness
Damiana leaf/herb	int: aphrodisiac, antidepressant	considered ineffective	*not recommended*	not recommended
Dandelion root/herb	int: digestive aid, diuretic, laxative	may increase bile production, acts as diuretic	*4 to 10 g of herb tid*	avoid in bile duct obstruction, ileus; may cause minor skin rash
Devil's Claw root	int: loss of appetite, dyspepsia	may increase bile production	*as directed*	avoid in peptic ulcer disease; use with caution with gallstones
DHEA	int: adrenal insufficiency, fatigue, sexual dysfunction	low DHEA levels associated with many diseases from Alzheimer's to SLE, but cause not determined; DHEA may be tested in blood or saliva	*as directed*	avoid if history of uterine, breast, cervical, or prostate cancer; avoid in pregnancy or if breastfeeding
Dill seed/herb	int: dyspepsia	may be antispasmodic, bacteriostatic; contains essential oil rich in carvone	*3 g or equivalent*	none known
Dong Quai root	int: PMS, amenorrhea, insomnia, anemia, HTN	may contain B-12, coumarin-like compounds	*as directed*	may cause photosensitization, bleeding, and rarely fever
Dyer's broom	int: emetic, bladder stones, gout, dyspepsia	limited scientific data	*1 to 2 cups infusion*	avoid during pregnancy/lactation
Echinacea Purpurea/ pallida/ augustfolia	int: supportive therapy for colds, flu-like illnesses; ext: wound healing	may act as immune stimulant by increasing phagocytosis; may induce TNF-alpha, IL-1, IL-6: may protect collagen	*as directed*	avoid with HIV, autoimmune diseases, Tb, MS; do not use for more than 8 weeks or during pregnancy; antibiotics may be given in addition; may cause GI symptoms if given IV
EDTA	used in chelation therapy for heavy metal toxicity and increasingly for heart disease, Parkinson's disease, arthritis	trials for CAD as alternative to surgery ongoing	*as directed*	must be given slowly (IV) in monitored setting; long-term effects unknown; overdose can cause organ failure
Elder flower	int: URIs	may increase bronchial secretion, cause sweating	*10 to 15 g drug or equivalent*	none known
Elecampane root	int: bronchitis, cough	may have antimicrobial, antihelminic effects	*1 g drug or equivalent*	severely irritating to mucous membranes; avoid during pregnancy; large amounts may cause vomiting, diarrhea, spasms, paralysis
English Chamomile	int: sluggishness of bowels, anxiety; ext: stomatitis, rhinitis, toothache	limited scientific data	*1.5 g drug tid or equivalent*	avoid during pregnancy; small risk of sensitization; used in manzanilla sherry (Spain) as flavoring agent

Herbs	Uses	Information	Daily Dose	Cautions
English Plantain	int: URIs, bronchitis, fevers, pharyngitis; ext: skin inflammation, wounds	has proven bactericidal effect - may increase blood clotting	*infusion with 2 to 4 g drug or equivalent; also syrups, lozenges, cough medications*	none known
Ephedra (Ma Huang)	int: mild bronchospasm, nasal decongestant	FDA issued warning in 1995	*equivalent of 15 to 30 mg total alkaloid (adults)*	contraindicated in glaucoma, HTN, thyroid dysfunction, BPH; may cause insomnia, motor restlessness, irritability, headaches, nausea/ vomiting, urinary dysfunction, tachycardia, arrhythmias; avoid with MAO-inhibitors, Parkinsonian agents, digoxin, antimigraine agents, antiarrythmics. Avoid in children. May be addictive.
Eryngo	int: UTIs, bronchitis, coughs	limited scientific data; no evidence of effectiveness	*tea as directed*	none known
Eucalyptus leaf	int: inflammation of respiratory tract	secretion, expectorant, weakly spasmolytic	*4 to 6 g of leaf or equivalent*	may rarely cause diarrhea, vomiting; may induce P450
Eucalyptus oil	int: inflammation of respiratory tract; ext: rheumatic complaints	secretomor, expectorant, weakly spasmolytic	*int: 0.3 to 0.6 g oil; ext: as directed*	avoid internally in liver disease, GI inflammation; avoid in young children; rare cause of vomiting and diarrhea; may induce P450
Evening Primrose oil	int: diverse complaints from GI sluggishness to PMS, mastalgia, dermatitis, chronic fatigue syndrome	gamma-linolenic acid (also found in fish) converted to PGE1 in vivo, has anti-inflammatory/ cell membrane stabilizing actions	*capsules 500 to 1,300 mg as directed*	may lower seizure threshold in patients with seizure disorders or on medications which do same: may require up to 3 months treatment
Eyebright	ext: eye inflammation, stye, coughs	limited scientific data	*tea or lotion as directed*	none known
Fennel seed/ oil/honey	int: mild dyspepsia, flatulence	stimulates GI motility	*0.1 to 0.6 g of herb or equivalent*	avoid in pregnancy; avoid fennel other than fennel honey in children; rare allergic reactions; avoid oil, as may cause vomiting or seizures
Fenugreek seed	int: anorexia, gout, diabetes, menstrual irregularity; ext: local inflammation	secretolytic, hyperemic	*int: 6 g drug or equivalent, ext: 50 g powder/l H2O*	avoid repeated external applications
Fever bark	int: fever, HTN	contains reserpine, echitamin	*infusion as directed*	alkaloid-type poisoning possible but rare
Feverfew	int: migraine, arthritis, rheumatism	contains parthenolide, which may inhibit thromboxane B2 and leukotriene B4; may inhibit platelet aggregation via serotonin	*200 to 250 mg qid (capsules) or equivalent*	may cause sensitization via skin contact; may cross-react with Tansy, Yarrow, Marguerite, Aster-Sunflower, Laurel, Liverwort; rebound headache, insomnia, muscle stiffness, and anxiety characterize post-feverfew syndrome in patients who stop taking drug abruptly; also reports of glossitis/stomatitis; may alter effects of anticoagulants or thrombolytics. Avoid during pregnancy.
Fish berry	int: scabies and similar infections, motion sickness/ dizziness	contains picotoxin, which acts as presynaptic inhibitor	*in combination preparations as directed with caution*	very toxic: may cause headache, dizziness, nausea, spasms, vomiting; two or three kernels may be fatal
Fish oils (Omega-3 Fatty Acids)	int: hypercholesterolemia	may decrease LDL while raising HDL	*no RDA: take as directed, but eating fish 3x/week preferred*	caution with anticoagulants; better to eat more fish, especially cod, mackerel, salmon; one serving usually gives 1-3 g omega-3's
Flaxseed	int: chronic constipation due to enteritis, IBS; heart disease; ext: local inflammation	contains albumin, alpha-linolenic acid, and other fatty acids; increases peristalsis and coats colonic mucosa	*as directed*	avoid with ileus; take with fluids; keep oil from heat and light; may affect coagulation studies in high doses
Folic Acid	vitamin found in leafy green vegetables, liver, other foods	essential for DNA replication and RBC production	*RDA (adults): 400 mg; 500 if breastfeeding; 800 mg if pregnant*	GI and CNS symptoms have been reported with very large doses
Frostwort	int: digestive disorders, especially peptic ulcer disease; ext: skin inflammation	limited scientific data	*liquid extract as directed*	none known
Fumitory	int: spastic discomfort of biliary and GI tracts	antispasmodic effect on GI tract	*6 g of herb or equivalent*	none known
Galangal	int: anorexia, dyspepsia	may inhibit prostaglandins, act as antispasmodic	*as directed*	none known
Gamboge	int: digestive disorders, especially constipation	contains mucilage, which confers strong laxative effect	*as directed, but use with caution*	abdominal pain and vomiting may occur with as little as 0.2 g drug; powdered resin may cause sneezing
Garlic	int: infections, hyperlipidemia, HTN, stroke prevention	contains allin, may enhance fibrinolysis, inhibit platelets, lower lipids; may have antiviral and antihelminic properties	*4 g fresh garlic or equivalent*	rare allergic reactions; may rarely cause changes to GI flora; avoid if on large amounts of ASA or anticoagulants

Herbs	Uses	Information	Daily Dose	Cautions
Gentian root	int: dyspepsia, anorexia, bloating, hepatitis, sexual infections	may increase saliva and gastric juice production; may have fungistatic and bacteriostatic effects	*as directed*	avoid in peptic ulcer disease, diarrhea, or obstruction; may rarely cause headaches
German Sarsaparilla root	int: gout, rheumatism, fever, UTIs	limited scientific data; no documented efficacy	*as directed*	none known
Ginger root	int: dyspepsia, prevention of motion sickness, antiemetic	may increase peristalsis, gastric juice/bile production	*2 to 4 g rhizome or equivalent*	caution with gallstones; no interactions known; do not use for morning sickness with pregnancy
Ginkgo Biloba leaf	int: vertigo/tinnitus, Alzheimer's disease, decreased cerebral blood flow, PVD, memory improvement	contains antioxidant flavones such as quercetin and kaempferol; may inhibit platelet-activating factor; may act as free-radical scavenger	*120 to 240 mg extract (dementia); 120 to 160 mg extract (PVD/ vertigo/tinnitus), 8 weeks minimum*	hypersensitivity- rare GI upset: may interfere with anticoagulants or alter PT/PTT
Ginseng root - American	int: diverse complaints, such as lethargy, atherosclerosis, DM, shock, sexual dysfunction	contains saponins, antioxidants, peptides, polysaccharides; may lower hyperglycemia in some diabetics	*1 to 2 g of root or equivalent*	may rarely cause insomnia, diarrhea, menopausal bleeding; note lack of standardized extracts; may slow heart and decrease oxygen needs
Siberian Ginseng root	int: general fatigue, lethargy	contains coumarin derivatives: may increase T-cells	*2 to 3 g of root or equivalent*	avoid with HTN: generally use for less than 3 months
Glucosamine	int: osteoarthritis, other degenerative diseases	sugar found in food and produced by body; stimulates production of proteoglycans	*usually 1000 to 2000 mg or as directed; dose may be affected by patient weight*	occasional mild GI side effects; often combined with chondroitin; does not affect NSAID efficacy
Glutamine	nonessential amino acid, found in many foods; used for many ailments including arthritis, autoimmune diseases, psychosis, GI inflammation, impotence, stress	any stress may deplete body's stores	*no RDA; 500 to 1500 mg often used*	contraindicated in kidney or liver disease or in hyperammonemia; take on empty stomach
Glutathione	primary intracellular antioxidant; used for liver disease, peptic ulcer disease, cataracts, cancer, Parkinson's disease, HIV, others	may be helpful in cystic fibrosis and post-chemotherapy, where oxidant stress is widespread; likely has immuno-stimulant, anti-carcinogenic effects	*no RDA; 500 mg bid often used*	little information; oral glutathione may not raise blood GSH levels: n-actetylcysteine (NAC) may be a better dietary source
Goat's Rue	int: UTIs, inflammation of urinary tract, hyperglycemia	contains galegin, which may lower blood sugar, although not documented in humans	*not recommended*	overdose in animals caused salivation, spasms, paralysis and death; theoretically could cause hypoglycemia; no demonstrated efficacy
Goldenrod	int: inflammation of urinary tract, prevention of nephrolithiasis	may act as diuretic	*6 to 12 g herb or equivalent*	avoid in edema from CHF or renal disease; drink large amounts of fluid
Goldenseal	int: URI, menorrhagia, mouth sores, diarrhea	increases saliva, gastric juice production	*as directed, often combined with echinacea*	may displace bilirubin from albumin; contraindicated in pregnancy or G-6-PD deficiency; may lower effectiveness of heparin; high doses have caused convulsions
Goldenthread	int: dyspepsia	contains berberine; limited scientific info	*as directed*	avoid during pregnancy
Gotu Kola	int: promote longevity, aphrodisiac, wound healing, hot flashes, rheumatism	Contains saponins that promote wound healing and decrease venous pressure insufficiency	*as directed*	none known
Grape seed/ leaf/fruit	int: hyperlipidemia, edema, venous insufficiency	contains proanthocyanidins (PCOs), antioxidants and LDL inhibitors, capillary wall stabilizers; may help poor vision due to retinal pathology	*many dosages of extract available, usually 150 to 600 mg daily*	none known
Greater Burnet	int: menopausal disorders, URIs, GI inflammation; ext: boils, wounds	limited scientific info	*as directed*	none known
Green Tea	int: diarrhea, indigestion, motion sickness	6x antioxidants as black tea; inhibit c. difficile, c. perfringens; may have cancer preventive effects; contains caffeine; may prevent dental caries	*many forms, as directed*	may cause GI symptoms; caution with renal disease, cardiovascular disease, anxiety, thyroid disease; avoid more than 5 cups daily if pregnant; avoid in nursing; reports of microcytic anemia in children
Guaiac wood	int: supportive therapy for rheumatic complaints		*4.5 g of drug or equivalent*	none known
Guarana	int: fatigue	contains caffeine, which has stimulatory and diuretic effects	*7 to 11 g powder or equivalent*	may lead to hypokalemia with chronic use; caution with thyroid disorders, anxiety, renal disease, cardiovascular disease; avoid in pregnancy/nursing

Herbs	Uses	Information	Daily Dose	Cautions
Gumweed herb	int: irritation of upper respiratory tract, cough	may have antibacterial properties	*4 to 6 g of drug or equivalent*	rare gastric irritation; no interactions known
Haronga bark/leaf	int: dyspepsia, mild exocrine pancreatic insufficiency	may increase bile production	*25 to 50 mg drug or equivalent*	avoid in gallstones, serious liver/biliary disease, ileus; may cause photosensitivity
Hawthorn leaf/flower	int: atherosclerosis, HTN	may act as positive inotrope, may increase coronary/myocardial perfusion	*as directed - 6 months minimum*	none known; avoid with MI or other serious heart disease; self-medication not recommended; leaf alone unproven
Hay flower	ext: anti-inflammatory, as in chronic arthritis	acts as topical hyperemic	*use as compress qid to bid*	avoid on open skin or with acute inflammation
Heart's Ease herb	ext: mild seborrheic skin ailments		*1.5 g of drug/ cup of water as tea*	none known
Heather herb/flower	int: prostate and urinary problems, liver/gallbladder disorders, gout, rheumatism	may have diuretic effect, although no proven efficacy	*add to water as directed*	none known
Hemp Nettle	int: mild respiratory inflammation	contains tannin and saponins	*6 g of herb or equivalent*	none known
Henbane leaf	int: spasms of GI tract, tremors	contains alkaloids such as hyoscyamine and scopolamine; inhibits ACh at muscarinic sites	*as directed*	avoid with tachyarrhythmias, BPH, narrow-angle glaucoma, acute pulmonary edema, GI obstruction, megacolon; may cause dry mouth, dry skin, tachycardia, tremor, difficult urination
Hibiscus	int: anorexia, URIs, constipation	may have laxative effect due to poorly absorbed fruit acids; may relax uterine muscle and vascular smooth muscle; no documented efficacy	*prepare tea as directed*	none known
Hollyhock flower	int: bronchitis, fever, cough; ext: wounds, ulcers	limited scientific info; no documented effects	*prepare tea as directed*	none known
Hops	int: restlessness, anxiety, anorexia	unknown efficacy or mechanism	*single dose: 0.5 g*	none known
Horehound	int: dyspepsia, bloating, flatulence	may increase bile production	*4.5 g of drug or equivalent*	none known
Horse Chestnut seed/leaf	int: chronic venous insufficiency, pruritus, edema	seeds contain aescin, which may have anti-exudative, vascular-tightening effect	*seed: 250 to 312.5 mg extract bid; leaf: prepare tea as directed*	seed may cause occasional GI complaints, hepatotoxicity, urticaria; leaf contains coumarins and may interact with warfarin, ASA, other anticoagulants
Horseradish	ext: minor muscle aches, inflammation of respiratory tract	may have antimicrobial, hyperemic properties	*20 g of fresh root or equivalent*	avoid with peptic ulcer disease or in children under 4
Horsetail	ext: wound healing; int: edema, irrigation therapy for urinary tract stones	contains silicic acid and flavonoids; may act as diuretic	*int: 6 g of herb or equivalent*	avoid with edema from CHF or renal disease; drink copious amounts of water
Hound's Tongue	ext: wounds; int: diarrhea	contains alkaloids which may be toxic	*avoid*	avoid folk medicinal preparations at all costs! hepatotoxic and hepatocarcinogenic
Hyssop	int: URIs, circulatory stimulation, liver/gallbladder dysfunction	may have antimicrobial, antiviral effects, especially vs. herpes simplex; no documented efficacy	*capsules 445 mg qid*	avoid during pregnancy; high doses may slightly increase seizure risk
Iceland Moss	int: anorexia, pharyngitis with cough, antiemetic, anemia	may act as demulcent	*4 to 6 g of herb or equivalent*	none known; avoid large amounts or chronic use due to possible lead content
Ignatius beans	int: faintness, anxiety, cramping (homeopathic doses)	contains strychnine and brucine, acts as psychoanaleptic	*avoid*	very toxic due to strychnine; avoid at all costs in allopathic doses; overdose may occur after one bean
Immortelle	int: dyspepsia	has antibacterial properties; increases bile production	*3 g of drug or equivalent*	avoid in biliary obstruction or cholethiasis
Indian Hemp	int: cardiac insufficiency, diuretic; ext: condylomas, warts	contains digitalis-like glycosides	*as directed, with caution*	causes irritation of mucous membranes, vomiting; use only if expert with this drug; overdose similar to digitalis
Indian Snakeroot	int: mild HTN, especially with anxiety	contains reserpine and alkaloids, which have alpha- and ß-blocking properties	*600 mg drug or equivalent*	avoid with depression, ulcers, pheochromocytoma, pregnancy, lactation; side effects may include stuffy nose, depressive mood, fatigue, reduction in sexual potency; may decrease ability to drive or operate machines; avoid with alcohol, digitalis, barbiturates, L-dopa, sympathomimetics

Herbs	Uses	Information	Daily Dose	Cautions
Indian Squill	int: cardiac insufficiency, cardiogenic edema, cough	contains cardioactive glycosides; may function as expectorant	*60 to 200 mg single dose or equivalent*	limited therapeutic range; may cause GI complaints; contraindicated with 1st or 2nd degree AV block, hypercalcemia, hypokalemia, hypertrophic cardiomyopathy, carotid sinus syndrome, ventricular tachycardia, aortic aneurysm, WPW; caution with anti-arrhythmics
Inositol	part of vitamin B complex; found in beans, fruit, meat; used for neurologic disorders, depression, diabetic neuropathy, hyperlipidemia	component of lecithin- may be important in nerve conduction: little scientific info	*no RDA: usually no more than 500 to 1000 mg*	none known, no information about pregnancy/nursing; may have dairy base
Iodine	mineral used in treating thyroid disease, fibrocystic breast disease, breast cancer, vaginitis, wounds	iodine deficiency rare in U.S.	*RDA: (adults): 150 mcg, 175 mcg if pregnant, 200 mcg if nursing*	iodine toxicity may affect thyroid; may interact with lithium; some foods such as cabbage and soybeans may inhibit iodine uptake in GI tract
Ipecac	int: emetic, expectorant, amebic dysentery		*tincture or extract as directed*	frequent contact may cause allergic reaction of skin; acts as emetic at higher doses
Iron	mineral, used for Fe-deficiency anemia	will not cause guaiac + stools	*RDA (men): 10 mg, (women): 18 mg; usually dose is 65 mg tid*	vitamin C increases absorption, calcium decreases absorption; iron inhibits absorption of drugs such as L-dopa, penicillamine, quinolones, tetracycline; antacids may decrease oral Fe absorption; can cause constipation; caution in first trimester of pregnancy
Ivy leaf	int: chronic respiratory inflammation. cough, bronchitis	contains saponins; may act as expectorant or antispasmodic; may have antibacterial/ antiviral effects	*0.3 g of drug or equivalent*	none known
Jambolan bark	int: nonspecific diarrhea, pharyngitis; ext: mild inflammation of skin	contains tannins; may act as astringent	*3 to 6 g of drug or equivalent*	none known
Java Tea	int: irrigation therapy for inflammation of urinary tract	contains lipophilic flavones, large amounts of potassium salts; may act as diuretic	*6 to 12 g herb or equivalent*	avoid with edema from CHF or renal disease; give with copious amounts of water
Jimsonweed leaf/seed	int: cough, bronchitis, pertussis, nervous system disorders such as Parkinson's	contains variable amounts of alkaloids such as scopolamine with anti-ACh effects similar to belladonna	*not recommended*	contraindicated in glaucoma, tachyarrhythmias, BPH/urinary retention, acute pulmonary edema, GI obstruction, atherosclerosis, megacolon; overdose similar to atropine; use not recommended due to non-standardization
Juniper berry	int: dyspepsia, diuretic	may increase urine output and stimulate smooth muscle contraction	*as directed*	chronic use may be nephrotoxic; avoid in pregnancy or nephritis
Kava Kava	int: anxiety, restlessness	may act as anxiolytic, antispasmodic, anticonvulsant	*60 to 120 mg kava pyrones or equivalent*	avoid in pregnancy, lactation, depression; may cause yellow skin, hair, or nails; may affect oculomotor function; may potentiate effects of alcohol, barbiturates, psychoactive drugs; may affect ability to drive or operate machinery; avoid use longer than 3 months
Kelp	int: regulation of thyroid function	contains various amounts of iodine	*no information*	allergic reactions may occur; may worsen hyperthyroidism, depending on iodine content
Knotweed	int: cough, bronchitis	contains tannins, silicic acid; may inhibit acetyl cholinesterase	*4 to 6 g of drug or equivalent*	none known
Lactobacillius acidophilus	int/ext: yeast and other sexual/GI infections, lactose intolerance, irritable bowel syndrome; found in yogurt, milk, and as supplement	helpful bacteria which produce lactase and lactic acid	*vaginitis: 1-2 billion live organisms; otherwise as directed*	mild GI upset in large doses; penicillins may deplete l. acidophilus; may affect sulfasalazine metabolism
Lady's Mantle	int: nonspecific diarrhea, anorexia, menstrual dysfunction	may act as astringent	*5 to 10 g of herb or equivalent*	rare hepatotoxicity
LaPacho	int: fungal and other infections	has antifungal, antiviral, and antibacterial properties as uncoupler of ox-phos; may have some antineoplastic effects	*as directed*	caution in children; avoid in pregnancy or if nursing; unrefined bark may be safest preparation; overdose may cause bleeding or vomiting
Larch Turpentine	ext: rheumatism, neurologic complaints, inflammation of respiratory tract	member of the Balsam family	*as directed*	topical administration may cause allergic reaction
Lavender flower	int: mood disturbances, anxiety, insomnia, abdominal complaints	may act as sedative, antiflatulent	*as directed*	may be used as bath therapy

Herbs	Uses	Information	Daily Dose	Cautions
Lecithin	int: hyperlipidemia	used by body to handle cholesterol and other fats; may help prevent atherosclerosis	*no RDA, as directed*	nicotinic acid (niacin) treatment for hyperlipidemia may deplete lecithin
Lemongrass	int: antipyretic, indigestion	limited scientific info; no proven effects	*prepare infusion as directed*	avoid inhalation of oil vapors, as may cause lung problems
Lesser Celandine	ext: bleeding wounds, swollen joints	contains tannins and large amounts of vitamin C	*as bath or extract*	extended contact to fresh plant may cause blisters; internal consumption may irritate GI and urinary tracts
Licorice root	int: inflammation of respiratory tract, peptic ulcers	contains coumarins, calcium, and potassium salts; may act as antitussive, anti-inflammatory agent; may have mineralocorticoid effects in high doses	*5 to 15 g of root or equivalent*	avoid in hypokalemia, pregnancy, heart disease, renal insufficiency, cirrhosis; hypokalemia with digitalis and diuretics may occur; do not use longer than 4-6 weeks without advice
Life root	int: uterine dysfunction, abortifacent, diuretic, urinary tract dysfunction	may contain toxic alkaloids		hepatotoxicity may occur; some experts do not recommend use of this drug
Lily of the Valley	int: mild CHF, chronic cor pulmonale	contains cardioactive glycosides, acting similar to digitalis	*as directed*	avoid with digitalis, hypokalemia; may cause nausea, vomiting, arrhythmias; may potentiate effects of quinidine, calcium, saluretics, laxatives, and glucocorticoids
Linden flower/ wood	int: URIs, cough (flower), liver/gallbladder disorders (wood)	little scientific data; contains tannins, glycosides, and flavonoids, which show anti-edema and antimicrobial effects in animals	*2 to 4 g of drug or equivalent*	none known
Lobelia	int: asthma, emetic, smoking addiction (homeopathic doses)	stimulates respiratory center but quickly metabolized	*homeopathic preparations only*	not used in allopathic doses; signs of overdose: dry mouth, vomiting, anxiety, sweating
Lovage root	int: irrigation therapy for urinary tract	contains essential oil and coumarin derivatives	*4 to 8 g of drug or equivalent*	avoid if edema due to CHF or renal disease
Lungwort	int: bronchitis, cough, diuretic; ext: wounds	contains polysaccharides and tannins with expectorant and soothing effects; limited efficacy documented	*prepare tea as directed*	none known
Lycium	int: fever, HTN, improving hepatic and renal circulation	may have immunoregulatory and hypoglycemic effects, especially L. barbarum; limited scientific data	*as directed*	avoid in chronic inflammatory states; avoid during pregnancy/ nursing
Lysine	essential amino acids, found in meat, cheese, soybeans, other foods; used in osteoporosis, cardiovascular disease, asthma, migraines	used in collagen production and fatty acid metabolism	*no RDA: recommended (adults): 12 mg/kg*	may in some cases increase cholesterol or triglycerides; otherwise nontoxic
Madder root	int: nephrolithiasis	contains inhibitor of calcium oxalate crystals in kidney; rubiadins are possibly carcinogenic	*not recommended*	lucidin is mutagenic; avoid this drug
Magnesium	found in green vegetables, fish, dairy products, nuts; used in constipation, Crohn's disease, HTN, stroke, preeclampsia, others	Important to normal bone structure and it plays an essential role in 300 fundamental cellular reactions	*RDA (men): 350 mg, (women): 300 mg*	avoid large doses while breastfeeding; toxicity includes GI and cardiovascular effects; avoid in kidney or heart disease; salt, sugar, caffeine, alcohol, fiber, riboflavin in high doses, insulin, diuretics, and digitalis may cause Mg loss; other ions such as Ca may interfere with Mg metabolism
Maidenhair	int: cough, bronchitis, menstrual disorders	may act as demulcent and expectorant	*prepare tea as directed*	avoid during pregnancy; no side effects known
Maitake	int: immune stimulant, HTN, diabetes	contains polysaccharide beta-D-glucan which may have immunostimulant properties	*may be eaten or taken as tea*	no information
Male Fern root/frond	int (root): liver fluke, band worms, viral infections; ext: (herb): muscle pains, neuralgia, toothache, earache, wounds	strongly antihelminic properties, but very toxic	*homeopathic preparations only*	highly toxic--avoid internal consumption!
Mallow flower/ leaf	int: pharyngitis associated with cough	may act as demulcent	*5 g of drug or equivalent*	none known
Manganese	mineral found in grains, nuts, beans, vegetables	needed for blood sugar control and in many other functions	*no RDA; recommended (adults): 2.5 to 5.0 mg*	overdose may include mood disorders; avoid in pregnancy/ nursing; may affect blood clotting
Manna	int: stool softener	contains mannitol	*adults: 20 to 30 g of drug or equivalent*	avoid in bowel obstruction; occasional nausea, flatulence; avoid chronic use

BOTANICAL

Herbs	Uses	Information	Daily Dose	Cautions
Marjoram	int: URIs, mild abdominal pain	may have antimicrobial, antiviral, and insecticidal effects	*prepare tea as directed*	none known
Marshmallow leaf/root	int: pharyngitis and cough	anti-inflammatory properties; root may stimulate phagocytosis and inhibit mucociliary activity	*5 g of leaf, 6 g of root or equivalent*	may decrease absorption of other drugs
Maté	int: mental and physical fatigue	contains caffeine; may have diuretic, lipolytic, glycogenolytic, positive chronotropic and inotropic effects	*3 g of drug or equivalent*	syrup may contain sugar, so diabetics should avoid
Mayapple root/resin	ext: removal of pointed condyloma	resin contains podophyllotoxin	*1.5 to 3 g root or equivalent*	avoid in pregnancy; treated area must be smaller than 25 cm2; protect adjacent area
Meadowsweet	int: supportive therapy for URIs	contains flavonoids, glycosides, and salicylates	*2.5 to 3.5 g flower or 4 to 5 g herb*	avoid if ASA-allergic
Melatonin	int: insomnia, jet lag, seasonal affective disorder	naturally produced by pineal gland from trytophan; low melatonin seen in many cancer patients; long-term effects unknown	*1 to 3 mg about 20 min before bedtime*	contraindicated in autoimmune diseases, HIV, heart disease, leukemia; avoid if you are trying to conceive; take only at bedtime; avoid driving; caution in patients on NSAIDs, steroids, ß-blockers, benzodiazepines; may test blood levels
Milk Thistle fruit	int: alone for dyspepsia, in formulations for hepatitis/ cirrhosis	contains silymarin, which may be hepatoprotective by altering hepatocyte cell membranes or protein synthesis	*12 to 15 g or equivalent*	none known; may have mild laxative effect; milk thistle herb is of doubtful benefit
Mint oil	int: flatulence, GI distress, liver/gallbladder complaints, URIs, fevers, pharyngitis; ext: myalgia, neuralgia	contains menthol, which cools skin; may increase bile production and have antibacterial properties	*as directed*	avoid internal use in biliary obstruction, cholecystitis, liver disease; avoid external use with children and on face; oil may exacerbate asthma; occasional GI upset as side effect
Molybdenum	trace mineral; found in vegetables, meats, other foods	deficiency can lead to tooth decay and anemia	*no RDA: recommended (adults): 15 to 50 mcg; supplement by prescription*	high doses can cause swollen joints; may decrease copper levels with supplementation
Monk's Hood	int: neuralgia, especially trigeminal; rheumatism, migraine; ext: skin inflammation	contains aconitin, which affects Na permeability in nerve ends; topically, has burning then anesthetizing effect	*not recommended*	highly toxic: signs of toxicity occur even with therapeutic doses; tingling of extremities is often first sign; may cause arrhythmias with overdose; drug is not recommended due to toxicity
Morning Glory	int: constipation, worm infections	contains resins with drastic laxative effects	*0.5 to 3.0 g drug or equivalent*	possibly teratogenic, so avoid during pregnancy; cramp-like pain is occasional side effect
Motherwort	int: used for cardiac disorders associated with anxiety, adjunct in hyperthyroidism	limited scientific data	*4.5 g herb or equivalent*	avoid with pregnancy; have uterine stimulating properties
Mountain Ash berry	int: kidney disease, diabetes, rheumatism, gout, diarrhea	contains vitamin C; little documented efficacy	*puree for diarrhea - otherwise no information*	popular ingredient in juices, jellies; cooking berries nearly eliminates incidence of GI side effects
Mugwort	int: GI infections, dyspepsia	may have antimicrobial effects; little documented efficacy	*not recommended for internal consumption*	avoid during pregnancy; used in Chinese technique of moxibustion, which is related to acupuncture
Muira Puama	ext: sexual disorders such as impotence; int: diarrhea, anorexia, sexual disorders	limited scientific data, no documented effect	*0.5 g drug or equivalent*	none known
Mullein flower	int: irritation of respiratory tract	contains saponins and mucopolysaccharides; may act as expectorant	*3 to 4 g of herb or equivalent*	none known
Myrrh	int: inflammation of respiratory tract, gingivitis, stomatitis	may act as antiseptic, astringent	*as directed as resin - tincture - gargle*	none known; used in commercial mouthwash, soaps, flavorings, cosmetics
Myrtle leaf/oil	int: bronchitis and other respiratory infections, diarrhea, cystitis, prostatitis	leaves show antimicrobial activity	*infusion as directed*	leaves contraindicated in chronic inflammatory states, liver disease, biliary stasis; avoid oil on face of children, as may trigger bronchial spasm; overdoses may be life-threatening
Nasturtium	int: UTIs, bronchitis, cough	contains benzyl mustard oil, which has antibacterial, antiviral, and antifungal effects	*tablets or infusion: add 30 g leaves to 1 L H2O*	contraindicated with peptic ulcers or renal disease; avoid in children; high or chronic doses can lead to mucous membrane or skin irritation
Niacin	water-soluble vitamin, used for tinnitus, PMS headaches, and in high doses for hyperlipidemia; found in meat, fish, poultry, other foods	important for DNA synthesis, many other functions	*RDA (men): 16 to 18 mg, (women): 14 mg, 18 mg if breastfeeding*	toxicity may include ulcers, GI symptoms, jaundice (only nicotinic acid form)

Herbs	Uses	Information	Daily Dose	Cautions
Niauli oil	ext./int: inflammation of respiratory tract, neuralgia, wounds, burns	contains cajeput oil; may act as antibacterial, circulatory stimulant; contains cineol, which may induce P450	*as directed*	rare GI distress with internal use; cajeput oil alone may cause life-threatening poisonings and should not be applied to faces of children; cajeput oil contraindicated in inflammation of GI tract, biliary tract, liver
Night-blooming Cereus	int: UTIs, angina, hemoptysis, menorrhagia	may have similar effect to digitalis	*fluid extract up to 0.6 ml to 10 times daily*	fresh juice may cause itching, rash, and vomiting; otherwise none known
Notoginseng root	int/ext: external bleeding, angina; ext: fractures, swelling, wounds	may have procoagulant properties	*no information*	occasional dry mouth, anxiety, insomnia, nausea; avoid during pregnancy, as may cause miscarriage
Nutmeg	int: indigestion, diarrhea/GI inflammation, liver disease	may decrease GI motility via effect on prostaglandins	*as directed*	avoid during pregnancy; may occasionally cause dermatitis; ingestion of "nuts" may produce amphetamine-like compounds; overdose may be signaled by red face, thirst, nausea, and occasional hallucinations
Nux Vomica	int: various GI complaints, anxiety/depression, migraine	contains strychnine and brucine, glycine antagonists	*not recommended in allopathic doses*	very toxic--do not use! similar to Ignatius beans
Oak bark	int: nonspecific diarrhea, anal/genital inflammation; ext: inflammation of skin	contains tannins; may have virustatic effects	*as directed*	ext: may cause skin damage in some cases; avoid baths with eczema, heart disease; may inhibit alkaloid-type drugs; use not recommended for more than 2-3 weeks
Oat straw/ herb/fruit	ext: inflammatory and itchy skin disease, warts (straw), hyperlipidemia (fruit)	fruit may have anti-lipid polysaccharides; limited data about herb and straw	*straw: bath as directed; others as directed*	none known
Oleander leaf	int: heart failure	similar to digitalis, with positive inotropic, negatively chronotropic effects	*no information - not recommended*	consumption has led to fatal poisonings; no longer used for nausea, vomiting, diarrhea, arrhythmias; avoid in pregnancy; may increase effects of quinidine, calcium salts, laxatives, diuretics, steroids; poisoning similar to digitalis
Olive leaf/oil	ext: (oil): psoriasis, eczema, sunburns, burns; int (oil): cholangitis, cholecystitis, atherosclerosis; (leaf) constipation	leaf may possess antiarrhythmic, spasmolytic, hypotensive effects; oil contains polyunsaturated, monounsaturated fatty acids	*various preparations*	contraindicated in gallstones
Omega-6 Fatty Acids	eye disease, heart disease, cancer; found in vegetable oils, oils of evening primrose, black currant, borage	gamma-lineolic acid may be important anti-inflammatory agent	*no RDA, often 1.4 g GLA for rheumatoid arthritis*	none known
Onion	int: anorexia, prevention of atherosclerosis	contains allein and similar sulfur compounds, essential oil, peptides, and flavonoids; may show anti-platelet, antibacterial effects	*50 g of fresh onions or equivalent*	none known
Oregano	int: cough, bronchitis	essential oil has antimicrobial properties; contains thymol (in commercial anti-cold medications)	*various preparations: infusions, gargles, powders*	none known
Orris root	int: cough, bronchitis	mild expectorant, may have antiulcer properties	*used primarily in homeopathic doses*	none known; juice of fresh plant may irritate skin and, if ingested, GI tract; avoid during pregnancy
Pancreatic enzymes	int: digestive disorders, autoimmune diseases, inflammatory diseases; ext: trauma	may affect fibrinolysis, complement cascade	*as directed*	contraindicated in coagulopathies, liver disease; may cause GI side effects, pale stools, allergic reactions, skin irritation with external application; no pregnancy studies
Papaya leaf	int: pancreatic enzyme deficiency, inflammation/ infection of GI tract; ext: skin ulcers (papain)	contains papain, used for healing of severe wounds and ulcers, as it dissolves dead tissue; may also have fibrinolytic effect	*ointments with papain by prescription*	avoid during pregnancy (teratogenic); documented interactions with warfarin, prolonging PT; allergic reactions known
Parsley herb/ root/seed	int: inflammation of urinary tract, urinary tract stones	may act as diuretic; seed may increase uterine tone	*herb/root: 6 g of prepared drug or equivalent*	avoid in pregnancy, nephritis; may cause photodermatitis; take copious amounts of fluid; essential oil may be toxic
Parsnip herb/root	int (herb): kidney, GI complaints, (root): kidney stones, fever	limited scientific data	*one handful/one liter H2O of tea as directed*	can increase photosensitivity in fair-skinned patients
Pasque flower	int: fever, GI inflammation, genital disorders, skin inflammation	may have antimicrobial, antipyretic, and GI spasmolytic effects	*use only with caution*	contraindicated during pregnancy; fresh plant may cause ulcers if contacts skin or GI distress if ingested; animals have died after large ingestions of similar plants

BOTANICAL

Herbs	Uses	Information	Daily Dose	Cautions
Passion Flower	int: anxiety, headaches, epilepsy, neuralgia, GI complaints associated with anxiety	may have both sedative and stimulant effects	*4 to 8 g of herb or equivalent*	none known
Pennyroyal	int: dyspepsia, liver/ gallbladder complaints; ext: skin inflammation	hepatotoxic effects preclude use	*external use only*	contraindicated during pregnancy; use oil externally only
Peony flower/ root	int: hemorrhoids, rheumatism	flower isolates may promote uterine contraction, GI relaxation, and hypotension	*infusion as directed*	overdoses may cause vomiting, abdominal pain; no efficacy demonstrated
Peppermint leaf	int: spasms of GI tract and gallbladder	may have direct antispasmodic effects on GI smooth muscle; may increase bile production	*3 to 6 g of leaf or equivalent*	avoid with gallstones or in small children due to possible choking sensation from menthol
Peppermint oil	int: spasms of GI tract and gallbladder, oral mucositis; ext: myalgia, neuralgia	may have similar actions to peppermint leaf; may have antimicrobial actions	*6 to 12 drops or equivalent*	avoid use on face of children: avoid in biliary obstruction- liver disease- gallstones
Perilla	int: cough, URIs, constipation, oral inflammation	may have antimicrobial and sedative effects; may lower serum lipids; little scientific data	*extract 3 to 10 g or equivalent*	avoid in pregnancy due to potential mutagenicity; one study showed pulmonary edema in sheep
Periwinkle	int: circulatory dysfunction (especially cerebral), hemorrhage; ext: skin inflammation	contains vincamine, which lowers BP and HR, also spasmolytic and hypoglycemic effects	*infusion or tea as directed*	flushing and GI symptoms may occur; overdose may cause severe hypotension
Peruvian Balsam	ext: hemorrhoids, wound healing, ulcers, burns	may have antiparasitic actions, especially for scabies; may promote granulation process	*as directed*	allergic skin reactions well known; use for more than one week not recommended
Petasites root/leaf	int: supportive therapy for pain associated with urinary stones	may have antispasmodic actions; may inhibit leukotrienes; pyrrolizidine alkaloids may be carcinogenic, hepatotoxic, and teratogenic; must check alkaloid content	*4.5 to 7 g drug or equivalent*	avoid with pregnancy or nursing; use for more than 4-6 weeks not recommended; check pyrrolizidine alkaloid content before using
Pheasant's Eye herb	int: mild cardiac insufficiency, especially with anxiety	contains cardioactive glycosides and flavonoids; may be positively inotropic	*0.6 g of standardized powder*	avoid with digitalis, hypokalemia; may cause nausea, vomiting, arrhythmias; may potentiate effects of quinidine, calcium, laxatives, and glucocorticoids
Phenylalanine	essential amino acid, as body cannot make enough; found in cheese, meat, eggs, fish, yeast, aspartame	converted by body to tyrosine	*no RDA: recommended (adults): 14 mg/kg*	may cause anxiety, headaches, HTN; contraindicated in PKU, pregnancy, breastfeeding; may compete with L-dopa; little pregnancy data about aspartame
Phosphatidyl-serine	phospholipid in brain, used for Alzheimer's disease and depression in elderly	critical layer in neurotransmitter release; semisynthetic prepared from soy; limited scientific data	*100 mg tid commonly used*	none known; pregnancy data unknown
Phosphorus	mineral found throughout body; found in meat, fish, milk; used for kidney stones as K-phos	innumerable functions in body, especially as ATP, and in tissue repair	*RDA (adults): 800 mg, 1200 mg if pregnant/nursing*	hyperphosphatemia
Phyllanthus	int: diabetes, gonorrhea, menstrual dysfunction, hepatitis B	may block enzyme crucial for hep B replication	*trials have used 900 to 2700 mg*	no information; used extensively in Indian medicine
Pimpinella root/herb	int: cough, bronchitis	contains essential oil and saponins	*6 to 12 g root or equivalent*	none known
Pine oil/ sprouts	int/ext: inflammation of respiratory tract; ext: rheumatic complaints	may decrease secretions	*as directed, oil may be applied or inhaled*	avoid in asthma, pertussis; skin and membrane irritation may occur
Plantain	int: inflammation of oral mucosa; ext: skin inflammation	may have astringent and antibacterial properties	*3 to 6 g of herb or equivalent*	none known; in 1997 FDA warned some products actually contained digitalis
Poke root/fruit	int: rheumatism, skin ulcers, pharyngitis, dyspepsia	fruit may have hepatoprotective, antiviral, and emetic effects; root may have anti-edema and immunostimulant effects; saponins and lectins are toxic	*use with caution*	symptoms of poisoning include diarrhea, hypotension, and vomiting; children particularly susceptible
Pollen	int: lethargy, anorexia	limited scientific data	*30 to 40 g of drug or equivalent*	avoid in pollen-allergic patients; rare GI side effects
Pomegranate	int: URIs, diarrhea, worm infections	contains alkaloids which are antihelminic	*as directed*	avoid in pregnancy; overdose may cause vomiting, dizziness, respiratory compromise
Poplar bud	ext: superficial skin inflammation, frostbite, sunburn	contains essential oil, flavonoids, and phenol glycosides; may promote wound healing with some antibacterial properties	*as directed*	occasional skin reactions

Herbs	Uses	Information	Daily Dose	Cautions
Poppyseed	int: cough, pain	contains morphine, codeine, papaverine	*as directed*	opium no longer used as medication; contraindicated in pregnancy, reduced respiratory function, elevated ICP, biliary colic; caution with Addison's disease and hypothyroidism; overdose may include respiratory failure, vomiting, edema, spasms
Potentilla	int: dysmenorrhea, nonspecific diarrhea	may increase uterine tone	*4 to 6 g of herb or equivalent*	may irritate GI tract
Primrose flower/root	int: bronchitis, cough	may act as secretolytic, expectorant	*flower: 2 to 4 g of drug or equivalent; root: 0.5 to 1.5 g of drug*	occasional GI upset; allergies to primrose documented
Psyllium seed/husk-black/blonde	int: chronic constipation, IBS, also secondarily for diarrhea associated with irritable bowel	FDA-approved as laxative; may promote peristalsis, may increase volume of stool	*as directed*	avoid in stenosis/obstruction of esophagus or GI tract; rare allergic reactions; blonde psyllium may create difficulty with diabetes management and may decrease absorption of other drugs; must take adequate amounts of fluids; may lower serum cholesterol
Pumpkin seed	int: irritated bladder, urinary dysfunction with mild BPH	contain scucurbitin, phytosterol in free and bound forms, s- and gamma-tocopherol, selenium	*10 g of seed or equivalent*	may relieve symptoms of BPH without treating BPH itself
Pygeum	int: BPH, male impotence	contains three types of compounds that may act against BPH by inhibition of prostaglandins, prolactin; less effective than saw palmetto when compared in one study	*extract: 50 to 100 mg bid*	may cause GI irritation; must allow 6-9 months for drug to work
Pyrethrum	ext: infections with scabies, lice, other insects	may have neurotoxic effects on lower insects	*liquid extract as directed*	none known; overdose may cause neurotoxicity; wash area after use
Pyruvate (with dihydroxy-acetone)	int: weight loss, endurance exercise-enhancer	product of glucose in glycolysis; may increase fat loss in addition to exercise in obese populations; limited data	*no information*	no information
Radish	int: dyspepsia, especially associated with biliary tract	contains mustard oil glycosides and essential oil; may act as secretagogue, promote GI motility	*50 to 100 ml pressed juice or equivalent*	avoid with gallstones
Raspberry leaf	int: menorrhagia, uterine stimulant, menstrual cramps, laxative	contains tannins that have astringent properties	*use with caution, as directed*	no information--use at own risk
Red Clover	ext: eczema, acne; int: bronchitis, cough	may have antispasmodic and expectorant effects; aids in skin healing	*4 g drug or equivalent*	none known; avoid fermented herb
Red Sandalwood	int: dyspepsia, diabetes, cough, toothache	extracts have hypoglycemic effects in animals; limited scientific info	*primarily as tea*	none known
Red Yeast Rice	int: high cholesterol	natural component, mevinolin, inhibits HMG-CoA reductase	*1200 mg or equivalent*	may be hepatotoxic in high doses; contraindicated in pregnancy or nursing; avoid during infections, post-surgery; rhabdomyolysis possible
Red-Rooted Sage	int: angina, menstrual dysfunction, furuncles, joint pain	increase in coronary blood flow noted; may also have antithrombotic, anti-inflammatory, and hepatoprotective effects; limited scientific info	*9 to 15 mg drug or equivalent*	none known
Reishi	int: asthma, cough, insomnia, HTN, hyperlipidemia, immunomodulator	may have sedative effect on CNS, may lower cholesterol; may enhance immune function via production of IL-2	*dried mushroom: 1.5 to 9 g or equivalent;: syrup: 4 to 6 ml*	caution with anticoagulants, as may heighten effects; avoid while pregnant or nursing
Rhatany root	int/ext: mild inflammation of pharyngeal/oral mucosa	may act as astringent; contains tannins	*as directed*	very rare allergic reactions; use greater than 2 weeks not recommended
Rhododendron-Rusty-leaved	int: rheumatism, gout, HTN, migraine, neuralgia	limited scientific data	*not recommended*	not recommended; overdose may cause arrhythmias, cold sweats, stupor, and death
Rhubarb root-	int: constipation	1-8-dihydroxy-anthracene derivatives have a laxative effect via increasing GI motility, increased Cl- secretion	*as directed*	may cause GI discomfort or hypokalemia, so caution with steroids, diuretics, glycosides; avoid during pregnancy and nursing; use only if diet/lifestyle not effective; avoid chronic use
Rose Flower	int: mild inflammation of oral, pharyngeal mucosa	contains tannins; may act as astringent	*1 to 2 g drug/cup H2O for tea*	none known

BOTANICALS

Herbs	Uses	Information	Daily Dose	Cautions
Rose Hip fruit/shell	Int: (fruit): immunostimulator; (shells): UTIs, kidney disease, gout	fruit contains pectin and acids which have diuretic and laxative effects; shells are source of vitamin C	*shell: prepared tea from powder as directed; fruit: found in vitamin supplements*	none known
Rosemary leaf	int: dyspepsia; ext: rheumatic complaints, circulatory dysfunction	may stimulate blood supply via irritation; may decrease spasms of biliary system; may be positively inotropic, may increase coronary perfusion	*as directed*	none known
Rue	int: PMS, menstrual disorders; ext: skin inflammation	may have fertility-inhibiting, spasmolytic effects	*tea or external application as directed*	generally avoid, due to toxicity which may include photosensitivity, abortion, GI complaints, renal failure, and death
Rupturewort	int: UTIs, respiratory inflammation, gout, rheumatism	limited data suggest possible diuretic and spasmolytic effects	*infusion or tea as directed*	none known
Sage leaf	int: dyspepsia, excessive sweating; ext: inflammations of membranes of nose-throat	contains thujone- cineol- and camphor: may inhibit viruses- fungi- and bacteria: may inhibit perspiration	*as directed*	essential oil and alcoholic extracts should not be used internally during pregnancy; some experts question if internal use is safe at all
Sandalwood	int: supportive therapy for UTI, URI, bronchitis	may be antibacterial and antispasmodic	*1 to 1.5 g essential oil or equivalent*	avoid in renal disease: may cause nausea or urticaria: use enteric-coated form: use for more than 6 weeks not recommended
Sanicle	int: inflammation of respiratory tract	contains saponins	*4 to 6 g of drug or equivalent*	none known
Sarsaparilla root	int: anabolic steroid, constipation, rheumatic complaints, URI, psoriasis	some evidence to support diuretic, expectorant, laxative effects: no evidence of steroid activity	*as directed*	none known
Savin Tops	ext: warts	very irritating to internal and external membranes: lignans and podophyllotoxins may have antiviral properties	*powder or ointment as directed*	avoid internal administration - may cause death; volatile oil may cause severe skin inflammation: avoid even external application during pregnancy
Saw Palmetto berry	int: urinary dysfunction in BPH stages I-II	may have antiandrogenic and anti-inflammatory effects: banned as drug in U.S. by FDA: first choice for mild BPH in some parts of Europe	*1 to 2 g berry or equivalent (tea ineffective)*	rare GI upset
Schisandra	int: liver disease, GI inflammation, insomnia, night sweats, fatigue	contains lignans which promote regeneration of hepatocytes: may also have antitumor and energy-boosting effects	*dried berries: 1 to 6 g or equivalent*	none known
Scopolia root	int: spasms of GI and urinary tracts	contains alkaloids similar in effect to scopolamine: acts as anti-ACh- with decreased spasms and tremors: caution in children	*as directed*	avoid with glaucoma, prostate adenoma, tachycardia, GI obstruction, megacolon: may cause dryness of mouth, decreased sweating, red skin, ocular dysfunction, hyperthermia-tachycardia, difficulties in urination, attacks of glaucoma: may potentiate tricycli
Scotch Broom herb	int: nonspecific cardiac and circulatory dysfunction	contains alkaloids; primarily sparteine	*1 to 1.5 g of drug or equivalent*	contains tryamine, so avoid with MAO-inhibitors
Scullcap	int: anxiety, insomnia	may have sedative effects: limited scientific data	*1 to 2 g dried herb or equivalent*	none known
Selenium	int: general health promoter; found in green vegetables, meat, eggs, milk	works with vitamin E as antioxidant: current trials as prostate cancer preventative	*no RDA: 70 mcg recommended for men; 55 mcg for women*	toxicity in very high doses can affect hair, nails, teeth
Seneca Snakeroot	int: respiratory tract irritation, decongestant	contain saponins: may act as expectorant, secretolytic	*1.5 to 3 g root or equivalent*	may cause GI upset
Senna leaf/pod	int: constipation	FDA-approved as laxative: 1-8-dihydroxy-anthracene derivatives have a laxative effect by stimulating GI motility	*titrate to soft stool*	avoid in chronic intestinal inflammation or obstruction: may cause cramping, hypokalemia with chronic use: avoid long-term use, no data on pregnancy or nursing
Shark/bovine cartilage	int: cancer, arthritis, SLE, others	Studies presently investigating utility in cancer: may have anti-angiogenic actions: turns out sharks really do get cancer!	*as directed*	long-term side effects or interactions unknown: certainly avoid in pregnant women or those with serious heart disease
Shepherd's Purse	int: mild menorrhagia and metrorrhagia, epistaxis; ext: superficial bleeding	may increase uterine tone: may have positive inotropic and chronotropic effects	*int: 10 to 15 g of drug or equivalents: ext: as directed*	none known
Shiitake	int: cancer, HIV and other infections	may stimulate T-cells; increase production of TNF	*soup, lentinan extract, or tincture as directed*	may cause GI complaints at high dosages

Herbs	Uses	Information	Daily Dose	Cautions
Slippery Elm	int: inflammation of respiratory tract	may act as anti-inflammatory: declared safe and effective demulcent by FDA	*as directed*	no information: found in some commercial throat lozenges
Soapwort root-red/white	int: upper respiratory tract inflammation	may act as expectorant by irritating gastric mucosa	*red: 1.5 g root or equivalent white: 30 to 150 mg drug or equivalent*	rare GI irritation
Solomon's seal	int: constipation, hyperlipidemia, atherosclerosis	may decrease absorption of dietary cholesterol: steroid saponins may have anti-inflammatory actions	*tablets as directed*	GI irritation in high doses; otherwise none known
Soy isoflavones	int: cancer prevention/ treatment especially gynecologic, breast, prostate: osteoporosis, cardiovascular disease	have wide range of effects on cell regulation: may have estrogenic partial agonist activity: may be anti-platelet and angiogenesis inhibitors: genistein has been conjugated with antibodies in clinical trials	*diet much preferred, no dosing information for supplements*	little information: estrogenic effects possible but unlikely: may have thyrotoxic, mutagenic, and even carcinogenic effects if large amounts of supplements taken: no data on pregnancy/nursing
Soy Lecithin/ phosphor-lipids	int: hyperlipidemia, chronic hepatitis or nutritional liver disease (e.g. TPN)	linolenic acid most predominant fatty acid: phospholipid may be hepatoprotective via membrane stabilization	*equivalent of 3.5 g (3-sn-phosphatidyl choline)*	occasional GI upset: use when dietary/lifestyle measures insufficient
Spearmint	int: dyspepsia, flatulence	may have antispasmodic, mild sedative effects	*oil or concentrate as directed*	rare allergic reactions: used as flavoring agent for commercial products
Speedwell	int: dyspepsia, UTIs, GI irritation; ext: skin inflammation	may have protective effect against ulcers- both internal and external	*prepare tea as directed*	none known
Spinach leaf	int: indigestion, anorexia, anemia, sluggish growth in children	contains vitamin C, oxalic acid, nitrates, and Fe	*no information*	high nitrate content; so do not eat frequently or give to infants
Spiny Restharrow root	int: wash-out therapy for inflammation or urinary tract	may act as diuretic: contains isoflavonoids	*6 to 12 g of drug or equivalent*	avoid if edema due to CHF or renal disease: drink large amounts of fluids
Spirulina	type of blue-green algae: used for HIV, cancer, skin diseases, candida, hypoglycemia	contains protein and vitamin A: effectiveness unproven: may have antiviral effect	*as directed - often 500 mg qid*	no information
Spruce shoots/oil	int: inflammation of respiratory tract; ext: neuralgia, rheumatic pain	Secretolytic, hyperemic	*as directed*	may exacerbate asthma - pertussis: avoid if acute skin infections - cardiac disease
Squill	int: mild cardiac insufficiency, renal insufficiency	contains glycosides of the bufadienolide type	*0.1 to 0.5 g of standardized sea onion or equivalent*	may cause diarrhea, vomiting, hypokalemia: arrhythmias: caution with steroids, diuretics, digitalis, quinine-like drugs, antiarrhythmic
St. John's Wort	int: depression, anxiety; ext: mild burns, myalgias, bruises	may have some mild antidepressant effect, although MAO-inhibitor like activity seems doubtful: may have some antiviral activity	*2 to 4 g of drug or equivalent*	may cause photosensitization in light-skinned patients: dermatitis has been reported: avoid with anti-HIV medications, cyclosporin: must take 4-6 weeks for depression
Star Anise seed	int: respiratory tract inflammation with cough, dyspepsia	may act as expectorant-antispasmodic of GI tract	*3 g of drug or equivalent*	none known: japanese star anise, a different herb, is poisonous
Stinging Nettle herb/leaf/root	int/ext: BPH (root), irrigation for lower urinary tract and prevention of nephrolithiasis (herb/leaf); ext: rheumatic complaints	contains calcium, potassium salts, and silicic acid: may increase urinary flow	*as directed*	avoid in heart or renal disease: take copious amounts of water: root may help urinary symptoms with BPH but does not treat BPH itself
Strawberry leaf	int: indigestion, diarrhea, gout, rheumatoid arthritis, urinary stones; ext: rashes	may have astringent and diuretic actions	*prepare infusion or extract as directed*	allergic reactions possible
Sulfur	mineral, used for skin complaints, arthritis, digestive disorders	found in many amino acids	*bath used for arthritis: tablets as directed*	none known, with exception of sulfa allergies: no pregnancy info
Sundew	int: cough, bronchitis	may have antispasmodic-antitussive actions	*3 g of herb or equivalent*	none known
Sweet Clover	int: venous insufficiency, thrombophlebitis, swelling; ext: contusions	contains coumarin and glycosides may increase wound healing	*3 to 30 mg coumarin or equivalent*	headaches and mild increase in LFTs are rare: to be safe, avoid during pregnancy
Sweet Violet herb/flower	int: cough, bronchitis, asthma, migraine	contains saponins, which have expectorant and secretolytic effects	*use leaf or flower for tea as directed*	none known
Sweet Woodruff	int: UTIs, insomnia, anxiety, edema	contains tiny amounts of coumarin: limited scientific data	*prepare tea as directed*	chronic use may cause reversible liver toxicity
Tangerine Peel	int: dyspepsia, nausea, diarrhea	limited scientific data	*no information*	none known

Herbs	Uses	Information	Daily Dose	Cautions
Tansy flower/ oil	int: (flower): GI infections, migraine neuralgia; (oil): PMS, intestinal worms	oil is antimicrobial, antihelminic, and repels insects: contains varying amounts of thujone, which is toxic	*not recommended*	avoid in allopathic doses, as may lead to spasms, arrhythmias, bleeding, and renal failure
Taurine	nonessential amino acid, as supplement for seizures, OCD, anxiety, angina, primary pulmonary HTN	important for muscle and CNS function: may be necessary for heart function	*no RDA: some use 500 mg bid*	occasional GI side effects reported
Tea tree leaf/oil	int: pharyngitis, colitis, sinusitis; ext: disinfectant, skin infections, acne	contains terpenes which have antibacterial and possibly antiviral actions	*primarily externally in skin ointments*	none known: overdose may lead to confusion if taken internally
Thuja oil/ branches	int: respiratory infections, cold sores, rheumatism, neuralgia, UTIs, conjunctivitis, other complaints	some preparations contain thujone, which is toxic: antiviral effects due to proliferation of T-cells, especially CD-4 cells	*follow doses carefully due to thujone content*	drug is misused as abortifacent, so avoid if pregnant: avoid essential oil: allopathic preparations do not contain thujone
Thyme- wild/ domestic	int: bronchitis, cough, pertussis	may have antibacterial and expectorant activity: contains thymol	*domestic: 1 to 2 g of herb /cup of tea or equivalent: wild: 6 g of herb or equivalent*	none known: found in commercial vapor, rubs and mouthwashes
Tree of Heaven bark	int: malaria, dysmenorrhea, cramps, asthma	trial vs. malaria presently ongoing limited scientific info	*6 to 9 g drug*	large doses may cause GI upset, headache, tingling
Turmeric root (Javanese/ regular)	int: dyspepsia	contains curcumin, which may increase bile flow: may have anti-inflammatory actions	*1.5 to 3 g of drug or equivalent*	occasional GI upset: avoid with gallstones, biliary obstruction
Turpentne oil- purified	ext/int: chronic bronchitis, cough: ext: rheumatic complaints, myalgias	may act as mucolytic, antiseptic	*several drops in hot water to be inhaled or rubbed on skin*	topic application to large areas may cause nephrotoxicity or neurotoxicity
Usnea	int: sore throat	may have antimicrobial effect	*take in lozenge form*	none known
Uva Ursi leaf	int: inflammation of urinary tract	may have antibacterial effect, especially against E. coli, Proteus, enterococcus, strep, and staph: contains arbutin, which is converted to hydroquinone	*as directed*	avoid in pregnancy, lactation, children: nausea and vomiting may occur: avoid using for more than one week: may decrease effectiveness of L-dopa: requires alkaline urine to function: may turn urine green (harmless)
Uzara	int: nonspecific diarrhea	contains glycosides: may inhibit intestinal motility: may cause digitalis,like effects in high doses	*as directed*	avoid with digitalis or other glycosides
Valerian root	int: restlessness, anxiety, insomnia, GI complaints	may act as sedative: generally viewed as effective	*as directed*	none known
Vanadium	trace mineral: no documented uses: found in vegetable oils, vegetables, meat	may affect blood sugar and cholesterol in animals, but scientific info lacking: Needed for bones and teeth	*no RDA: supplementation rarely necessary*	toxicity may include depression, liver/kidney disease: avoid taking with chromium: vitamin C may decrease levels
Vervain	int: cough, bronchitis, sore throat; ext: edema, bruising, arthritis	contains iridoid glycosides, which act as astringent: limited scientific info	*prepare extract or infusion as directed*	none known
Walnut leaf/ hull	ext: mild skin inflammation, excessive sweating	has astringent and fungistatic properties	*2 to 3 g herb per 100 ml water or equivalent*	topical use of hulls has been linked to leukoplakia and cancer of oral region
Watercress	int: inflammation of respiratory tract	contains glycosides and mustard oil	*4 to 6 g dried herb or equivalent*	avoid in peptic ulcer disease, nephrolithiasis, in young children: rarely causes GI distress
Whey protein	int: protein source of choice for anaerobic exercise	contains albumin, lactoglobulin, and immunoglobulins: Substrate for glutathione, which is depleted in exercise	*as directed, usually post-exercise*	allergic reactions possible: contains lactose: contains bovine albumin (BSA) which may be linked to IDDM (link unclear)
White bryony	int: laxative, emetic, diuretic	contains cucurbitanes which have strong toxic and cytotoxic effects	*not recommended*	high toxicity, not recommended: toxicity decreases with storage: avoid skin contact
White Mustard seed	ext: URIs, bronchitis, rheumatism	contains mustard oil glycosides and mustard oils: may be bacteriostatic	*poultice prepared as directed*	chronic use may cause nerve and skin damage
White Nettle herb/flower	ext/int: inflammation of mucous membranes, respiratory tract	contains tannin, mucilage and saponins	*3 g of drug or equivalent or sitz bath*	none known
White Willow bark	int: fever, rheumatic complaints, headaches	contains salicylate-like compounds: may have antipyretic, analgesic properties	*dose corresponding to 60 to 120 mg total salicin*	may cause ASA-like effects, although few if any reported
Wild Cherry	int: bronchitis, cough, indigestion	acts as astringent, antitussive, sedative: contains small amounts of cyanogenic glycosides	*syrup or tincture as directed*	risk of cyanide-like poisoning small

Herbs	Uses	Information	Daily Dose	Cautions
Wild Yam root	int: hyperlipidemia, GI inflammation, dysmenorrhea, rheumatism	contains diosgenin, which may increase cholesterol excretion: may also have estrogenic effect on mammary cells, but no progesterone effects	*capsules: 200 to 400 mg; 505 to 535 mg usually 1 pill tid or as directed*	may decrease anti-inflammatory effect of NSAIDs such as indomethacin: caution with other estrogen-like drugs
Wintergreen	int: GI irritation, bloating; ext: rheumatism, myalgias, inflammation, neuralgia	limited scientific data	*as directed*	has been largely replaced by synthetic version, methyl salicylate, found in many commercial products: avoid oral intake of essential oil, which may be fatal
Witch Hazel leaf/bark	ext: minor wounds, skin inflammation, hemorrhoids, varicose veins	FDA-approved as astringent: contains tannins and other constituents: may have anti-inflammatory- hemostatic properties	*as directed*	none known
Woody Nightshade stem	internal/ext: as supportive therapy for chronic eczema, acne, warts, furuncles	contains tannins, steroid alkaloids and steroid saponins may have anti-Ach, antimicrobial, cortisone-like properties	*int: 1 to 3 g of drug or equivalent; ext: as directed*	contraindicated in pregnancy and nursing: avoid unripe berries with children
Wormwood	int: anorexia, biliary dysfunction	approved for food use with thujone-free products	*2 to 3 g of herb as water infusion or equivalent*	none known: avoid essential oil alone as may be poisonous
Yarrow	int: dyspepsia, GI discomfort; ext: female pelvic cramps	may have antibacterial, bile-producing properties	*4.5 g herb or equivalent or as sitz bath*	allergic reactions known
Yeast-Brewer's	int: anorexia, acne and skin infections: related type S. boulardii (Hansen CBS 5926) may be used for diarrhea	contains vitamins, particularly B complex, glucans and mannans: may be antibacterial via phagocytosis stimulation	*6 g or equivalent*	occasionally migraine-type headaches, flatulence, or itching: avoid with MAO-inhibitors
Yellow Dock root	int: constipation, liver/ gallbladder dysfunction	may have mild laxative effects	*capsules 500 mg as directed*	avoid eating large amounts of leaves: fresh root may cause GI upset
Yohimbe	int: sexual dysfunction, primarily non-organic: xerostomia	contains Yohimbe, which is a selective alpha-2-adrenergic antagonist: increases salivary flow, epinephrine/NE	*as directed (smaller doses for xerostomia)*	contraindicated in liver and kidney disease: may exacerbate anxiety or HTN: avoid with ethanol, naltrexone, morphine: generally less safe than sildenafil: overdoses have been fatal
Yucca root	ext: arthritis, sprains, inflammation	FDA-approved food additive: in-vitro studies showed hemolysis after addition of one of yucca's components, but never seen in vitro	*as directed*	may cause loose stools
Zedoary	int: anorexia, liver/gallbladder dysfunction	may increase bile flow and have a spasmolytic effect: Fungicial and antitumor effects also shown	*prepare tea as directed*	avoid chronic use
Zinc	mineral, needed for enzymes, insulin function, wound healing, found in meat, milk, soybeans: supplement may help with URIs (gluconate or acetate may be best)	data on URIs mixed	*RDA (adults): 15 mg to 25 mg if breast feeding*	GI toxicity or lack of coordination rare

Source: *Natural Medicines Comprehensive Database*, 4th Edition, Therapeutic Research Faculty, 2002. *The Complete Guide to Herbal Medicines*, Charles Fetrow, Juan Avila, Simon & Schuster, 2000.

TOP 50 MEDICATIONS & USAGE

Top 50 Most Prescribed Prescriptions & Usage (2007)

	Drug	Usage
1	Lipitor	Lowers cholesterol levels in the blood. Helps prevent certain heart and blood vessel diseases in people who are at higher risk for these diseases.
2	Singulair	Helps prevent and control asthma attacks and treats seasonal allergies.
3	Lexapro	A selective serotonin reuptake inhibitor (SSRI) that treats severe depression and generalized anxiety disorder (GAD).
4	Nexium	Treats GERD and conditions associated with stomach acids. Also used with antibiotics to treat certain types of ulcers. Prevents stomach ulcers and stomach irritation in clients taking pain and arthritis drugs, such as aspirin or ibuprofen, for long periods of time.
5	Synthroid	Treats hypothyroidism and other associated thyroid disorders.
6	Plavix	A blood thinner that Helps reduce strokes, heart attacks, and other heart problems caused by atherosclerosis.
7	Toprol XL	A beta-blocker that treats high blood pressure and angina and lowers the risk of repeated heart attacks.
8	Prevacid	Treats stomach ulcers, GERD, esophagitis, and other conditions caused by too much stomach acid.
9	Vytorin	Lowers cholesterol levels in the blood. Helps prevent certain heart and blood vessel diseases in people who are at higher risk for these diseases.
10	Advair Diskus	A steroid and a bronchodilator that prevents the symptoms of asthma or COPD and chronic bronchitis.
11	Zyrtec	An antihistamine that treats hay fever and allergy symptoms, hives, and itching.
12	Effexor XR	A selective serotonin reuptake inhibitor (SSRI) that treats depression, panic disorder, social anxiety disorder, and generalized anxiety disorder.
13	Protonix	Decreases stomach acid. Treats inflammation and ulcers of the esophagus and acid regurgitations.
14	Diovan	Treats high blood pressure and heart failure. May also prolong life after a heart attack.
15	Fosamax	Treats and prevents osteoporosis and other bone disorder.
16	Zetia	A statin drug that lowers cholesterol in your blood.
17	Crestor	Lowers cholesterol and triglycerides in the blood. Helps prevent certain heart and blood vessel diseases in people who are at higher risk for these diseases.
18	Levaquin	An antibiotic that treats infections that are caused by certain kinds of bacteria.
19	Diovan HCT	A diuretic that treats high blood pressure.
20	Klor-Con	A diuretic that treats potassium loss from the body.
21	Cymbalta	A selective serotonin reuptake inhibitor (SSRI) that treats severe depression and generalized anxiety disorder (GAD), and chronic pain.
22	Actos	Treats type 2 diabetes and used together with diet and exercise to help control your blood sugar.
23	Premarin	Treats menopausal symptoms including hot flashes, severe dryness, itching, and burning, in and around the vagina area and to help reduce your chances of getting osteoporosis.
24	ProAir HFA	Inhalation aerosol that treats or prevents breathing problems in clients who have asthma or certain other airway diseases.
25	Celebrex	An NSAID that treats pain, including pain caused by arthritis, ankylosing spondylitis, or menstrual cramps.
26	Flomax	An alpha-blocker that treats problems with urination caused by an enlarged prostate or BPH.
27	Seroquel	An antipsychotic used for schizophrenia and bipolar disorder (manic depression).
28	Norvasc	A calcium channel blocker that treats high blood pressure and chest pain.
29	Nasonex	Treats and prevents nasal symptoms such as congestion, sneezing, and runny nose caused by seasonal or year-round allergies.
30	Tricor	Lowers cholesterol and triglycerides in the blood. Helps prevent certain heart and blood vessel diseases in people who are at higher risk for these diseases..
31	Lantus	Treats type 2 diabetes and used together with diet and exercise to help control your blood sugar.
32	Viagra	Treats erectile dysfunction and also treats a lung condition and pulmonary arterial hypertension.
33	Altace	An ACE inhibitor that treats high blood pressure. Treats congestive heart failure after a heart attack. Reduces risk of heart attack, stroke, and death in people 55 years of age or older who have heart disease.
34	Yasmin	Prevents pregnancy.
35	Levoxyl	Treats hypothyroidism, enlarged thyroid gland, goiter and thyroid associated problems.
36	Adderall XR	A stimulant that treats attention deficit hyperactivity disorder (ADHD).
37	Lotrel	An ACE inhibitor and a calcium channel blocker that treats high blood pressure.
38	Actonel	Treats and prevents osteoporosis in women who have gone through menopause.
39	Ambien	Treats insomnia.
40	Cozaar	Used alone or with other medicines to treat high blood pressure. Reduces the risk of stroke in clients with high blood pressure and enlargement of the heart. Treats kidney disease in clients with Type 2 diabetes and a history of high blood pressure.
41	Coreg	A beta-blocker that treats high blood pressure and angina and lowers the risk of repeated heart attacks.
42	Valtrex	Antiviral used to treat to control the spread of herpes, shingles, and genital herpes and cold sores.
43	Lyrica	An anticonvulsant used to slow down impulses of the brain that causes seizures and epilepsy.
44	Concerta	Treats attention deficit hyperactivity disorder (ADHD) and narcolepsy.
45	Ambien	Treats insomnia.
46	Risperdal	An antipsychotic used for schizophrenia and bipolar disorder (manic depression).
47	Digitek	Used to treat heart failure and slowed heart rate by making heart beat stronger and with a more regular rhythm.
48	Topamax	Anticonvulsant used to treat seizures and epilepsy.
49	Chantix	Used as a smoking cessation medicine or treatment.
50	Avandia	Treats type 2 diabetes and used together with proper diet and exercise to help control your blood sugar.

Source: Verispan VONA, Full year 2007

Drugs	Effects and Precautions
Antibiotics	
Cephalosporins, penicillin	Take on an empty stomach to speed absorption of the drugs.
Erythromycin	Don't take with fruit juice or wine, which decrease the drug's effectiveness.
Sulfa drugs	Increase the risk of Vitamin B-12 deficiency.
Antifungal	Best taken with food. Can cause skin rash and increase sun sensitivity.
Tetracycline	Dairy products reduce the drug's effectiveness. Lowers Vitamin C absorption.
Anticonvulsants	
Dilantin, phenobarbital	Increase the risk of anemia and nerve problems due to deficiency of folate and other B vitamins.
Antidepressants	
Fluoxetine	Reduce appetite and can lead to excessive weight loss.
Lithium	A low-salt diet increases the risk of lithium toxicity; excessive salt reduces the drug's efficacy.
MAO Inhibitors	Foods high in tyramine (aged cheeses, processed meats, legumes, wine, beer, among others) can bring on a hypertensive crisis.
Antipsychotic	Do not take if you have blood problems and liver damage.
Tricyclics	Many foods, especially legumes, meat, fish, and foods high in Vitamin C, reduce absorption of the drugs.
Antihypertensive, Heart Medications	
ACE inhibitors	Take on an empty stomach to improve the absorption of the drugs.
Alpha blockers	Take with liquid or food to avoid excessive drop in blood pressure.
Antiarrhythmic drugs	Avoid caffeine, which increases the risk of irregular heartbeat.
Beta blockers	Take on an empty stomach; food, especially meat, increases the drug's effects and can cause dizziness and low blood pressure.
Digitalis	Avoid taking with milk and high fiber foods, which reduce absorption, increasing potassium loss.
Diuretics	Increase the risk of potassium deficiency. Do not take if you have any known allergies to sulfa drugs, or oral diabetes medicine. Avoid sudden changes in posture and use caution when driving or operating machinery that requires alertness.
Nitrates	Not usually used on their own, but may be added with other medications.
Potassium sparing diuretics	Unless a doctor advises otherwise, don't take diuretics with potassium supplements or salt substitutes, which can cause potassium overload.
Thiazide diuretics	Increase the reaction to MSG.
Asthma Drugs	
Pseudoephedrine	Avoid caffeine, which increases feelings of anxiety and nervousness.
Bronchodilators	Do not use if solution turns brown or contains sold particles and follow inhaler instructions closely.
Steroids	May be risky in cases of serious infections.
Theophylline	Charbroiled foods and high protein diet reduce absorption. Caffeine increases the risk of drug toxicity.
Cholesterol Lowering Drugs	
Cholestyramine	Increases the excretion of folate and vitamins A, D, E, and K.
Gemfibrozil	Avoid fatty foods, which decrease the drug's efficacy in lowering cholesterol.
Heartburn and Ulcer Medications	
Antacids	Interfere with the absorption of many minerals; for maximum benefit, take medication 1 hour after eating.
Cimetidine, Fanotidine, Sucralfate	Avoid high protein foods, caffeine, and other items that increase stomach acidity.

DRUG EFFECTS & PRECAUTIONS

Drugs	Effects and Precautions
Hormone Preparations	
Oral contraceptives	Salty foods increase fluid retention. Drugs reduce the absorption of folate, vitamin B-6, and other nutrients; increase intake of foods high in these nutrients to avoid deficiencies.
Steroids	Salty foods increase fluid retention. Increase intake of foods high in calcium, vitamin K, potassium, and protein to avoid deficiencies.
Thyroid drugs	Iodine-rich foods lower the drug's efficacy.
Digestives Drugs	
Stomach acid reducers	Higher doses can cause constipation, diarrhea, headaches, dizziness, and rashes.
Kaolin-pectin	Takes 1 to 4 hours to work.
Loperamide	Do not use if you have blood in diarrhea or excess temperature and use caution if you have ulcerative colitis.
Antiemetic	Do not use if you have breathing problems, emphysema, bronchitis, and difficult urination due to enlarged prostrate.
Saline laxative	Do not take if you have kidney disease, abdominal pain, nausea or vomiting.
Stool softeners	Long-term usage should be avoided.
Mineral Oils	Overuse can cause a deficiency of vitamins A, D, E, and K.
Painkillers	
Acetaminophen	Excessive amounts can cause liver disease.
Aspirin and stronger NSAIDs	Always take with food to lower the risk of gastrointestinal irritation; avoid taking with alcohol, which increases the risk of bleeding. Frequent use of these drugs lowers the absorption of folate and vitamin C.
Codeine	Increase fiber and water intake to avoid constipation.
Sleeping Pills, Tranquilizers	
Benzodiazepines	Never take with alcohol. Caffeine increases anxiety and reduces drug's effectiveness.
Cold and Allergy Drugs	
Antihistamine	Use caution if you have glaucoma, cardiovascular disease, high blood pressure, or asthma. Can have a sedative effect.
Decongestant	Take 30 minutes to 1 hour prior to work and use caution if you have heart disease or high blood pressure.
Suppressants	Drink plenty of fluids while taking these drugs.

Brand	Generic	Usage
Accupril	*quinapril*	ACE inhibitor Rx: HTN - CHF
Accurbron	*theophylline*	Bronchodilator - Rx: COPD - asthma
Accutane	*isotretinoin*	Rx: severe cystic acne
Acebutolol	*sectral*	B-blocker - Rx: HTN - angina - arrhythmias
Acetaminophen	*tylenol*	Non-narcotic analgesic
Acetazolamide	*diamox*	Diuretic / anticonvulsant - Rx: glaucoma - CHF - epilepsy - mountain sickness
Acetylcysteine	*mucomyst*	Mucolytic - Rx: asthma
Achromycin V	*tetracycline*	Antibiotic
Aclovate	*alclometasone*	Steroid anti-inflammatory
Actibine	*yohimbine*	Alpha-2 blocker - Rx: male impotence
Actidil	*triprolidine*	Antihistamine - Rx: allergies
Actifed	*triprolidine + pseudoephedrine*	Antihistamine /decongestant - Rx: allergies
Actigall	*ursodiol*	Bile acid - Rx: dissolves gall stones
Adalat	*nifedipine*	Calcium blocker - Rx: angina - hypertension
Adapin	*doxepin*	Cyclic antidepressant
Adipex-P	*phentermine*	Appetite suppressant / stimulant
Adrenalin	*epinephrine*	Bronchodilator - Rx: asthma
Advil	*ibuprofen*	NSAID analgesic
Aerobid	*flunisolide*	Steroid anti-inflammatory inhaler - Rx: asthma - bronchitis
Aerolate - Aerolate Iii - Aerolate Jr.	*theophylline*	Xanthine bronchodilator - Rx: asthma - COPD
Aerolone	*isoproterenol*	B-2 -bronchodilator - Rx: asthma
Aerosporin	*polymycin*	Antibiotic
Akineton	*biperiden*	Antiparkinsonian - Rx: prophylaxis of EPS
Albuterol	*proventil*	B-2 bronchodilator - Rx: asthma - COPD
Aldactazide	*hctz - spironolactone*	Antihypertensive /diuretic
Aldactone	*spironolactone*	Potassium-sparing diuretic
Aldochlor	*methyldopa + chlorothiazide*	Antihypertensive / diuretic compound
Aldomet	*methyldopa*	Antihypertensive
Aldoril	*methyldopa + hctz*	Antihypertensive compound
Alfenta	*alfentanil*	Narcotic analgesic / anesthetic
Allopurinol	*zyloprim*	Reduces serum uric acid - Rx: gout
Alprazolam	*xanax*	Benzodiazepine hypnotic
Altace	*ramipril*	ACE inhibitor - Rx: hypertension
Alupent	*metaproterenol*	B-2 bronchodilator - Rx: COPD - asthma
Alurate	*aprobarbital*	Barbiturate - Rx: insomnia
Ambenyl Cough Syrup	*codeine - bromodiphenhydramine*	Narcotic antitussive / antihistamine - Rx: colds - allergies
Ambien	*zolpidem*	Hypnotic - Rx: insomnia
Amcill	*ampicillin*	Antibiotic
Amikin	*amikacin*	Antibiotic
Amiloride	*midamor*	Potassium-sparing diuretic - Rx: CHF - hypertension
Aminophylline	*mudrane*	Bronchodilator - Rx: COPD - asthma
Amitril	*amitriptyline*	Tricyclic antidepressant
Amitriptyline	*elavil*	Tricyclic antidepressant
Amoxicillin	*amcill*	Antibiotic
Amoxil	*amoxicillin*	Antibiotic
Amphotericin B	*fungizone*	Antifungal agent
Amytal	*amobarbital*	Barbiturate sedative / hypnotic
Anadrol-50	*oxymetholone*	Androgen / steroid - Rx: anemia
Anafranil	*clomipramine*	Tricyclic antidepressant
Anaprox -	*naproxen*	NSAID analgesic / anti-inflammatory agent
Ancobon	*flucytosine*	Antifungal agent
Android	*methyltestosterone*	Androgen / steroid - Rx: hypogonadism
Anexsia	*hydrocodone - apap*	Narcotic analgesic
Anhydron	*cyclothiazide*	Antihypertensive / diuretic
Ansaid	*flurbiprofen*	NSAID analgesic - Rx: arthritis
Antabuse	*disulfiram*	Inhibits metabolism of alcohol - Rx: alcohol addiction
Antivert	*meclizine*	Anti-nausea - Rx: vertigo
Anturane	*sulfinpyrazone*	Uricosuric - Rx: gouty arthritis
Apap	*acetaminophen*	Non-narcotic analgesic
Apresazide	*hydralazine - hctz*	Antihypertensive / diuretic
Apresoline	*hydralazine*	Antihypertensive / diuretic
Aquatensen	*methyclothiazide*	Antihypertensive / diuretic
Aralen	*chloroquine*	Anti-malarial agent
Aristocort	*triamcinolone*	Steroid anti-inflammatory
Artane	*trihexyphenidyl*	Anti-parkinsonian - Rx: prophylaxis of EPS
Asa	*acetylsalicylic acid*	Aspirin - NSAID analgesic
Asbron-G	*theophylline - guaifenesin*	Xanthine bronchodilator - expectorant compound Rx: asthma - copd
Asendin	*amoxapine*	Tricyclic antidepressant
Astramorph Pf	*morphine*	Narcotic analgesic
Atarax	*hydroxyzine*	Tranquilizer / antihistamine - Rx: urticaria - anxiety
Ativan	*lorazepam*	Benzodiazepine hypnotic
Atromid-S	*clofibrate*	Antilipidemic. Rx: hyperlipidemia
Atrovent	*ipratropium*	Anticholinergic bronchodilator - Rx: copd
Augmentin	*amoxicillin - clavulanate potassium*	Antibiotic
Aventyl	*nortriptyline*	Tricyclic antidepressant

Note: The following information is for therapists who want educational tools and knowledge beyond typical massage scope of practice.

Brand	Generic	Usage
Axld	*nizatidine*	Histamine-2 antagonist - which inhibits gastric acid secretion - Rx: ulcers
Axotal	*butalbital - asa*	Anxiolytic / analgesic Rx: Tension H/A
Azdone	*hydrocodone - asa*	Narcotic analgesic compound
Azmacort	*triamcinolone*	Steroid anti-inflammatory - Rx: asthma - bronchitis
Azo Gantanol	*sulfamethoxazole - phenazopyridine*	Antibiotic/analgesic - Rx: urinary tract infection
Azt	*zidovudine*	Antiviral agent - Rx: HIV AIDS virus
Azulfidine	*sulfasalazine*	Anti-infective - Rx: colitis
Bactocill	*oxacillin*	Antibiotic
Bactrim - Bactrim Ds	*trimethoprim - sulfamethoxazole*	Antibacterial - Rx: UTI - ear infection - bronchitis
Bancap Hc	*hydrocodone - apap*	Narcotic analgesic
Beclovent	*beclomethasone*	Steroid anti-inflammatory agent - Rx: COPD - asthma
Beconase	*beclomethasone*	Steroid anti-inflammatory
Beepen-Vk	*penicillin*	Antibiotic
Belladonna	*belladenal*	Antispasmodic - Rx: irritable bowel syndrome
Bellergal	*phenobarbital - ergotamine - belladonna*	Rx: menopause - headaches - uterine cramps
Benadryl	*diphenhydramine*	Antihistamine - Rx: allergies
Benemid	*probenecid*	Uricosuric - Rx: gout. Also prolongs effects of penicillin
Bentyl	*dicyclomine*	GI tract antispasmodic
Benylin	*diphenhydramine*	Antihistamine
Benzamycin	*erythromycin - benzoyl peroxide*	Topical antibiotic / keratolytic compound - Rx: acne
Benzthiazide	*exna*	Antihypertensive / diuretic
Bepadin	*bepridil*	Calcium channel blocker - Rx: angina
Bepridil	*bepadin*	Calcium channel blocker - Rx: angina
Betaloc	*metoprolol*	B -blocker - Rx: HTN - angina - arrhythmias
Betapace	*sotalol*	B-blocker - Rx: angina - HTN - arrhythmias
Betaseron	*interferon*	Immunologic agent - Rx: Multiple Sclerosis
Betaxolol	*kerlone*	Beta blocker - Rx: HTN
Bethanechol	*urecholine*	Vagomimetic agent which increases bladder tone - Rx: urinary retention
Betoptic	*betaxolol*	Beta-1 blocker eye drops - Rx: glaucoma
Biaxin	*clarithromycin*	Antibiotic
Bicillin	*penicillin*	Antibiotic
Biphetamine	*dextroam-phetamine - amphetamine*	Stimulants
Blocadren	*timolol*	O-blocker - Rx: angina - HTN - arrhythmias
Brethaire	*terbutaline*	B-2 bronchodilator - Rx: asthma - COPD
Brethine	*terbutaline*	B-2 bronchodilator - Rx: asthma - COPD
Brevicon		Oral contraceptive
Bricanyl	*terbutaline*	B-2 bronchodilator - Rx: asthma - COPD
Bronitin Mist	*epinephrine*	B-2 bronchodilator - Rx: asthma
Bronkaid Mist	*epinephrine*	B-2 bronchodilator - Rx: asthma
Bronkaid Tablets	*ephedrine - theophylline - guaifenesin*	Bronchodilator / expectorant compound
Bronkephrine	*ethylnorepinephrine*	Bronchodilator - Rx: asthma
Bronkodyl	*theophylline*	Bronchodilator - Rx: COPD - asthma
Bronkolixir	*ephedrine - guaifenesin - theophylline - phenobarbital*	Xanthine bronchodilator / expectorant
Bronkometer	*isoetharine*	B-2 bronchodilator - Rx: COPD - asthma
Bronkosol	*isoetharine*	B-2 bronchodilator - Rx: COPD - asthma
Bronkotabs	*ephedrine - theophylline - phenobarbital - guaifenesin*	Bronchodilator / expectorant - Rx: COPD - asthma
Bucladin-S	*buclizine*	Piperazine antiemetic
Bumex	*bumetanide*	Diuretic - Rx: CHF - edema
Buprenex	*buprenorphine*	Narcotic analgesic
Butalbital	*fiorinal*	Barbiturate muscle relaxant / sedative
Butazolidin	*phenylbutazone*	NSAID analgesic - Rx: arthritis
Buticaps	*butabarbital*	Barbiturate sedative - Rx: insomnia
Butisol	*butabarbital*	Barbiturate sedative - Rx: insomnia
Clidinium	*librex*	Antispasmodic - Rx: peptic ulcers
Cafergot	*ergotamine - caffeine*	Cranial vasoconstrictor - Rx: migraine & vascular headaches
Cafergot P-B Suppository	*ergotamine - caffeine - belladonna - pentobarbital*	Cranial vasoconstrictor /antiemetic / sedative - Rx: migraine & vascular H/A
Calan - Calan Sir	*verapamil*	Calcium blocker - Rx: angina - hypertension - PSVT prophylaxis - headache
Calcidrine	*codeine - calcium iodide*	Narcotic antitussive /expectorant compound
Caldecort	*hydrocortisone*	Steroid anti-inflammatory
Capital W/ Codeine	*apap - codeine*	Narcotic analgesic
Capoten	*captopril*	Ace inhibitor - Rx: HTN - CHF
Capozide	*captopril - hctz*	Antihypertensive / diuretic
Carafate	*sucralfate*	Anti-ulcer agent
Carbamazepine	*tegretol*	Anticonvulsant - Rx: epilepsy
Carbidopa & Levodopa	*sinemet*	Dopamine precursors - Rx: Parkinson's disease
Cardene	*nicardipine*	Calcium blocker - Rx: angina - HTN
Cardilate	*erythrityl tetranitrate*	Vasodilator - Rx: angina
Cardioquin	*quinidine*	Antiarrhythmic - Rx: cardiac dysrhythmias
Cardizem - Cardizem Cd - Cardizem Sr	*diltiazem*	Calcium blocker - Rx: angina - HTN - PSVT
Cardura	*doxazosin*	Ace inhibitor alpha blocker - Rx: HTN
Carisoprodol	*soma*	Muscle relaxant / analgesic
Carteolol	*cartrol*	Beta blocker - Rx: HTN - angina
Cartrol	*carteolol*	Nonselective b-blocker - Rx: HTN - angina
Cataflam	*diclofenac*	NSAID analgesic

Brand	Generic	Usage
Catapres	clonidine	Antihypertensive agent
Catapres Tts	transdermal clonidine	Antihypertensive
Ceclor	cefaclor	Antibiotic
Ceftin	cefuroxime	Antibiotic
Cefzil	cefprozil	Antibiotic
Celestone	betamethasone	Steroid anti-inflammatory
Celontin	methsuximide	Anticonvulsant - Rx: absence SZ
Centrax	prazepam	Benzodiazepine hypnotic
Cephalexin	keflex	Antibiotic
Cephradine	anspor	Antibiotic
Chardonna-2	belladonna alkaloids - phenobarbital	Antispasmodic compound - Rx: ulcers
Chlor-Trimeton	chlorpheniramine	Antihistamine
Chlordiazepoxide	librium	Benzodiazepine hypnotic
Cipro	ciprofloxacin	Antimicrobial agent
Claforan	cefotaxime	Antibiotic
Claritin	ioratadine	Non-sedating antihistamine - Rx: allergies
Cleocin	clindamycin	Antibiotic
Clindamycin	cleocin	Antibiotic
Clomipramine	anafranil	Tricyclic antidepressant
Clonidine	catapres	Antihypertensive agent
Cloxapen	cloxacillin	Antibiotic
Clozaril	clozapine	Psychotropic - Rx: schizophrenia
Codalan	codeine - apap - salicylamide - caffeine	Narcotic analgesic compound
Codeine	codeine	Narcotic analgesic / antitussive
Codiclear Dh	hydrocodone - guaifenesin	Narcotic antitussive/expectorant - Rx: coughs
Codimal Dh	hydrocodone - phenylephrine - pyrilamine	Narcotic antitussive / decongestant - Rx: colds - allergies
Codimal Expectorant	phenypropanolamine - guaifenesin	Decongestant / expectorant - Rx: colds - allergies
Codimal La	chlorpheniramine - pseudoephedrine	Antihistamine / decongestant compound - Rx: colds - allergies
Codimal Ph	codeine - phenylephrine - pyrilamine	Narcotic antitussive / decongestant compound - Rx: colds - allergies
Cogentin	benztropine	Antiparkinsonian - Rx: EPS
Cogesic	hydrocodone - apap	Narcotic analgesic compound
Cognex	tacrine	Cholinomimetic / Ach-ase inhibitor - Rx: Alzheimer's disease
Colace	docusate	Stool softener
Colbenemid	probenecid - colchicine	Uricosuric - Rx: gout
Colchicine	colbenemid	Reduces incidence of gout attacks
Colestid	colestipol	Reduces serum cholesterol
Combipres	clonidine - chlorthalidone	Antihypertensive/diuretic
Compazine	prochlorperazine	Phenothiazine antiemetic

Brand	Generic	Usage
Congess Jr/Sr	guaifenesin - pseudoephedrine	Expectorant / decongestant compound - Rx: colds - asthma
Conjugated Estrogens	premarin	Rx: menopause
Constant-T	theophylline	Bronchodilator - Rx: asthma - COPD
Cordarone	amiodarone	Ventricular antiarrhythmic
Corgard	nadolol	Beta blocker - Rx: angina - hypertension
Corzide	nadolol - bendroflumethiazide	B-blocker / antihypertensive / diuretic compound
Cotrim	sulfamethoxazole - trimethoprim	Antibacterial
Coumadin	warfarin	Anticoagulant - Rx: thrombosis prophylaxis
Cromolyn	intal	Antiallergenic - Rx: asthma prophylaxis
Crystodigin	digitoxin	Cardiac glycoside - Rx: CHF - SVT
Cutivate	fluticasone	Topical steroid anti-inflammatory - Rx: dermatoses
Cyanocobalamin	vitamin b-12	Rx: anemia
Cyclacillin	none	Antibiotic
Cyclobenzaprine	flexeril	Skeletal muscle relaxant
Cyclospasmol	cyclandelate	Vasodilator - Rx: cerebral & peripheral ischemia
Cycrin	medroxyprogesterone	Hormone - Rx: uterine bleeding
Cylert	pemoline	Stimulant - Rx: attention deficit disorder in children
Cyproheptadine	periactin	Antihistamine
Cystospaz - Cystospaz-M	hyoscyamine	Urinary tract antispasmodic
Cytotec	misoprostol	Prevents gastric ulcers caused by nsaids
Cytovene	ganciclovir	Antiviral - Rx: cytomegalovirus - ARC - AIDS
Dalgan	dezocine	Narcotic analgesic
Dallergy	chlorpheniramine - phenylephrine - methscopolamine	Antihistamine / decongestant - Rx: allergies
Dalmane	flurazepam	Hypnotic - Rx: insomnia
Damason-P	hydrocodone - asa - caffeine	Narcotic analgesic
Dantrium	dantrolene	Skeletal muscle antispasmodic - Rx: multiple sclerosis - cerebral palsy
Daranide	dichlorphenamide	Carbonic anhydrase inhibitor-lowers intraocular pressure - Rx: glaucoma
Darvocet-N	propoxyphene - apap	Narcotic analgesic
Darvon	propoxyphene	Narcotic analgesic
Darvon Compound	propoxyphene - asa - caffeine	Narcotic analgesic compound
Darvon W/Asa	propoxyphene - aspirin	Narcotic analgesic
Daypro	oxaprozin	NSAID - Rx: arthritis.
Ddavp	desmopressin	Antidiuretic hormone - Rx: nocturia - diabetes insipidus
Decadron	dexamethasone	Steroid anti-inflammatory
Declomycin	demeclocycline	Antibiotic
Deconamine	chlorpheniramine - pseudoephedrine	Antihistamine / decongestant compound - Rx: colds - allergies
Delsym	dextromethorphan	Cough suppressant
Deltasone	prednisone	Steroid anti-inflammatory agent

DRUGS

Brand	Generic	Usage
Demadex	*torsemide*	Diuretic - Rx: HTN - edema - CHF - kidney disease - liver disease.
Demerol	*meperidine*	Narcotic analgesic
Demerol Apap	*meperidine - apap*	Narcotic analgesic
Demi-Regroton	*chlorthalidone - reserpine*	Antihypertensive / diuretic compound
Demser	*metyrosine*	Antihypertensive - Rx: pheochromocytoma
Depakote	*divalproex*	Antiepileptic - Rx: absence seizures
Depen	*penicillamine*	Chelating agen - Rx: Wison's disease, RA
Deponit	*nitroglycerin*	Transdermal nitrate Rx: angina
Deprol	*meprobamate - benactyzine*	Antidepressant/ tranquilizer compound
Desoxyn	*methamphetamine*	Stimulant
Desyrel	*trazodone*	Antidepressant
Detensol	*propranolol*	B-blocker - Rx: HTN - angina - arrhythmias
Dexamethasone	*decadron*	Steroid anti-inflammatory agent
Dexedrine	*dextroamphetamine*	Stimulant
Dextromethorphan	*delsym*	Cough suppressant
Diabeta	*glyburide*	Oral hypoglycemic - Rx: diabetes
Diabinese	*chlorpropamide*	Oral hypoglycemic agent - Rx: diabetes
Dialose	*docusate*	Stool softener
Diamox	*acetazolamide*	Diuretic / anticonvulsant - Rx: glaucoma - CHF - epilepsy - mountain sickness
Diazepam	*valium*	Benzodiazepine hypnotic
Dibenzyline	*phenoxybenzamine*	Alpha blocker - Rx: HTN - sweating
Dicloxacillin	*dynaden*	Antibiotic
Dicumarol	*bishydroxycoumarin*	Anticoagulant
Dicyclomine	*bentyl*	Anticholinergic - Rx: colitis
Didrex	*benzphetamine*	Stimulant - Rx: obesity
Diethylpropion	*tepanil*	Stimulant
Diflucan	*fluconazole*	Antifungal agent
Diflunisal	*dolobid*	NSAID analgesic
Digitoxin	*crystodigin*	Cardiac glycoside - Rx: CHF - supraventricular dysrhythmias
Digoxin	*lanoxin*	Cardiac glycoside - Rx: CHF - supraventricular dysrhythmias
Dihydrocodeine	*synalgos-dc*	Narcotic analgesic
Dilacor	*diltiazem*	Calcium blocker - Rx: angina - HTN - PSVT
Dilacor Xr	*diltiazem*	Calcium blocker - Rx: HTN
Dilantin	*phenytoin*	Anticonvulsant
Dilatrate Sr	*isosorbide dinitrate*	Long-acting nitrate - Rx: angina prophylaxis
Dilaudid	*hydromorphone*	Narcotic analgesic
Dilor - Dilor-200 - Dilor-400 - Dilor Elixir	*dyphylline*	Xanthine bronchodilator - Rx: asthma - COPD
Dilor-G	*dyphylline - guaifenesin*	Bronchodilator / expectorant
Diltiazem	*cardizem*	Calcium blocker - Rx: angina - HTN - PSVT
Dimetane-Dc	*codeine - brompheniramine - phenylpropanol-amine*	Narcotic antitussive - antihistamine - decongestant
Dimetapp	*brompheniramine - phenylpropanolamine*	Antihistamine / decongestant - Rx: allergies
Diphenhydramine	*benadryl*	Antihistamine
Dipyridamole	*persantine*	Vasodilator - Rx: angina
Disalcid	*salsalate*	NSAID - Rx: arthritis
Disopyramide	*norpace*	Antiarrhythmic - Rx: pvc's
Disulfiram	*antabuse*	Inhibits metabolism of alcohol - Rx: alcohol addiction
Ditropan	*oxybutynin*	Anticholinergic / antispasmodic - Rx: urinary frequency - incontinence - dysuria
Diucardin	*hydroflumethiazide*	Antihypertensive / diuretic
Diuchlor-H	*hydrochlorothiazide*	Antihypertensive / diuretic
Diupres	*chlorothiazide - reserpine*	Antihypertensive / diuretic
Diuril	*chlorothiazide*	Antihypertensive / diuretic
Diutensen	*cryptenamine - meclothiazide*	Antihypertensive / diuretic compound
Diutensen-R	*methyclothiazide - reserpine*	Antihypertensive / diuretic compound
Dizac	*diazepam*	Anxiolytic - antianxiety agent
Docusate	*dialose*	Stool softener
Dolene	*propoxyphene*	Narcotic analgesic
Dolobid	*diflunisal*	NSAID analgesic
Dolophine	*methadone*	Narcotic analgesic
Dolprn # 3	*codeine - apap - asa - mgoh2 - aioh3*	Buffered narcotic analgesic compound
Donnagel	*kaolin - pectin - belladonna alkaloids*	Antispasmodic / stool binder - Rx: diarrhea
Donnagel Pg	*kaolin - pectin - belladonna alkaloids - opium*	Narcotic antispasmodic / stool binder - Rx: diarrhea
Donnatal	*phenobarbital - belladonna alkaloids*	Barbiturate sedative - antispasmodic - Rx: ulcers
Doral	*quazepam*	Benzodiazepine hypnotic - Rx: insomnia
Doryx	*doxycycline*	Antibiotic
Dovonex	*calciporiene*	Topical agent Rx: psoriasis
Doxepin	*sinequan*	Tricyclic antidepressant
Doxidan	*docusate - danthron*	Stool softener
Doxycycline	*vibramycin*	Antibiotic
Dramamine	*dimenhydrinate*	Anti-nausea
Drixoral	*dexbrompheniramine - pseudoephedrine*	Antihistamine / decongestant - Rx: allergies
Dss	*docusate*	Stool softener
Dulcolax	*bisacodyl*	Laxative
Duo-Medihaler	*isoproterenol - phenylephrine*	Bronchodilator - decongestant - Rx: asthma - COPD
Duocet	*hydrocodone - apap*	Narcotic analgesic compound

Brand	Generic	Usage
Duotrate	*pentaerythritol tetranitrate*	Long-acting nitrate - Rx: angina prophylaxis
Duradyne	*hydrocodone - apap*	Narcotic analgesic
Duragesic	*fentanyl*	Narcotic analgesic
Duramorph	*morphine*	Narcotic analgesic
Duraquin	*quinidine*	Rx: cardiac dysrhythmias
Duratuss	*hydrocodone - pseudoephedrine - guaifenesin*	Antitussive - decongestant - expectorant - Rx: colds - allergies
Duretic	*methyclothiazide*	Antihypertensive / diuretic
Duricef	*cefadroxil*	Antibiotic
Dyazide	*hctz - triamterene*	Antihypertensive / diuretic - Rx: HTN
Dycill	*dicloxacillin*	Antibiotic
Dymelor	*acetohexamide*	Oral hypoglycemic
Dynacirc	*isradipine*	Calcium blocker - Rx: HTN - angina
Dynapen	*dicloxacillin*	Antibiotic
Dyphylline	*lufyllin*	Bronchodilator - Rx: COPD - asthma
Dyrenium	*triamterene*	Potassium-sparing diuretic - Rx: CHF
E-Mycin	*erythromycin*	Antibiotic
Easprin	*asa*	NSAID analgesic - Rx: arthritis
Ecotrin	*aspirin*	Enteric coated aspirin - NSAID analgesic
Edecrin	*ethacrynic acid*	Diuretic - Rx: CHF
Ees	*erythromycin*	Antibiotic
Effexor	*venlafaxine*	Antidepressant
Elavil	*amitriptyline*	Tricyclic antidepressant
Eldepryl	*selegiline*	MAO inhibitor - Rx: Parkinson's disease
Elimite	*permethrin*	Topical scabicidal agent - Rx: scabies - lice
Elixophyllin	*theophylline*	Bronchodilator - Rx: asthma - COPD
Elocon	*mometasone*	Topical steroid anti-inflammatory
Emetrol	*glucose - fructose - phosphoric acid*	Anti-nausea
Empirin W/ Codeine	*asa - codeine*	Narcotic analgesic
Endep	*amitriptyline*	Tricyclic antidepressant
Enduron	*methyclothiazide*	Antihypertensive / diuretic
Enduronyl	*methyclothiazide - daserpidine*	Antihypertensive / diuretic compound
Enkaid	*encainide*	Ventricular antiarrhythmic
Enovid	*norethynodrel - mestranol*	Oral contraceptive
Entex La	*phenylpropanolamine - guaifenesin*	Decongestant / expectorant compound
Ephed Ii	*ephedrine*	Bronchodilator - decongestant
Ephedrine	*tedral*	Bronchodilator - Rx: asthma - COPD
Epi-Pen	*epinephrine*	Bronchodilator - vasoconstrictor - Rx: allergic reaction
Epinephrine	*bronkaid-mist*	Bronchodilator - Rx: asthma
Equagesic	*meprobamate - asa*	Tranquilizer / analgesic
Equanil	*meprobamate*	Tranquilizer
Ergo-Stat	*ergotamine*	Cerebral vasoconstrictor - Rx: migraines
Ery-Tab	*erythromycin*	Antibiotic
Eryc	*erythromycin*	Antibiotic
Erythrityl Tetranitrate	*cardilate*	Long-acting nitrate
Erythrocin	*erythromycin*	Antibiotic
Esgic	*apap - caffeine - butalbital*	Analgesic / muscle relaxant / antianxiety compound - Rx: headache
Esgic C Codeine	*apap - caffeine - butalbital - codeine*	Analgesic / muscle relaxant / anxiolytic compound
Esidrix	*hctz*	Antihypertensive / diuretic
Esimil	*guanethidine - hctz*	Antihypertensive / diuretic
Eskalith	*lithium*	Tranquilizer - Rx: mania - depression
Esp	*erythromycin - sulfisoxazole*	Antibiotic compound
Estrace	*estradiol*	Estrogen - Rx: menopause
Estraderm	*estradiol*	Topical estrogen - Rx: menopause
Estropipate	*ogen*	Estrogens - Rx: menopause
Ethatab	*ethaverine*	Smooth muscle relaxant / vasodilator - Rx: vascular insufficiency - GI & GU tract spasm.
Ethmozine	*moricizine*	Antiarrhythmic - Rx: severe ventricular dysrhythmias
Etrafon	*perphenazine - amitriptyline*	Major tranquilizer - tricyclic antidepressant - Rx: anxiety with depression
Eutonyl	*pargyline*	MAO inhibitor - Rx: hypertension
Eutron	*pargyline - methyclothiazide*	MAO inhibitor / antihypertensive / diuretic - Rx: hypertension
Exna	*benzthiazide*	Antihypertensive/diuretic
Extendryl	*phenylephrine - methscopolamine - chlorpheniramine*	Antihistamine - decongestant - Rx: allergies
Famvir	*famciclovir*	Antiviral - Rx: shingles
Fastin	*phentermine*	Stimulant - Rx: appetite suppression
Felbatol	*felbamate*	Antiepileptic Rx: seizures
Feldene	*piroxicam*	NSAID analgesic
Felodipine	*renedil*	Calcium blocker - Rx: HTN - angina
Femcet	*apap - butalbital - caffeine*	Analgesic / anxiolytic - Rx: tension headaches
Feosol	*ferrous sulfate*	Iron supplement
Fergon	*ferrous gluconate*	Iron supplement
Fevernol	*apap*	Antipyretic/analgesic suppository
Fioricet	*butalbital - apap - caffeine*	Analgesic - Rx: h/a
Fiorinal	*butalbital - asa - caffeine*	Non-narcotic analgesic
Fiorinal W/ Codeine	*butalbital - asa - caffeine - codeine*	Narcotic analgesic compound
Flagyl	*metronidazole*	Antimicrobial agent
Flatulex	*simethicone - activated charcoal*	Anti-flatulent
Flexeril	*cyclobenzaprine*	Skeletal muscle relaxant

DRUGS

Brand	Generic	Usage
Florone	diflorasone	Steroid anti-inflammatory agent
Floropryl	isoflurophate	Topical miotic - Rx: glaucoma
Floxln	ofloxacin	Antibiotic
Flumadine	rimantadine	Antiviral - Rx: influenza A
Fortaz	ceftazidime	Antibiotic
Fulvicin	griseofulvin	Antifungal agent
Furadantin	nitrofurantoin	Antibacterial agent - Rx: UTI
Furosemide	lasix	Diuretic - Rx: CHF - hypertension
Gantanol	sulfamethoxazole	Antibacterial agent - Rx: UTI
Gantrisin	sulfisoxazole	Antibacterial agent - Rx: UTI
Garamycin	gentamicin	Antibiotic
Gemnisyn	apap - asa	Non-narcotic analgesic
Genora	ethinyl estradiol	Oral contraceptive
Gentamicin	garamycin	Antibiotic
Geocillin	carbenicillin	Antibiotic
Geopen	carbenicillin	Antibiotic
Glucagon	glucoagon	Hormone which releases glucose from the liver - Rx: hypoglycemia
Glucophage	metformin	Oral hypoglycemic - Rx: diabetes
Glucotrol	glipizide	Oral hypoglycemic - Rx: diabetes
Glynase	glyburide	Oral hypoglycemic - Rx: diabetes
Grifulvin V	griseofulvin	Antifungal - Rx: ringworm
Grisactin	griseofulvin	Antifungal agent
Guaifed - Guaifed-Pd	guaifenesin - pseudoephedrine	Expectorant / decongestant
Guanethidine	ismelin	Sympatholytic antihypertensive agent
Gyne-Lotrimin	clotrimazole	Antifungal agent
Halcion	triazolam	Benzodiazepine hypnotic - Rx: insomnia
Haldol	haloperidol	Major tranquilizer
Harmonyl	daserpidine	Sedative / antihypertensive
Hctz	hydrochlorothiazide	Antihypertensive / diuretic - Rx: HTN
Hexadrol	dexamethasone	Steroid anti-inflammatory
Hismanal.	astemizole	Antihistamine - Rx: allergies
Hivid	zalcitabine	Antiviral - Rx: AIDS
Humorsol	demecarium	Topical miotic - Rx: glaucoma
Hycodan	hydrocodone - homatropine	Narcotic antitussive
Hycomine Compound	hydrocodone - chlorpheniramine - apap - caffeine - phenylephrine	Narcotic antitussive / antihistamine / decongestant - Rx: colds - URI
Hycomine Syrup	hydrocodone - phenylpropanolamine	Narcotic antitussive /decongestant - Rx: cough - nasal congests.
Hycotuss	hydrocodone - guaifenesin	Narcotic antitussive / expectorant
Hydergine	ergoloids	Rx: improves mentation in the elderly
Hydralazine	apresoline	Antihypertensive agent
Hydrex	benzthiazide	Antihypertensive / diuretic
Hydro Diuril	hctz	Antihypertensive / diuretic
Hydro-Chlor	hydrochlorothiazide	Antihypertensive / diuretic
Hydro-D	hydrochlorothiazide	Antihypertensive / diuretic
Hydrocet	hydrocodone - apap	Narcotic analgesic compound
Hydrochlorothiazide	hctz	Antihypertensive / diuretic
Hydrocodone	vicodin	Narcotic analgesic / antitussive
Hydrocodone W! Apap	t-gesic	Narcotic analgesic
Hydrocortisone	cortef	Steroid anti-inflammatory agent
Hydroflumethiazide	salutensin	Antihypertensive / diuretic
Hydromorphone	dilaudid	Narcotic analgesic / antitussive
Hydromox	quinethazone	Diuretic - Rx: hypertension
Hydropres	hctz - reserpine	Antihypertensive / diuretic
Hydroxyzine	atarax	Antiemetic / antitussive agent
Hygroton	chlorthalidone	Antihypertensive / diuretic
Hylorel	guanadrel	Sympatholytic antihypertensive
Hyoscyamine	cystospaz	Antispasmodic - Rx: lower UTI & GI tract spasm
Hytrin	terazosin	Antihypertensive agent
Iletin	insulin	Insulin preparations - Rx: diabetes mellitus
Ilosone	erythromycin	Antibiotic
Imdur	isosorbide mononitrate	Long-acting nitrate - Rx: angina prophylaxis.
Imipramine	tofranil	Tricyclic antidepressant
Imitrex	sumatriptan	Auto-injectible drug - Rx: migraine H/A
Imodium	loperamide	Slows peristalsis - Rx: diarrhea
Imuran	azathioprine	Immunosuppressant - Rx: organ transplants - ulcerative colitis - lupus - severe arthritis
Inapsine	droperidol	Major tranquilizer
Inderal	propranolol	Beta blocker - Rx: HTN - prophylaxis of: angina - cardiac dysrhythmias - AMI - migraine H/A
Inderal La	propranolol	Long-acting B-blocker - Rx: HTN; prophylaxis of: angina - cardiac dysrhythmias - AMI - & migraine H/A
Inderide	propranolol - hctz	Beta blocker - antihypertensive / diuretic compound - Rx: hypertension
Indocin	indomethacin	NSAID analgesic - Rx: arthritis
Indomethacin	indocin	NSAID analgesic - Rx: arthritis
Inn	isoniazid	Antibiotic - Rx: TB
Intal	cromolyn	Antiallergic - Rx: asthma prophylaxis
Inversine	mecamylamine	Antihypertensive agent
Ionamin	phentermine	Stimulant - Rx: appetite suppression
Ismelin	guanethidine	Sympatholytic antihypertensive agent

Brand	Generic	Usage
Iso-Bid	*isosorbide dinitrate*	Long-acting nitrate - Rx: angina
Isoclor Expectorant	*codeine - pseudoephedrine - guaifenesin*	Narcotic antitussive / decongestant / expectorant compound - Rx: cough - colds
Isocom	*isometheptene - dichloralphenazone - apap*	Cerebral vasoconstrictor - sedative - analgesic - Rx: headaches
Isoniazid	*inh*	Antibiotic - Rx: TB
Isoproterenol	*isuprel*	B-bronchodilator - Rx: asthma - COPD
Isoptin - Isoptin Sr	*verapamil*	Calcium blocker - Rx: angina - hypertension - PSVT prophylaxis - headache
Isordil	*isosorbide dinitrate*	Long-acting nitrate - Rx: angina
Isosorbide Dinitrate	*isordil*	Long-acting nitrate - Rx: angina
Isoxsuprine	*vasodilan*	Beta vasodilator - Rx: cerebral & peripheral ischemia
Isuprel	*isoproterenol*	Bronchodilator - Rx: asthma
K-Dur	*kcl*	Potassium supplement
K-Lor	*kcl*	Potassium supplement
K-Lyte	*kcl*	Potassium supplement
K-Norm	*kcl*	Potassium supplement
Kaolin - Pectin	*kaopectate*	Stool binder - Rx: diarrhea
Kaopectate	*kaolin-pectin*	Stool binder - Rx: diarrhea
Kenalog	*triamcinolone*	Steroid anti-inflammatory agent
Kerlone	*betaxolol*	Beta-1 blocker - Rx: HTN
Ketoprofen	*orudis*	NSAID - Rx: arthritis
Klonopin	*clonazepam*	Benzodiazepine hypnotic
Klor-Con	*kcl*	Potassium supplement
Klorvess	*kcl*	Potassium supplement
Klotrix	*kcl*	Potassium supplement
Kolyum	*potassium chloride*	Potassium supplement
Labetalol	*normodyne*	Beta blocker - Rx: HTN - angina
Lamictal	*lamotrigine*	Antiepileptic - Rx: absence seizures
Lanoxicaps	*digoxin*	Cardiac glycoside - Rx: CHF - supraventricular dysrhythmias
Lanoxin	*digoxin*	Cardiac glycoside - Rx: CHF - dysrhythmias
Larodopa	*levodopa - carbidopa*	Dopamine precursors - Rx: Parkinson's disease
Lasix	*furosemide*	Diuretic - Rx: CHF - hypertension - edema
Laudanum	*tincture of opium*	Narcotic analgesic
Ledercillin	*penicillin*	Antibiotic
Lescol	*fluvastatin*	Cholesterol reducer
Levatol	*penbutolol*	Beta blocker - Rx: hypertension
Levo-Dromoran	*levorphanol*	Narcotic analgesic
Levorphan	*levorphanol*	Narcotic analgesic
Levorphanol	*levorphan*	Narcotic analgesic
Levothroid	*levothyroxine*	Thyroid hormone
Levoxine	*levothyroxine*	Thyroid hormone
Levsin	*hyoscyamine*	Antispasmodic - Rx: ulcers
Librax	*chlordiazepoxide - clidinium*	Benzodiazepine hypnotic - antispasmodic compound - Rx: ulcers
Libritabs	*chlordiazepoxide*	Benzodiazepine hypnotic
Librium	*chlordiazepoxide*	Benzodiazepine hypnotic
Limbitrol - Limbitrol Ds	*chlordiazepoxide - amitriptyline*	Benzodiazepine hypnotic / tricyclic antidepressant - Rx: depression with anxiety
Lithane	*lithium*	Anti-manic agent - Rx: depression - mania
Lithium Carbonate	*lithobid*	Anti-manic - Rx: depression - mania
Lithobid	*lithium*	Anti-manic agent - Rx: depression - mania
Lithonate	*lithium*	Anti-manic agent - Rx: depression - mania
Lithotabs	*lithium*	Anti-manic agent - Rx: depression - mania
Lo-Ovral	*ethinyl estradiol*	Oral contraceptive
Lodine	*etodolac*	NSAID - analgesic
Lomotil	*diphenoxylate - atropine*	Narcotic anti-diarrhea / antispasmodic compound
Loniten	*minoxidil*	Vasodilator - Rx: hypertension - baldness
Lopid	*gemfibrozil*	Lowers serum lipids
Lopressor	*metoprolol*	Beta-1 blocker - Rx: hypertension
Lopurin	*allopurinol*	Reduces uric acid in gout
Lorazepam	*ativan*	Benzodiazepine hypnotic
Lorcet Hd - Lorcet Plus	*hydrocodone - apap*	Narcotic analgesic compound
Lorelco	*probucol*	Reduces serum cholesterol
Lortab	*hydrocodone - apap*	Narcotic analgesic
Lortab Asa	*hydrocodone - asa*	Narcotic analgesic
Lotensin	*benazepril*	Ace inhibitor - Rx: HTN
Lotrimin	*clotrimazole*	Antifungal agent
Lotrisone	*clotrimazole - betamethasone*	Topical antifungal / steroid anti-inflammatory compound
Loxitane	*loxapine*	Tranquilizer
Lozol	*indapamide*	Antihypertensive / diuretic
Ludiomil	*maprotiline*	Tetracyclic antidepressant
Lufyllin	*dyphylline*	Bronchodilator - Rx: COPD - asthma
Luminal	*phenobarbital*	Barbiturate sedative / anticonvulsant
Lurline PMS	*apap - pamabrom - pyridoxine*	Analgesic / diuretic / vitamin B-6 - Rx: premenstrual syndrome
Luvox	*fluvoxamine*	Rx: obsessive compulsive disorder
Macrobid	*nitrofurantoin*	Antibacterial - Rx: UTI
Macrodantin	*nitrofurantoin*	Antibacterial - Rx: UTI
Magan	*magnesium salicylate*	NSAID - Rx: arthritis
Magonate	*magnesium gluconate*	Electrolyte sedative - Rx: alcoholism - HTN - asthma
Mandelamine	*methylamine*	Antibacterial - Rx: UTI

Brand	Generic	Usage
Marax	*ephedrine - theophylline - hydroxyzine*	Bronchodilator compound - Rx: asthma
Marinol	*dronabinol*	Appetite stimulant - Rx: weight loss in AIDS - chemotherapy
Marplan	*isocarboxazid*	Mad inhibitor - Rx: depression
Materna	*prenatal vitamin*	Vitamin supplement
Maxair	*pirbuterol*	Beta-2 stimulant - Rx: asthma - COPD
Maxzide	*triamterene - hctz*	Anti-hypertensive / diuretic
Mebaral	*mephobarbital*	Barbiturate sedative / anticonvulsant
Meclizine	*antivert*	Anti-nausea - Rx: vertigo
Meclomen	*meclofenamate*	NSAID - Rx: arthritis - pain - dysmenorrhea - heavy menstrual blood loss
Medihaler-Epi	*epinephrine*	B-bronchodilator - Rx: asthma
Medrol	*methylprednisolone*	Steroid anti-inflammatory
Mefoxin	*cefoxitin*	Antibiotic
Megace	*megestrol*	Appetite stimulant - Rx: anorexia with AIDS
Mellaril	*thioridazine*	Major tranquilizer
Menrium	*chlordiazepoxide - estrogens*	Anxiolytic / hormone compound - Rx: menopause symptoms
Mepergan	*meperidine - promethazine*	Narcotic analgesic - phenothiazine sedative/antiemetic
Meperidine	*demerol*	Narcotic analgesic
Meprobamate	*meprospan*	Tranquilizer
Mepron	*atovaquone*	Antibiotic - Rx: pneumocystis carinii pneumonia in AIDS
Meprospan	*meprobamate*	Tranquilizer
Mesantoin	*mephenytoin*	Anticonvulsant
Mestinon	*pyridostigmine*	Anticholinesterase - Rx: myasthenia gravis
Metahydrin	*trichlormethiazide*	Antihypertensive / diuretic
Metaprel Inhaler	*metaproterenol*	Bronchodilator - Rx: COPD - asthma
Metastron	*strontium*	Non-narcotic analgesic - Rx: bone ca
Metatensin	*trichlormethiazide - reserpine*	Antihypertensive / diuretic
Methadone	*dolophine*	Narcotic analgesic
Methergine	*methylergonovine*	Uterotonic - Rx: postpartum hemorrhage
Methocarbamol	*robaxin*	Skeletal muscle antispasmodic
Methyclothiazide	*aquatensen*	Antihypertensive / diuretic
Methyldopa	*aldomet*	Antihypertensive
Methylprednisolone	*medrol*	Steroid anti-inflammatory
Metoclopramide	*reglan*	Improves gastric emptying - Rx: heartburn - ulcers
Metoprolol	*lopressor*	Cardio selective beta blocker - Rx: HTN - angina - arrhythmias
Metronidazole	*flagyl*	Antimicrobial agent
Mevacor	*lovastatin*	Lowers serum cholesterol
Mexitil	*mexiletine*	Antiarrhythmic
Micro-K	*kcl*	Potassium supplement
Micronase	*glyburide*	Oral hypoglycemic - Rx: diabetes
Midamor	*amiloride*	Potassium-sparing diuretic
Midol 200	*ibuprofen*	NSAID - Rx: menstrual cramps
Midol PMS	*apap - pamabrom - pyrilamine*	Analgesic - diuretic - antihistamine/ sedative - Rx: premenstrual syndrome
Milontin	*phensuximide*	Anticonvulsant - Rx: absence Sz
Miltown	*meprobamate*	Tranquilizer
Minipress	*prazosin*	Alpha-1 blocker - Rx: hypertension
Minizide	*prazosin - polythiazide*	Antihypertensive
Minocin	*minocycline*	Antibiotic
Minoxidil	*loniten*	Vasodilator / antihypertensive / topical hair growing agent - Rx: HTN - baldness
Moban	*molindone*	Tranquilizer
Moduretic	*amiloride - hctz*	Antihypertensive / diuretic
Monistat 7	*micronazole*	Antifungal agent
Monitan	*acebutolol*	B-blocker - Rx: HTN - angina - arrhythmias
Mono-Gesic	*salsalate*	NSAID - Rx: arthritis
Monoclate-P	*factor viii*	Antihemophilic factor
Monoket	*isosorbide mononitrate*	Nitrate - Rx: angina
Monopril	*fosinopril*	Ace inhibitor - Rx: HTN
Morphine Sulfate	*morphine*	Narcotic analgesic
Motofen	*difenoxin - atropine*	Narcotic antidiarrheal agent
Ms Contin	*morphine*	Narcotic analgesic
Msir	*morphine*	Narcotic analgesic
Mucomyst	*acetylcysteine*	Mucolytic - Rx: asthma
Myambutol	*ethambutol*	Chemotherapeutic - Rx: TB
Mycobutin	*rifabutin*	Antibiotic - Rx: AIDS
Mycolog li	*nystatin - triamcinolone*	Antifungal / steroid
Mycostatin	*nystatin*	Antifungal agent
Mykrox	*metolazone*	Antihypertensive / diuretic
Mysoline	*primidone*	Anticonvulsant - Rx: epilepsy
Nadolol	*corgard*	B-blocker - Rx: HTN - angina - arrhythmias
Naftin	*naftifine*	Topical antifungal agent
Naldecon	*phenylpropanolamine - phenylephrine - phenyltoloxamine - chlorpheniramine*	Antihistamine / decongestant compound - Rx: colds - allergies
Nalfon	*fenoprofen*	NSAID analgesic
Naprosyn	*naproxen*	NSAID analgesic
Naproxen	*anaprox*	NSAID analgesic
Naqua	*trichlormethiazide*	Antihypertensive / diuretic
Naquavil	*trichlormethiazide - reserpine*	Antihypertensive / diuretic
Nardil	*phenelzine*	MAO inhibitor - Rx: depression

DRUGS

Brand	Generic	Usage
Nasalcrom	*cromolyn*	Antiallergic - Rx: allergic rhinitis
Nasalide	*flunisolide*	Steroid anti-inflammatory agent
Naturetin	*bendroflumethiazide*	Antihypertensive / diuretic
Navane	*thiothixene*	Major tranquilizer
Nebupent	*pentamidine*	Anti-protozoal agent - Rx: pneumocystis carinii infection in AIDS
Nembutal	*pentobarbital*	Barbiturate sedative / hypnotic
Neo-Codima	*hydrochlorothiazide*	Antihypertensive / diuretic
Neosporin	*polymycin - bacitracin - neomycin*	Antibiotic
Neothylline	*dyphylline - guaifenesin*	Xanthine bronchodilator compound - Rx: COPD - asthma
Neptazane	*methazolamide*	Reduces intraocular pressure - Rx: glaucoma
Neurontin	*gabapentin*	Antiepileptic
Neutrexin	*trimetrexate*	Antineoplastic - Rx: Ca & pneumocystis pneumonia in AIDS.
Nia-Bid	*niacin*	Reduces serum cholesterol
Niacels	*nicotinic acid*	Reduces serum cholesterol niacin
Nicobid	*niacin*	Reduces serum cholesterol
Nicolar	*niacin*	Reduces serum cholesterol
Nifedipine	*procardia*	Calcium blocker - Rx: angina - HTN
Nilstat	*nystatin*	Antifungal agent
Nimotop	*nimodipine*	Calcium channel blocker - improves neurological deficits after subarachnoid hemorrhage
Nisentil	*alphaprodine*	Narcotic analgesic
Nitro-Bid	*nitroglycerin*	Long-acting nitrate - Rx: angina prophylaxis
Nitro-Dur	*nitroglycerin*	Long-acting nitrate - Rx: angina prophylaxis
Nitrodisc	*nitroglycerin*	Long-acting nitrate - Rx: angina prophylaxis
Nitrofurantoin	*furadantin*	Antibacterial agent - Rx: UTI
Nitrogard	*nitroglycerin*	Long-acting nitrate - Rx: angina prophylaxis
Nitroglycerin	*nitrostat*	Vasodilator - Rx: angina
Nitrol	*nitroglycerin*	Nitrate ointment - Rx: angina
Nitrolingual Spray	*nitroglycerin*	Nitrate - Rx: angina
Nitrong	*nitroglycerin*	Nitrate - Rx: angina prophylaxis
Nitrostat	*nitroglycerin*	Vasodilator - Rx: angina
Nix	*permethrin*	Parasiticide - Rx: head lice
Nizoral	*ketoconazole*	Antifungal agent - Rx: yeast infections
Nolamine	*phenindamine - chlorpheniramine - phenylpropanolamine*	Antihistamine / decongestant
Nolvadex	*tamoxifen*	Anticancer agent - Rx: breast ca
Nordette	*ethinyl estradiol*	Oral contraceptive
Norflex	*orphenadrine*	Non-narcotic analgesic
Norgesic	*orphenadrine*	Non-narcotic analgesic
Norinyl	*ethinyl estradiol*	Oral contraceptive
Norisodrine Aerotrol	*isoproterenol*	B-bronchodilator -Rx: asthma - COPD
Norlestrin	*ethinyl estradiol*	Oral contraceptive
Normodyne	*labetalol*	Beta blocker - Rx: HTN - angina
Noroxin	*norfloxacin*	Urinary tract antibiotic
Norpace	*disopyramide*	Antiarrhythmic - Rx: pvc's
Norpramin	*desipramine*	Tricyclic antidepressant
Norvasc	*amlodipine*	Calcium blocker - Rx: HTN - angina
Novahistine Dh	*codeine - pseudoephedrine - chlorpheniramine*	Narcotic antitussive / decongestant / antihistamine
Novahistine Expectorant	*codeine - pseudoephedrine - guaifenesin*	Narcotic antitussive / decongestant / expectorant
Novo-Hydrazide	*hydrochlorothiazide*	Antihypertensive /diuretic
Novolin	*insulin*	Rx: diabetes mellitus
Novopranol	*propranolol*	Beta blocker - Rx: HTN - angina - arrhythmias
Novosalmol	*albuterol*	B-2 bronchodilator - Rx: asthma - COPD
Nubain	*nalbuphine*	Narcotic analgesic
Nucofed	*codeine. pseudoephedrine*	Narcotic antitussive / decongestant
Numorphan	*oxymorphone*	Narcotic analgesic
Nuprin	*ibuprofen*	NSAID analgesic
Nylidrin	*arlidin*	Beta vasodilator - Rx: peripheral ischemia
Nystatin	*mycostatin*	Antifungal agent
Octamide	*metoclopramide*	Improves gastric emptying - Rx: heartburn - ulcers
Ogen	*estropipate*	Estrogen - Rx: menopause
Omnipen	*ampicillin*	Antibiotic
Optimine	*azatadine*	Antihistamine - Rx: urticaria - rhinitis
Oramorph	*morphine sulfate*	Narcotic analgesic
Orap	*pimozide*	Antipsychotic - Rx: meter & phonic tics
Oretic	*hydrochlorothiazide*	Antihypertensive / diuretic
Oreticyl	*hctz - deserpidine*	Antihypertensive
Orinase	*tolbutamide*	Oral hypoglycemic - Rx: diabetes
Orlaam	*levomethadyl*	Opiate agonist - Rx: narcotic addition
Ornade	*chlorpheniramine - phenylpropanolamine*	Antihistamine/ decongestant compound
Ortho-Novum	*ortho*	Oral contraceptive
Orudis	*ketoprofen*	NSAID - Rx: arthritis
Oruvail	*ketoprofen*	NSAID analgesic
OsCal	*calcium carbonate*	Calcium & Vitamin D supplement
Ovcon	*ethinyl estradiol*	Oral contraceptive
Ovide	*malathion*	Organophosphate insecticide - Rx: lice
Ovral	*ethinyl estradiol*	Oral contraceptive

Brand	Generic	Usage
Oxacillin	*antibiotic*	Antibiotic
Oxazepam	*serax*	Benzodiazepine hypnotic
Oxistat	*oxiconazole*	Topical antifungal agent
Oxprenolol	*trasicor*	B-blocker - Rx: HTN - angina - arrhythmias
Oxycodone	*percodan*	Narcotic analgesic
Oxycodone W/Apap	*tylox*	Narcotic analgesic compound
Pabalate	*salicylate - aminobenzoate*	Analgesic
Pamelor	*nortriptyline*	Tricyclic antidepressant
Panmycin	*tetracycline*	Antibiotic
Pantopon	*opium alkaloids*	Narcotic analgesic
Panwarfarin	*warfarin*	Anticoagulant
Panwarfin	*warfarin*	Anticoagulant
Papaverine	*pavabid*	Vasodilator - Rx: cerebral & peripheral vascular ischemia
Paradione	*paramethadione*	Antiepileptic agent - Rx: absence seizures
Paraflex	*chlorzoxazone*	Skeletal muscle antispasmodic - Rx: sprains - strains
Parafon Forte	*chlorzoxazone - acetaminophen*	Muscle relaxant / analgesic compound
Paregoric	*tincture of opium*	Narcotic - Rx: diarrhea
Parepectolin	*opium - pectin*	Narcotic analgesic / stool binder compound - Rx: diarrhea
Parlodel	*bromocriptine*	Ergot - Rx: Parkinson's disease; also decreases milk production in the postpartum female
Parnate	*tranylcypromine*	MAO inhibiter - Rx: depression
Pavabid	*papaverine*	Vasodilator - Rx: cerebral & peripheral vascular disease
Paxil	*paroxetine*	Antidepressant.
Paxipam	*halazepam*	Benzodiazepine hypnotic
Pce	*erythromycin*	Antibiotic
Pediaprofen	*ibuprofen*	NSAID analgesic / antipyretic
Pediazole	*erythoromycin*	Antibiotic compound
Peganone	*ethotoin*	Antiepileptic - Rx: seizures
Pen-Vee K	*penicillin*	Antibiotic
Penbutolol	*levatol*	Beta blocker - Rx: HTN - angina
Penicillin	*penicilin*	Antibiotic
Pentam 300	*pentamidine*	Antimicrobial - Rx: pneumocystis carinii pneumonia
Pentasa	*mesalamine*	For ulcerative colitis
Pentids	*penicillin*	Antibiotic
Pentritol	*pentaerythritol tetranitrate*	Long-acting nitrate - Rx: angina prophylaxis
Pepcid	*famotidine*	Histamine-2 blocker which inhibits gastric acid production - Rx: ulcers
Percocet	*oxycodone - apap*	Narcotic analgesic
Percodan	*oxycodone - aspirin*	Narcotic analgesic
Percodan-Demi	*oxycodone - aspirin*	Narcotic analgesic

Brand	Generic	Usage
Periactin	*cyproheptadine*	Antihistamine
Peritrate	*pentaerythritol tetranitrate*	Long-acting nitrate - Rx: angina prophylaxis
Permax	*pergolide*	Dopamine receptor stimulator - Rx: Parkinson's disease
Perphenazine	*trilafon*	Phenothiazine major tranquilizer
Persantine	*dipyridamole*	Cerebral & coronary vasodilator - Rx: CVA - angina
Pertofrane	*desipramine*	Tricyclic antidepressant
Phazyme	*simethicone*	Anti-gas agent
Phenaphen With Codeine	*apap - codeine*	Narcotic analgesic
Phenergan	*promethazine*	Phenothiazine sedative / antiemetic
Phenobarbital	*luminal*	Barbiturate sedative / anticonvulsant
Phenurone	*phenacemide*	Antiepileptic
Phenylbutazone	*butazolidin*	NSAID - Rx: arthritis
Phenylpropanolamine W/ Guaifenesin	*entex la*	Decongestant / expectorant compound
Phenytoin	*dilantin*	Anticonvulsant - Rx: epilepsy
Phrenilin	*butalbital - apap*	Analgesic compound
Pindolol	*visken*	Bata blocker - Rx: HTN - angina
Placidyl	*ethchlorvynol*	Hypnotic - Rx: insomnia
Plaquenil	*hydroxychloroquine*	Antimalarial agent
Plendil	*felodipine*	Calcium blocker - Rx: HTN - angina
Pmb 200 & 400	*estrogens - meprobamate*	Rx: s/s menopause
Polaramine	*dexchlorpheniramine*	Antihistamine - Rx: allergies
Poly-Vi-Flor	*multivitamin*	Vitamins with fluoride
Polycillin	*ampicillin*	Antibiotic polymycin
Pondimin	*fenfluramine*	Stimulant - Rx: appetite suppression
Ponstel	*mefenamic acid*	NSAID analgesic
Potassium	*potassium supplement*	K-tab
Pravachol	*pravastatin*	Cholesterol reducer
Prazosin	*minipress*	Alpha-1 blocker - vasodilator - Rx: HTN
Prednisolone	*prelone*	Steroid anti-inflammatory agent
Prednisone	*deltasone*	Steroid anti-inflammatory agent
Prelone Syrup	*prednisolone*	Steroid anti-inflammatory agent
Preludin	*phenmetrazine*	Stimulant - Rx: appetite suppression Rx: ulcers - esophagitis
Primatene Mist	*epinephrine*	Bronchodilator - Rx: asthma
Primatene Tablets	*theophylline - ephedrine - phenobarbital*	Xanthine bronchodilator - Rx: asthma
Primidone	*mysoline*	Anticonvulsant - Rx: epilepsy
Principen	*ampicillin*	Antibiotic
Prinivil	*lisinopril*	Ace inhibitor - Rx: HTN - CHF
Prinzide	*lisinopril - hctz*	Antihypertensive compound

Brand	Generic	Usage
Pro-Banthine	*propantheline*	Anticholinergic - Rx: ulcers
Probenecid	*benemid*	Increases uric acid secretion in gout; also slows the elimination of penicillin from the body
Procainamide	*procan*	Antiarrhythmic - Rx: pvc's
Procan	*procainamide*	Antiarrhythmic - Rx: pvc's
Procardia - Procardia XI	*nifedipine*	Calcium channel blocker - Rx: angina - hypertension
Prochlorperazine	*compazine*	Phenothiazine antiemetic
Proglycem	*diazoxide*	Increases blood glucose - Rx: hypoglycemia
Prograf	*tacrolimus*	Immunosuppressant - Rx: liver transplant
Prolixin	*fluphenazine*	Major tranquilizer
Proloid	*thyroglobulin*	Thyroid hormones
Promet	*promethazine*	Phenothiazine antiemetic
Promethazine	*phenergan*	Phenothiazine sedative/ antiemetic
Pronestyl	*procainamide*	Antiarrhythmic - Rx: pvc's
Propacet	*propoxyphene - apap*	Narcotic analgesic compound
Propagest	*phenylpropanolamine*	Nasal decongestant
Propoxyphene	*darvon*	Narcotic analgesic
Propranolol	*inderal*	Beta blocker - Rx: HTN - prophylaxis of: angina - cardiac dysrhythmias - AMI - migraine H/A
Propulsid	*cisapride*	Increases gastric emptying
Proscar	*finasteride*	Rx: prostatic hypertrophy
Prosom	*estazolam*	Hypnotic - Rx: insomnia
Prostigmin	*neostigmine*	Anticholinesterase - Rx: myasthenia gravis
Protropin	*somatrem*	Human growth hormone
Proventil	*albuterol*	Beta-2 bronchodilator - Rx: asthma
Provera	*medroxyprogesterone*	Hormone - Rx: amenorrhea
Prozac	*fluoxetine*	Heterocyclic antidepressant
Pulmozyme	*domase alfa or dnase*	Lyric enzyme which dissolves infected lung secretions - Rx: cystic fibrosis
Pyridium	*phenazopyridine*	Urinary tract analgesic
Quadrinal	*ephedrine - phenobarbital - theophylline - potassium iodide*	Bronchodilator / sedative / expectorant - Rx: COPD
Questran	*cholestyramine*	Lowers serum cholesterol
Quibron	*theophylline - guaifenesin*	Xanthine bronchodilator compound - Rx: COPD - asthma
Quinaglute	*quinidine*	Antiarrhythmic - Rx: supraventricular & ventricular dysrhythmias
Quinidex	*quinidine*	Antiarrhythmic - Rx: supraventricular & ventricular dysrhythmias
Quinidine Gluconate	*quinidine*	Antiarrhythmic - Rx: supraventricular & ventricular dysrhythmias
Quinidine Sulfate	*quinidine*	Antiarrhythmic - Rx: supraventricular & ventricular dysrhythmias
Rauzide	*rauwolfia - bendroflumethiazide*	Antihypertensive / diuretic compound
Reglan	*metoclopramide*	Improves gastric emptying - Rx: heartburn - ulcers
Regroton	*chlorthalidone - reserpine*	Antihypertensive / diuretic compound
Relafen	*nabumetone*	NSAID - Rx: arthritis
Renedil	*felodipine*	Calcium channel blocker - Rx: HTN - angina
Renese	*polythiazide*	Antihypertensive / diuretic
Renese-R	*polythiazide - reserpine*	Antihypertensive / diuretic compound - Rx: hypertension
Renormax	*spirapril*	Ace inhibitor - Rx: hypertension
Rescudose	*morphine*	Oral narcotic analgesic
Reserpine	*serpasil*	Antihypertensive / tranquilizer
Respbid	*theophylline*	Bronchodilator - Rx: asthma - COPD
Restoril	*temazepam*	Benzodiazepine hypnotic
Retin-A	*tretinoin*	Anti-acne - anti-wrinkle agent
Retrovir	*zidovudine*	Antiviral agent - Rx: HIV/AIDS
Rid	*pyrethrins*	Parasiticide - Rx: lice
Ridaura	*auranofin*	Gold compound - Rx: arthritis
Rifadin	*rifampin*	Antibiotic - Rx: TB - meningitis
Rifamate	*rifampin - isoniazid*	Antibiotics - Rx: TB
Rifater	*isoniazid - rifampin - pyrazinamide*	Antibiotic - Rx: TB
Risperdal	*risperidone*	Antipsychotic - Rx: schizophrenia
Ritalin - Ritalin-Sr	*methylphenidate*	Stimulant - Rx: attention deficit disorder in children
Rms	*morphine sulfate*	Narcotic analgesic suppositories
Robaxin	*methocarbamol*	Skeletal muscle antispasmodic
Robaxisal	*methocarbamol - aspirin*	Skeletal muscle antispasmodic / analgesic compound
Robitet	*tetracycline*	Antibiotic
Rocephin	*ceftriaxone*	Antibiotic
Roferon-A	*interferon*	Immunoadjuvant - Rx: hairy cell leukemia - AIDS-related Karposi's sarcoma
Rogaine	*minoxidil*	Topical hair growing agent - Rx: baldness
Roxanol 100	*morphine*	Narcotic analgesic
Roxicet	*oxycodone - apap*	Narcotic analgesic compound
Roxicodone	*oxycodone*	Narcotic analgesic
Rynatan	*phenylephrine - chlorpheniramine - pyrilamine*	Antihistamine / decongestant compound
Rynatuss		Antitussive / decongestant / antihistamine
Rythmol	*propafenone*	Antiarrhythmic - Rx: severe ventricular dysrhythmias such as ventricular tachycardia
Sabril	*vigabatrin*	Anticonvulsant
Salbutamol	*albuterol*	Bronchodilator - Rx: asthma - COPD
Salflex	*salsalate*	NSAID analgesic - Rx: arthritis
Saluron	*hydroflumethiazide*	Antihypertensive / diuretic
Salutensin - Salutensin Demi	*hydroflumethiazide - reserpine*	Antihypertensive / diuretic compound
Sandimmune	*cyclosporine*	Immunosuppressant agent - Rx: prophylaxis of rejection of transplanted organs
Sansert	*methysergide*	Serotonin inhibitor - Rx: headaches

DRUGS

Brand	Generic	Usage
Scopolamine	*plexonal*	Antispasmodic / sedative
Secobarbital	*seconal*	Barbiturate sedative / hypnotic
Seconal	*secobarbital*	Barbiturate sedative / hypnotic
Sectral	*acebutolol*	B-blocker - Rx: HTN - cardiac dysrhythmias
Sedapap # 3	*codeine - apap - butalbital*	Narcotic analgesic
Sedapap - Sedapap # 10	*butalbital - apap*	Sedative / analgesic compound - Rx: tension headaches
Seldane	*terfenadine*	Antihistamine - Rx: allergies
Selenium	*selsun blue*	Trace mineral - Rx: seborrhea - dandruff
Senokot	*senna fruit extract*	Laxative
Septra	*trimethoprim - sulfamethoxazole*	Antibacterial compound - Rx: UTI - ear infection - bronchitis
Ser-Ap-Es	*reserpine - hydralazine - hctz*	Antihypertensive / diuretic compound
Serax	*oxazepam*	Benzodiazepine hypnotic
Serentil	*mesoridazine*	Major tranquilizer
Serevent	*salmeterol*	B-2 bronchodilator - Rx: asthma - COPD
Seromycin	*cycloserine*	Antibiotic - Rx: TB - UTI
Serpasil	*reserpine*	Antihypertensive / tranquilizer
Serpasil-Apresoline	*reserpine - hydralazine*	Antihypertensive compound
Serpasil-Esidrix	*reserpine - hctz*	Antihypertensive
Serzone	*nefazodone*	Antidepressant - Rx: depression
Silvadene	*silver sulfadiazine*	Topical antimicrobial agent - Rx: infection prophylaxis for burns of the skin
Sinemet	*carbidopa - levodopa*	Dopamine precursors - Rx: Parkinson's disease
Sinequan	*doxepin*	Tricyclic antidepressant
Sinubid	*apap - phenylpropanolamine - phenyltoloxamine*	Analgesic / decongestant compound
Sinulin	*apap - phenylpropanolamine - chlorpheniramine*	Analgesic / decongestant / antihistamine - Rx: colds - allergies
Slo-Bid	*theophylline*	Bronchodilator - Rx: COPD - asthma
Slo-Phyllin	*theophylline*	Bronchodilator - Rx: COPD - asthma
Slow-Trasicor	*oxprenolol*	Beta blocker - Rx: HTN - angina - arrhythmias
Sofarin	*warfarin*	Anticoagulant
Solfoton	*phenobarbital*	Barbiturate sedative/hypnotic
Soma	*carisoprodol*	Sedative / antispasmodic
Soma Compound	*carisoprodol - aspirin*	Sedative / antispasmodic / analgesic - Rx: muscle spasm
Sorbitrate	*isosorbide dinitrate*	Nitrate - Rx: angina
Sotacor	*sotalol*	B-blocker - Rx: HTN - angina - arrhythmias
Sotalol	*betapace*	B-blocker - Rx: HTN - angina - arrhythmias
Sparine	*promazine*	Major tranquilizer
Spectazole	*econazole*	Antifungal agent
Spectrobid	*bacampicillin*	Antibiotic
Spironolactone	*aldactone*	Potassium-sparing diuretic

Brand	Generic	Usage
Sporanox	*itraconazole*	Antifungal
Spt	*pork thyroid hormone*	Rx: hypothyroidism
Sski	*potassium iodide*	Expectorant
Stadol	*butorphanol*	Narcotic analgesic
Stelazine	*trifluoperazine*	Major tranquilizer
Sublimaze	*fentanyl*	Narcotic analgesic
Sufenta	*sufentanil*	Narcotic analgesic / anesthetic
Sulfamethoxazole	*gantanol*	Bacteriostatic - Rx: UTI
Sulfisoxazole	*gantrisin*	Bacteriostatic agent - Rx: UTI
Sulindac	*clinoril*	NSAID analgesic - Rx: arthritis
Sumycin	*tetracycline*	Antibiotic
Supac	*apap - asa - caffeine - calcium*	Analgesic compound - Rx: colds - headache - arthritis
Suprax	*cefixime*	Broad spectrum antibiotic
Surfak	*docusate*	Stool softener
Surmontil	*trimipramine*	Tricyclic antidepressant
Symmetrel	*amantadine*	Antiparkinsonian / antiviral
Synalgos	*aspirin - promethazine - caffeine*	Analgesic - sedative/ antiemetic compound
Synalgos-Dc	*dihydrocodeine - aspirin - caffeine*	Narcotic analgesic compound
Synthroid	*levothyroxine*	Thyroid hormone
T-Gesic	*apap - hydrocodone*	Narcotic analgesic
T-Phyl	*theophylline*	Bronchodilator - Rx: asthma - COPD
Tagamet	*cimetidine*	Histamine-2 blocker which inhibits gastric acid secretion - Rx: ulcers
Talacen	*pentazocine + apap*	Narcotic analgesic
Talwin	*pentazocine*	Narcotic analgesic
Talwin Compound	*pentazocine - asa*	Narcotic analgesic
Talwin Nx	*pentazocine - naloxone*	Narcotic analgesic
Tambocor	*flecainide*	Ventricular antiarrhythmic
Tamoxifen	*nolvadex*	Anticancer agent - Rx: breast ca
Taractan	*chlorprothixene*	Major tranquilizer
Tavist	*clemastine*	Antihistamine - Rx: allergies
Tavist-D	*clemastine - phenylpropanolamine*	Antihistamine /decongestant - Rx: allergies
Tazicef	*ceftazidime*	Antibiotic
Tazidime	*ceftazidime*	Antibiotic
Tedral	*theophylline - ephedrine - phenobarbital*	Bronchodilator compound - Rx: asthma - bronchitis
Tegretol	*carbamazepine*	Anticonvulsant - Rx: epilepsy
Teldrin	*chlorpheniramine*	Antihistamine
Temaril	*trimeprazine*	Phenothiazine antipyretic / antihistamine - Rx: urticaria
Ten-K	*potassium*	Potassium supplement

Brand	Generic	Usage
Tenex	*guanfacine*	Antihypertensive agent
Tenodmin	*atenolol*	Beta-1 blocker - Rx: dysrhythmias - HTN - angina - MI prophylaxis
Tenuate	*diethylpropion*	Stimulant / appetite suppressant
Terazol	*terconazole*	Antimicrobial - Rx: candidiasis
Terazosin	*hytrin*	Alpha-1 blocker antihypertensive
Terpin Hydrate	*codeine*	Expectorant
Terramycin	*oxtetracycline*	Antibiotic
Teslac	*testolactone*	Antineoplastic - Rx: breast cancer
Tessalon	*benzonatate*	Non-narcotic cough suppressant
Tetracycline	*achromycin*	Antibiotic
Thalitone	*chlorthalidone*	Antihypertensive / diuretic - Rx: HTN - CHF
Theo-24	*theophylline*	Bronchodilator - Rx: asthma - COPD
Theo-Dur	*theophylline*	Bronchodilator - Rx: asthma - COPD
Theo-Organidin	*theophylline - glycerol*	Bronchodilator/ expectorant compound - Rx: asthma - COPD
Theobid	*theophylline*	Bronchodilator - Rx: asthma - COPD
Theochron	*theophylline*	Bronchodilator - Rx: asthma - COPD
Theoclear	*theophylline*	Bronchodilator - Rx: asthma - COPD
Theolair	*theophylline*	Bronchodilator - Rx: asthma - COPD
Theophyl-Sr	*theophylline*	Bronchodilator - Rx: asthma - COPD
Theophylline	*theodur*	Bronchodilator - Rx: asthma - COPD
Theox	*theophylline*	Bronchodilator - Rx: asthma - COPD
Thiosulfil-A	*phenazopyridine - sulfamethizole*	Urinary tract analgesic / antibiotic
Thorazine	*chlorpromazine*	Major tranquilizer
Thyrolar	*liotrix*	Thyroid hormone
Tigan	*trimethobenzamide*	Antiemetic
Timentin	*ticarcillin / clavulanate*	Antibiotic compound
Timolide	*timolol - hctz*	B-blocker / antihypertensive / diuretic
Timoptic	*timolol*	Beta blocker - Rx: glaucoma
Tobrex	*tobramycin*	Antibiotic
Tofranil	*imipramine*	Tricyclic antidepressant
Tolazamide	*tolinase*	Oral hypoglycemic - Rx: diabetes
Tolbutamide	*orinase*	Oral hypoglycemic - Rx: diabetes
Tolectin	*tolmetin*	NSAID analgesic
Tolinase	*tolazamide*	Oral hypoglycemic - Rx: diabetes
Tonocard	*tocainide*	Ventricular antiarrhythmic
Toprol-Xl	*metoprolol*	Cardio selective beta blocker - Rx: HTN - angina - arrhythmias
Toradol	*ketorolac*	NSAID analgesic
Torecan	*thiethylperazine*	Phenothiazine antiemetic
Trancopal	*chlormezanone*	Anxiolytic agent
Trandate	*labetalol*	Beta blocker - Rx: hypertension
Trandate Hct	*labetalol - hctz*	Alpha & beta blocker/ antihypertensive / diuretic compound - Rx: hypertension
Transderm Nitro	*nitroglycerin*	Nitrate vasodilator - Rx: angina prophylaxis
Transderm-Scop	*scopolamine*	Anticholinergic antiemetic - Rx: motion sickness prophylaxis
Tranxene T-Tab - Tranxene-Sd	*clorazepate*	Benzodiazepine hypnotic - Rx: anxiety - seizures
Trasicor	*oxprenolol*	B-blocker - Rx: HTN - angina - arrhythmias
Trazodone	*desyrel*	Antidepressant
Trecator-Sc	*ethionamide*	Bacteriostatic - Rx: TB
Trental	*pentoxifylline*	Reduces blood viscosity - improves circulation in peripheral vascular disease
Trexan	*naltrexone*	Opioid antagonist - Rx: maintenance of narcotic-free state for detoxified addicts
Tri-Levlen		Oral contraceptive
Trialodine	*trazodone*	Antidepressant
Triamcinolone	*azmacort*	Steroid anti-inflammatory
Triamterene C Hctz	*dyazide*	Antihypertensive / diuretic
Triavil	*amitriptyline - perphenazine*	Tricyclic antidepressant / major tranquilizer combination
Trichlorex	*trichlormethiazide*	Antihypertensive / diuretic
Trichlormethiazide	*metahydrin*	Antihypertensive / diuretic
Tridione	*trimethadione*	Antiepileptic - Rx: absence seizures
Trifluoperazine	*stelazine*	Major tranquilizer
Trihexyphenidyl	*artane*	Antispasmodic - Rx: Parkinson's disease
Trilafon	*perphenazine*	Major tranquilizer
Trilisate	*salicylate*	Anti-inflammatory / analgesic
Trimethoprim	*bactrim*	Antibiotic
Trimethoprim-Sulfamethoxazole	*bactrim*	Antibacterial - Rx: UTI - ear infection - bronchitis
Trimox	*amoxicillin*	Antibiotic
Trinalin	*azatadine - pseudoephedrine*	Antihistamine / decongestant compound
Triphasil	*ethinyl estradiol*	Oral contraceptive
Triprolidine	*actidil*	Antihistamine - Rx: allergies
Tuinal	*secobarbital - amobarbital*	Barbiturate/sedative
Tussar -Sf	*codeine - chlorpheniramine - guaifenesin*	Narcotic antitussive / antihistamine / expectorant - Rx: colds
Tussar-2	*codeine - chlorpheniramine - guaifenesin*	Narcotic antitussive / antihistamine / expectorant - Rx: colds
Tussend	*hydrocodone*	Narcotic antitussive agent
Tussi-Organidin	*glycerol - codeine*	Narcotic antitussive / expectorant compound
Tussi-Organidin Dm	*dextromethorphan - iodinated glycerol*	Antitussive / mucolytic - Rx: COPD - asthma - colds
Tussigon	*hydrocodone - homatropine*	Narcotic antitussive
Tussionex	*hyde - chlorpheniramine*	Narcotic antitussive / antihistamine compound
Tylenol W/ Codeine	*apap - codeine*	Narcotic analgesic
Tylox	*oxycodone - acetaminophen*	Narcotic analgesic

DRUGS

Brand	Generic	Usage
Ultracef	cefadroxil	Antibiotic
Uniphyl	theophylline	Bronchodilator - Rx: asthma - COPD
Unipres	hydralazine - hctz - reserpine	Antihypertensive / diuretic compound
Unitensen	cryptenamine	Antihypertensive
Urecholine	bethanechol	Vagomimetic agent which increases bladder tone - Rx: urinary retention
Uridon	chlorthalidone	Antihypertensive / diuretic
Urispas	flavoxate	Urinary tract antispasmodic - Rx: urinary incontinence
Urozide	hydrochloro-thiazide	Antihypertensive / diuretic
V-Cillin	penicillin	Antibiotic
Valisone	betamethasone	Steroid anti-inflammatory
Valium	diazepam	Benzodiazepine hypnotic
Valmid	ethinamate	Sedative
Valrelease	diazepam	Benzodiazepine hypnotic
Valtrex	valaciclovir	Antiviral - Rx: herpes
Vancenase - Vancenase Ac	beclomethasone	Steroid anti-inflammatory agent - Rx: allergic rhinitis - nasal polyps
Vanceril Inhaler	beclomethasone	Steroid - Rx: asthma
Vancocin	vancomycin	Antibiotic
Vantin	cefpodoxime	Antibiotic
Vapo-Iso	isoproterenol	B-bronchodilator - Rx: asthma - COPD
Vaponephrine	racepinephrine	Bronchodilator - Rx: asthma
Vascor	bepridil	Calcium blocker - Rx: angina prophylaxis
Vaseretic	enalapril - hctz	Antihypertensive / diuretic
Vasodilan	isoxsuprine	Beta vasodilator - Rx: peripheral & cerebral ischemia
Vasotec	enalapril	Ace inhibitor - Rx: hypertension - CHF
Veetids	penicillin	Antibiotic
Velosef	cephradine	Antibiotic
Venlafaxine	effexor	Antidepressant
Ventolin	albuterol	B-2 bronchodilator - Rx: asthma - COPD
Verapamil	calan	Calcium blocker - Rx: angina - PSVT - HTN - H/A
Verelan	verapamil	Calcium blocker - Rx: angina - hypertension - PSVT - prophylaxis - headache
Vermox	mebendazole	Anthelminthic - Rx: intestinal worms
Versed	midazolam	Benzodiazepine hypnotic
Vesprin	triflupromazine	Major tranquilizer
Vibramycin	doxycycline	Antibiotic
Vibratabs	doxycycline	Antibiotic
Vicodin	hydrocodone - apap	Narcotic analgesic
Vicodin Es	hydrocodone - apap	Narcotic analgesic
Vicon-C	multivitamin	Vitamins
Videx	didanosine	Antiviral - Rx: aids
Virazole	ribavirin	Antiviral drug - Rx: chronic hepatitis C
Visken	pindolol	Beta blocker - Rx: HTN - angina
Vistaril	hydroxyzine	Antiemetic / antihistamine / sedative
Vivactil	protriptyline	Tricyclic antidepressant
Voltaren	diclofenac	NSAID analgesic - Rx: arthritis
Vontrol	diphenidol	Antiemetic - Rx: N&V - vertigo
Wellbutrin	bupropion	Antidepressant
Westcort	hydrocortisone	Topical steroid - Rx: dermatoses
Wigraine	ergotamine - caffeine	Alpha blocker / cranial vasoconstrictor - Rx: migraine headache
Winstrol	stanozolol	Anabolic steroid / androgen - Rx: hereditary angioedema
Wycillin	penicillin	Antibiotic
Wygesic	propoxyphene - apap	Narcotic analgesic
Wymox	amoxicillin	Antibiotic
Wytensin	guanabenz	Antihypertensive
Xanax	alprazolam	Benzodiazepine hypnotic
Yocon	yohimbine	Sympathicolytic / cholinergic agent - Rx: male erectile impotence
Yodoxin	iodoquinol	Amebicide - Rx: intestinal amebiasis
Yohimex	yohimbine	Sympathicolytic / cholinergic agent - Rx: male erectile impotence
Yutopar	ritodrine	Beta-2 stimulant which decreases uterine activity - prevents labor & prolongs gestation
Zantac	ranitidine	Histamine-2 blocker which inhibits gastric acid secretion - Rx: ulcers
Zarontin	ethosuximide	Anticonvulsant - Rx: absence SZ
Zaroxolyn	metolazone	Antihypertensive/diuretic
Zebeta	bisoprolol	Beta blocker antihypertensive
Zefazone	cefmetazole	Antibiotic
Zerit	stavudine	Anti-HIV antibiotic
Zestoretic	lisinopril - hctz	Ace inhibitor / diuretic - Rx: HTN
Zestril	lisinopril	Ace inhibitor - Rx: HTN - CHF
Ziac	bisoprolol - hctz	Antihypertensive/diuretic - Rx: HTN.
Zidovudine	azt	Antiviral agent - Rx: HIV aids virus
Zithromax	azithromycin	Antibiotic
Zocor	simvastatin	Cholesterol reducer
Zoladex	goserelin	Gonadotropin-releasing hormone agonist - Rx: endometriosis.
Zoloft	sertraline	Antidepressant
Zorprin	aspirin	NSAID analgesic
Zostrix	capsaicin	Topical analgesic - Rx: herpes
Zovirax	acyclovir	Antiviral agent - Rx: herpes - shingles
Zydone	apap - hydrocodone	Narcotic analgesic
Zyloprim	allopurinol	Reduces serum uric acid - Rx: gout

Herb	Interaction
Astragalus	**Immunosuppressants** - astragalus ↓ the efficacy of these medications
Bilberry	**Warfarin, aspirin, anti-platelet drugs** - bilberry (at very high doses) ↑ the risk of bleeding
Black cohosh	**Chemotherapeutic agents** - black cohosh may affect the cytotoxicity of some drugs used in breast cancer treatment
	Tamoxifen - evidence regarding the effect of black cohosh on tamoxifen efficacy and breast cancer cell growth is conflicting
Celery	**Thyroid hormone** - celery ↓ blood levels of this medication
Coleus	**Antihypertensive medication** - coleus may have additive hypotensive effects
Cranberry	**Warfarin** - cranberry juice ↑ or ↓ the anticoagulant effect of this medication
Dong quai	**Warfarin** - dong quai ↑ the risk of bleeding
Echinacea	**Immunosuppressants** - echinacea ↓ the efficacy of these medications
Evening primrose oil	**Phenothiazines** - EPO ↑ the risk of seizures in patients receiving phenothiazines
Fenugreek	**Hypoglycemic therapy** - fenugreek ↓ blood glucose levels
Garlic	**Protease inhibitors** - garlic ↓ blood levels of protease inhibitors
	Warfarin, aspirin, anti-platelet drugs - garlic ↑ the risk of bleeding with these medications
Ginkgo	**Haloperidol, olanzapine** - ginkgo may enhance the therapeutic effect of these medications in the treatment of schizophrenia
	Hypoglycemic therapy - ginkgo may affect blood glucose levels
	Nifedipine - ginkgo ↑ blood levels and side effects of this medication
	Warfarin, aspirin, anti-platelet drugs - ginkgo ↑ the risk of bleeding with these medications
Ginseng (Korean)	**Digoxin** - Korean ginseng may affect digoxin assays
	Hypoglycemic therapy - Korean ginseng may affect blood glucose levels
	Phenelzine - Korean ginseng ↑ side effects of phenelzine or other MAOIs
	Warfarin - Korean ginseng ↓ the anticoagulant effect of warfarin
Ginseng (Siberian)	**Digoxin** - Siberian ginseng may affect digoxin assays
	Phenelzine - Siberian ginseng ↑ side effects of phenelzine or other MAOIs
Hawthorn	**Antihypertensive medication** - hawthorn may have an additive hypotensive effect with these medications
Kelp	**Thyroid hormone** - kelp (at very high doses) may precipitate or exacerbate hyper- or hypothyroidism

Herb	Interaction
Licorice	**Antihypertensive medication** - licorice may have a hypertensive effect
	Digoxin - licorice ↑ the risk of digoxin toxicity (possibly via hypokalaemia)
	Diuretics, laxatives - licorice (at high doses) ↑ the risk of electrolyte disturbances, especially hypokalemia, with the use of these medications
	Prednisolone - licorice ↑ blood levels of prednisolone
Milk thistle/ St. Mary's thistle	**Metronidazole** - milk thistle ↓ blood levels of this medication
	Paracetamol and other hepatotoxic medications - milk thistle protects and stimulates the regeneration of normal liver cells
Pau d'arco	**Warfarin, aspirin, anti-platelet drugs** - pau d'arco (at very high doses) ↑ the risk of bleeding with these medications
Psyllium husk	**Lithium, other orally administered drugs** - psyllium ↓ the absorption of lithium and other oral drugs unless doses are taken at least one hour before
Red clover/ isoflavones	**Tamoxifen** - evidence regarding the effect of red clover on tamoxifen efficacy and breast cancer cell growth is conflicting
St John's wort	**St John's wort has been noted to increase the action of the hepatic enzyme system, which ↓ the efficacy of these medications**: oral contraceptives, warfarin, protease inhibitors, reverse transcriptase inhibitors, simvastatin, verapamil, irinotecan, imatinib, methadone, cyclosporin, tacrolimus, midazolam, omeprazole
	Digoxin - St John's wort ↓ blood levels of this medication
	Prescription antidepressants - tricyclics & SSRIs - St John's wort may cause serotonergic syndrome with SSRIs; St John's wort ↓ blood levels of tricyclic antidepressants
Slippery elm	**Orally administered drugs** - slippery elm may reduce the absorption of some medications unless doses are separated by 2-3 hours
Soy/ isoflavones	**Tamoxifen** - evidence regarding the effect of soy on tamoxifen efficacy and breast cancer cell growth is conflicting
	Thyroid hormone - soy protein ↓ absorption and efficacy of this medication unless doses are separated by at least 2 hours
	Warfarin - soy protein ↓ the anticoagulant effect of this medication
Willow	**Warfarin, aspirin, anti-platelet drugs** - willow ↑ the risk of bleeding with these medications

Nutrient	Interaction
L. acidophilus	**Antibiotics -** probiotics such as L. acidophilus restore gut flora and reduce diarrhea secondary to antibiotic therapy
Calcium	**Bisphosphonates, tetracycline and quinolone antibiotics, thyroid hormones** - calcium ↓ the absorption and efficacy of these medications unless doses are separated by at least 2 hours
	Calcium channel blockers - calcium ↓ the hypotensive and antiarrhythmic effects of verapamil
	Thiazide diuretics - calcium ↑ the risk of hypercalcaemia with these medications
Co-enzyme Q10	**HMG-CoA reductase inhibitors (statins)** - CoQ10 levels may be depleted by statin medications
	Hypoglycemic therapy - CoQ10 ↓ blood glucose levels
	Warfarin - CoQ10 ↓ the anticoagulant effect of warfarin
Fish oil	**Hypoglycemic therapy** - fish oils (at high doses) ↑ blood glucose levels and/or affect insulin levels
Flaxseed oil	**Warfarin, aspirin, anti-platelet drugs -** flaxseed oil ↑ the risk of bleeding with these medications
Folic acid	**Anticonvulsant medication -** folic acid ↓ the efficacy of phenytoin. Phenytoin and folic acid should be commenced at the same time
	Co-trimoxazole, sulphasalazine, phenytoin, phenobarbital, primidone and methotrexate - ↓ efficacy of folic acid supplements
	Fluorouracil - folic acid ↑ the toxicity of fluorouracil
Glucosamine	**Hypoglycemic therapy -** glucosamine may affect blood glucose levels in diabetics
Iodine	**Lithium carbonate -** iodine (at high doses) ↑ the hypothyroid activity of lithium carbonate
	Thyroid hormone - iodine (at very high doses) may precipitate or exacerbate hyper- or hypothyroidism
Iron	**Bisphosphonates, tetracycline and quinolone antibiotics, thyroid hormone, methyldopa, carbidopa, levodopa and penicillamine -** iron ↓ the absorption and efficacy of these medications unless doses are separated by at least 2 hours
Magnesium	**Tetracycline and quinolone antibiotics -** magnesium ↓ the absorption and efficacy of these medications unless doses are separated by at least 2 hours
L-Methionine	**Levodopa -** L-Methionine ↓ the efficacy of levodopa in Parkinson's disease
Nicotinic acid	**Antihypertensive medication -** nicotinic acid may have additive hypotensive effects with antihypertensive
	HMG-CoA reductase inhibitors (statins) - nicotinic acid ↑ the risk of rhabdomyolysis and myopathy with statins
	Hypoglycemic therapy - nicotinic acid ↓ the efficacy of these medications
Para-aminobenzoic acid (PABA)	**Sulphonamides** - PABA ↓ the efficacy of these medications
	Dapsone - PABA ↓ activity of dapsone
Policosanol	**Aspirin -** policosanol (at very high doses) ↑ the risk of bleeding with aspirin
	Beta blockers - policosanol ↑ the hypotensive effect of beta blockers. Only systolic BP is affected, not diastolic BP or heart rate. Not usually clinically significant
Potassium	**ACE inhibitors -** potassium ↑ the risk of hyperkalemia
	Potassium-sparing diuretics - potassium ↑ the risk of hyperkalemia
Vitamin B6	**Anticonvulsant medication -** vitamin B6 ↓ blood levels of phenytoin and phenobarbitone
Vitamin C	**Aluminum-containing antacids -** vitamin C increases aluminum absorption
	Desferrioxamine - vitamin C may cause transient deterioration of cardiac function with desferrioxamine
	Indinavir - vitamin C ↓ blood levels of indinavir
Vitamin D3	**Thiazide diuretics -** vitamin D3 ↑ the risk of hypercalcemia if taken with calcium supplements and/or thiazide diuretics (note: cod liver oil contains 85 IU vitamin D per 1 g)
Vitamin E	**Warfarin, aspirin, anti-platelet drugs -** vitamin E (at doses over 400 IU) daily ↑ the risk of bleeding with these medications
Vitamin K	**Warfarin -** vitamin K decreases the activity of warfarin and other coumarin (oral) anticoagulants. Avoid changes in vitamin K intake whilst taking these medications
Zinc	**Tetracycline and quinolone antibiotics -** zinc ↓ the absorption and blood levels of these medications unless doses are separated by at least 2 hours

Drug	Interaction
Aluminum-containing antacids	**Vitamin C** - increases aluminum absorption
Antibiotics/antimicrobials	
Cotrimoxazole and sulphasalazine	↓ the efficacy of folic acid supplements
Dapsone	**Para-aminobenzoic acid -** ↓ the efficacy of dapsone
General	**Probiotics therapy such as L. acidophilus -** helps restore gut flora and reduces diarrhea secondary to antibiotic therapy
Metronidazole	**Milk thistle** - ↓ blood levels of metronidazole
Sulphonamides	**Para-aminobenzoic acid** - ↓ the efficacy of sulphonamides
Tetracyclines & quinolones	**Calcium, iron, magnesium and zinc -** ↓ absorption and blood levels unless doses are separated by at least 2 hours
Anticonvulsants	**Folic acid -** ↓ the efficacy of phenytoin. Phenytoin and folic acid should be commenced at the same time to avoid risk of adverse effects
	Phenytoin, phenobarbital and primidone - ↓ the efficacy of folic acid
	Vitamin B6 - ↓ blood levels of phenytoin and phenobarbitone
Antidepressants	
Monoamine oxidase inhibitors (MAOIs)	**Korean or Siberian ginseng -** ↑ side effects of phenelzine or other MAOIs
SSRIs (selective serotonin reuptake inhibitors)	**St John's wort -** may cause serotonergic syndrome with SSRIs
Tricyclics	**St John's wort -** ↓ blood levels of tricyclic antidepressants
Antihypertensives/ Cardiovascular medications	
ACE inhibitors	**Potassium -** ↑ the risk of hyperkalemia
Antihypertensives	**Coleus -** may have additive hypotensive effects with these medications
	Hawthorn - may have an additive hypotensive effect with these medications
	Licorice - may have a hypertensive effect
	Nicotinic acid - may have an additive hypotensive effect with these medications
Beta blockers	**Policosanol -** ↑ the hypotensive effect of beta blockers. Only systolic BP is affected, not diastolic BP or heart rate. Not usually clinically significant
Calcium channel blockers	**Calcium -** ↓ the hypotensive and antiarrhythmic effects of verapamil
Digoxin	**Licorice -** ↑ the risk of digoxin toxicity (possibly via hypokalemia)
	Korean or Siberian ginseng - may affect digoxin assays
	St John's wort - ↓ blood levels of digoxin
Methyldopa	**Iron -** ↓ absorption and blood levels unless doses are separated by at least 2 hours
Verapamil	**St John's Wort -** ↓ blood levels of verapamil
Antineoplastic agents	
Antineoplastic agents	**Black cohosh -** may affect the cytotoxicity of some drugs used in breast cancer treatment
Cisplatin	**Vitamin E -** ↓ the incidence and severity of neurotoxicity caused by cisplatin
Fluorouracil	**Folic acid -** ↑ the toxicity of fluorouracil
Imatinib mesylate	**St John's wort** - ↓ blood levels of imatinib mesylate
Irinotecan	**St John's wort -** ↓ blood levels of irinotecan
Methotrexate	**Folic acid -** ↓ the efficacy of methotrexate. Efficacy of methotrexate may be reduced by folic acid
Tamoxifen	Evidence regarding the effect of black cohosh on tamoxifen and breast cancer cell growth is conflicting
	Evidence regarding the effect of red clover on tamoxifen efficacy and breast cancer cell growth is conflicting
	Evidence regarding the effect of soy on tamoxifen efficacy and breast cancer cell growth is conflicting
Anti-platelet drugs Anticoagulants	
Aspirin	**Policosanol** (at very high doses) - ↑ the risk of bleeding with aspirin
Aspirin, warfarin	**Bilberry** (at very high doses) - ↑ the risk of bleeding with these medications
	Flaxseed oil - ↑ the risk of bleeding with these medications
	Garlic - ↑ the risk of bleeding with these medications
	Ginkgo - ↑ the risk of bleeding with these medications
	Pau d'arco (at very high doses) - ↑ the risk of bleeding with these medications
	Vitamin E (at doses over 400 IU daily) - ↑ the risk of bleeding with these medications
	Willow - ↑ the risk of bleeding with these medications
Warfarin	**CoQ10** - ↓ the anticoagulant effect of warfarin
	Cranberry - ↑ or ↓ the anticoagulant effect of warfarin
	Dong quai - ↑ the risk of bleeding with warfarin
	Korean ginseng - ↓ the anticoagulant effect of warfarin
	Soy protein - ↓ the anticoagulant effect of warfarin
	St John's wort - ↓ blood levels and efficacy of warfarin
	Vitamin K - ↓ the activity of warfarin and other coumarin (oral) anticoagulants. Avoid changes in vitamin K intake whilst taking these medications

Drug	Interaction
Anti-psychotics	
Haloperidol, olanzapine	**Ginkgo** - may enhance the therapeutic effects of haloperidol and olanzapine in the treatment of schizophrenia
Lithium	**Iodine** (at high doses) - ↑ the hypothyroid activity of lithium carbonate
	Psyllium - ↓ the absorption of lithium unless doses are separated by at least 1 hour
Phenothiazines	**Evening primrose oil** - ↑ the risk of seizures in patients receiving phenothiazines
Anti-rheumatoids	
Methotrexate	**Folic acid** - ↓ the efficacy of methotrexate. Efficacy of methotrexate may be reduced by folic acid
Penicillamine	**Iron** - ↓ absorption and efficacy of penicillamine unless doses are separated by at least 2 hours
Antiviral agents	
Protease inhibitors	**Garlic** - ↓ blood levels of protease inhibitors
	Vitamin C - ↓ blood levels of protease inhibitors
Protease inhibitors, reverse transcriptase inhibitors	**St John's wort** - ↓ blood levels of protease inhibitors and reverse transcriptase inhibitors
Bisphosphonates	**Calcium** - ↓ absorption of alendronate and clodronate unless doses are separated by at least 30 minutes
	Iron - ↓ absorption of bisphosphonates unless doses are separated by at least 2 hours
Corticosteroids	**Licorice** - ↑ blood levels of prednisolone
Desferrioxamine	**Vitamin C** - may cause transient deterioration of cardiac function with desferrioxamine
Diabetic medication	See 'Hypoglycemics'
Diuretics	
Loop and thiazide (potassium-depleting) diuretics	**Licorice** - ↑ the risk of electrolyte disturbances, especially hypokalemia
Potassium-sparing diuretics	**Potassium** - ↑ the risk of hyperkalemia
Thiazide diuretics	**Calcium** - ↑ the risk of hypercalcemia with thiazide diuretics
	Vitamin D3 - ↑ the risk of hypercalcemia if taken with calcium and/or thiazide diuretics
HIV medications	See 'Antiviral agents'
HMG-coa reductase inhibitors	See 'Statins'
Hypoglycemics - oral and insulin	**CoQ10** - ↓ blood glucose levels
	Fenugreek - ↓ blood glucose levels
	Fish oil (at high doses) - ↑ blood glucose levels and/or affect insulin levels
	Ginkgo - may affect blood glucose levels
	Glucosamine - may affect blood glucose levels in diabetics
	Korean ginseng - may affect blood glucose levels
	Nicotinic acid - ↓ the efficacy of these medications
Hypolipidamics	See 'Statins'
Immunomodifiers	**Astragalus** - ↓ the efficacy of immunosuppressants
	Echinacea - ↓ the efficacy of immunosuppressants
	St John's wort - ↓ the efficacy of cyclosporin, and other immunosuppressants
Methadone	**St John's wort** - may reduce blood levels of methadone and cause withdrawal symptoms
Midazolam	**St John's wort** - ↓ blood levels of midazolam
Omeprazole	**St John's wort** - ↓ blood levels of omeprazole
Paracetamol	**Milk thistle** - protects and stimulates the regeneration of normal liver cells
Oral contraceptives	**St John's wort** - ↓ the efficacy of oral contraceptives
Parkinson's medications	**Iron** - ↓ the absorption and efficacy of levodopa and carbidopa unless doses are separated by at least 2 hours
	L-methionine - ↓ the efficacy of levodopa
Penicillamine	See 'Anti-rheumatoids'
Statins	**CoQ10** - levels may be depleted by statins
	Nicotinic acid - ↑ the risk of rhabdomyolysis and myopathy if taken with HMG-CoA reductase inhibitors
	St John's wort - ↓ levels of simvastatin (but not pravastatin)
Thyroid hormone	**Calcium** - ↓ absorption and efficacy of thyroid hormone unless doses are separated by at least 2 hours
	Celery - ↓ blood levels of this medication by at least 2 hours
	Kelp and iodine supplements (at very high doses) - may precipitate or exacerbate hyper- or hypothyroidism
	Soy protein - ↓ absorption and efficacy unless doses are separated by at least 2 hours

Prefixes and Suffixes

The following is a list of medical prefixes and suffixes, along with their meanings and example(s).

Pre-/Suffix	Meanings	Example(s)
a-, an-	denotes an absence of	apathy, analgia
ab-	away from	abduction
abdomin(o)-	of or relating to the abdomen	abdomen
-ac	pertaining to	cardiac
acanth(o)-	thorn or spine	acanthocyte
acous(io)-	of or relating to hearing	
acr(o)-	extremity, topmost	acromegaly
-acusis	hearing	
-ad	toward, in the direction of	dorsad
ad-	increase, adherence, motion toward, very	adduction
aden(o)-, aden(i)-	of or relating to a gland	adenology
adip(o)-	of or relating to fat or fatty tissue	adipocyte
adren(o)-	of or relating to adrenal glands	adrenal artery
-aemia	blood condition	anaemia
aer(o)-	air, gas	aerosinusitis
aesthesio-	sensation	anesthesia
-al	pertaining to	abdominal
alb-	denoting a white or pale color	albino
alge(si)-	pain	analgesic
-algia	pain	myalgia
alg(i)o-	pain	myalgia
allo-	denoting something as different, or as an addition	alloantigen, allopathy
ambi-	denoting something as positioned on both sides; describing both of two	ambidextrous
amnio-	pertaining to the membraneous fetal sac (amnion)	amniocentesis
an-	not, without	analgesia
an(o)-	anus	
andr(o)-	pertaining to a man	andrology, android
angi(o)-	blood vessel	angiogram
aniso-	describing something as unequal	anisotropic
ankyl(o)-, ancyl(o)-	denoting something as crooked or bent	ankylosis
ante-	describing something as positioned in front of another thing	antepartum
anti-	describing something as 'against' or 'opposed to' another	antibody, antipsychotic
apo-	separated from, derived from	apoptosis
arteri(o)-	of or pertaining to an artery	artery, arteriole
arthr(o)-	of or pertaining to the joints, limbs	arthritis
articul(o)-	joint	articulation
-ary	pertaining to	billary tract
-ase	enzyme	lactase
-asthenia	weakness	myasthenia gravis
-ation	process	
aur(i)-	of or pertaining to the ear	aural

Pre-/Suffix	Meanings	Example(s)
aut(o)-	self	autoimmune
axill-	of or pertaining to the armpit (uncommon as a prefix)	axilla
balano-	of the glans penis or glans clitoridis	balanitis
bi-	twice, double	bilateral
bio-	life	biology
blast(o)-	germ or bud	blastomere
blephar(o)-	of or pertaining to the eyelid	blepharoplast
brachi(o)-	of or relating to the arm	brachium
brachy-	indicating 'short' or less commonly 'little'	brachycephalic
brady-	indicating 'slow'	bradycardia
bronch(i)-	bronchus	bronchiolitis obliterans
bucc(o)-	of or pertaining to the cheek	buccolabial
burs(o)-	bursa	bursitis
capit-	pertaining to the head (as a whole) or pertaining to hair	capitation
carcin(o)-	cancer	carcinoma
cardi(o)-	of or pertaining to the heart	cardiology
carp(o)-	of or pertaining to the wrist.	carpopedal
cata-	down	cataract
-cele	pouching, hernia	hydrocele
-centesis	surgical puncture for aspiration	amniocentesis
cephal(o)-	of or pertaining to the head (as a whole)	cephalalgy
cerat(o)-	of or pertaining to the cornu; a horn	ceratoid
cerebell(o)-	of or pertaining to the cerebellum	cerebellum
cerebr(o)-	of or pertaining to the brain	cerebrology
cervic-	of or pertaining to the neck, the cervix	cervicodorsal
chem(o)-	chemistry, drug	chemotherapy
chir(o)-, cheir(o)-	of or pertaining to the hand	chiropractor
chlor(o)-	denoting a green color	chlorophyll
chol(e)-	of or pertaining to bile	cholemia
cholecyst(o)-	of or pertaining to the gallbladder	cholecystectomy
chondr(i)o-	cartilage, gristle, granule, granular	chondrocalcinosis
chrom(ato)-	color	hemachromatosis
-cidal, -cide	killing, destroying	
cili-	of or pertaining to the cilia, the eyelashes; eyelids	ciliary
circum-	denoting something as 'around' another	circumcision
cis-	on this side	
clast	break	
co-	with, together, in association	
col-, colo-, colono-	colon	colonoscopy
colp(o)-	of or pertaining to the vagina	colposcopy
com-	with, together	
contra	against	contraindicate

WESTERN

Pre-/Suffix	Meanings	Example(s)
cor-	with, together	
cor-, core-, coro-	of or pertaining to eye's pupil	corectomy
cordi-	of or pertaining to the heart (uncommon as a prefix)	commotio cordis
cornu-	applied to processes and parts of the body describing them likened or similar to horns	
cost(o)-	of or pertaining to the ribs	costochondral
cox-	of or relating to the hip, haunch, or hip-joint	coxopodite
crani(o)-	belonging or relating to the cranium	craniology
-crine	to secrete	endocrine
cry(o)-	cold	cryoablation
cutane-	skin	subcutaneous
cyan(o)-	denotes a blue color	cyanopsia
cyst(o)-, cyst(i)-	of or pertaining to the urinary bladder	cystotomy
cyt(o)-	cell	cytokine
-cyte	cell	leukocyte
dacryo-	tear	
dactyl(o)-	of or pertaining to a finger, toe	dactylology
de-	away from, cessation	
dent-	of or pertaining to teeth	dentist
dermat(o)-, derm(o)-	of or pertaining to the skin	dermatology
-desis	binding	arthrodesis
dextr(o)-	right, on the right side	dextrocardia
di-	two	
di-	apart, separation	
dia-	(same as greek meaning)	diacetyl
dif-	apart, separation	
digit-	of or pertaining to the finger (rare as a root)	digit
dis-	separation, taking apart	dissection
dors(o)-, dors(i)-	of or pertaining to the back	dorsal, dorsocephalad
duodeno-	duodenum, twelve: upper part of the small intestine (twelve inches long on average), connects to the stomach	duodenal atresia
dynam(o)-	force, energy, power	
-dynia	pain	
dys-	bad, difficult	dysphagia, dysphasia
eal-	pertaining to	
ec-	out, away	
ect(o)-	outer, outside	ectopic pregnancy
-ectasis	expansion, dilation	bronchiectasis
-ectomy	denotes a surgical operation or removal of a body part	mastectomy
-emesis	vomiting condition	hematemesis
-emia	blood condition	anemia
encephal(o)-	of or pertaining to the brain. also see cerebro.	encephalogram

Pre-/Suffix	Meanings	Example(s)
endo-	denotes something as 'inside' or 'within'	endocrinology, endospore
enter(o)-	of or pertaining to the intestine	gastroenterology
epi-	(same as greek meaning: on, upon)	epistaxis, epicardium, episclera, epidural
episi(o)-	of or pertaining to the pubic region, the loins	episiotomy
erythr(o)-	denotes a red color	erythrocyte
-esophageal, -esophago	gullet	
esthesio-	sensation	
eu-	true, good, well, new	eukaryote
ex-	out of, away from	
exo-	denotes something as 'outside' another	exoskeleton
extra-	outside	
faci(o)-	of or pertaining to the face	facioplegic
fibr(o)	fiber	fibroblast
filli-	fine, hair like	
-form, -iform	used to form adjectives indicating 'having the form of'	cuneiform
front-	of or pertaining to the forehead	frontonasal
galact(o)-	milk	galactorrhea
gastr(o)-	of or pertaining to the stomach	gastric bypass
-gen	1. denotes the sense 'born in, from' 2. denotes the sense 'of a certain kind'	1. endogen; 2. heterogenous
-genic	formative	cardiogenic shock
genu-	of or pertaining to the knee	genu valgum
gingiv-	of or pertaining to the gums	gingivitis
glauc(o)-	denoting a grey, bluish-grey color	glaucoma
gloss(o)-, glott(o)-	of or pertaining to the tongue	glossology
gluco-	glucose	glucocorticoid
glyco-	sugar	glycolysis
gnath(o)-	of or pertaining to the jaw	gnathodynamometer
gon(o)-	seed, semen; also, reproductive	gonorrhea
-gram	record or picture	angiogram
-graph	record or picture	electrocardiograph
-graphy	process of recording	angiography
gyn(aec)o- , gyn(ec)o-	woman	gynecomastia
halluc-	to wander in mind	hallucinosis
hemat-, haemato- (haem-, hem-)	of or pertaining to blood	hematology, older form haematology
hema or hemo-	blood	hematological malignancy
hemi-	one-half	cerebral hemisphere
hepat- (hepatic-)	of or pertaining to the liver	hepatology
heter(o)-	denotes something as 'the other' (of two), as an addition, or different	heterogeneous
hidr(o)-	sweat	hyperhidrosis

WESTERN

Pre-/Suffix	Meanings	Example(s)
hist(o)-, histio-	tissue	histology
home(o)-	similar	homeopathy
hom(o)-	denotes something as 'the same' as another or common	homosexuality
humer(o)-	of or pertaining to the shoulder (or [rarely] the upper arm)	humerus
hydr(o)-	water	hydrophobe
hyper-	denotes something as 'extreme' or 'beyond normal'	hypertension
hyp(o)-	denotes something as 'below normal'	hypovolemia,
hyster(o)-	of or pertaining to the womb, the uterus	hysterectomy
-i-asis	condition	mydriasis
iatr(o)-	of or pertaining to medicine, or a physician (uncommon as a prefix; common as a suffix, see -iatry)	iatrochemistry
-iatry	denotes a field in medicine of a certain body component	podiatry, psychiatry
-ic	pertaining to	hepatic artery
-icle	small	ovarian follicle
-ics	organized knowledge, treatment	
idio-	self, one's own	idiopathic
ileo-	ileum	ileocecal valve
infra-	below	infrahyoid muscles
inter-	between, among	interarticular ligament
intra-	within	intracranial hemorrhage
irid(o)-	iris	iridectomy
ischio-	of or pertaining to the ischium, the hip-joint	ischiorrhogic
-ism	condition, disease	dwarfism
-ismus	spasm, contraction	
iso-	denoting something as being 'equal'	isotonic
-ist	one who specializes in	pathologist
-ite	the nature of, resembling	hermaphrodite
-itis	inflammation	tonsillitis
-ium	structure, tissue	pericardium
isch-	restriction	ischemia
karyo-	nucleus	eukaryote
kerat(o)-	cornea (eye or skin)	keratoscope
kin(e)-, kin(o)-, kinesi(o)-	movement	kinesthesia
koil(o)-	hollow	koilocyte
kyph(o)-	humped	kyphoscoliosis
labi(o)-	of or pertaining to the lip	labiodental
lacrim(o)-	tear	lacrimal canaliculi
lact(i)-, lact(o)-	milk	lactation
lapar(o)-	of or pertaining to the abdomen-wall, flank	laparotomy
laryng(o)-	of or pertaining to the larynx, the lower throat cavity where the voice box is	larynx
latero-	lateral	lateral pectoral nerve
lei(o)-	smooth	leiomyoma

Pre-/Suffix	Meanings	Example(s)
-lepsis, -lepsy	attack, seizure	epilepsy, narcolepsy
lept(o)-	light, slender	
leuc(o)-, leuk(o)-	denoting a white color	leukocyte
lingu(a)-, lingu(o)-	of or pertaining to the tongue	linguistics
lip(o)-	fat	liposuction
lith(o)-	stone, calculus	lithotripsy
log(o)-	speech	
-logist	denotes someone who studies a certain field: _____-logy	oncologist, pathologist
-logy	denotes the academic study or practice of a certain field	hematology, urology
lymph(o)-	lymph	lymphedema
lys(o)-, -lytic	dissolution	lysosome
-lysis	destruction	paralysis
macr(o)-	large, long	macrophage
-malacia	softening	osteomalacia
mamm(o)-	of or pertaining to the breast	mammogram
mammill(o)-	of or pertaining to the nipple	
manu-	of or pertaining to the hand	manufacture
mast(o)-	of or pertaining to the breast	mastectomy
meg(a)-, megal(o)-, megaly	enlargement	splenomegaly
melan(o)-	denoting a black color	melanin
mening(o)-	membrane	meningitis
mero-	part	merocrine, meroblastic
mes(o)-	middle	mesoderm
meta-	after, behind	metacarpus
-meter	measurement	sphygmomanometer
-metry	process of measuring	optometry
metr(o)-	pertaining to conditions or instruments of the uterus	metrorrhagia
micro-	denoting something as small, or relating to smallness	microscope
mon(o)-	single	infectious mononucleosis
morph(o)-	form, shape	morphology
muscul(o)-	muscle	musculoskeletal system
my(o)-	of or relating to muscle	myoblast
myc(o)-	fungus	onychomycosis
myel(o)-	of or relating to bone marrow	myeloblast
myring(o)-	eardrum	myringotomy
myx(o)-	mucus	myxoma
narc(o)-	numb, sleep	narcolepsy
nas(o)-	of or pertaining to the nose	nasal
necr(o)-	death	necrotizing fasciitis
neo-	new	neoplasm
nephr(o)-	of or pertaining to the kidney	nephrology

Pre-/Suffix	Meanings	Example(s)
nerv-	of or pertaining to nerves and the nervous system (uncommon as a root: neuro- mostly always used)	nerve
neur(i)-, neur(o)-	of or pertaining to nerves and the nervous system	neurofibromatosis
normo-	normal	normocapnia
ocul(o)-	of or pertaining to the eye	oculist
odont(o)-	of or pertaining to teeth	orthodontist
odyn(o)-	pain	stomatodynia
-oesophageal, oesophago-	gullet	
-oid	resemblance to	sarcoidosis
ole-	small or little	
olig(o)-	denoting something as 'having little, having few'	oligotrophy
om(o)-	of or pertaining to the shoulder	omoplate
-oma (singular), -omata (plural)	tumor	sarcoma, teratoma
omphal(o)-	of or pertaining to the navel, the umbilicus	omphalotomy
onco-	tumor, bulk, volume	oncology
onych(o)-	of or pertaining to the nail (of a finger or toe)	onychophagy
oo-	of or pertaining to the an egg, a woman's egg, the ovum	oogenesis
oophor(o)-	of or pertaining to the woman's ovary	oophorectomy
ophthalm(o)-	of or pertaining to the eye	ophthalmology
optic(o)-	of or relating to chemical properties of the eye	opticochemical
or(o)-	of or pertaining to the mouth	oral
orchi(o)-, orchido-	testis	orchiectomy, orchidectomy
orth(o)-	denoting something as straight or correct	orthodontist
-osis	a condition, disease or increase	harlequin type ichthyosis
osseo-	bony	
ossi-	bone	peripheral ossifying fibroma
ost(e)-, oste(o)-	bone	osteoporosis
ot(o)-	of or pertaining to the ear	otopathy
-ous	pertaining to	
ovari(o)-	of or pertaining to the ovaries	ovariectomy
ovo-, ovi-, ov-	of or pertaining to the eggs, the ovum	ovogenesis
oxo-	addition of oxygen	
oxy-	sharp, acid, acute, oxygen	
pachy-	thick	pachyderma
palpebr-	of or pertaining to the eyelid (uncommon as a root)	palpebra

Pre-/Suffix	Meanings	Example(s)
pan-, pant(o)-	denoting something as 'complete' or containing 'everything'	panophobia, panopticon
papill-	of or pertaining to the nipple (of the chest/ breast)	papillitis
papul(o)-	indicates papulosity, a small elevation or swelling in the skin, a pimple, swelling	papulation
para-	alongside of, abnormal	
-paresis	slight paralysis	hemiparesis
path(o)-	disease	pathology
-pathy	denotes (with a negative sense) a disease, or disorder	sociopathy, neuropathy
ped-, -ped-, -pes	of or pertaining to the foot; -footed	pedoscope
pelv(i)-, pelv(o)-	hip bone	pelvis
-penia	deficiency	osteopenia
peo-	of or pertaining to the penis	peotomy
-pepsia	denotes something relating to digestion, or the digestive tract.	dyspepsia
per-	through	
peri-	denoting something with a position 'surrounding' or 'around' another	periodontal
-pexy	fixation	nephropexy
phaco-	lens-shaped	
-phage, -phagia	forms terms denoting conditions relating to eating or ingestion	sarcophagia
-phago-	eating, devouring	phagocyte
phagist-	forms nouns that denote a person who 'feeds on' the first element or part of the word	lotophagis
-phagy	forms nouns that denotes 'feeding on' the first element or part of the word	anthropophagy
phallo-	phallus	aphallia
pharmaco-	drug, medication	pharmacology
pharyng(o)-	of or pertaining to the pharynx, the upper throat cavity	pharyngitis, pharyngoscopy
-phil(ia)	attraction for	hemophilia
phleb(o)-	of or pertaining to the (blood) veins, a vein	phlebography, phlebotomy
phob(o)-	exaggerated fear, sensitivity	arachnophobia
phon(o)-	sound	
phos-	of or pertaining to light or its chemical properties, now historic and used rarely. see the common root phot(o)- below.	phosphene
phot(o)-	of or pertaining to light	photopathy
phren(i)-, phren(o)-, phrenico	diaphragm	phrenic nerve
-plasia	formation, development	achondroplasia

WESTERN

Pre-/Suffix	Meanings	Example(s)
-plasty	surgical repair, reconstruction	rhinoplasty
-plegia	paralysis	paraplegia
pleur(o)-, pleur(a)	of or pertaining to the ribs	pleurogenous
-plexy	stroke or seizure	cataplexy
pneum(o)-	of or pertaining to the lungs	pneumonocyte, pneumonia
pneumat(o)-	air, lung	
pod-, -pod-, -pus	of or pertaining to the foot, -footed	podiatry
-poiesis	production	hematopoiesis
polio-	denoting a grey color	poliomyelitis
poly-	denotes a 'plurality' of something	polymyositis
por(o)-	pore, porous	
porphyr(o)-	denotes a purple color	porphyroblast
post-	denotes something as 'after' or 'behind' another	postoperation, postmortem
pre-	denotes something as 'before' another (in [physical] position or time)	prematurity
presby(o)-	old age	presbyopia
prim-	denotes something as 'first' or 'most-important'	primary
pro-	denotes something as 'before' another (in [physical] position or time)	procephalic
proct(o)-	anus, rectum	proctology
prot(o)-	denotes something as 'first' or 'most-important'	protoneuron
pseudo-	denotes something false or fake	
psych(e)-, psych(o)-	of or pertaining to the mind	psychology, psychiatry
-ptosis	falling, downward placement, prolapse	apoptosis
-ptysis	(a spitting), spitting, hemoptysis, the spitting of blood derivied from the lungs or bronchial tubes	
pulmon-, pulmo-	of or relating to the lungs.	pulmonary
pyel(o)-	pelvis	pyelonephritis
pyo-	pus	pyometra
pyro-	fever	antipyretic
quadr(i)-	four	quadriceps
radio-	radiation	
re-	again, backward	
rect(o)-	rectum	
ren(o)-	of or pertaining to the kidney	renal
reticul(o)-	net	
retro-	backward, behind	retroverted
rhabd(o)-	rod shaped, striated	
rhachi(o)-	spine	
rhin(o)-	of or pertaining to the nose	rhinoceros, rhinoplasty
rhod(o)-	denoting a rose-red color	rhodophyte
-rrhage	burst forth	hemorrhage
-rrhagia	rapid flow of blood	
-rrhaphy	surgical suturing	

Pre-/Suffix	Meanings	Example(s)
-rrhea	flowing, discharge	galactorrhea
-rrhexis	rupture	
-rrhoea	flowing, discharge	diarrhoea
rubr(o)-	of or pertaining to the red nucleus of the brain	rubrospinal
salping(o)-	of or pertaining to the fallopian tubes	salpingectomy
sangui-, sanguine-	of or pertaining to blood	sanguine
sarco-	muscular, fleshlike	sarcoma
schist(o)-	split, cleft	
schiz(o)-	denoting something 'split' or 'double-sided'	schizophrenia
scler(o)-	hardness	atherosclerosis
scoli(o)-	twisted	scoliosis
-scope	instrument for viewing	stethoscope
-scopy	use of instrument for viewing	endoscopy
semi-	one-half, partly	
sial(o)-	saliva, salivary gland	sialagogue
sigmoid(o)-	sigmoid, sigmoid colon	
sinistr(o)-	left, left side	
sinus-	of or pertaining to the sinus	sinusitis
-sis	condition of	osteoporosis
sito-	food, grain	
somat(o)-, somatico-	body, bodily	
spasmo-	spasm	
sperma-, spermo-, spermato-	semen, spermatozoa	spermatogenesis
splanchn(i)-, splanchn(o)-	viscera	
splen(o)-	spleen	splenectomy
spondyl(o)-	of or pertaining to the spine, the vertebra	spondylitis
squamos(o)-	denoting something as 'full of scales' or 'scaly'	squama
-stasis	stop, stand	
-staxis	dripping, trickling	
sten(o)-	denoting something as 'narrow in shape' or pertaining to narrow-ness	stenography
steth(o)-	of or pertaining to the upper chest, chest, the area above the breast and under the neck	stethoscope
stheno-	strength, force, power	
stom(a)-	mouth	stomatognathic system
stomat(o)-	of or pertaining to the mouth	stomatogastric
-stomy	creation of an opening	colostomy
sub-	beneath	subcutaneous tissue
super-	in excess, above, superior	superior vena cava
supra-	above, excessive	supraorbital vein

Pre-/Suffix	Meanings	Example(s)
sy(l)-, sym-, syn-, sys-	indicates similarity, likeness, or being together; assimilates before some consonants: before l to syl-, s to sys-, before a labial to sym-.	synalgia, synesthesia, syssarcosis
tachy-	denoting something as fast, irregularly fast	tachycardia
-tension, -tensive	blood pressure	hypertension
thel(e)-, thel(o)-	of or pertaining to a nipple (uncommon as a prefix)	theleplasty
thely-	denoting something as 'relating to a woman, feminine'	thelygenous
therm(o)-	heat	
thorac(i)-, thorac(o)-, thoracico-	of or pertaining to the upper chest, chest; the area above the breast and under the neck	thorax
thromb(o)-	of or relating to a blood clot, clotting of blood	thrombus, thrombocytopenia
thyr(o)-	thyroid	
-tic	pertaining to	
toco-	childbirth	
-tome	cutting instrument	
-tomy	cutting operation	cystotomy
tono-	tone, tension, pressure	
-tony	tension	
top(o)-	place, topical	
tox(i)-, tox(o)-, toxico-	toxin, poison	toxoplasmosis
trache(o)-	trachea	
trachel(o)-	of or pertaining to the neck	tracheotomy
trans-	denoting something as moving or situated 'across' or 'through'	transfusion
trich(i)-, trichia-, trich(o)-	of or pertaining to hair, hair-like structure	trichotomy
-tripsy	crushing	lithotripsy
-trophy	nourishment, development	
tympan(o)-	eardrum	
-ula, -ule	small	nodule
ultra-	beyond, excessive	
umbilic-	of or pertaining to the navel, the umbilicus	umbilical
ungui-	of or pertaining to the nail, a claw	unguiform, ungual
un(i)-	one	unilateral hearing loss
ur(o)-	of or pertaining to urine, the urinary system; (specifically) pertaining to the physiological chemistry of urine	urology
uri(c)-, urico-	uric acid	
urin-	of or pertaining to urine, the urinary system	uriniferous
uter(o)-	of or pertaining to the uterus or womb	uterus
vagin-	of or pertaining to the vagina	vagina
varic(o)-	swollen or twisted vein	varicose
vas(o)-	duct, blood vessel	vasoconstriction
vasculo-	blood vessel	
ven-	of or pertaining to the (blood) veins, a vein (used in terms pertaining to the vascular system)	vein, venospasm
ventr(o)-	of or pertaining to the belly; the stomach cavities	ventrodorsal
vesic(o)-	of or pertaining to the bladder	vesica
viscer(o)-	of or pertaining to the internal organs, the viscera	viscera
xanth(o)-	denoting a yellow color, an abnormally yellow color	xanthopathy
xen(o)-	foreign, different	xenograft
-y	condition or process of	surgery
zo(o)-	animal, animal life	
zym(o)-	fermentation, enzyme	

Body Parts and Components
(Internal Anatomy, External Anatomy, Body Fluids, Body Substances)

Parts	Roots	Roots
abdomen	lapar(o)-	abdomin-
aorta	aort(o)-	aort(o)-
arm	brachi(o)-	-
armpit	-	axill-
artery	arteri(o)-	-
back	-	dors-
big toe	-	allic-
bladder	cyst(o)-	vesic(o)-
blood	haemat-, hemat- (haem-, hem-)	sangui-, sanguine-
blood clot	thromb(o)-	-
blood vessel	angi(o)-	vascul-, vas-
body	somat-, som-	corpor-
bone	oste(o)-	ossi-
bone marrow, marrow	myel(o)-	medull-
brain	encephal(o)-	cerebr(o)-
breast	mast(o)-	mamm(o)-
chest	steth(o)-	-
cheek	-	bucc-
ear	ot(o)-	aur-
eggs, ova	oo-	ov-
eye	ophthalm(o)-	ocul(o)-
eyelid	blephar(o)-	cili-; palpebr-
face	-	faci(o)-
fallopian tubes	salping(o)-	-
fat, fatty tissue	lip(o)-	adip-
finger	dactyl(o)-	digit-
forehead	-	front(o)-
gallbladder	cholecyst(o)-	fell-
genitals, sexually undifferentiated	gon(o)-, phall(o)-	-
gland	aden(o)-	-
glans *penis* or *clitoridis*	balan(o)-	-

Body Parts and Components (cont.)

Parts	Roots	Roots
gums	-	gingiv-
hair	trich(o)-	capill-
hand	cheir(o)-, chir(o)-	manu-
head	cephal(o)-	capit(o)-
heart	cardi(o)-	cordi-
hip, hip-joint	-	cox-
horn	cerat(o)-	cornu-
intestine	enter(o)-	-
jaw	gnath(o)-	-
kidney	nephr(o)-	ren-
knee	gon-	genu-
lip	cheil(o)-, chil(o)-	labi(o)-
liver	hepat(o)- (hepatic-)	jecor-
loins, pubic region	episi(o)-	pudend-
lungs	pneumon-	pulmon(i)- (pulmo-)
marrow, bone marrow	myel(o)-	medull-
mind	psych-	ment-
mouth	stomat(o)-	or-
muscle	my(o)-	-
nail	onych(o)-	ungui-
navel	omphal(o)-	umbilic-
neck	trachel(o)-	cervic-
nerve; the nervous system	neur(o)-	nerv-
nipple, teat	thele-	papill-, mammill-
nose	rhin(o)-	nas-
ovary	oophor(o)-	ovari(o)-
pelvis	pyel(o)-	pelv(i)-
penis	pe(o)-	-
pupil (of the eye)	cor-, core-, coro-	-
rib	pleur(o)-	cost(o)-
rib cage	thorac(i)-, thorac(o)-	-
shoulder	om(o)-	humer(o)-
sinus	-	sinus-
skin	dermat(o)- (derm-)	cut-, cuticul-
skull	crani(o)-	-
stomach	gastr(o)-	ventr(o)-
testis	orchi(o)-, orchid(o)-	-
throat (upper throat cavity)	pharyng(o)-	-
throat (lower throat cavity/ voice box])	laryng(o)-	-
thumb	-	pollic-
tooth	odont(o)-	dent(i)-
tongue	gloss-, glott-	lingu(a)-
toe	dactyl(o)-	digit-
tumour	cel-, onc(o)-	tum-
ureter	ureter(o)-	ureter(o)-
urethra	urethr(o)-, urethr(a)-	urethr(o)-, urethr(a)-
urine, urinary System	ur(o)-	urin(o)-
uterine tubes	sarping(o)-	sarping(o)-
uterus	hyster(o)-, metr(o)-	uter(o)-
vagina	colp(o)-	vagin-
vein	phleb(o)-	ven-
vulva	episi(o)-	vulv-
womb	hyster(o)-, metr(o)-	uter(o)-
wrist	carp(o)-	carp(o)-

Roots of Description
(Size, Shape, Strength, etc.)

Description	Roots	Roots
bad, incorrect	cac(o)-, dys-	mal(e)-
bent, crooked	ankyl(o)-	prav(i)-
big	mega-, megal(o)-	magn(i)-
biggest	megist-	maxim-
broad, wide	eury-	lat(i)-
cold	cry(o)-	frig-
dead	necr(o)-	mort-
equal	is(o)-	equ(i)-
false	pseud(o)-	fals(i)-
female, feminine	thely-	-
flat	platy-	plan(i)-
good, well	eu-	ben(e)-, bon(i)-
great	mega-, megal(o)-	magn(i)-
hard	scler(o)-	dur(i)-
heavy	bar(o)-	grav(i)-
hollow	coel(o)-	cav-
huge	megal(o)-	magn(i)-
incorrect, bad	cac(o)-, dys-	mal(e)-
large; extremely large	mega-	magn(i)-
largest	megist-	maxim-
long	macr(o)-	long(i)-
male, masculine	arseno-	vir-
narrow	sten(o)-	angust(i)-
new	neo-	nov(i)-
normal, correct; straight	orth(o)-	rect-
old	paleo-	veter-
sharp	oxy-	ac-
short	brachy-	brev(i)-
small	micr(o)-	parv(i)- (rare)
smallest	-	minim-
slow	brady-	tard(i)-
fast	tachy-	celer-
soft	malac(o)-	moll(i)-
straight, normal, correct	orth(o)-	rect(i)-
thick	pachy-	crass(i)-
varied, various	poikilo-	vari-
well, good	eu-	ben(e)-
wide, broad	eury-	lat(i)-

Cranial Nerve Examination

Nerve	Test	Lesion
I-Olfactory	***Sensory:*** smell; Can the patient smell coffee or soap with each nostril?	Anosmia (loss of smell)
II-Optic	***Sensory***: vision; Examine both retinas carefully with an ophthalmoscope and test for visual acuity, visual field, color vision, and optic disc appearance.	Visual field deficits
III-Oculomotor	***Motor & parasympathetic***: constrictor pupillae, ciliary muscles (lens shape): rectus superior, inferior, medial; inferior oblique, levator palpebra; Record the pupil size and shape at rest. Next, note the *direct response*, meaning constriction of the illuminated pupil, as well as the *consensual response*, meaning constriction of the opposite pupil.	Dilated pupil, ptosis, eye turned down & lateral loss of pupillary light reflex on lesion side
IV-Trochlear	***Motor***: superior oblique; Check extraocular movements (eye movements) by having the patient look in all directions without moving their head and ask them if they experience any double vision.	Inability to look down when eye is adducted
V-Trigeminal	***Sensory:*** V1(opthalmic), V2(maxillary), V3(mandibular), sensation anterior 2/3 tongue. ***Motor:*** V3-masseter, temporalis, lat & med pterygoid, anterior belly digastric, mylohyoid, tensor, tympani/veli palatini; Test facial sensation using a cotton wisp and a sharp object.	Paresthesia (pain & touch) mandible deviation to side of lesion when mouth is opened, masseter & temporalis do not contract
VI-Abducens	***Motor:*** lateral rectus muscle; Test smooth pursuit by having the patient follow an object moved across their full range of horizontal and vertical eye movements. Test convergence movements by having the patient fixate on an object as it is moved slowly toward a point right between the patient's eyes. Also, observe the eyes at rest to see if there smooth tracking, nystagmus, or any abnormalities.	No abduction if ipsilateral eye medial strabismus, diplopia
VII-Facial	***Sensory***: taste – anterior 2/3 of tongue; Look for asymmetry in facial shape or in depth of furrows such as the nasolabial fold. Also look for asymmetries in spontaneous facial expressions and blinking. Ask patient to smile, puff out their cheeks, clench their eyes tight, wrinkle their brow, and so on. ***Motor:*** frontalis, occipitalis, orbicularis, buccinator, zygomaticus, mentalis, post. Belly digastric, stapedius, stylohyoid. ***Parasympathetic***: lacrimal, nasal & palatine, sublingual, lingual submandibular, labial.	Loss of taste anterior 2/3 of tongue. Paralysis of facial muscles, hyperacousis (stapedius paralysis). ↓ salivation, lacrimation
VIII-Acoustic (vestibulocochlear)	***Sensory***: hearing & equilibrium; Can the patient hear fingers rubbed together or words whispered just outside of the auditory canal and identify which ear hears the sound?	Unilateral hearing loss of balance problems
IX-Glosso-pharyngeal	***Sensory:*** sensation & taste posterior 1/3 of tongue, pharynx, tympanic cavity, carotid baro/chemo receptors; Say aah. Does the patient gag when the posterior pharynx is brushed? ***Motor:*** stylopharyngeus muscle. ***Parasympathetic:*** parotid gland.	Loss of taste on posterior 1/3 of tongue. Loss of sensation on affected side of soft palate. ↓ salivation
X-Vagus	See IX Test - ***Sensory:*** pinna of ear, GI distention. ***Motor:*** muscles of palate, pharynx & larynx. ***Parasympathetic:*** heart, esophagus, GI tract up to distal 2/3 of transverse colon.	Ipsilateral: uvula deviates to opposite side of lesion, dyspnea, hoarse voice
XI-Accessory	***Motor:*** SCM, Trapezius; Ask the patient to shrug their shoulders, turn their head in both directions, and raise their head from the bed, flexing forward against the force of your hands.	Paralysis of SCM & superior fibers of trapezius → drooping of shoulder
XII-Hypoglossal	***Motor:*** intrinsic muscle of tongue, genioglossus, styloglossus, hyoglossus; Ask the patient to stick their tongue straight out and note whether it curves to one side or the other. Ask the patient to move their tongue from side to side and push it forcefully against the inside of each cheek.	Tongue deviates toward side of lesion on protrusion (action of genioblossus)

Dermatomes are specific areas on the skin that represent sensory innervations from a specific root level. Dermatomes are useful in neurology for finding the site of damage to the spine. Abnormally functioning dermatomes provide important clues about injury to the spinal cord or specific spinal nerves. If a dermatome is stimulated but no sensation is perceived, it can be inferred that the nerve to that specific dermatome has been injured.

Refer to the dermatome chart on the following page for specific areas. Testing is usually done with a blunt object (paperclip) or a pin. Compare same area on opposite side and ask the client if it is the same, increased (hypersensitive) or reduced (hyposensitive).

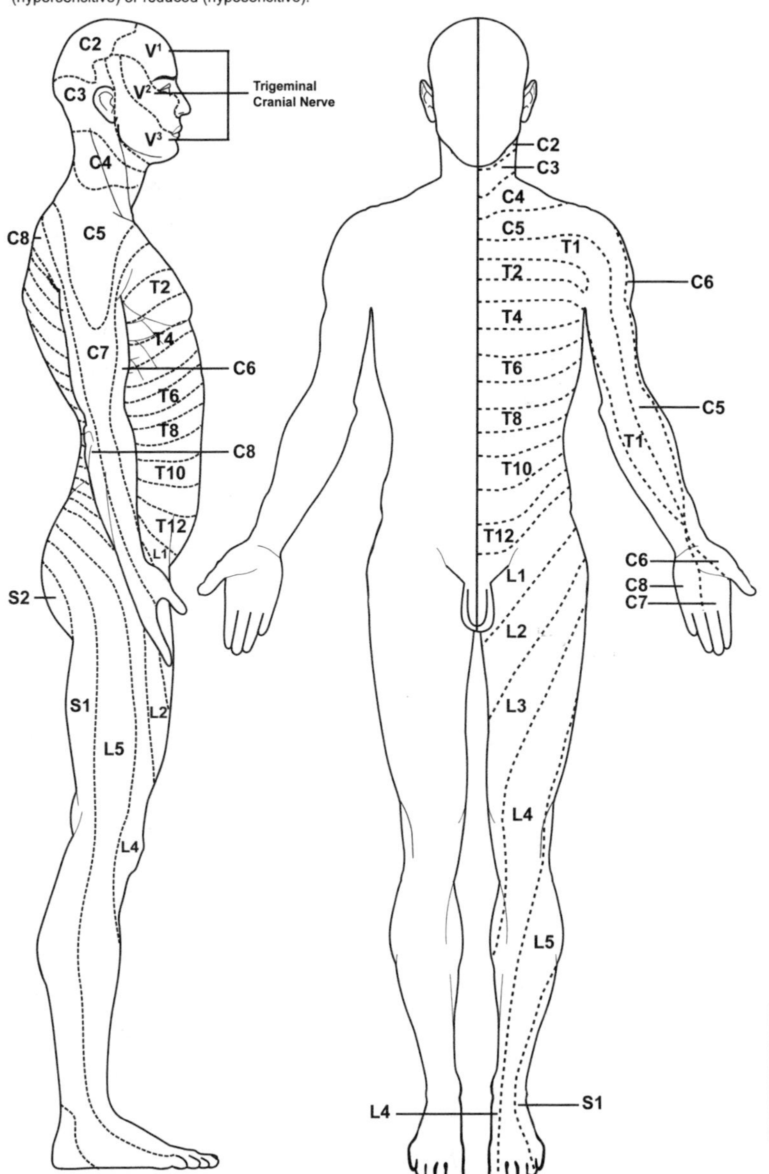

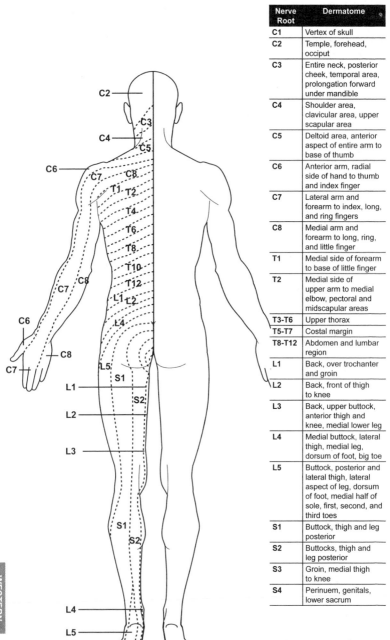

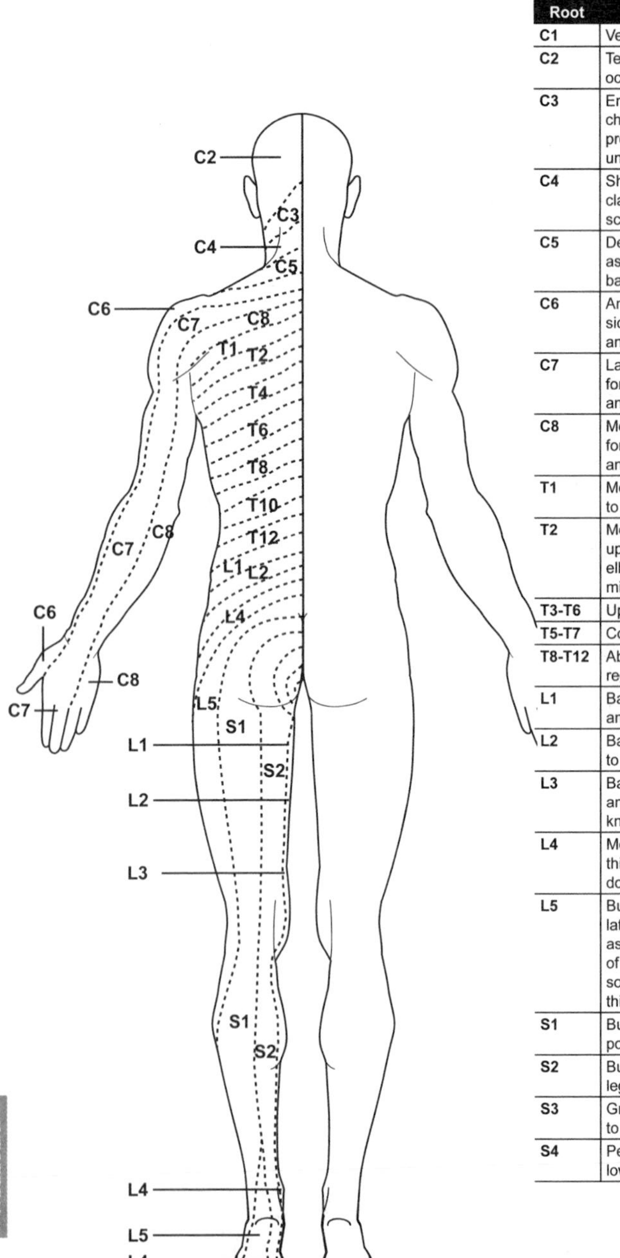

Nerve Root	Dermatome
C1	Vertex of skull
C2	Temple, forehead, occiput
C3	Entire neck, posterior cheek, temporal area, prolongation forward under mandible
C4	Shoulder area, clavicular area, upper scapular area
C5	Deltoid area, anterior aspect of entire arm to base of thumb
C6	Anterior arm, radial side of hand to thumb and index finger
C7	Lateral arm and forearm to index, long, and ring fingers
C8	Medial arm and forearm to long, ring, and little finger
T1	Medial side of forearm to base of little finger
T2	Medial side of upper arm to medial elbow, pectoral and midscapular areas
T3-T6	Upper thorax
T5-T7	Costal margin
T8-T12	Abdomen and lumbar region
L1	Back, over trochanter and groin
L2	Back, front of thigh to knee
L3	Back, upper buttock, anterior thigh and knee, medial lower leg
L4	Medial buttock, lateral thigh, medial leg, dorsum of foot, big toe
L5	Buttock, posterior and lateral thigh, lateral aspect of leg, dorsum of foot, medial half of sole, first, second, and third toes
S1	Buttock, thigh and leg posterior
S2	Buttocks, thigh and leg posterior
S3	Groin, medial thigh to knee
S4	Perinuem, genitals, lower sacrum

Manual Muscle Testing & Myotomes

Procedure: When conducting muscle tests, be sure to assess for asymmetry of the muscle groups (for example, atrophy on one side but not the other) and landmarks before testing.

General screening: check muscle in middle of range of motion (ROM) or through ADLs.

Specific muscle testing: estimate origin and insertion of muscle as accurately as possible.

Muscle testing is suggested for anyone with suspected or actual impaired muscle function, including strength, power or endurance. Impairments in muscle performance may be the effects of cardiovascular, pulmonary, musculoskeletal or neuromuscular disease or disorders. It is imperative to know how much resistance a **"normal"** muscle can endure to recognize when a muscle is not operating to its potential. All tests must be done bilaterally and the unaffected side should be tested before the other. This is crucial because the tester can then develop an accurate idea of the amount of resistance the unaffected side can take and what would be deemed normal for the client. The scale below is composed of both subjective and objective factors.

Muscles should be tested on a regular basis in order to determine improvement or deterioration of function. It should be noted that the unaffected side should always be tested as well as the affected side for contrast. Identification of specific muscles or muscle groups with compromised function gives information for appropriate treatment, which may include strengthening exercises, functional drills, bracing, or compensatory muscle use.

1. Place client in most pain-free and most favorable stance for testing
2. Use best testing position and body biomechanics
3. Show client the motion you want him/her to oppose
4. Ask client to hold position and rest when test is finished ("hold, hold, hold & relax")

- Normally, s/he holds position for 3 seconds
- If there is a high index of suspicion of injury or neurological compromise:
  - Hold for 5-10 seconds or,
  - Repeat for up to 10 repetitions (e.g. chart as 3/5 at 8x) or,
  - Test at various angles through ROM, eccentric, concentric, isometric
- Joint should only be moved ~10° or through ~10% of range of motion
  - Typical mistake is to move joint too much, thereby examining many different muscles and affecting reliability & validity
  - Consider testing in positions or with actions that give client mild discomfort to help get a true sense of specific limitations and actual muscle impairment or splinting

5. Compare results bilaterally and remember dominant vs. non-dominant extremity

Muscle strength grading system

Grade			
5	**Normal**	**100%**	Complete ROM against gravity with full resistance
4	**Good***	**75%**	Complete ROM against gravity with some resistance *(reduced fine movements & motor control)*
3	**Fair***	**50%**	Complete ROM against gravity but no resistance
2	**Poor***	**25%**	Complete ROM with gravity eliminated
1	**Trace**	**~5%**	Evidence of slight contractility; *no joint motion or inability to achieve complete ROM with gravity eliminated*
0	**Zero**	**0%**	No evidence of contractility *(flaccid)*

% = % normal strength, ROM = range of motion, *Muscle spasm or contracture may limit ROM; Place question mark after grading a movement that is incomplete from this cause; Chart as a rating out of 5; e.g. 5/5, 4/5, 3/5, 2/5, 1/5, 0/5

Blood Type Diet

The blood type diet is a diet advocated by Peter D'Adamo and outlined in his book *Eat Right 4 Your Type*. Its basic premise is that ABO blood type is the most important factor in determining a healthy diet.

According to blood type diet, the program shows you how to:

- Avoid many common viruses and infections
- Lose weight as your body rids itself of toxins and fats
- Gain body energy which will speed up healing
- Determine your genetic susceptibility to certain diseases
- Avoid many factors which cause cell deterioration, thus slowing down the aging process

The Blood Type Diet is the restoration of your natural genetic rhythm. D'Adamo groups those thirteen races together by ABO blood group, each type within this group having unique dietary recommendations:

- **Blood Type O** = hunter, protein meat was the main food staple, strong immune system as it builds antibodies to anything than looks like A or B. It has no blood antigens, allowing compatibility of a specific range of food.

- **Blood Type A** = grains and livestock cultivation, community effort required, planning and networking, more resistance to infection (highest in Western Europe). Has A antigen and best allows "A" marker foods.

- **Blood Type B** = historical people are Indian, Mongolian, Asian, & later western European (German & Austrian). Strong in meat and cultured diary products. Has B antigen and best allows "B" marker foods.

- **Blood Type AB** = rare, in less than 5% of the population, have enhanced ability to make antibodies to microbial infections, lowered susceptibility to allergies, arthritis, inflammation and lupus. Has both A and B antigen.

Blood type determines strength of your immune system. The immune system works to define "self" (matching indicators) and destroys non-self invaders or conditions. Protects us by recognizing our own cells and keeping them safe.

Below is a summary of the various Blood Type Diets and detailed plan of each one according to Dr. D'Adamo.

Blood Types	Diet Profile	Beneficial Foods	Limited Foods	Foods to avoid for Weight Loss purpose	Foods that help with Weight Loss
Type O	High Proteins	Meat Fish Vegetables Fruit	Grains Beans Legumes	Wheat Corn Kidney Beans Navy Beans Lentils Cabbage Brussels Sprouts Cauliflower Mustard Greens	Kelp Seafood Salt Liver Red Meat Kale Spinach Broccoli
Type A	Meat eaters	Vegetables Tofu Seafood Grains Beans Legumes Fruit		Meat Dairy Kidney Beans Lima Beans Wheat	Vegetable Oil Soy Foods Vegetables Pineapple
Type B	Vegetarian	Meat (no chicken) Dairy Grains Beans Legumes Vegetables Fruit		Corn Lentils Peanuts Sesame Seeds Buckwheat Wheat	Greens Eggs Venison Liver Licorice Tea
Type AB	Balanced omnivore	Meat Seafood Dairy Tofu Beans Legumes Grains Vegetables Fruits		Red Meat Kidney Beans Lima Beans Seeds Corn Buckwheat	Tofu Seafood Dairy Greens Kelp Pineapple

pH for health

Healthcare practitioners understand that disease often results from acid/alkaline imbalances, weakened body systems, creating an ideal environment where bacteria and viruses can thrive, and making it difficult for the body to resist disease. The combination of massage and the proper balance of acidity and alkalinity in your body allow essential chemical reactions to take place in cells and tissues for crucial for health and vitality. Balancing the pH is a major step toward well-being and greater health. Research has discovered that the body fluids of healthy people are alkaline **(high pH)** whereas the body fluids of sick people are acidic **(low pH)** - below **7.30.**

Your body operates ideally within a narrow pH range of **7.35 and 7.45** and will do so at all costs. It is naturally more alkaline than acidic; even though some of the systems (like the digestive system) are more acidic. If the pH levels get too acidic, a condition called acidosis can occur. Fatigue and stress can contribute to acidosis. Acidosis occurs when your blood pH level falls below **7.30**. Most health problems occur when the body becomes acidic. Chronic acidity hinders all cellular activities and forces the body to borrow minerals, sodium, calcium, potassium and magnesium from vital organs and bones to neutralize the acid resulting in mineral deficiencies. The balances are maintained via various proteins, minerals, and kidney and lung functions. In addition, everything you eat or drink affects pH balance, for good or for ill. Your body must maintain the proper pH levels.

Energy habits, stress, toxicity, improper elimination, prescription medications and the inability to excrete acids all contribute to an over-acid state. The biggest factor is a diet with acid-producing foods such as meat, eggs and dairy, white flour, coffee, tea, milk, soft drinks, and fruit juice. The chief culprits in mineral depletion within our body are the acid-forming foods we eat and what we drink (almost all of the fluids we drink on a daily basis are acidic). For example, a carbonated beverage has a pH of 2, orange juice is pH of 3, and average tap water is 4.5. However, bottled water is typically a pH of only 6. The other major cause of acidity is stress. In addition, antibiotics which can destroy friendly bacteria create a problem because the bacteria that 'grow back' are often acid forming and can potentially create a problem that could drain the body of health-enhancing electrolyte minerals. Some other causes of electrolyte loss might be: strenuous exercise, sickness, infection, or even fasting.

How to test your own pH

You can have clients test their own pH simply and inexpensively by using pH test strips. Tear off two three-inch strips. As they awaken, before drinking or eating anything, have them excrete saliva onto the test strip. Compare the color to a pH color chart that comes with the test strips. Next, measure the pH of your second urination of the morning. To do this, urinate on the strip or collect the urine in a plastic or glass (not paper) cup and dip the test strip. Again, compare the color to the pH color chart. If your urinary pH fluctuates between **6.0 and 6.5** in the morning and between **6.5 and 7.0** in the evening, your body is functioning within a healthy range. If your saliva stays between **6.5 and 7.5** all day long, your body is functioning within a healthy range. The best time to test your pH is about one hour before a meal and two hours after a meal. Test your pH two days a week. Optimum health cannot occur when the body is too acidic.

Acid

An acidic balance will decrease the body's ability to absorb minerals and other nutrients, decrease the energy production in the cells, decrease its ability to repair damaged cells, decrease its ability to detoxify heavy metals, make tumor cells thrive, and make it more susceptible to fatigue and illness. Chronic acidity hinders cellular activities and forces the body to borrow minerals, including sodium, potassium and magnesium from vital organs and bones, resulting in mineral deficiencies.

An acidic pH can occur from an acid-forming diet, emotional stress, toxic overload, and/or immune reactions or any process that deprives the cells of oxygen and other nutrients. The body will try to compensate for acidic pH by using alkaline minerals. If the diet does not contain enough minerals to compensate, a build-up of acids in the cells will occur. Acidosis is the primary indicator of calcium deficiency disease which lead to more severe and chronic problems.

Acidosis can cause such problems as:

- Cardiovascular damage, including the constriction of blood vessels and the reduction of oxygen
- Weight gain, obesity and diabetes
- Bladder and kidney conditions, including kidney stones
- Immune deficiency
- Acceleration of free radical damage, possibly contributing to cancerous mutations
- Hormone concerns
- Premature aging
- Osteoporosis, weak, brittle bones, hip fractures and bone spurs
- Joint pain, aching muscles and lactic-acid buildup
- Low energy and chronic fatigue
- Slow digestion and elimination
- Yeast/fungal overgrowth

pH BALANCE

Alkaline

Alkalinity is relatively rare. Healthier people tend to be more alkaline than acidic. Be sure to monitor your progress with easy-to-use pH test strips. The balancing nature of the human body tends to bring the pH back toward normal no matter which direction it has gone.

Foods

Proper pH levels are essential to good health. Blood that is too acidic or too alkaline can trigger defense mechanisms that may compensate for the problem at hand, but could potentially cause other problems. We can protect ourselves, and possibly turn these problems around, by eating foods with the proper pH.

Most diets cause an unhealthy acid pH. In fact, diet appears to be the major influence in maintaining appropriate pH levels throughout the body. Research demonstrates that when food is metabolized and broken down, it leaves certain chemical and metallic residues, a noncombustible "ash", when combined with our body fluids, yields either acid or alkali potentials of pH. Certain foods are "acid-forming" in nature, whereas others are known to be "alkali-forming."

Correcting the pH balance is quickly and easily accomplished through foods. The following is a list of foods and beverages you can consume on a regular basis that will assist you in balancing your pH levels. Start simple.

Alkaline Foods

Sample alkaline foods to comprise most (75-80%) of your diet. Eat salads, fresh vegetables, healthy nuts and oils, and plenty of raw foods. Drink at least 2-3 liters of clean, pure water daily.

Vegetables	Fruits	Seeds, Nuts, Grains	Drinks
Asparagus	Avocado	Almonds	Green Drinks
Beetroot	Grapefruit	Buckwheat	Fresh vegetable juice
Broccoli	Lemon	Cumin	Pure water (distilled,
Brussels Sprouts	Lime	Flax	reverse osmosis,
Cabbage	Rhubarb	Lentils	ionized)
Carrot	Tomato	Pumpkin	Lemon water (pure water
Cauliflower	Watermelon (neutral)	Sesame	+ fresh lemon or lime).
Celery		Spelt	Herbal Tea
Courgettes	**Fats & Oils**	Sprouts/sprouted seeds	Vegetable broth
Cucumber	Avocado	Alfalfa	Non-sweetened Soy Milk
Garlic	Borage	Mung bean	Almond Milk
Grasses (e.g. wheat,	Evening Primrose	Wheat	
barley)	Flax	Hummus	
Green Beans	Hemp	Tahini	
Lettuce	Olive & Oil Blends	Sunflower	
Onion			
Peas			
Radish			

Acidic Foods

Sample acid-forming foods to comprise the remainder (20-25%) of your diet. Avoid fatty meats, dairy, cheese, sweets & candy, chocolates, alcohol and tobacco. Beware of hidden content of packaged foods and microwave meals. Don't overcook meals - this removes all of the nutrition.

Meats	Dairy Products	Drinks	Seeds & Nuts
Beef	Cheese	Beers	Cashew Nuts
Chicken	Cream	Carbonated Drinks	Peanuts
Crustaceans	Ice Cream	Coffee	Pistachio Nuts
Seafood (apart from	Milk	Dairy Smoothies	
occasional oily fish and	Yogurt	Fruit Juice	**Others**
salmon)		Milk	Artificial Sweeteners
Lamb	**Fats & Oils**	Spirits	Biscuits
Pork	Corn Oil	Tea	Condiments (tomato
Turkey	Hydrogenated Oils		sauce, mayonnaise etc.)
Fruits	Margarine	**Convenience Foods**	Eggs
All fruits not listed in the	Saturated Fats	Candy/Sweets	Honey
alkaline table	Vegetable Oil	Canned/Tinned Foods	Soy Sauce
	Sunflower Oil	Chocolate	Tamari
		Fast Food	Vinegar
		Instant Meals	White Bread
		Microwave Meals	White Pasta
		Powdered Soups	Wholemeal Bread

Body Mass Index (BMI)

Body mass index is the measurement of choice for many physicians and researchers studying obesity. BMI uses a mathematical formula that takes into account both a person's height and weight. BMI equals a person's weight in kilograms divided by height in meters squared. (BMI=kg/m2).

Risk of Associated Disease According to BMI and Waist Size

	BMI	Waist less than or equal to 40 in. (men) or 35 in. (women)	Waist greater than 40 in. (men) or 35 in. (women)
Underweight	18.5 or less	--	--
Normal	18.5 - 24.9	--	--
Overweight	25.0 - 29.9	Increased	High
Obese	30.0 - 34.9	High	Very High
Obese	35.0 - 39.9	Very High	Very High
Extremely Obese	40 or greater	Extremely High	Extremely High

Source: National Heart, Lung and Blood Institute

Determining Your Body Mass Index (BMI)

The table below has already done the math and metric conversions. To use the table, find the appropriate height in the left-hand column. Move across the row to the given weight. The number at the top of the column is the BMI for that height and weight. Or, use our BMI calculator.

	BMI (kg/m^2)	19	20	21	22	23	24	25	26	27	28	29	30	35	40
Height (feet)	**Height (in.)**	**Weight (lb.)**													
4'10"	**58**	91	96	100	105	110	115	119	124	129	134	138	143	167	191
4'11"	**59**	94	99	104	109	114	119	124	128	133	138	143	148	173	198
5'0"	**60**	97	102	107	112	118	123	128	133	138	143	148	153	179	204
5'1"	**61**	100	106	111	116	122	127	132	137	143	148	153	158	185	211
5'2"	**62**	104	109	115	120	126	131	136	142	147	153	158	164	191	218
5'3"	**63**	107	113	118	124	130	135	141	146	152	158	163	169	197	225
5'4"	**64**	110	116	122	128	134	140	145	151	157	163	169	174	204	232
5'5"	**65**	114	120	126	132	138	144	150	156	162	168	174	180	210	240
5'6"	**66**	118	124	130	136	142	148	155	161	167	173	179	186	216	247
5'7"	**67**	121	127	134	140	146	153	159	166	172	178	185	191	223	255
5'8"	**68**	125	131	138	144	151	158	164	171	177	184	190	197	230	262
5'9"	**69**	128	135	142	149	155	162	169	176	182	189	196	203	236	270
5'10"	**70**	132	139	146	153	160	167	174	181	188	195	202	207	243	278
5'11"	**71**	136	143	150	157	165	172	179	186	193	200	208	215	250	286
6'0"	**72**	140	147	154	162	169	177	184	191	199	206	213	221	258	294
6'1"	**73**	144	151	159	166	174	182	189	197	204	212	219	227	265	302
6'2"	**74**	148	155	163	171	179	186	194	202	210	218	225	233	272	311
6'3"	**75**	152	160	168	176	184	192	200	208	216	224	232	240	279	319
6'4"	**76**	156	164	172	180	189	197	205	213	221	230	238	246	287	328

Weight

lb/2.2 = Kg		Kg x 2.2 = lb	
lb	**Kg**	**Kg**	**lb**
1	0.5	1	2.2
2	0.9	2	4.4
3	1.4	3	6.6
4	1.8	5	11
10	4.5	10	22
50	22.7	20	110
100	45.5	80	176
150	68.2	90	198
200	90.9	100	220

Units of Measurement

°F – 32 x 0.5555 = °C		°C X 1.8 + 32 = °F	
°F	**°C**	**°C**	**°F**
0	-17.8	0	32.0
95	35.0	35.0	95.0
96	35.6	35.5	95.0
97	36.1	36.0	96.8
98	36.7	36.5	97.7
99	37.2	37.0	98.6
100	37.8	37.5	99.5
101	38.3	38.0	100.4
102	38.9	38.5	101.3
103	39.4	39.0	102.2
104	40.0	39.5	103.1
105	40.6	40.0	104.0

HEIGHT TO WEIGHT RATIO

Height to Weight Ratio Averages

It is essential to maintain height and weight balance to prevent any health risks. Height and weight ratio is important because it relates to your present and future health. Moreover, height and weight charts in combination with body mass index will help you determine whether you are overweight or obese and thus have a health risk. Calculating ideal weight for height is one way of determining whether one is over or underweight. This method also takes into account the frame size of a person.

People who exercise and are physically fit tend to have more lean muscle mass and lower levels of fat tissue than people who are not physically fit. Muscle tissue weighs more, and this does not necessarily affect the actual frame of the person, but will affect weight. In order to get an ideal weight for height, one may need to do a body-fat composition test to more accurately measure the good tissue "muscle" versus the "bad" fat tissue. Remember that height-to-weight ratio are averages and needs to take into account with BMI and muscle mass. Avoid rigid interpretations of the perfect height-to-weight ratios. There is no such thing; rather it should be used as another diagnostic tool or indicator for health risk since individual variations are going to affect ideal weight figures for each person.

This height to weight guideline as follows:

Female Height to Weight Ratio			
Height	Small Frame	Medium Frame	Large Frame
4' 10"	100	115	131
4' 11"	101	117	134
5' 0"	103	120	137
5' 1"	105	122	140
5' 2"	108	125	144
5' 3"	111	128	148
5' 4"	114	133	152
5' 5"	117	136	156
5' 6"	120	140	160
5' 7"	123	143	164
5 '8"	126	146	167
5' 9"	129	150	170
5' 10"	132	153	173
5' 11"	135	156	176
6' 0"	138	159	179

Male Height to Weight Ratio			
Height	Small Frame	Medium Frame	Large Frame
5' 1"	123	134	145
5' 2"	125	137	148
5' 3"	127	139	151
5' 4"	129	142	155
5' 5"	131	145	159
5' 6"	133	148	163
5" 7"	135	151	167
5' 8"	137	154	171
5' 9"	139	157	175
5' 10"	141	160	179
5' 11"	144	164	183
6' 0"	147	167	187
6' 1"	150	171	192
6' 2"	153	175	197
6' 3"	157	179	202

Equivalents of Measurement

Metric (volume)	Apothecary	Household
1ml	15 minims	15 drops
15 ml	4 fluid grams	1 tablespoon
30 ml	1 fluid ounce	2 tablespoons
240 ml	8 fluid ounces	1 cup
480 ml (approx. 0.5L)	1 pint	1 pint
960 ml (approx. 1.0 L)	1 quart	1 quart
3840 ml	1 gallon	1 gallon

RICE

"RICE" is a pneumonic for rest, ice, compression, and elevation. RICE refers to the basic course of treatment that is appropriate immediately after a minor injury. It can help relieve pain and prevent swelling. When there is an injury, interstitial fluid can collect in the area of the injury. This extra fluid causes swelling, redness, and, possibly, pain. RICE can be used for minor injuries such as bruises, sprains, strains, and pulled muscles. The earlier the RICE treatment is started after an injury, the better it works.

R-Rest
Rest the injured area. Moving the injured area causes pain because the body needs rest to heal itself. Do not use the area or bear weight (such as standing or walking) until the injury is evaluated by a healthcare provider. Sometimes resting an injured area means not participating in any physical activity, or just the activity that caused the injury. For example, walking may be allowed, but no running. If necessary, you may suggest using crutches or a cane so that less weight is put on an injured foot or leg.

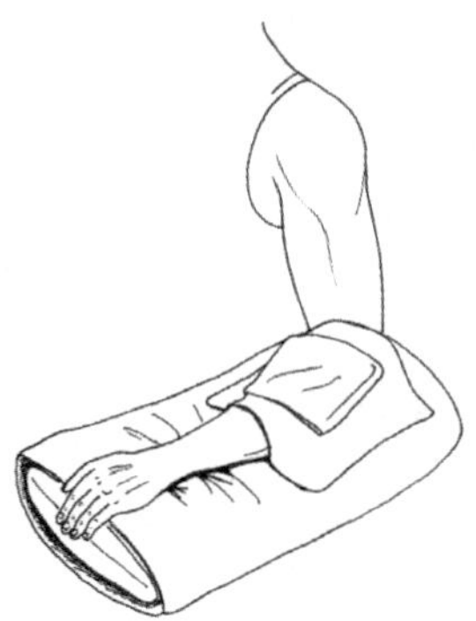

I-Ice
Ice applied to the injured area helps prevent or reduce swelling. Swelling causes pain and can slow healing. Apply a cloth-covered ice pack to the injured area for no more than 20 minutes at a time, four to eight times a day. Applying ice more than 20 minutes may cause cold injury. A one-pound package of frozen corn or peas makes a good ice pack. It is lightweight, conforms to the injured area, and is inexpensive and reusable. When making an ice pack with a plastic bag, make sure all the air is out of the bag before closing it. Areas with little fat and muscle, such as fingers or toes, should only have ice on them for about 10 minutes. Frozen gel packs are colder than ice, so they should be removed 10 minutes sooner.

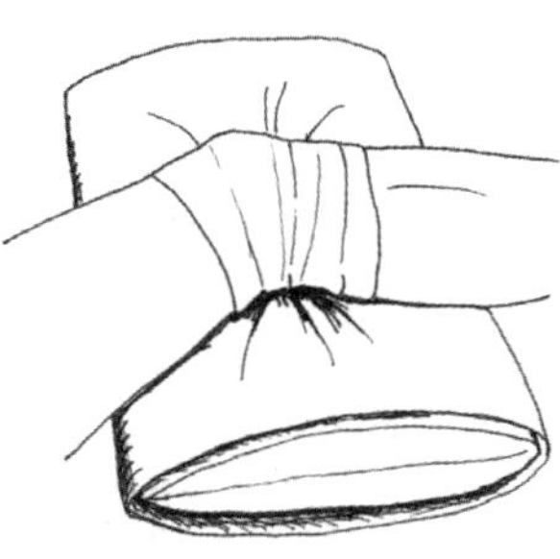

C-Compression
Compression, most often as a pressure bandage, also helps prevent and reduce swelling. Wrap the injured area with an elastic bandage, but not so tightly that the blood is cut off. It should not hurt or throb. Fingers or toes beyond the bandage should remain pink and not become "tingly." The elastic bandage should be taken off every 4 hours, and then reapplied as necessary.

E-Elevation
Elevation means raising the injured area above the level of the heart. The affected area should be elevated so it is 12 inches above the heart. Prop up a leg or arm while resting it. It may be necessary to lie down to get the area above heart level. Elevation can be done with several pillows.

Anyone with Raynaud's, diabetes, sensitivity to cold or any medical condition with reduced blood flow to the arms or legs should not use RICE therapy. These people need to see their primary care provider for care of minor and more serious injuries.

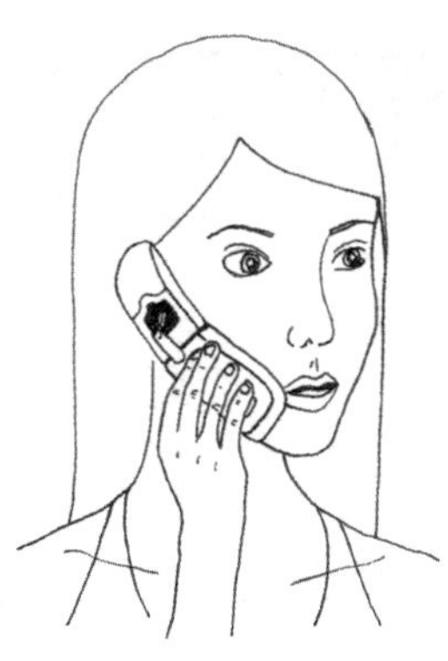

Call Doctor
Do all four parts of the RICE treatment together. If there is still pain when using the injured part after 1 or 2 days, consult your healthcare provider or if the injury is serious, such as internal bleeding or a broken bone, go to the nearest emergency room.

Caution
- Fingers or toes feel numb, are cold to the touch, or change color
- Skin looks shiny or tight
- Pain, swelling, or bruising worsens and is not improved with elevation

Heat Therapy

Heat is usually used as therapy for chronic injuries or injuries that have no inflammation or swelling. It can take the form of a hot pack, hot cloth, hot water, ultrasound, heating pad, hydrocollator packs, heat lamps, hyperthermia blankets, whirlpool baths, and many others. Heat therapy can be beneficial to those with arthritis, stiff muscles or injuries to the deep tissue of the skin. The use of heat therapy causes the injured muscles to relax by opening the capillaries and improving circulation to the treated area. Therefore, it is recommended that heat therapy be avoided for already inflamed joints. Heat appears to be best for untightening muscles and increasing overall flexibility. The proper tissue temperature for vigorous heating is between 104° F and 113° F (40° to 45° C), and the correct duration of temperature elevation is about 5 to 30 minutes.

It is generally recommended to use heat therapy for muscular pain and general relaxation in conjunction with a therapeutic massage. Heat increases blood circulation to the area and speeds recovery by transporting fresh blood cells and removing wastes. Because heat increases circulation and raises skin temperature, you should not apply heat to acute injuries or injuries that show signs of inflammation.

Sore, stiff, nagging muscle or joint pain is ideal for the use of heat therapy. Athletes with chronic pain or injuries may use heat therapy *before* exercise to increase the elasticity of joint connective tissues and to stimulate blood flow. Heat can also help relax tight muscles or muscle spasms. Do not apply heat after exercise. After a workout, ice is the better choice on a chronic injury.

Physiologic Effects

- Muscle relaxation
- Local increase in temperature, metabolism, phagocytosis, perspiration
- Less sensation in sensory nerve endings
- Local vasodilatation with hyperemia (due to increase in metabolism and histamine release)
  - Heat penetrates only a few millimeters deep
  - Deeper reactions are due to reflexes and require more than 15 minutes of heat application
- For deeper blood vessels, vasoconstriction then vasodilatation
  - Undesirable for cancer or infection
- Increase in capillary pressure, cell permeability: can cause edema
- Improves lymphatic flow and pliability of collagen
- Long-term effects include increase in body temperature, respiration, pulse rate and lower BP to disperse heat
- Repeated strong doses, chronic use over time may cause *erythema ab igne*

Indications	Contraindications
• Sub acute, chronic traumatic and inflammatory conditions of superficial muscles and joints • Improves range of motion • Promotes tissue healing by increasing blood circulation and nutrients to the area • Indirect heating for peripheral vascular disease or infection • Less muscle contraction	• Acute Inflammatory Conditions • Open wounds • Dermatitis • Non-inflammatory edema • Circulatory issues • Fever • Skin illness with redness or blisters • DVT, peripheral vascular disease • Bleeding • Those with cardiac insufficiency may not endure more stress on the heart • Malignant tumors and infections • For adults 60 and older and children under four- unreliable thermoregulation, might get fever

Cautions

• Preexisting edema might be aggravated by heat
  – Acute edema: painful, puffy, clearly circumscribed
  – Chronic edema: not clearly circumscribed, pitting
• Patient with sensory loss should be watched closely
• Confused clients should be watched closely

Application

Hydrocollator Packs (hot packs)

- 140° F to 170° F (60°to 77 °C)
- Fill canvas with silica gel, heat in water. Presoak packs for about 20 minutes in hot water

Process:

- Look closely at area to be treated
- Wrap pack in cover, then add three to five layers of towels
- Tell client to indicate if it is too hot
- Recheck frequently to avoid burns or remove layer of towel for more heat
- Treatment should be 15 to 20 minutes

Electric Heating Pads

- Most often used by individuals as a home remedy
- Treatment time should be from 10 to 20 minutes
- Instructions for client:
  - Use a medium setting- not high
  - Stay awake while pad is applied
  - Use a timer to prevent application going too long

Paraffin Bath

- 118° F to 130° F (48° to 54° C)
- Use a six-to-one mixture of paraffin and mineral oil
- Oil lowers the melting point of the wax, helping to remove it from the skin more easily
- Delivers heat to difficult-to-reach areas
- Use for non-acute arthritis, Raynaud's, osteoarthritis, Dupuytren's contracture
- Not for open wounds, infections, burns, or fungal infections
- Process:
  - After removing jewelry, wash and examine area
  - Prepare two towels plus wax paper/plastic wrap
  - Patient dips the part in paraffin about six times, letting wax solidify between dips
  - Wrap the part in wax paper and towel to preserve heat
  - Patient should sit for about 20 to 30 minutes
  - Peel paraffin off

Infrared

- Heat lamp should be positioned 18 to 30 inches from treatment area
- Treatment time should be 10 minutes to an hour
- Use when superficial heat is indicated (provides dry heat)
- Should not be used on clients with light-sensitive skin ailments

Cold Therapy

Cold is generally used for acute and chronic injuries to reduce pain, inflammation, and swelling. It can take the form of ice bags, cold packs, ice massage, cooling sprays or bags of frozen vegetables. It can be beneficial to those with edema and swelling. Cold therapy is used for reducing pain and inflammation, and slowing metabolic action. During an injury, the blood vessels around the injured tissues open up, rushing blood, nutrients and fluids to the area to help tissues heal. The problem is that the increased blood flow often causes the healthy tissues surrounding the injury to swell and become inflamed. If swelling and inflammation are not slowed, more extensive tissue damage may occur and the injury may take longer to heal. The additional fluids in the swollen tissues may press on nerves around the injury site, increasing pain.

By cooling the surface of the skin and the underlying tissues, cold therapy causes the narrowing of blood vessels, a process known as vasoconstriction. This vasoconstriction leads to a decrease in the amount of blood being delivered to the area and subsequently lessens the amount of swelling and constricts blood vessels, which permits fluid drainage and reduces pain.

Physiologic Effects

- Local vasoconstriction
  - After the cold item is removed, there is instant vasodilation
- Decrease in local inflammation, edema, hemorrhage, metabolism and oxygen demand
- Decrease of nerve conduction velocity
- Reduced heart rate and respiratory rate
- Muscle spasm relief
- Because of decreased cellular nutrition, there may be decreased tissue healing
- Extended exposure to cold will bring about an increased metabolism in order to produce heat and maintain homeostasis
- When cooling is excessive (lower than 50° F for more than 10 minutes) the body will respond with regular bursts of vasodilatation then vasoconstriction; this is the only time the application of cold can cause edema

Indications	Contraindications
• Intense injury, inflammation or edema • Lowering of fever • New burns • Inhibits bleeding • Muscle spasticity due to UMNL • Acute or chronic pain from muscle spasm	• Open wounds over 48 to 72 hours post-injury • Peripheral vascular disease • Patients with angina pectoris, cardiac dysfunctions or arterial insufficiency • Hypersensitivity to cold (Raynaud's, uticaria, MS) • Patients with areas of cutaneous anesthesia

Cautions
• Cold applied longer than two to three days after injury may delay healing time • Patients with significant medical problems, slow healing wounds and diminished circulation • Monitor client carefully if they show confusion • Elderly typically prefer heat to cold

Application
Cold Packs

Hydrocollator packs (cold packs)
- Cover area with a layer of moist towel, then place cold pack over towel
- Cover other side of cold pack with layers of dry towel
- Keep on for 10 to 20 minutes for pain, edema or bleeding
  - For emergencies, treatment time may be several hours
- Goal is to reduce edema and inflammation
- Usually applied right after acute musculoskeletal injuries

Ice Bags
- Inexpensive and easy application that is ideal for home usage
- Apply for 10 to 20 minutes for acute pain, edema or bleeding
- RICE treatments call for 20 minutes on and 40 minutes off and repeated as necessary for 24 to 48 hours after injury

Ice Massage
- Examine area where ice massage will be applied
- Do not use on client with history of frostbite or open wound. Do not use directly on bone
- Apply ice directly to skin, then repeatedly move ice over the treatment area
  - Application will produce reactive hyperemia, increased pain threshold (decreased sensation), decreased nerve conduction
  - Ice massage won't reduce edema (needs application of cold pack at least 10 minutes)
- Treat for five minutes or until client feels numbness over the treatment area
- During ice massage treatment, client should feel: cold, burning, aching, then numbness

Vapocoolant Spray (spray and stretch)
- Vapocoolant spray (also known as fluoromethane) is applied to the skin, and cooling is achieved through evaporation
- Physiologic effects will include temporary analgesia, reflexive muscle relaxation below the treatment area
- Indications include myofascial trigger points (MFTP), spasms, reduced ROM, stretching
- Contraindications include contact with mucous membranes, eyes and the client's history of frostbite
- Application
  - Find MFTP, direction of muscle fibers, area of pain
  - Starting 15 to 24 inches from the skin, sweep area three times in direction of muscle fibers
  - Stretch muscle
  - Repeat process three or four times
  - Apply hot pack for five to 15 minutes when finished
  - Instruct client to move area through active range of motion

Alternating Hot/Cold Therapy

Heat therapy expands blood vessels, filling them with blood, and cold therapy constricts the blood vessels, forcing the blood to move on to other parts of the body. Heat and cold can be applied to any part of the body that is inflamed, congested, or injured. The time for each cold or hot treatment is one to five minutes with a total treatment time of 15 to 25 minutes. Treatment normally consists of applying hot to cold, alternating to the client's comfort level. The amount of time the hot and cold are applied may vary as long as the cold application is of shorter duration than the hot. You may repeat this cycle two to three times or more, but always end on a short hot or warm application to remove or neutralize any remaining chills.

Physiologic Effects
- This is used as vascular exercise which produces alternating vasodilatation and vasoconstriction
- Stimulates peripheral blood flow and soft tissue healing
- Reduces edema during subacute stages of healing

Indications	Contraindications
• During transition between acute and subacute phases • Chronic edema and impaired venous circulation • Sinus and congestive headaches, apply to hands and feet • Musculoskeletal conditions: OA, RA, sprains, strains	• All contraindications for heat and cold alone, but adverse effects are generally less • Small vessel disease (advanced diabetes complications) • Patients with insufficient thermoregulatory systems, children or elderly • Reduced cutaneous sensation (local anesthesia)

Application
- Examine treatment area
- Begin and end treatment with heat
- Length of time for treatment:
  - Heat, four to six minutes
  - Cold, one to two minutes
  - The hot-to-cold ratio should be three-to-one or four-to-one (minutes)
  - Apply heat first, approximately 100° to 112°F
- Then apply cold, at about 50° to 65°F
- At end of treatment, apply warm to neutralize any remaining chills
- Treatment should last 20 to 30 minutes

Hydrotherapy

Hydrotherapy treatments are used as a means of physical therapy, both to promote relaxation and to relieve minor aches and pains. It can take the form of whirlpools, tanks, sitz bath, saunas, steam baths, or hot baths. Warm water expands blood vessels, which can temporarily increase circulation, help to relax muscles, and reduce pain and inflammation in arthritis and other rheumatologic conditions. It also reduces the effects of stress by increasing endorphin production.

Physiologic Effects
- Thermal effects include elevated temperature, metabolism, leukocytosis, perspiration
- Mechanical effects include massaging, stimulation, removal of debris from open wounds
- Buoyancy (relieving the stress of weight bearing)
- Viscosity (use as resistance for exercise)
- Extended exposure to heated water may cause:
  - Increase in heart rate
  - Slight increase in body temperature and hyperemia
  - Mild rise in alkalinity of tissues, blood and urine

Indications	Contraindications
• Promotes tissue healing by increasing blood circulation • RA, OA, fibromyalgia, general body muscle and joint soreness • Hypothermia • Sub acute, chronic traumatic and inflammatory conditions	• Young or elderly with inefficient thermoregulation • Immersion in pregnancy • Heart and vascular conditions, hypertension • Diabetes • Rashes, dermatological conditions (anything contagious) • Dizziness, nausea, weakness

Sitz Baths

- In a sitz bath, only the hips and buttocks are soaked in water or saline solution
- Indications:
  - For clients who have had surgery in rectal area
  - Pilonidal cysts, decreased pain from hemorrhoids, uterine cramps, prostate infections, painful ovaries, testicles, infections of the bladder, prostate, vagina, inflammatory bowel diseases
- Some clients get dizzy when standing after sitting in hot water
- Application:
  - Treatment should be for 15 to 25 minutes
  - Bath should be filled with three to four inches of water
  - Warm sitz bath can be used to address pain of hemorrhoids, genital herpes, uterine cramps
  - For prostate pain, clients should take two hot sitz baths daily for about 15 minutes each
  - A cool, 10-minute sitz bath can help ease inflammation, constipation, vaginal discharge
  - Some conditions are better treated by a contrasting bath of both hot and cold
    * One tub of hot water and one tub of ice water
    * Patient sits in the hot water for three to four minutes, then in the cold water for 30 to 60 seconds
    * Repeat cycle three to five times

Whirlpools/Hubbard tanks

- Whirlpools are most often used to treat the distal body segments of the upper and lower extremities
- Hubbard tanks are used to treat one or both of the upper or lower extremities, as well as the trunk
- Both may give pain relief and an increased range of motion
- 99° to 104°F for full body immersion
- Consider cold for acute musculoskeletal problems
- Treatment should last 15 to 20 minutes

Steam Tent/Sauna

- Steam tents use 100-percent humidity while saunas are relatively dry
- Steam tents operate at a lower temperature than saunas
- Specific indications: upper respiratory congestion, sinusitis
- Heat water, add white vinegar, peppermint, wintergreen or eucalyptus oil
- Have client inhale through nose
- Warn client to stay awake in steam tent or sauna
- It is important to check on client regularly and pay close attention to heart rate

Foot or Hand Baths

- Treatment should be for 15 to 30 minutes
- Hot foot bath for congested pelvis
- Hot hand bath for congestive headache, nosebleeds

Vital Signs

Pulse	
Descriptors: regular, irregular, strong or weak	
Adult	60 to 100 bpm
Children - age 1 to 8 years	80 to 100 bpm
Infants - age 1 to 12 months	100 to 120 bpm
Neonates - age 1 to 28 days	120 to 160 bpm

Blood pressure			
	Systolic	**Diastolic**	**Average**
Adult	90 to 130	60 to 90	80 to 120
Children	80 to 110	50 to 70	60 to 100
Infants	70 to 95	40 to 80	60 to 90
Neonates	>60		

Respirations	
Descriptors: normal, shallow, labored, noisy	
Adult (normal)	12 to 20 bpm
Children - 1 to 8 years	15 to 30
Infants - 1 to 12 months	25 to 50
Neonates - 1 to 28 days	40 to 60

Common Lab Values

There are some basic rules which hold true for nearly all laboratory tests

1. Different laboratories can get different results on the same sample of blood.
2. Laboratories can make mistakes. If your results have changed dramatically from your previous test, have it run again.
3. Most lab values need to be interpreted along with other clinical and laboratory data in order to develop a meaningful diagnosis. Very seldom will only one value give all of the answers.
4. Laboratory values differ according to age, sex, current medications, etc. Therefore, the interpretation of these values needs to be done with these other parameters in mind.

Clinical laboratory test are used by the practioner to aid in the diagnostic process; screen for early recognition of preventable health problems; and to monitor patient progress and outcomes. It is recommended that the practioner who used the services of a laboratory should be aware of laboratory's scope of services, recognition, and reputation. A listing of diagnostic labs can be found on page 404.

Test	Reference Range (conventional units)
17 Hydroxyprogesterone (Men)	0.06-3.0 mg/L
17 Hydroxyprogesterone (Women) Follicular phase	0.2-1.0 mg/L
25-hydroxyvitamin D (25(OH)D)	8-80 ng/mL
Acetoacetate	<3 mg/dL
Acidity (pH)	7.35 - 7.45
Alcohol	0 mg/dL (more than 0.1 mg/dL normally indicates intoxication) (ethanol)
Ammonia	15 - 50 µg of nitrogen/dL
Amylase	53 - 123 units/L
Ascorbic Acid	0.4 - 1.5 mg/dL
Bicarbonate	18 - 23 mEq/L (carbon dioxide content)
Bilirubin	Direct: up to 0.4 mg/dL Total: up to 1.0 mg/dL
Blood Volume	8.5 - 9.1% of total body weight
Calcium	8.5 - 10.5 mg/dL (normally slightly higher in children)
Carbon Dioxide Pressure	35 - 45 mm Hg
Carbon Monoxide	Less than 5% of total hemoglobin
CD4 Cell Count	500 - 1500 cells/µL
Ceruloplasmin	15 - 60 mg/dL
Chloride	98 - 106 mEq/L

Test	Reference Range (conventional units)
Complete Blood Cell Count (CBC)	Tests include: hemoglobin, hematocrit, mean corpuscular hemoglobin, mean corpuscular hemoglobin concentration, mean corpuscular volume, platelet count, white blood cell count
Copper	Total: 70 - 150 µg/dL
Creatine Kinase (CK or CPK)	Male: 38 - 174 units/L Female: 96 - 140 units/L
Creatine Kinase Isoenzymes	5% MB or less
Creatinine	0.6 - 1.2 mg/dL
Electrolytes	Test includes: calcium, chloride, magnesium, potassium, sodium
Erythrocyte Sedimentation Rate (ESR or Sed-Rate)	Male: 1 - 13 mm/hr Female: 1 - 20 mm/hr
Glucose	Tested after fasting: 70 - 110 mg/dL
Hematocrit	Male: 45 - 62% Female: 37 - 48%
Hemoglobin	Male: 13 - 18 gm/dL Female: 12 - 16 gm/dL
Iron	60 - 160 µg/dL (normally higher in males)
Iron-binding Capacity	250 - 460 µg/dL
Lactate (lactic acid)	Venous: 4.5 - 19.8 mg/dL Arterial: 4.5 - 14.4 mg/dL
Lactic Dehydrogenase	50 - 150 units/L
Lead	40 µg/dL or less (normally much lower in children)
Lipase	10 - 150 units/L
Zinc B-Zn	70 - 102 µmol/L
Lipids	
Cholesterol	Less than 225 mg/dL (for age 40-49 yr; increases with age)
Triglycerides	10 - 29 years; 53 - 104 mg/dL
	30 - 39 years; 55 - 115 mg/dL
	40 - 49 years; 66 - 139 mg/dL
	50 - 59 years; 75 - 163 mg/dL
	60 - 69 years; 78 - 158 mg/dL
	> 70 years; 83 - 141 mg/dL
Liver Function Tests	Tests include bilirubin (total), phosphatase (alkaline), protein (total and albumin), transaminases (alanine and aspartate), prothrombin (PTT)
Magnesium	1.5 - 2.0 mEq/L
Mean Corpuscular Hemoglobin (MCH)	27 - 32 pg/cell

Test	Reference Range (conventional units)
Mean Corpuscular Hemoglobin Concentration (MCHC)	32 - 36% hemoglobin/cell
Mean Corpuscular Volume (MCV)	76 - 100 cu µm
Osmolality	280 - 296 mOsm/kg water
Oxygen Pressure	83 - 100 mm Hg
Oxygen Saturation (arterial)	96 - 100%
Phosphatase, Prostatic	0 - 3 units/dL (Bodansky units) (acid)
Phosphatase	50 - 160 units/L (normally higher in infants and adolescents) (alkaline)
Phosphorus	3.0 - 4.5 mg/dL (inorganic)
Platelet Count	150,000 - 350,000/mL
Potassium	3.5 - 5.0 mEq/L
Prostate-Specific Antigen (PSA)	0 - 4 ng/mL (likely higher with age)
Proteins	
Total	6.0 - 8.4 gm/dL
Albumin	3.5 - 5.0 gm/dL
Globulin	2.3 - 3.5 gm/dL
Prothrombin (PTT)	25 - 41 sec
Pyruvic Acid	0.3 - 0.9 mg/dL
Red Blood Cell Count (RBC)	4.2 - 6.9 million/µL/cu mm
Sodium	135 - 145 mEq/L
Thyroid-Stimulating Hormone (TSH)	0.5 - 6.0 µ units/mL
Transaminase	
Alanine (ALT)	1 - 21 units/L
Aspartate (AST)	7 - 27 units/L
Urea Nitrogen (BUN)	7 - 18 mg/dL
BUN/Creatinine Ratio	5 - 35
WBC (leukocyte count and white Blood cell count)	4.3-10.8 × 103/mm3
White Blood Cell Count (WBC)	4,300 - 10,800 cells/µL/cu mm
Vitamin A	30 - 65 µg/dL
Uric Acid	Male - 2.1 to 8.5 mg/dL (likely higher with age)
	Female - 2.0 to 7.0 mg/dL (likely higher with age)

Complete Blood Count

Tests	Ranges	Calculations	Significance
RBC count	4.2 - 5.9 million cells/cmm	Absolute # of circulating RBCs per unit volume of blood • Indirect measure of the amount of circulating hemoglobin (i.e. oxygen carrying capacity of the blood) ↑ → polycythemia vera; ↓ → anemia	Decreased with anemia; increased when too many made and with fluid loss due to diarrhea, dehydration, burns
Hemoglobin Concentration	14.0-18.0 g/dl for men and 12.0-16.0 g/dl for women	Direct measure of weight of hemoglobin/unit volume of blood • Most sensitive measurement for existence of anemia • Used medically to judge need for transfusion ↑ → dehydration, polycythemia vera; ↓ → anemia, pregnancy	Hemoglobin measures the amount of oxygen-carrying protein in the blood.
HCT (Hematocrit)	Men are 40- 54% and for women 37-47%	PCV (Packed Cell Volume), ratio of the volume of the RBCs (after centrifugation) to that of whole blood ↑ → polycythemia vera, Addison's disease, acute pancreatitis ↓ → anemia, cystic fibrosis, CHF, pregnancy	Measures the amount of space red blood cells take up in the blood. It is reported as a percentage.
MCV (Mean Corpuscular Volume)	Normal range is 80 - 100	Calculated measure of the size of the average circulating RBC **MCV = HCT/RBC x 10** (Normocytic: 80 – 100 μm3 (fL); → iron deficiency anemia, leukocytosis; **Macrocytic:** > 100 μm3; → chronic alcoholism, methanol poisoning	Increased with B12 and folate deficiency; decreased with iron deficiency and thalassemia
MCH (Mean Corpuscular Hb Concentration)	Normal range is 27 - 32 picograms	Calculated weight of hemoglobin in the average circulating RBC **MCH = HGB/RBC x 10** (Normochromic: 27 – 32 pg) • **Hypochromic:** < 27 pg, **Hyperchromic:** > 32 pg	
MCHC (Mean Corpuscular Hb Concentration)	Normal range is 32 - 36%	Average concentration of Hb in a given volume of packed cells **MCHC = HGB/HCT x 100** (Normochromic: 330 – 370 g/L) • **Hypochromic:** < 330 g/L → hemolytic anemia; • **Hyperchromic:** > 370 g/L → polycythemia vera, malignancy, leukemia, rheumatoid arthritis	May be decreased when MCV is decreased; increases limited to amount of Hgb that will fit inside a RBC
RBC morphology		Microscope determinations from Wright's stained peripheral blood smear; **Microcytosis:** small MCV, **Macrocytosis:** large MCV, **Poikilocytosis:** different shapes	
WBC count (Leukocyte count)	4,300 and 10,800	Absolute quantification of total circulating WBC/unit volume blood • **Leukocytosis:** ↑ total WBC count → infection, inflammation, leukemia, bacterial infection • **Leukopenia:** ↓ total WBC count → aplastic anemia, pernicious anemia, severe infections, viral infections	May be increased with infections, inflammation, cancer, leukemia, decreased with some medications, some autoimmune conditions, some severe infections, bone marrow failure
WBC differential count -cytosis/-philia= ↑ -penia = ↓	Normal PMNs is 55-80%. Normal lymphocytes is 25-33% Normal for monocytes is 3-7%	**Neutrophilia** → Hodgkin's disease, infection **Lymphocytosis** → pertussis, mono, mumps, measles, TB **Monocytosis** → chronic infection, leukemia, protozoan infection **Eosinophilia** → allergies, parasitic infections, scarlet fever **Basophilia** → polycythemia vera, leukemia, chicken or small pox	
Platelet count	150,000-350,000/ cmm	Absolute quantification of circulating thrombocytes/volume	

→ may indicate/suggests/seen in, ↑ = increase, ↓ = decrease, TB = tuberculosis

Test interpretation

CBC - The Complete Blood Count (CBC) is one of the most common tests ordered by most provider. It is a routine test used to evaluate the blood and general health.

RBC Count - The RBC count is the number of RBCs in a cubic millimeter of blood. The RBCs are the cells produced in the bone marrow that carry oxygen to your tissues. The normal range is 4.5 - 5.9 million/mm3 for men and 4.0-5.3 million/mm3 for women. A person with a significantly low RBC count can have symptoms of fatigue, shortness of breath, and appear pale in color. A low RBC count can be due to progression of illness or to certain medications, or both. A decrease in the RBC count usually causes a decrease in the hemoglobin and hematocrit values.

WBC Count - The WBC count is the number of WBCs in a cubic millimeter of blood. The primary function of these cells is to prevent and fight infections. There are many different types of white blood cells that play specific roles in fight infections. These specific types of WBCs can be measured in the white cell differential. Normal WBC count is from 4,300 to 10,800. The WBC count can be decreased for a variety of reasons: certain medications decease the production of WBCs in the bone marrow, minor viral infections which you may not even be aware of, stress, and opportunistic infections. Values markedly decreased should be cause for concern, since during this situation one is more susceptible to other infections.

Hemoglobin - Oxygen is carried to the tissues via hemoglobin in the RBC. A normal hemoglobin level is 14.0-18.0 g/dl for men and 12.0-16.0 g/dl for women. Any drug which causes a suppression of the bone marrow will decrease the hemoglobin level. In most cases it's a matter of balancing the effects of the drug with its potential side effects. When the side effects become too great, either the drug must be removed or the dose reduced to a tolerable level.

Hematocrit - The hematocrit (HCT) is the percent of the cellular components in your blood to the fluid or blood plasma. This test is one of the truest markers of anemia. Normal values for men are 40- 54% and for women 37-47%. A decrease in hematocrit is always seen with a decrease in the hemoglobin. These two values are linked to one another.

MCV - The mean cell volume or MCV is the most important of the RBC indices. It is a measure of the average size of the RBC. Normal MCV levels are 80-100. Vitamin B12 and Folic Acid deficiencies cause increases in MCV.

The other 2 indices are not so important. They are the MCH and the MCHC and are used to help diagnose various anemias and leukemias.

Platelets - Platelets are cellular fragments which are necessary for the blood to clot. When activated by "trauma," platelets migrate to the site of injury where they become "sticky," adhering to the injured site and subsequently used in the developing fibrin clot (scab). Normal platelet values are 150,000-350,000.

White Cell Differential - The white cell differential counts 100 white cells and differentiates them by type. This gives a percent of the different kinds of white cells in relation to one another. The three main types are: polymorphonuclear cells (or PMNs), lymphocytes, and monocytes. PMNs are increased during bacterial infections while lymphocytes are decreased with viral infections. Increased monocytes are sometimes seen in chronic infections. Normal percent of PMNs is 55-80%, 25-33% is the normal number of lymphocytes, and 3-7% is normal for monocytes.

Liver function Tests - Liver Function Tests include 5-6 individual tests which collectively can help determine the status of ones liver, detect liver damage or disease. Elevated liver enzymes are most often caused by certain medications or hepatitis. Therefore compound factors can be at work. The names of these liver function tests include SGOT, SGPT, alkaline phosphate, total bilirubin and LDH.

Kidney Function Tests - Two tests which measure kidney function are the BUN and creatinine. The usefulness of these tests usually relates to toxicity of the kidneys. Hence kidney function is monitored in this way. Normal BUN levels are 10-20 mg/dl. Normal levels of creatinine are 0.6-1.2 mg/dl.

ALT - the enzyme mainly found in the liver and is the ideal test for detecting hepatitis and evaluating patient who has symptoms of a liver disorder.

ALP - an enzyme related to the bile ducts; often increased when they are blocked. It helps check for liver disease or damage to the liver.

AST - an enzyme found in the liver and a few other places, particularly the heart and other muscles in the body. AST test is requested with several other tests to help evaluate a patient who has symptoms of a liver disorder.

Test Interpretation (cont.)

Amylase - amylase is an enzyme that is secreted in the mouth by the salivary glands and also in the pancreas. It can be an early warning sign of acute Pancreatitis when elevated. DDL can cause problems with the pancreas in a small number of patients taking the drug. Normal amylase levels are 25-125 milliunits/ml.

Cholesterol - Normal cholesterol levels are 150-250 mg/dl.

CPK - CPK or CK is an enzyme that's found in the brain and the muscles of the body. Strenuous exercise as well as a heart attack can cause increases in CPK. This makes clear the point of evaluating an abnormal test result in the context of other factors. Myopathy, dysfunction/distress with the muscles, can sometimes be confirmed with an elevated CPK. Normal levels of this enzyme are 12-80 milliunits/ml (30 degrees) or 55-170 milliunits/ml (37 degrees). Values will be slightly lower for women.

Total bilirubin - measures all the yellow bilirubin pigment in the blood. Another test, direct bilirubin, measures a form made in the liver and is often requested with total bilirubin in infants with jaundice.

Albumin – measures the main protein made by the liver and tells how well the liver is making this protein.

Blood Enzyme Tests

Enzyme	Source	Significance	
ALP Alkaline phosphatase	Bone Liver Placenta Intestine Malignant tissue	**↑ALP** Primary biliary tract disorders Bone disorders (osteoblastic) Healing fractures Paget's disease	↓ALP Malnutrition Hypophosphatasia Hypothyroidism
ALT - alanine aminotransferase **SGPT** - serum glutamate-pyruvate transaminase	Liver (99%) Heart Muscle Kidney	**↑ALT** Liver disease Myocardial Infarction (MI) Skeletal muscle disease	
AST - aspartate aminotransferase	Liver, Heart, Skeletal Muscle	**↑AST** Hepatobiliary inflammation Myocardial pathology Cirrhosis; Neoplasm Skeletal muscle condition	
CGT - gamma glutamyl transferase	Liver Kidney	**↑CGT** Liver disorders: all forms Hepatotoxic drugs - ETOH (alcoholics), Acetaminophen; Diabetes mellitus, Renal disease, Neurological disorders	
LDH or LD - lactate dehydrogenase	LDH_1 Heart, RBCs LDH_2 Heart, RBCs LDH_3 Lungs LDH_4 Liver, Sk. Muscle LDH_5 Liver, Sk. Muscle	**↑LDH** Hematological conditions, liver inflammation or disorders, disseminated cancer, cardiopulmonary conditions, muscular pathology	
CK - creatine kinase **CPK** - creatine phosphokinase	CK_1 Brain, smooth muscle, GI, genitourinary CK_2 Cardiac muscle CK_3 Cardiac, Sk. Muscle	**↑CK** Myocardial Infarction, skeletal muscle abnormalities, trauma, severe exercises, cholesterol lowering medication, brain trauma	

Selected Conditions Labs

Allergic Reactions
- Eosinphilia, increased total IgG
- RAST testing - sneezing, itchy eyes, runny/ congested nose, swollen sinuses, coughing, and wheezing

Atherosclerosis
- Cholesterol (HDL, LDL, VLDL)
- Triglycerides, glucose, uric acid, thyroxine

Bacterial Infections
- Neutrophilia, high total WBC

Bone Cancer
- Anemia is usually normocytic anemia
- Elevated serum ALP; also indicative of osteomalacia or celiac sprue

Hepatitis
- AST, ALT, ALP; leukopenia, bilirubinuria
- Specific serological viral markers for individual types
- Anti-HAV (IgM), HbsAg (surface antigen), Anti-HCV, Anti-HBc (core antigen)

Kidney Function
- BUN, albumin, globulins, uric acid, creatine

Metastatic Cancer
- Check with levels of enzymes are highest
- Increase WBC, ALP, pancytopenia
- Consider bone scan

Mononucluceis
- Leukocytosis, lymphocytes comprise > 50%
- (+) HA monspot, anti-VCA IgM, IgG

Multiple Myeloma
- IgG (monoclonal antibody), Rouleaux formation, Bence-Jones proteins
- Increased total protein, increase globulin, decreased A/G ratio
- Definitive bone marrow aspiration

Myocardial Infarction
- SGOT, LDH, CPK

Obstructive Liver Disease
- Bilirubin (best) - total, indirect, or direct
- ALP (best)
- ALT (mild increase) AST (mild increase)
- CGT/GGTP (increase), LDH if severe

Prostate Cancer
- Digital Rectal Exam (DRE)
- PSA - may also be increased in benign prostatic hypertrophy (BPH)
- May be falsely elevated post-prostatic massage/ exam

Rheumatoid Arthritis
- Rheumatoid factor - IgM type
- N/N anemia
- ESR, CRP, & other acute phase reactant proteins may be increased
- Involves PIP joint & MCP joints

SLE (Lupus)
- ANA or FANA (Anti-Nuclear Antibodies)
- Anti-DNA (only do this if ANA/FANA is positive)
- CBC - N/N anemia, leukocytopenia, lymphocytopenia
- Possible thrombocytopenia
- UA - hematuria, proteinuria, casts

Thyroid Disease
- Free T4, T3
- TSH - best test for general screen
- THBR (thyroid hormone binding ratio)
- Serum calcium, PTH

Viral Infections
- Lymphocytosis (normal 20-40%)
- Possible decreased WBC count or neutrophils (neutropenia)

Warning Signs of Cancer (General)
- Insidious onset with no known mechanism of injury
- A change in bowel or bladder habits
- A sore that does not heal
- Unusual bleeding or discharge from any place
- A lump in the breast or other parts of the body
- Chronic indigestion or difficulty in swallowing
- Obvious changes in a wart or mole
- Persistent coughing or hoarseness

Prostate
- A need to urinate frequently, especially at night
- Difficulty starting urination or holding back urine
- Inability to urinate
- Weak or interrupted flow of urine
- Painful or burning urination
- Painful ejaculation
- Blood in urine or semen
- Frequent pain or stiffness in the lower back, hips, or upper thighs

Bladder
- Blood in the urine
- Burning with urination
- Bladder spasms/pain
- Intense urge to urinate

Skin
- A sore that does not heal
- A new growth
- Spread of pigment from the border of a spot to surrounding skin
- Redness or a new swelling beyond the border
- Change in sensation—itchiness, tenderness or pain
- Change in the surface of a mole - scaliness, oozing, bleeding or the appearance of a bump or nodule

Breast
- Lump or mass in breast(s)
- Enlarged lymph nodes (lumps) in the armpit(s)
- Nipple symptoms: bleeding or discharge, retraction, elevation, eczema
- Skin symptoms: dimpling, redness, edema (swelling), ulceration

Lung
- Nagging cough
- Coughing up blood
- Recurrent attacks of pneumonia or bronchitis
- Chest and arm pain
- Unexplained weight loss
- Increased shortness of breath upon exertion
- Increase in the amount of sputum
- Swelling of the face and arms

Liver
- Pain in the upper abdomen on the right side; the pain may extend to the back and shoulder
- Swollen abdomen (bloating)
- Weight loss
- Loss of appetite and feelings of fullness
- Weakness or feeling very tired
- Nausea and vomiting
- Yellow skin and eyes and dark urine from jaundice
- Fever

Leukemia
- Fevers or night sweats
- Frequent infections
- Feeling weak or tired
- Headache
- Bleeding and bruising easily
- Pain in the bones or joints
- Swelling or discomfort in the abdomen
- Swollen lymph nodes, especially in the neck or armpit
- Weight loss

Ovarian
- General abdominal discomfort and/or pain (gas, indigestion, pressure, swelling, bloating, cramps)
- Nausea, diarrhea, constipation, or frequent urination
- Loss of appetite
- Feeling of fullness even after a light meal
- Weight gain or loss with no known reason
- Abnormal bleeding from the vagina

Colon and Rectal
- A change in bowel habits
- Diarrhea, constipation or feeling that the bowel does not empty completely
- Blood (either bright red or very dark) in the stool
- Stools that are narrower than usual
- General abdominal discomfort (frequent gas pains, bloating, fullness and/or cramps)
- Weight loss with no known reason
- Constant tiredness
- Vomiting

Thyroid
- A lump in the front of the neck near the Adam's apple
- Hoarseness or difficulty speaking in a normal voice
- Swollen lymph nodes, especially in the neck
- Difficulty swallowing or breathing
- Pain in the throat or neck

Stomach
- A loss of appetite
- Difficulty swallowing, particularly difficulty that increases over time
- Vague abdominal fullness
- Nausea and vomiting
- Vomiting blood
- Abdominal pain
- Excessive belching
- Breath odor
- Excessive gas (flatus)
- Weight loss
- A decline in general health
- Abdominal fullness prematurely after meals

Uterine
- Unusual vaginal bleeding or discharge, including in women older than 40: extremely long, heavy or frequent episodes of bleeding
- Difficult or painful urination
- Pain during intercourse
- Lower abdominal pain or cramping in the pelvic area

The ABCD Rule for Early Detection of Melanoma

Almost everyone has moles. The vast majority of moles are perfectly harmless. A change in a mole's appearance is a warning sign to your client to get it checked by their general practitioner. Here is the simple ABCD rule to help you remember the important signs of melanoma and other skin cancers.

- **A is for ASYMMETRY:** One-half of a mole or birthmark does not match the other.
- **B is for BORDER:** The edges are irregular, ragged, notched or blurred.
- **C is for COLOR:** The color is not the same all over, but may have differing shades of brown or black, sometimes with patches of red, white or blue.
- **D is for DIAMETER**: The area is larger than 6 millimeters (the size of a pencil eraser) or is growing larger.

Source: National Cancer Institute; www.cancer.gov and the American Cancer Society; www.cancer.org

Red Flag Cases to Refer to a Physician

Here is a list of the more common conditions that require immediate or prompt referral to a Western medical doctor or treatment facility. Remember that when urgently referring a client to a hospital, a practitioner must make direct voice-to-voice contact with the person who will receive the client.

- **Sudden chest pain** (coronary artery occlusion, spontaneous pneumothorax, pulmonary embolism, dissecting thoracic aneurysm)
- **Persistent cough** (could be benign, such as postnasal drip or even acid reflux, but might be lung cancer, lymphoma, heart failure, pleural effusion, etc.)
- **Severe abdominal pain** (appendicitis, ruptured duodenal or gastric ulcer, acute pancreatitis, Chrohn's disease or ulcerative colitis with intestinal rupture or abscess, acute cholecystitis, acute diverticulitis, or many other conditions)
- **Upper GI or lower GI bleeding** (bleeding duodenal or gastric ulcer, ulcerative colitis, gastrointestinal cancer, bleeding from intestinal polyps or vascular malformations, esophageal or gastric varices, or many other conditions)
- **New onset of severe headaches** (always worrisome; could be any number of severe neurological conditions, possibly a brain tumor)
- **Impending or actual gangrene of a finger, toe or foot in a client** (advanced arteriosclerosis, diabetes mellitus, Raynaud's disease or syndrome, or many other possible causes)
- **Tender swelling in a calf or thigh** (impending or actual deep thrombophlebitis, with the risk of potentially fatal pulmonary embolism)
- **Redness in the whites of the eye**, especially with pain and alteration of vision (may be benign, but could be uveitis, glaucoma, or a foreign body in the eye)
- **Change in level of consciousness** (impending or actual stroke, diabetic coma, intracerebral bleeding from ruptured cerebral aneurysm or trauma, brain tumor, hydrocephalus, others)
- **Pain with weight loss** (possible cancer, often missed by practitioners in the early stages when it can still be cured)
- **Suspicious breast lumps; abdominal masses; axillary, neck or groin masses** (may be cancer)
- **Vaginal bleeding after menopause, or excessive bleeding before menopause** (may be benign, but might be cancer, large fibroids, endometriosis)
- **New onset of neurological symptoms** such as weakness, numbness, visual changes, sudden mood swings, irrational or reckless behavior (could be a degenerative disease, brain infection, stroke, cancer, etc.)
- **Fever of unknown origin**
- **Frequent episode of dizziness or light-headedness** (may be benign, but might be an impending stoke, heart trouble, or possible brain tumor)
- **Unexplained weight loss** or failure to thrive in a normal fashion

This list is necessarily incomplete and cannot take into account every conceivable urgent clinical situation you might encounter. Cancer in any form is best treated in conjunction with a Western physician or hospital, and a practitioner who takes on the role of primary provider of a cancer patient can expose himself or herself to medical liability. Of course, there is much that complementary medicine can do to improve the outcome of Western medical cancer treatments and reduce the morbidity of such modalities as chemotherapy and radiation.

More Red Flags According to Body Systems

Cancer
- Persistent night pain
- Constant pain anywhere in body
- Unexplained weight loss
- Loss of appetite
- Unusual lumps or growth

Cardiovascular
- Shortness of breath
- Dizziness
- Pain or feeling of heaviness in the chest
- Pulsating pain anywhere in the body
- Constant and severe pain in lower leg or arm
- Discolored or painful feet
- Swelling (without history of injury)

Gastrointestinal / Genitourinary
- Frequent or severe abdominal pain
- Frequent heartburn or indigestion
- Frequent nausea or vomiting
- Change in or problems with bladder function
- Unusual menstrual irregularities

Miscellaneous
- Fever or night sweats
- Recent severe emotional disturbances
- Swelling or redness in any joint (without history of injury)
- Pregnancy

Neurological
- Changes in hearing
- Frequent or severe headaches (without history of injury)
- Problems with swallowing or changes in speech
- Changes in vision (blurriness, loss of sight)
- Problems with balance, coordination, or falling
- Fainting spells
- Sudden weakness

It's good to remember the old adage, "If in doubt, check it out." Talk with a Western doctor if you are uncertain about what is going on with one of your clients and are concerned it might be serious or even potentially life-threatening.

WESTERN

Source: Bruce Robinson, Acupuncture Today.com and Stith, J. S, S. A. Sahrmann, K.K Dixion, and B.J. Norton, *Ciurriculum to prepare diagnostics in physical therapy*. J. Phys. Ther. Educ. 9:50, 1995

The ABC's of CPR

Establish responsiveness: Gently shake the victim and shout, "Are you OK?" If the person answers;

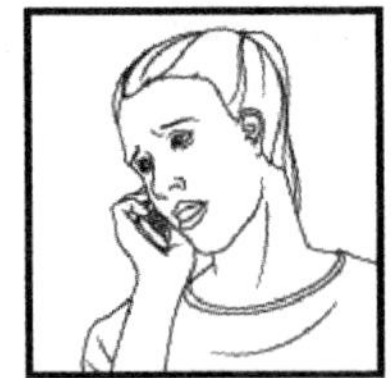

Call 911 or have someone with you call 911; If the person is unresponsive or conscious and showing signs of a stroke or heart attack;

Immediately initiate the ABCs of life support:

A-Airway – Open Airway: If the person is unresponsive, open the airway as soon as you've called 911. If the victim has no head or neck injuries, gently tilt the head back by lifting the chin with one hand and pushing down on the forehead with the other. Place your ear near the mouth and listen and feel for breath while looking at the chest to see if it is rising and falling.

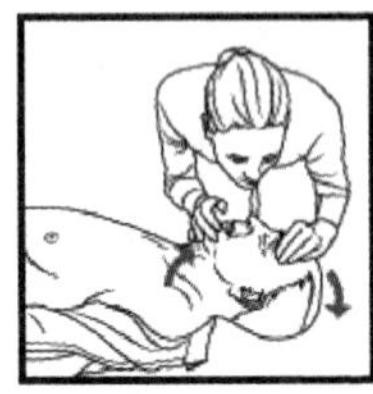

B-Breaths – Check Breath: If the person is not breathing normally, **give two rescue breaths**. Keeping the victim's head tilted, pinch the nose closed and place your mouth around their mouth. Give two slow, full breaths (about two seconds each), while watching to see that the chest rises with each breath. After delivering two breaths, check for signs of circulation, such as breathing, coughing, movement or responsiveness. Keeping the head tilted, once again place your ear near the mouth and listen, feel, and look for signs of breathing while you watch for movement.

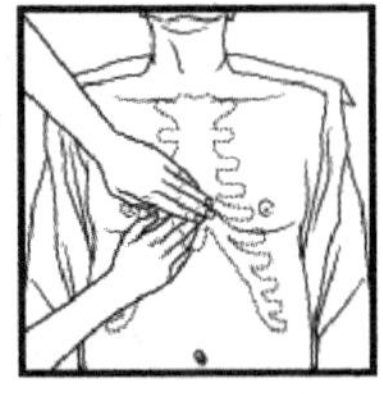

C-Chest – Compressions: If no pulse is detected, begin chest compressions immediately. Place the heel of one hand in the center of the chest (right between the nipples), with the heel of the second hand on top. Position your body directly over your hands, elbows locked. **Give 15 compressions** by pushing the breastbone down about two inches, allowing the chest to return to normal between compressions. Use the full weight of your body and DO NOT bend your elbows. **After 15 compressions, make sure the victim's head is tilted, and give two more rescue breaths**. Repeat this "pump and blow" cycle three more times, for a total of 60 compressions.

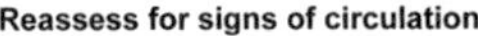

Reassess for signs of circulation

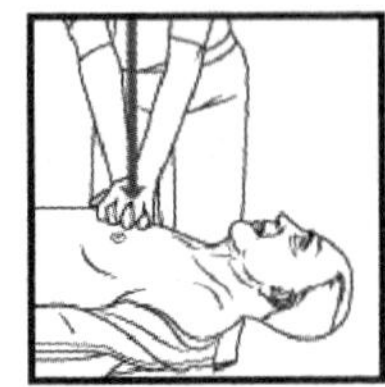

If no signs of circulation, repeat the pump-and-blow cycle until circulation resumes or help arrives.

When performing CPR, keep in mind that the person you are working on is clinically dead: You cannot make the situation any worse. Don't be afraid to put your whole weight behind each compression - a cracked rib can be repaired, dead brain cells cannot.

Where to find a course

Call 1-877-AHA-4CPR or visit www.americanheart.org/cpr. Or, call your local American Heart Association office for a list of training sites. Some states require current CPR card for licensing or renewal.

Dr. Fred Lerner and Lerner Education provides post-graduate education courses for licensed health professionals in training in clinical skills and education regarding primary care as it relates to neuromusculoskeletal disorders. A helpful resource for therapists interested in learning more about orthopedics and muscle testing. For more information www.lernereducation.com.

Head Examination

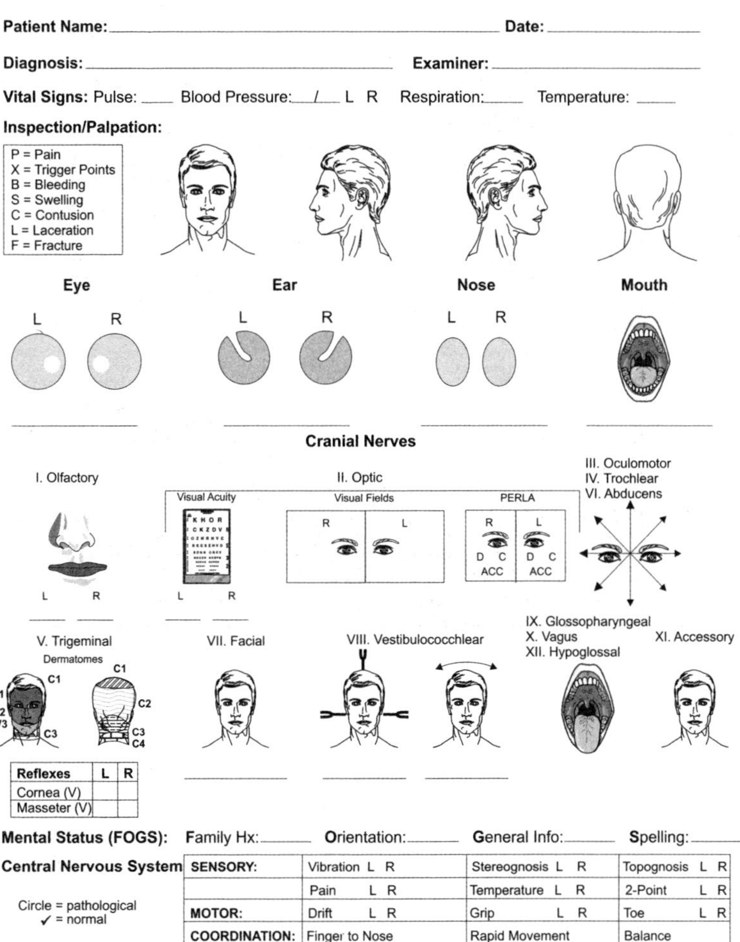

Patient Name: ________________ **Date:** ________

Diagnosis: ________________ **Examiner:** ________

Vital Signs: Pulse: ____ Blood Pressure: ___/___ L R Respiration: ____ Temperature: ____

Inspection/Palpation:

P = Pain
X = Trigger Points
B = Bleeding
S = Swelling
C = Contusion
L = Laceration
F = Fracture

Eye L R

Ear L R

Nose L R

Mouth

Cranial Nerves

I. Olfactory — L R

II. Optic — Visual Acuity (L R); Visual Fields (R L); PERLA (R L; D C ACC; D C ACC)

III. Oculomotor
IV. Trochlear
VI. Abducens

V. Trigeminal — Dermatomes: V1, V2, V3, C1, C2, C3, C4

VII. Facial

VIII. Vestibulocochlear

IX. Glossopharyngeal
X. Vagus
XII. Hypoglossal

XI. Accessory

Reflexes	L	R
Cornea (V)		
Masseter (V)		

Mental Status (FOGS): Family Hx: ____ Orientation: ____ General Info: ____ Spelling: ____

Central Nervous System

Circle = pathological
✓ = normal

SENSORY:	Vibration L R	Stereognosis L R	Topognosis L R
	Pain L R	Temperature L R	2-Point L R
MOTOR:	Drift L R	Grip L R	Toe L R
COORDINATION:	Finger to Nose	Rapid Movement	Balance
PATHOLOGICAL:	Babinski L R	Hoffman: L R	Ankle Jerk L R

WESTERN

Source: Reproduced with the permission of Lerner Education. Forms can be downloaded at www.lernereducation.com

Test Name	Structures	Description of Test	Positive Test
ANKLE			
Anterior Drawer Test	*Anterior Talofibular Ligament, Medial Deltoid ligament*	Patient in sitting or supine position, knee flexed and relaxed, therapist stabilizes the tibia and fibula and grasps the foot or calcaneus, therapist draws the foot anteriorly.	Anterior shift of the foot relative to the stabilized tibia/fibula, if lateral side of ankle translates forward, lateral ligament damage is suspected, if both medial and lateral sides of the ankle translate forward, damage is suspected to the deltoid ligament as well.
External Rotation Test	*Distal tibiofibular joint (syndesmosis)*	Patient seated, knee hanging from edge of bed, therapist holds foot with ankle in slight dorsiflexion, therapist passively externally rotates the lower leg slowly but forcefully.	Pain between tibia and fibula either anteriorly or posterior.
Distal Tibiofibular Compression Test	*Distal Tibiofibular joint*	Patient in seated, leg hanging over edge of bed, therapist applied a compression force to both malleoli of the same ankle (squeezing them together), Therapist may ALSO apply an anterior force to one and a posterior force on the other malleolus, shearing them gently.	Compression Test-pain on compression, indicating a problem with the syndesmosis at the distal tibiofibular joint, Shear Test-Pain on shear and/or significant displacement, indicating possible ligament rupture.
Homan's sign (Test for DVT)	*DVT*	Therapist passively dorsiflexes ankle with knee extended.	Pain in calf suggests possible DVT. Other signs and symptoms must be taken into consideration, history, coloration, pulses and swelling.
Posterior Drawer Test	*Posterior talofibular ligament, medial deltoid ligament (posterior elements)*	Patient in sitting or supine position, knee flexed and relaxed, therapist stabilizes the tibia and fibula and grasps the foot or calcaneus, therapist pushes the foot posterior, examining for change of position of the ankle relative to the tibia and fibula.	Posterior shift of the foot relative to the stabilized tibia/fibula, if lateral side of ankle translates backward, lateral ligament damage is suspected, if both medial and lateral sides of the ankle translate backward, damage is suspected to the deltoid ligament as well.
Talar Tilt Test	*Calcaneofibular ligament, medial deltoid ligament (middle element)*	Patient in side lying or supine, foot and ankle relaxed, knee bent. Foot is placed into 90° relative to the tibia; talus is tilted from side to side into adduction and abduction. If foot is plantar flexed, the ATF is more likely to be tested.	Laxity and elicited pain.
Thompson's Sign	*Achilles Tendon rupture*	Patient lies prone or kneels in a chair, foot and ankle relaxed, therapist squeezes calf muscle.	Absence of plantar flexion when calf is squeezed.
Tinel's Sign	*Anterior branch of deep peroneal nerve, Posterior tibial nerve*	Therapist taps on the peripheral nerve being tested, anterior branch of the deep peroneal nerve-anterio portion of ankle (dorsum of foot), slightly lateral to the EHL tendon, posterior tibial nerve-behind medial malleoli, tap for 30 sec.	Anterior branch of deep peroneal nerve-parasthesia on dorsum of foot, posterior tibial nerve-parasthesia on plantar aspect of foot.

Source: David J. Magee, *Orthopedic Physical Assessment Enhanced Edition, 4th Edition,* 2006, W.B. Saunders Company, NY, NY.

Ankle & Foot Examination

Patient Name:____________________ **Date:**__________

Diagnosis:____________________ **Examiner:** __________

Vital Signs: Pulse: ____ Blood Pressure:___/___ L R Respiration:____ Temperature: ____

Inspection/Palpation:

P = Pain
X = Trigger Points
B = Bleeding
S = Swelling
C = Contusion
L = Laceration
H = Hot

Range of Motion:

Activity	Normal	Active	Passive
Plantar Flexion	50		
Dorsiflexion	20		
Inversion	45-60		
Eversion	15-30		
Great Toe Extension	70		
Great Toe Flexion	45		

Nerve Supply (Skin):

Anterior **Posterior**

L4
L5
Saphenous
S1
L5
Deep Peroneal
Superficial Peroneal
Sural
Saphenous
Tibial
S2
S1
L5

Pulses	L	R
Dorsalis Pedis		
Post. Tibial		

Muscle Testing/Myotomes:

Muscle	Strength L	Strength R
Hamstrings (L5):		
Medial		
Lateral		
Quadriceps (L2-4):		
Rectus Femoris		
Vastus Lateralis		
Vastus Medialis		
Sartorius (L2-3)		
Gracilis (L3)		
Tensor Fascia Lata (L5)		
Gluteus Min/Med (L5)		
Adductors (L4)		
Tibialis Anterior (L4)		
Tibialis Posterior (L4)		
Peroneus Long/Brev (L5)		
Peroneus Tertius (L5)		
Gastrocnemius (S1)		
Soleus (S1)		

Circumferential	L	R
Thigh		
Calf		

Functional Assessment	✓
Squatting	
Squatting on Toes	
Squatting & Bouncing	
Standing on One Foot At A Time	
Standing on Toes, 1 Foot At A Time	
Going Up & Down Stairs	
Walking on Toes	
Running Straight Ahead	
Running & Twisting	
Jumping	
Jumping & Full Squatting	

Orthopedic: ____________________

____

Neurological: ____________________

Antalgia: __________ **Special:** __________

WESTERN

Test Name	Structures	Description of Test	Positive Test
CERVICAL			
Cranial Nerve Tests	*Cranial Nerves*	**CN1:** (olfactory): Smell coffee or a similar substance with eyes closed. **CN2:** (optic): Read something with one eye closed. **CN3, 4, 6**: Eye movements - note any ptosis. **CN5:** (trigeminal): Contract muscles of mastication (masseter and temporalis). **CN7:** (facial): Move eyebrows up and down, purse lips, bare teeth; Bell's Palsy common - esp. if patient unable to whistle or wink on one side. **CN8:** (auditory): Have patient repeat what you say with eyes closed. **CN9**: Patient swallows. **CN10:** (vagus): Patient swallows. **CN11:** (spinal accessory): Have patient contract SCM. **CN12**: Patient sticks out tongue & moves left/right.	Inability to perform actions above.
Distraction Test	*IVF, IV Disc, Spinal nerve root*	Patient in sitting, lying or standing position. Therapist places one hand under chin, the other under the occiput and provides an axial traction to the head. If symptoms are referred to the shoulder, a further reduction in symptoms can be achieved by abducting the arms while traction is applied.	Reduction of radicular symptoms.
Spurling's Test	*Cervical Foramen, IVF*	Patient seated. First stage, therapist provides a compression force on the head in neutral. Second stage, patient extends head and therapist applies axial compression. Third stage, patient extends head and rotates to unaffected side first, then affected side while therapist applies axial compression. Spurling's version simply applies axial compression with side flexion, first to the unaffected side, then to the affected side.	Radicular pain which peripheralizes on the side when the head is flexed sideways or rotated. Traction should alleviate the peripheral symptoms.
Hautant's Test	*Vertebral artery*	Patient sits, forward flexes both arms to 90°, closes eyes and therapist watches for any loss of arm position, Patient rotates or extends and rotated neck while holding arm position and eyes are closed again, hold each position for 10-30 sec.	If arms move when neck is NOT rotated, cause is non-vascular. If wavering of arms occurs with cervical motion (rotation), likely vascular problem to brain.
Hoffman's Sign	*Upper Motor Neuron Lesion*	Patient lying, sitting or standing position. Therapist holds patient's middle finger and gently "flicks" the distal phalanx.	IP joint of thumb on hand flexes.
Romberg's Test	*Upper Motor Neuron Lesion*	Patient standing. Ask patient to close eyes and remain still for 30 seconds.	Patient begins to sway excessively or loses balance.
Stability -Lateral Shear Test-Coronal Stability	*Dens integrity*	Patient in supine position. Supporting the occiput, therapist places radial side of 2nd MCP on transverse processes of atlas, on one side and on axis on other side, Therapist stabilizes the axis while providing a lateral force on the Atlas and occiput.	Soft end feel, cord signs, lump-in-throat feeling, excessive movement or reproduction of patient symptoms. **Pain is a normal sensation and does not indicate a positive test**
Stability- Alar Ligament Rotational Test	*Alar Ligament*	Patient sitting, clinician fixes C2 using a grip over the lamina. Clinician rotates the head.	More than 20-30 degrees of rotation indicates damaged contra lateral alar ligament. If excessive rotation occurs ipsilaterally to the side of excessive lateral flexion in the lateral flexion test, this points to alar ligament damage. If the excessive motions are in opposite directions, this suggests joint instability at C0-C1.
Stability- Anterior translation- atlas on axis	*Atlanto-axial joint*	With the patient supine, the clinician fixes C2. (using thumb pressure over the anterior aspect of the transverse processes) and then lifts the head and atlas vertically.	Excessive movement. cord signs, symptom reproduction.
Stability- Sharp-Purser Test-Saggital Stability	*Transverse Ligament of C1-2*	Patient flexes head and neck in seated position. Therapist places on hand over patient's forehead and stabilizes C2 posteriorly at the spinous process with thumb of other hand, therapist applies a gentle posterior force to patient's forehead.	Relief of patient's symptoms, relief of cord signs, Clunk of posterior slide of occiput (less reliable).
Stability-Alar Ligament Side Flexion Test	*Alar ligament*	Patient supine head in neutral, therapist stabilizes C2 with wide pinch grip around spinous process and lamina, Therapist attempts to side flex head away from side being stabilized (ie. contralateral side flexion). REPEAT test in flexion and extension of upper C-spine.	Significant side flexion possible in ALL three positions.

Test Name	Structures	Description of Test	Positive Test
Stability-Anterior-atlanto-occipital joint	*Atlanto-occipital joint*	Patient supine, clinician applies a posterior force bilaterally to the anterolateral aspect of the transverse processes of the atlas and axis on occiput.	Excessive movement, cord signs.
Stability-Distraction Test-Longitudinal Stability	*Tectoral membrane, Upper cervical ligaments.*	Patient supine, therapist applies traction to the occiput, if no symptoms, reposition head in flexion and reapplies traction.	Pain or parasthesia, cord signs.
Stability-Posterior Test-Atlanto-occipital joint	*Atlanto-Occipital Joint*	Patient supine, clinician applies an anterior force bilaterally to the atlas and axis on the occiput.	Excessive Movement, cord signs.
Upper Limb Tension Test (Genera)	*Median Nerve, C5, C6, C7, Anterior Interosseous Nerve*	Patient in supine lying position. Scapular depression and shoulder abduction to 110° without rotation. Forearm supination and wrist extension are applied. The fingers and thumb are also extended. Finally, the elbow is moved into full extension. An additional sensitizing motion that can be used is cervical side flexion to the contralateral side.	Reproduction of patient's symptoms, significant differences between sides.
Upper Limb Tension Test (Median Nerve)	*Median Nerve, Musculocutaneous Nerve, Axillary Nerve*	Patient lying supine. Shoulder depression and slight abduction (10°) with full lateral rotation. Position forearms into supination with wrist extension and extend the thumb and fingers. Elbow is then moved into extension. The test can be sensitized further by side flexing the cervical spine to the contralateral side.	Reproduction of patient's symptoms, significant differences between sides.
Upper Limb Tension Test (Radial Nerve)	*Radial Nerve*	Patient lying supine. Shoulder depression and slight abduction (10°) with full medial rotation. Position forearm into pronation with wrist flexion and ulnar deviation and flex the thumb and fingers. Elbow is then moved into extension. The test can be sensitized further by side flexing the cervical spine to the contralateral side.	Reproduction of patient's symptoms, significant differences between sides.
Upper Limb Tension Test (Ulnar-ULTT4)	*Ulnar Nerve, C8, T1*	Patient lying supine. Shoulder depression and abduction (90°) in lateral rotation with elbow flexion, as though they were placing their hand on their ear. Position forearms into pronation with wrist extension and radial deviation and extend the thumb and fingers. The test can be sensitized further by side flexing the cervical spine to the contralateral side.	Reproduction of patient's symptoms, significant differences between sides.
Cervical kineasthesia	*Proprioceptors in cervical spine*	Use ROM measure at start to measure position then move patient out of position and ask them to go back to the start position. Record amount of change from initial and final measure.	N/A

Neck Examination

Patient Name: ______________________ **Date:** __________

Diagnosis: ______________________ **Examiner:** __________

Vital Signs: Pulse: ____ Blood Pressure: __/__ L R Respiration: ____ Temperature: ____

Inspection/Palpation:

P = Pain
X = Trigger Points
B = Bleeding
S = Swelling
C = Contusion
L = Laceration
H = Hot

Range of Motion:

Activity	Normal	Active
Flexion	50	
Extension	60	
Right Lateral Bend	45	
Left Lateral Bend	45	
Right Rotation	80	
Left Rotation	80	

Nerve Supply (Skin):

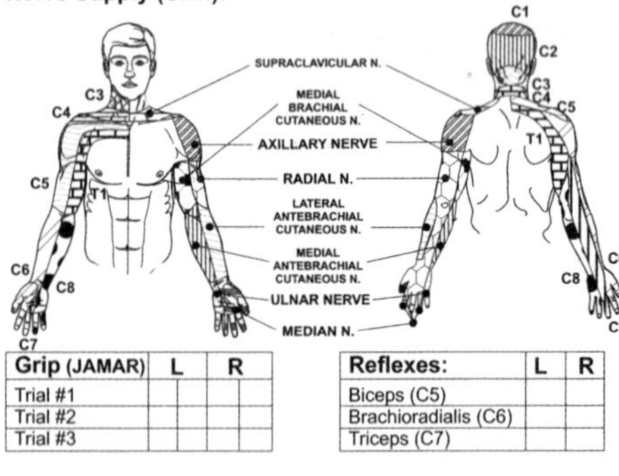

Grip (JAMAR)	L		R	
Trial #1				
Trial #2				
Trial #3				

Reflexes:	L	R
Biceps (C5)		
Brachioradialis (C6)		
Triceps (C7)		

Muscle Testing/Myotomes:

Muscle	Strength L	Strength R
Scalenes (C4-8)		
SCM (C2)		
Trapezius (C3-4)		
Upper		
Middle		
Lower		
Rhomboid (C5)		
Levator Scapula (C4-5)		
Serratus Anticus (C6)		
Latissimus Dorsi (C6-8)		
Pectoralis Major:		
Clavicular (C5-7)		
Sternal (C6-8)		
Deltoid: (C5-6)		
Anterior		
Middle		
Posterior		
Supraspinatus (C5)		
Teres Minor (C5-6)		
Infraspinatus (C5-6)		
Subscapularis (C5-6)		
Teres Major (C6)		
Coracobrachialis (C6-7)		
Biceps (C5-6)		
Triceps (C7-8)		
Wrist Extensors (C7)		
Finger Flexors (C8)		
Interossei (T1)		

Orthopedic: ______________________

Neurological: ______________________

Gait: ____________ **Special:** ____________

WESTERN

Source: Reproduced with the permission of Lerner Education. Forms can be downloaded at www.lernereducation.com

Test Name	Structures	Description of Test	Positive Test
ELBOW			
Lateral Epicondylitis Test 1 (Cozen's Test)	*Lateral Epicondylitis*	Patient seated. Therapist stabilizes elbow with one hand, thumb resting on lateral epicondyle. Patient actively makes a fist, pronates the forearm, radially deviates, and then extends the wrist. Therapist applies a force to the wrist, resisting the above motions.	Pain at the lateral epicondyle.
Lateral Epicondylitis Test 2 (Mill's Test)	*Lateral Epicondylitis, Radial Nerve*	Patient seated. Therapist palpates the lateral epicondyle while passively pronating the forearm, flexing the wrist fully and extending the elbow.	Pain at the lateral epicondyle is positive for lateral epicondylitis or radial nerve compression.
Lateral Epicondylitis Test 3 (Tennis Elbow Test)	*Lateral Epicondylitis*	Patient seated. Therapist resists extension of the 3rd digit distal to the PIP joint, stressing extensor carpi digitorum.	Pain over the lateral epicondyle.
Medial Epicondylitis Test	*Medial Epicondylitis*	Patient seated. Therapist palpates medial epicondyle while the forearm is passively supinated and the elbow and wrist are extended.	Pain over medial epicondyle.
Pinch Grip Test	*Anterior interosseous nerve*	Patient is asked to pinch tip of the index finger together with the tip of the thumb.	Patient is unable to touch tip-to-tip and instead touches the pad of each digit together. May indicate median nerve or anterior interosseous nerve pathology. May also be indicative of pronator teres syndrome or entrapment.
Posterolateral Pivot-shift Apprehension Test	*Olecranon dislocation, subluxation, Posterolateral stability*	Patient in supine position lying with arm overhead. Therapist grasps forearm at the elbow and proximal to the wrist. A slight supination force is applied to the forearm. Therapist flexes elbow while applying a valgus force and axial compression force.	Subluxation or clunk between 40-70° as elbow is flexed.
Pronator Teres Syndrome Test	*Pronator Teres*	Patient sits with elbow flexed 90° and supinated. Therapist strongly resists active pronation while the elbow is actively extended.	Tingling or parasthesia in a median nerve distribution.
Wartenberg's Sign	*Ulnar nerve*	Patient sitting with hands resting on table. Therapist passively spreads fingers apart and asks the patient to actively bring them together.	Unable to adduct little finger indicates positive test for ulnar neuropathy.

Elbow Examination

Patient Name: ______________________________ **Date:** ____________

Diagnosis: ______________________________ **Examiner:** ____________

Vital Signs: Pulse: ____ Blood Pressure: ___/___ L R Respiration: ____ Temperature: ____

Inspection/Palpation:

P = Pain
X = Trigger Points
B = Bleeding
S = Swelling
C = Contusion
L = Laceration
F = Fracture

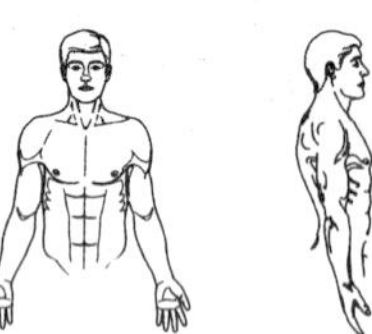
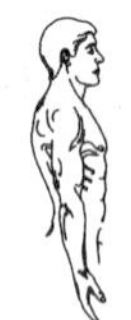
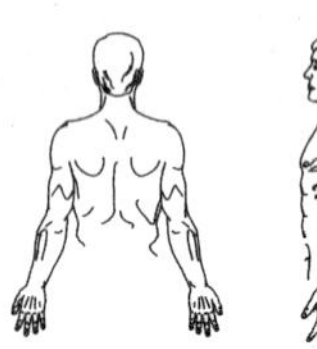

Range of Motion:

Activity	Normal	Active	Passive
Flexion	140-150		
Extension	0-10		
Supination	90		
Pronation	80-90		

Muscle Testing/Myotomes:

Muscle	Strength L	Strength R
Triceps/Anconeus (C7-8)		
Biceps/Brachialis (C5-6)		
Brachioradialis (C5-6)		
Supinator (C6)		
Pronator Teres (C6-7)		
Forearm Extensors (C7-8)		
Forearm Flexors (C7-T1)		

Nerve Supply (Skin):

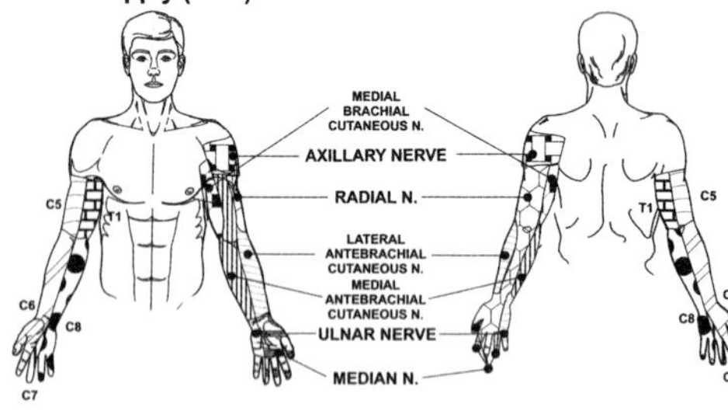

Orthopedic: ______________________________

Neurological: ______________________________

Antalgia: ____________ **Special:** ____________

WESTERN

Test Name	Structures	Description of Test	Positive Test
HIP			
90-90° SLR	*Hamstrings length*	Patient lies supine and flexes hips to 90° and holds both legs up with arms. Patient actively extends knees one at a time to full extension, maintaining hip flexion, then relaxes and attempts the other side.	Knee should extend to at least 20° from full extension, if not, indicates hamstring tightness.
Anatomical Leg Length Test	*Femoral, tibial leg length*	Patient lies supine. Therapist has patient perform a Weber-Barstow maneuver, measure with tape measure from ASIS to lateral malleolus, compare bilaterally.	Should be no more than 1.5 cm difference between legs.
Craig's Test	*Femoral Neck position*	Patient lies prone, knee flexed to 90°. Therapist palpates posterior aspect of greater trochanter, then rotates it medially and laterally until the greater trochanter is parallel with the examining table. Degree of retro or ante version can be estimated based on the angle of the lower leg from vertical.	Ante version is indicated by internal hip rotation in the final position (tibia falls laterally due to 90 degrees of knee flexion in prone).
FABER (Patrick) Test	*Sacroiliac joint, hip flexor muscles, hip joint*	Patients lie supine. Therapist places patient's leg with foot of test leg on top of the knee of opposite leg, therapist slowly lowers knee toward examining table.	Test leg knee remains above opposite straight leg.
Functional Leg Length Test	*Pelvis effect on leg position*	Patient lies supine. Therapist has patient perform a Weber-Barstow maneuver, measure with tape measure from umbilicus or xyphoid process to lateral malleolus, compare bilaterally.	Should be no more than 1.5 cm difference between sides
Modified Ober's Test	*Iliotibial band, tensor fascia latae*	Patient in side lying position. Therapist stands behind patient, flexes hip slightly with the knee nearly straight and abducts fully, stabilizing pelvis. Therapist then extends hip, allowing no internal or external rotation, therapist then slowly lowers leg into adduction while patient relaxes.	Leg "hangs" in abduction or does not fall below horizontal.
Quadrant (Scouring) Test	*Hip Joint Play*	Patient lies supine. Therapist flexes hip and adducts so that knee points to opposite shoulder, therapist maintains slight resistance while the hip is moved passively towards abduction forming an arc of motion, therapist notes any lack of smoothness in the motion, pain or apprehension. Test is done with hip in internal rotation (tests anterior femoral head and superior acetabulum), then external rotation (tests superior acetabulum and posterior femoral head). Also repeat test in extension.	Pain, irregular motion pattern, "bump" in the movement pattern, apprehension, crepitus.
Rectus Femoris Test	*Rectus femoris*	Patient lies supine with legs hanging over edge of table. Therapist flexes one hip and knee similar to Thomas Test, patient holds bent knee towards chest (not all the way), therapist observes the "hanging" knee. Knee flexion should not change (remain at 90°), if knee straightens, therapist should passively flex the knee to see if it will remain in flexion.	Knee straightens, indicating tight rectus femoris.
Sign of the Buttock	*Hip pathology versus neurological tissue lesion or hamstring tension*	Patient lies supine. Therapist performs a Straight Leg Raise. Once maximum SLR is reached, therapist flexes knee and attempts to further flex the hip.	If hip continues to flex once knee is flexed (stretch taken off hamstrings and dura), pathology is likely in the neurological structures or the hamstrings. If the hip will not flex further, the pathology is likely in the hip structures.
Thomas Test	*Hip flexors, rectus femoris*	Patient lies supine. Therapist checks for excessive lordosis, therapist raises one hip and flexes that knee, bringing the knee towards the chest (but not all the way) to flatten the lordosis, patient holds this leg with both hands locked, the straight leg is examined.	Straight leg lifts off table, when leg is pushed down, increased pelvic tilt or lordosis becomes evident.
Trendelenburg	*Gluteus medius, gluteus minimus, superior gluteal nerve, L4, L5, S1 nerve roots*	Patient in standing position. Therapist behind patient, patient lift leg on test side off ground, therapist assesses PSIS for symmetry.	Pelvis drops on side of test leg.
Weber-Barstow Maneuver	*Reset pelvic position while lying supine*	Patient lies in supine position, knees bent so feet are flat on treatment bed, patient pushes down with heels to raise buttocks off of bed, patient then drops buttocks down onto the table, allowing a natural position to be assumed, therapist then passively straightens legs and pulls gently to "take up slack".	Examine medial malleolus for asymmetry.

Hip Examination

Patient Name: ______________________ **Date:** __________

Diagnosis: ______________________ **Examiner:** __________

Vital Signs: Pulse: ____ Blood Pressure: __/__ L R Respiration: ____ Temperature: ____

Inspection/Palpation:

P = Pain
X = Trigger Points
B = Bleeding
S = Swelling
C = Contusion
L = Laceration
H = Hot

Muscle Testing/Myotomes:

Muscle	Strength L	Strength R
Psoas (L2,3)		
Iliacus (L2,3)		
Piriformis (S1,2)		
Abdominals		
Hamstrings (L5):		
Medial		
Lateral		
Quadriceps (L2-4):		
Rectus Femoris		
Vastus Lateralis		
Vastus Medialis		
Sartorius (L2-3)		
Gracilis (L3)		
Tensor Fascia Lata (L5)		
Gluteus Min/Med (L5)		
Adductors (L4)		
Gluteus Maximus (S1)		

Range of Motion:

Activity	Normal	Active	Passive
Flexion	110-120		
Extension	10-15		
Abduction	30-50		
Adduction	30		
Internal Rotation	30-40		
External Rotation	40-60		

Circumferential	L	R
Thigh		

Nerve Supply (Skin):

Anterior

Posterior

Orthopedic: ______________________

____

Neurological: ______________________

Antalgia: ______________ **Special:** ______________

WESTERN

Test Name	Structures	Description of Test	Positive Test
KNEE			
Anterior Drawer Test	*Anterior Cruciate Ligament, posterolateral capsule, posteromedial capsule, MCL, Iliotibial Band, posterior oblique ligament, arcuate-popliteus complex*	Patient lying supine, with knee bent to 90°, foot flat on testing surface. Therapist palpates posterior aspect of tibia and fibula, grasps tibia posteriorly and draws it anteriorly. Test is done in neutral, then repeated in lateral tibial rotation, then medial tibial rotation to test two-plane instability.	Greater than 6 mm of anterior tibial translation, soft "mushy" end feel.
Apley's Compression Test	*Lateral and medial menisci*	Patient lies prone on the examining table, knees flexed 90°, and soles of his feet are parallel to the ceiling. Therapist places hands on the foot or heel, presses down firmly on the lower limb, axially loading it, and rotate it back and forth thus applying a compressive grinding force to the meniscus.	More pain on compression than on distraction indicates a meniscal injury rather than a ligament tear. The location of injury can be hard to determine.
Apley's Distraction Test	*LCL, MCL, ACL, PCL, ITB, Patellar tendon*	Patient lies prone on the examining table, knees flexed 90°, and soles of his feet are parallel to the ceiling. Therapist places hands on the ankle and stabilizes the patient's thigh with their knee. Therapist then lifts the tibia upwards, distracting the joint, and rotates the tibia internally and externally.	More pain on distraction than on compression indicates a ligamentous injury rather than a meniscal tear. The location of injury is determined by location of pain.
Lachman Test	*Anterior Cruciate Ligament, Posterior Oblique Ligament, Arcuate-popliteus complex*	Patient lying supine. Therapist holds patient's knee and passively bends to 20-30° of flexion. Therapist stabilizes the anterior femur with outside hand and applies a P-A force to the posterior tibia with the inside hand.	Soft end feel, significant anterior translation.
McMurray Test-Lateral Meniscus	*Lateral Meniscus*	Patient in supine lying position, knee completely flexed (heel to butt), therapist applies a varus stress to the knee, medially rotates the tibia fully and extends knee slowly feeling for any snapping or clicking, indicating a lateral meniscal tear.	Clunk, snapping, or reproduction of patient's typical pain. Popping or snapping is NOT necessary for a positive sign.
McMurray Test-Medial Meniscus	*Medial meniscus*	Patient in supine lying position, knee completely flexed (heel to butt), therapist applies a valgus stress to the knee, laterally rotates the tibia fully and extends knee slowly feeling for any snapping or clicking, indicating a medial meniscal tear.	Clunk, snapping, or reproduction of patient's typical pain. Popping or snapping is NOT necessary for a positive sign.
Patellar Tap Test	*Knee Effusion*	Patient in supine position. Knee positioned in extension and relaxed. Therapist applies a thumb and forefinger lightly to each side of the patella, the therapist then strokes downward on the suprapatellar pouch with the other hand.	Separation of the thumb and forefinger due to fluid expanding the area.
Posterior Drawer Test	*Posterior Cruciate Ligament*	Patient lies supine, knee bent to 90°, foot flat on testing surface. Therapist palpates anterior aspect of tibia and fibula, grasps tibia anteriorly and draws it posteriorly. Test is done in neutral, then repeated in lateral tibial rotation, then medial tibial rotation to test two-plane instability.	Greater than 6 mm of posterior translation, soft "mushy" end feel.
Posterior Sag sign	*Single Plane Posterior Instability, PCL, Posterior oblique ligament, ACL*	Patient lies supine, hip flexed 45° and knee flexed to 90°, foot flat on table. Therapist observes position of tibia relative to femur.	Tibia "sags" backward on femur with gravity. Normally, the medial tibial plateau extends 1cm anteriorly beyond the femoral condyle when the knee is flexed 90°. If this step-off is lost, the test is considered positive.
Q Angle Measurement	*Femoral/tibial alignment*	Therapist ensures that the lower limbs are at a right angle to a line drawn through both ASIS. On a single side, draw a line from ASIS through the mid-point of the patella. Then draw a line from the midpoint of the patella through the tibial tuberosity. The angle between the two lines is the Q angle.	In Males, Q angle is approximately 10° (13° in Magee) and in females, approximately 15° (18° in Magee). Increased Q angle may be indicative of femoral neck ante version and lateral tibial torsion and may lead to lateral tracking of the patella (common). Decreased Q angle may be indicative of femoral neck retroversion and medial tibial torsion and this tends to centralize patellar tracking.
Quadriceps Active Test	*PCL, joint capsule*	Subject is supine with knee flexed to 90° in the drawer-test position. The foot is stabilized by the therapist, and the subject is asked to slide the foot gently down the table.	Contraction of the quadriceps muscle in the PCL-deficient knee results in an anterior shift of the tibia of >2mm.
Reverse Lachman	*Posterior Cruciate Ligament*	Patient lying prone, knee flexed to 30°. Therapist grasps tibia with one hand and stabilizes femur with the other. Therapist pulls tibia posteriorly.	Soft end feel and/or significant posterior translation.

Test Name	Structures	Description of Test	Positive Test
Slocum Test (Anterolateral/ medial Instability)	*Anterolateral instability, Anteromedial instability, ACL, Posterolateral capsule, Arctuate-Popliteus complex, PCL, LCL, ITB*	Patient in supine lying, hip flexed 45° and knee bend 90°, test starts with 30° internal tibial rotation with therapist sitting on foot to stabilize, therapist performs an anterior drawer test. This assesses anterolateral instability. If positive, foot is moved into 15° external tibial rotation and the test is repeated.	First test-positive is movement occurring primarily on the lateral portion of the knee. Second test-positive is movement primarily on the medial side of the knee.
Valgus (MCL) Stress Test	*MCL*	Patient supine on the examination table. Flex the knee to 30° over the side of the table, place 1 hand about the lateral aspect of the knee, and grasp the ankle with the other hand. Apply abduction (valgus) stress to the knee. The test must also be performed in full extension.	Excessive motion, joint gapping on medial side.
Varus (LCL) Stress Test	*LCL*	Patient supine on the examination table. Flex the knee to 30° over the side of the table, place 1 hand about the medial aspect of the knee, and grasp the ankle with the other hand. Apply adduction (varus) stress to the knee. The test must also be performed in full extension.	Excessive movement, pain reproduction.

Knee Examination

Patient Name:________________ **Date:**________

Diagnosis:________________ **Examiner:**________

Vital Signs: Pulse: ____ Blood Pressure: ___/___ L R Respiration: _____ Temperature: _____

Inspection/Palpation:

P = Pain
X = Trigger Points
B = Bleeding
S = Swelling
C = Contusion
L = Laceration
H = Hot

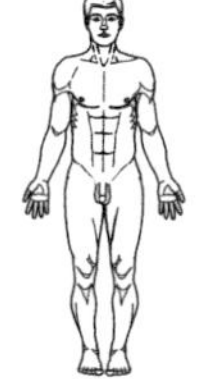
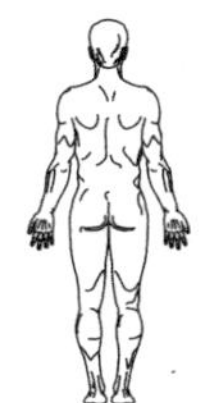

Muscle Testing/Myotomes:

Muscle	Strength L	Strength R
Hamstrings (L5):		
Medial		
Lateral		
Quadriceps (L2-4):		
Rectus Femoris		
Vastus Lateralis		
Vastus Medialis		
Sartorius (L2-3)		
Gracilis (L3)		
Tensor Fascia Lata (L5)		
Gluteus Min/Med (L5)		
Adductors (L4)		
Tibialis Anterior (L4)		
Tibialis Posterior (L4)		
Peroneus Long/Brev (L5)		
Peroneus Tertius (L5)		
Gastrocnemius (S1)		
Soleus (S1)		

Range of Motion:

Activity	Normal	Active	Passive
Flexion	135		
Extension	0 - 15		
Medial Rotation	20 - 30		
Lateral Rotation	30 - 40		

Circumferential	L	R
Thigh		
Calf		

Functional Assessment	✓
Squatting	
Squatting & Bouncing	
Ascend Stairs	
Descend Stairs	
Running Straight Ahead	
Running & Twisting	
Jumping	
Jumping & Full Squatting	

Nerve Supply (Skin):

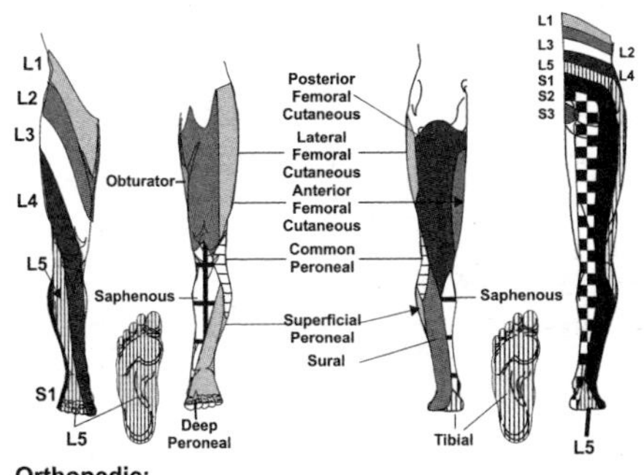

Orthopedic: ________________

Neurological: ________________

Antalgia: ________________ **Special:** ________________

Test Name	Structures	Description of Test	Positive Test
LUMBAR			
Anterior Lumbar Stability Test	*Anterior Spinal Stability*	Patient in side lying position, hips flexed 70°, knees flexed to 90°. Therapist palpates Spinous process at desired level and stabilizes SP above, therapist pushes patient's knees posteriorly along the line of the femur, lower segment moves posteriorly with stabilized segment remaining (flexion).	Reproduction of symptoms, significant motion compared to other segments.
Bowstring Test	*Sciatic Nerve*	Perform a Straight Leg Raise, once dural stretch has been attained, the hip is maintained in position and the knee is slightly flexed until stretch disappears, therapist then pushes their thumb in to the popliteal fossa against the sciatic nerve to re-establish dural tension.	Reproduction of symptoms.
Crossed Straight Leg Raise	*Sciatic nerve, L5, S1, and S2 nerve roots*	Performed in similar manner to straight leg raising, except the non-symptomatic leg is raised.	Reproduction of symptoms in contralateral leg.
Farfan Test	*Facet joints, joint capsule, supraspinous and interspinous ligaments, neural arch, longitudinal ligaments, intervertebral disc*	Patient in prone lying, therapist stabilizes ribs and spine at T12, therapist places other hand on anterior aspect of ilium, therapist pulls ilium backwards, rotating spine.	Reproduction of symptoms.
H and I Stability Test	*Hypo/ Hypermobility, Disc, Z-joints*	H Test-Patient in standing position, pain-free side tested first, patient flexes to side as far as possible, then move into flexion, then extension (or reverse if flexion is painful), patient returns to neutral and attempts on opposite side. I Test-Patient in standing position, pain-free side tested first, patient fully flexes as far as possible (or reverse if flexion painful). Therapist stabilizes while patient side bends to right and left, patient returns to neutral and repeats in extension.	Hypo-mobility indicated by 2 movements into the same quadrant would be limited. If hypermobility (instability) one quadrant will be affected with only one of the movements (H or I but not both).
Lateral Lumbar Stability Test	*Lateral Spinal Stability*	Patient in side lying position. Therapist places forearm over the side of thorax at L3, therapist applies downward pressure to L3 Transverse process.	Reproduction of symptoms.
Posterior Lumbar Stability Test	*Posterior Spinal Stability*	Patient in sitting position at edge of table. Therapist stands in front, patient places pronated forearms on therapist's shoulders; therapist puts both hands around the patient below the desired level (ie. place on sacrum if L5 being assessed), patient is asked to push through their forearm while maintaining lordosis.	Reproduction of symptoms, excessive movement.
Prone Knee Bend (Nachlas) Test	*L2 or L3 nerve root, femoral nerve*	Patient lying prone. Therapist passively flexes the knee as far as possible so patients heel rests against the buttocks. Ensure patient's hip is not rotated. Test may also be performed by passive extension of the hip while the knee is flexed as much as possible.	Unilateral pain in the lumbar, buttock, and/or posterior thigh may indicate an L2 or L3 nerve root lesion. Pain in anterior thigh may indicate femoral nerve or quadriceps lesion/tightness.
Quadrant Test	*Intervertebral foramen, Z joints*	Patient in standing position. Therapist stands behind. Patient extends spine while therapist stabilizes (can also support head on their shoulder), overpressure is applied while the patient sideflexes and rotates to the side of pain.	Reproduction of symptoms.
Repeated Extension movements	*Z-joints (Facet joints), anterior longitudinal ligament, pars interarticularis, Spinous processes of vertebrae and intervertebral foramen*	Patient in standing position. Therapist stands near to assist if needed, patient places hands on buttocks or hips and bends backward, keeping knees straight, repeat up to 10 times, therapist asks what symptoms are doing during test.	Increased localized pain, increased peripheralization, peripheral parasthesia, crepitus.
Repeated Flexion movements	*Intervertebral Disc, posterior longitudinal ligament, ligamentum flavum, erector spinae, thoracolumbar fascia*	Patient in standing position. Therapist stands near to assist if needed, patient slowly bends forward with knees straight to fully flex as far as tolerated, then return to start position, repeat up to 10 times, therapist asks patient what symptoms are doing during the test, repeat in lying position after standing extension is performed.	Peripheralization of pain, increase in localized pain (weaker indicator).
Slump Test	*Spinal cord, cervical and lumbar nerve roots, sciatic nerve*	Patient in short sitting position. Patient slumps lumbar and thoracic spine, therapist pushes down on shoulders, patient flexes head, therapist applies over pressure to cervical spine, therapist extends patient's knee, therapist dorsiflexes foot, patient extends head.	If symptoms are reproduced further movements are not attempted.

Test Name	Structures	Description of Test	Positive Test
Specific Lumbar Spine Torsion Test	*Rotary torsion of specific spinal levels, Z-joints*	Patient in side lying position and in slight extension. Therapist "winds" up the patient by pulling bottom arm towards them (rotates patient's chest towards ceiling until movement is felt at the tested segment), thus locking all vertebrae above, therapist stabilizes segment while rotating pelvis forward to detect motion.	Minimal movement and normal capsular end feel.
Straight Leg Raise	*Sciatic nerve, L5, S1, S2 nerve roots*	Patient in supine position. Hip medially rotated and adducted, knee fully extended. Therapist passively flexes hip until radicular symptoms are precipitated. Leg is lowered slowly until pain is relieved, therapist then dorsiflexes foot, cervical spine can also be flexed.	Radicular symptoms with straight leg raise, and return of symptoms with foot dorsiflexion. Most important is to compare findings bilaterally to determined if a difference exists.
Pelvic Stability	*Pelvic and spinal stability, musculature*	Patient lying prone. Therapist palpates PSIS first and asks patient to extend arm overhead, then other arm followed by each leg in turn, therapist feels for any rotation of pelvis with movement, repeat test, palpating ASIS.	Movement which cannot be controlled by patient. Posterior rotation/side flexion indicates possible weakness of the opposite back extensors or hip flexor tightness. Drop in ASIS may indicate hip flexor tightness or abs weakness or same side back extensor weakness .
SACROILIAC			
Gillett Test	*Sacroiliac mobility*	Patient standing. Therapist behind. Therapist palpates PSIS and sacral spine at level of PSIS, patient is asked to flex ipsilateral hip, PSIS should move inferiorly at the start, then the SI will lock and the PSIS and sacrum move together. Following this, patient is asked to flex the contralateral hip while maintaining the same landmarks, in this case, the sacrum should not move until the end of hip flexion, at which time it will move inferiorly while the ipsilateral PSIS remains fixated.	No PSIS movement individually, or on contralateral leg, no sacral movement.
Long Sitting Test (Supine to Sit)	*Sacroiliac joint-clearing test*	Patient lying supine. Therapist notes symmetry of medial malleoli relative to one another, patient sits up into long sitting position, therapist re-examines levels of malleoli.	Change in symmetry of malleoli from supine lying position to long sitting position.
Prone Knee Flexion Test	*Sacroiliac joint-clearing test*	Patient lying prone. Therapist compares position of medial malleoli. Therapist passively flexes both knees and compares height of medial malleoli.	Asymmetry of malleolus when knees are extended indicates either femoral or pelvic involvement regarding leg length. Asymmetry when knees are bent indicates tibial or foot shortening.
PSIS in Sitting	*Sacroiliac joint-clearing test*	Patient in sitting. Therapist palpates and compares PSIS bilaterally.	PSIS asymmetry.
Sacral Apex Pressure (Sacral P-A)	*Anterior & Posterior ligaments, A-P joint stability, Rotational shift of SI, Sacral shearing force*	Patient Prone, therapist applies anteriorly directed force directly to sacrum.	Elicited pain over SI joint.
SI Compression (Transverse Anterior Stress) Test	*Anterior joint gapping, posterior joint compression*	Patient supine. Therapist applies a cross arm pressure to the ASIS bilaterally, therapist pushes down and out with his arms.	Unilateral gluteal or posterior leg pain.
SI Distraction (Approximation Test)	*Anterior joint compression, posterior ligament stretch*	Patient side-lying. Therapist stabilizes and ensures no rotation of pelvis, therapist applies a downward force on the upper portion of the topmost iliac crest, force is directly straight downward towards lower iliac crest.	Increase pain or pressure feeling in SI area.
Standing Flexion Test	*Sacroiliac joint-clearing test*	Patient standing. Therapist palpates PSIS, examines for symmetry, patient flexes, therapist re-examines symmetry.	Asymmetry between PSIS.

Lumbosacral Examination

Patient Name: ______________________ **Date:** __________

Diagnosis: ______________________ **Examiner:** __________

Vital Signs: Pulse: ____ Blood Pressure: ___/___ L R Respiration: _____ Temperature: _____

Inspection/Palpation:

P = Pain
X = Trigger Points
B = Bleeding
S = Swelling
C = Contusion
L = Laceration
H = Hot

Range of Motion:

Activity	Normal	Active
Flexion	60	
Extension	25	
Left Lateral	25	
Right Lateral	25	
Right Rotation	0	
Left Rotation	0	

Nerve Supply (Skin):

Anterior

Posterior

Muscle Testing/Myotomes:

Muscle	Strength L	Strength R
Quadratus Lumborum		
Psoas (L2,3)		
Iliacus (L2,3)		
Piriformis (S1,2)		
Abdominals		
Hamstrings (L5):		
Medial		
Lateral		
Quadriceps (L2-4):		
Rectus Femoris		
Vastus Lateralis		
Vastus Medialis		
Sartorius (L2-3)		
Gracilis (L3)		
Tensor Fascia Lata (L5)		
Gluteus Min/Med (L5)		
Adductors (L4)		
Gluteus Maximus (S1)		
Tibialis Anterior (L4)		
Tibialis Posterior (L4)		
Peroneus Long/Brev (L5)		
Peroneus Tertius (L5)		
Gastrocnemius (S1)		
Soleus (S1)		

Reflexes:	L	R
Patella (L4)		
Achilles (S1)		

Circumferential	L	R
Thigh		
Calf		

Orthopedic: ______________________

____

Neurological: ______________________

Antalgia: __________ **Special:** __________

WESTERN

Source: Reproduced with the permission of Lerner Education. Forms can be downloaded at www.lernereducation.com

Test Name	Structures	Description of Test	Positive Test
SHOULDER			
AC Crossover Test/Horizontal Adduction Test	*AC Joint*	Patient in standing or sitting position. Therapist passively flexes the shoulder to 90° and horizontally adducts it across body as far as possible.	Localized pain over AC joint indicates AC joint problem. Localized pain over sternoclavicular joint indicates pathology there.
AC Sheer Test	*AC Joint*	Patient in sitting position. Therapist clasps hands over the anterior and posterior aspects of the AC joint, one hand on the clavicle and the other on the spine of the scapula. Therapist slowly squeezes the heels of the hands together, providing a sheer force on the AC joint.	Pain or abnormal movement at the AC joint.
Active Compression Test of O'Brian	*SLAP lesions in labrum*	Patient in standing position. Patient forward flexes arm to 90° with elbow straight and shoulder adducted 15° from midline, thumb pointed down. Therapist applies a downward force on the forearm. The test is then repeated with the palm facing up, fully supinated.	Pain during the first portion of the test with reduced symptoms during the second portion.
Apprehension (Crank) Test	*Joint capsule, G-H ligaments, rotator cuff*	Patient in supine lying position. Therapist passively abducts arm to 90°. Therapist then slowly laterally rotates patient's arm watching for facial grimacing or apprehension. Therapist can add sensitivity by placing the hand or fist under the posterior humeral head to increase the postero-anterior force. This is termed the Fulcrum test. Conversely, the therapist can also place an antero-posterior force on the humeral head to reduce it back into the glenoid fossa. This is termed the relocation test and should reduce the patient's symptoms.	Apprehension and Fulcrum tests-apprehension or pain before 90° of lateral rotation. Relocation test-able to move further into lateral rotation without apprehension than during the Apprehension or Fulcrum tests.
Biceps Tension Test (Biceps Load Test I and II)	*Biceps Tendon, SLAP lesion*	Patient in standing or sitting position actively abducts to 90° and laterally rotates fully with the elbow extended and forearm supinated. If apprehension occurs, patient is asked to flex elbow against resistance (therapist supports arm and isolated elbow flexion is performed by patient). The test may be repeated in 120° of abduction (Biceps Load Test II).	Reproduction of typical symptoms may indicate a SLAP lesion. Use Speed's Test to rule out biceps tendon pathology. If patient becomes MORE apprehensive with resisted elbow flexion occurs, SLAP lesion can be suspected.
Clunk Test	*Labrum*	Patient lying supine. Therapist places hand on posterior aspect of shoulder over humeral head. Therapist's other hand grasps the humerus above the elbow. Therapist provides a P-A force on the humeral head while the other hand rotates the shoulder into lateral rotation. Therapist may alter the position of the shoulder to test various areas of the labrum.	Clunking or grinding sound through movement.
Coracoclavicular Ligament Test	*Coracoclavicular Ligament*	Patient in side lying position facing therapist. Therapist stabilizes clavicle while pulling the inferior angle of the scapula away from the chest wall. This tests the coracoid portion of the ligament. The trapezoid portion of the ligament may be tested by pulling the medial border of the scapula away from the chest wall.	Pain under the anterior clavicle between outer one-third and inner two-thirds of the clavicle.
Crank Ligament Test	*GH Ligaments-Superior, middle, inferior*	Patient sitting with arms at side and elbow bent to 90°. Therapist passively externally rotates humerus at 0° (superior GH Ligament), 45-60° (middle GH Ligament), over 90° (inferior GH ligament).	Significant GH joint laxity or pain.
Drop Arm Test	*Rotator Cuff*	Patient in standing position. Therapist passively abducts the patients arm to 90°. Patient is instructed to slowly lower the arm actively to the side.	Patient unable to lower arm slowly, significant pain.
Empty Can/Full Can Test	*Supraspinatus*	Patient in sitting or standing position. Patient abducts arm to 90° and resistance is applied by therapist. Shoulder is then medially rotated fully and angled forward 30° from the saggital plane, the patient's thumbs pointing to the floor. Resistance is applied again. Finally, the shoulder is laterally rotated so the thumbs are pointing up and resistance is applied again.	Pain or weakness unilaterally.
Faegin Test (Sulcus)	*Glenohumeral joint, joint capsule*	Patient in sitting or standing position. Therapist passively abducts shoulder to 90°, elbow extended and resting on top of the therapist's shoulder. Therapist clasps hands over the patient's humerus at the upper third and applies inferiorly and anteriorly.	Appearance of a sulcus above the corocoid process, apprehension.
Hawkins-Kennedy Test for Impingement	*Supraspinatus, biceps tendon*	Patient standing while therapist forward flexes the arm to 90° and medially rotates the humerus. Test may also be performed.	Pain or apprehension in superior/anterior aspect of shoulder.
Infraspinatus Spring Back Test	*Infraspinatus, Teres minor*	Patient in sitting or standing position with arm at side and elbow flexed to 90°. Therapist passively abducts the arm to 90° in scapular plane and laterally rotates shoulder to end range.	Patient cannot hold the position and hand "springs back" out of lateral rotation.

Test Name	Structures	Description of Test	Positive Test
Load and Shift Test	*Glenohumeral instability, joint capsule*	Patient in sitting position. Therapist stands slightly behind patient and stabilizes the scapula and clavicle from the top. Therapist grasps the head of the humerus with thumb over the posterior aspect and fingers over the anterior humeral head. Therapist feels for the seating of the humeral head in the glenoid to determine postural position. Therapist then moves the humeral head anteriorly and posteriorly to determine proper seating position within the glenoid, ie. the "start" position. This is the LOAD part of the test to seat the head fully in the glenoid fossa. To complete the SHIFT part of the test, the therapist glides the humeral head anteriorly or posteriorly, noting the amount of displacement from the seated position.	Translation greater than 25% of the humeral head width either posteriorly or anteriorly from the seated position.
Neer's Test for Impingement	*Supraspinatus, biceps tendon*	Patient in sitting or standing position. Therapist passively elevates shoulder in the scapular plane (scaption) with arm medially rotated. Therapist controls scapular and clavicular movement. The test is repeated in lateral rotation, which should be negative.	Pain in superior or anterior aspect of the shoulder. If positive in lateral rotation, suspect an AC joint problem.
Norwood Test for Posterior Instability	*Posterior Capsule, Infraspinatus, Teres Minor*	Patient lying supine with shoulder abducted 60-100° and laterally rotated 90° with elbow flexed to 90°. Therapist stabilizes the scapula at the AC joint, palpating the posterior humerus head with fingers. The therapist then passively moves the arm into horizontal adduction until the forward flexed position is reached.	Humeral head translating posteriorly in relation to the glenoid.
Posterior Apprehension Test	*Posterior Capsule, Infraspinatus, Teres Minor*	Patient in supine lying (can be done in sitting) position with elbow bent 90° and shoulder flexed to 90°. Therapist applies an axial load along the arm and passively medially rotates and horizontally adducts the arm, feeling on the posterior aspect of the GH joint for posterior dislocation or excessive translation. This should be repeated in 90° of abduction with one hand palpating the head of the humerus and the other hand providing a posterior force to the humeral head.	More than 50% of the humeral head width translation is considered positive.
Posterior Inferior Glenohumeral Ligament Test	*Posterior Inferior Glenohumeral Ligament, Posterior joint capsule*	Patient in sitting position. Therapist flexes shoulder to 90° then horizontally adducts the shoulder 40° with medial rotation. Therapist palpates the posteroinferior region of the glenoid during movement.	Humerus protrudes or pain in posteroinferior glenoid area. Restriction in motion indicates tight posterior capsule.
Posterior Internal Impingement Test	*Infraspinatus*	Conducted similarly to the Crank test. Patient in supine lying position. Therapist passively abducts shoulder to 90° with 15-20° of forward flexion and full external rotation.	Posterior shoulder pain.
Push-Pull Test	*Posterior Capsule*	Patient lying supine. Therapist holds patient's arm at wrist and abducts shoulder to 90° and flexes to 30°. Therapist places other hand over the humeral head. Therapist then pulls up on wrist while pushing down on the humeral head, placing a posterior force on the humerus.	Greater than 50% translation of the humeral head width is considered positive.
Reverse Impingement Sign	*Supraspinatus, biceps tendon*	Conduct impingement, test then provide an inferior force on the humeral head.	Relief of symptoms with the inferior force indicates that supraspinatus impingement is relieved with the application of force.
Speed's Test	*Biceps tendon, possible Labral involvement if SLAP lesion is present*	Patient in sitting or standing position, elbow fully extended. Patient flexes arm to 90° and therapist provides an eccentric force on the forearm. Testing is done both in full pronations, followed by full supination.	Increased symptoms in the bicipital groove when the forearm is supinated.
Lift Off Test	*Subscapularis*	Patient in standing position, hand behind back against mid-lumbar spine. Patient lifts hand away from low back. Therapist can apply an external load to further test subscapularis.	Inability to lift hand off low back. Abnormal scapular motion may indicate scapular instability.
Sulcus Sign	*Glenohumeral joint, joint capsule*	Patient stands with arm by their side and muscles relaxed. Therapist grasps patient's forearm below the elbow and pulls inferiorly.	Appearance of a sulcus above the corocoid process or below the AC joint.
Wall Pushup Test	*Scapular stability*	Patient in standing arms length from wall. Patient is asked to do a push-up against the wall 15-20 times.	Weakness of the scapular stabilizers may occur with 5-10 push ups and presents as winging or changes in elevation or depression.
Yergason's Test	*Transverse Humeral Ligament*	Patient in sitting or standing position. Patient's elbow flexed to 90°, arm stabilized against the side, forearm pronated. Therapist provides resistance against supination while the patient laterally rotates. Therapist palpates the biceps tendon in the bicipital groove to feel if the tendon "pops out."	Biceps tendon is felt to "pop out" of the groove.

Shoulder Examination

Patient Name:____________________ **Date:** __________

Diagnosis:____________________ **Examiner:** __________

Vital Signs: Pulse: ____ Blood Pressure:__/__ L R Respiration:____ Temperature: ____

Inspection/Palpation:

P = Pain
X = Trigger Points
B = Bleeding
S = Swelling
C = Contusion
L = Laceration
F = Fracture

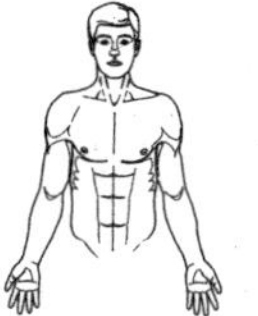
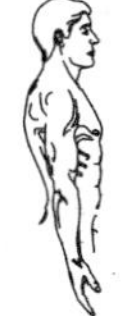
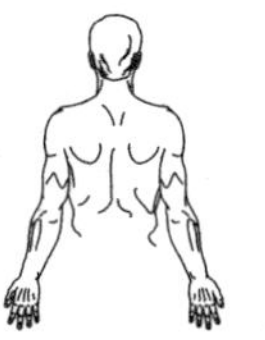
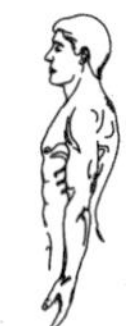

Range of Motion:

Activity	Normal	Active	Passive
Flexion	170		
Extension	50		
Abduction	170		
Adduction	45		
External Rotation	110		
Internal Rotation	80		

Muscle Testing/Myotomes:

Muscle	Strength L	Strength R
Trapezius (C3-4)		
Upper		
Middle		
Lower		
Rhomboid (C5)		
Levator Scapula (C4-5)		
Serratus Anticus (C6)		
Latissimus Dorsi (C6-8)		
Pectoralis Major:		
Clavicular (C5-7)		
Sternal (C6-8)		
Pectoralis Minor (C7-8)		
Subclavius (C5-6)		
Deltoid: (C5-6)		
Anterior		
Middle		
Posterior		
Supraspinatus (C5)		
Teres Minor (C5-6)		
Infraspinatus (C5-6)		
Subscapularis (C5-6)		
Teres Major (C6)		
Coracobrachialis (C6-7)		
Biceps (C5-6)		
Triceps (C7-8)		

Nerve Supply (Skin):

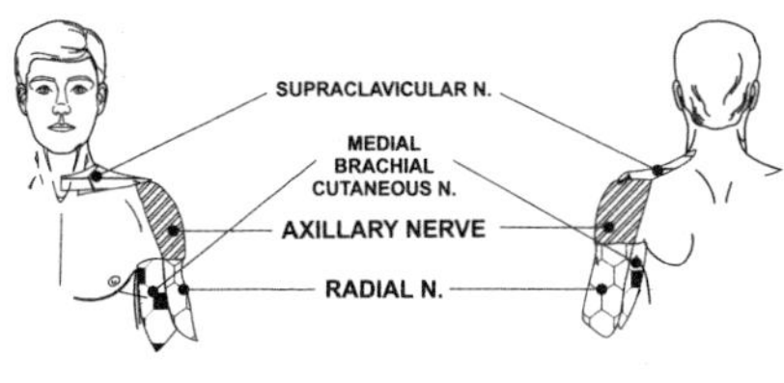

Orthopedic: ____________________

Neurological: ____________________

Antalgia:__________ **Special:** __________

WESTERN

Test Name	Structures	Description of Test	Positive Test
THORACIC			
Adson's Test	*Thoracic Outlet Syndrome*	Patient in sitting position. Therapist palpates the radial pulse. Patient rotates the head to the test side, and then extends head while therapist laterally rotates and extends the shoulder. Patient is instructed to take a deep breath and hold it.	Disappearance of the radial pulse.
Allen Maneuver	*Thoracic Outlet Syndrome*	See Wright test.	
EAST (Roos) Test	*Thoracic Outlet syndrome*	Patient in sitting or standing position. Patient abducts both arms to 90°, laterally rotates fully, flexes the elbows to 90° and horizontally extends the shoulder so the elbows are slightly behind the frontal plane. The patient is asked to slowly open and close the hands for up to 3 min.	Fatigue or distress is NOT positive tests. Profound weakness, ischemic symptoms, whitening of the arms or numbness/tingling of the hand are considered positives.
Halstead Test	*Thoracic Outlet Syndrome*	Therapist palpates radial pulse and applies an inferior traction on the test extremity while the patient's neck is extended and rotated AWAY from the test side.	Disappearance of the radial pulse.
Wright Test (Allen Maneuver)	*Thoracic Outlet Syndrome*	Patient in sitting position. Therapist flexes the elbow to 90° and horizontally extends the shoulder and fully rotates it laterally. Patient then rotates the head AWAY from the test side. Therapist then palpates the radial pulse. Therapist may also have the patient take a deep breath and hold it or extend the cervical spine.	Radial pulse disappears.

Thoracic Examination

Patient Name: ____________________ **Date:** __________

Diagnosis: ____________________ **Examiner:** __________

Vital Signs: Pulse: ____ Blood Pressure: ___/___ L R Respiration: ____ Temperature: ____

Inspection/Palpation:

P = Pain
X = Trigger Points
B = Bleeding
S = Swelling
C = Contusion
L = Laceration
H = Hot

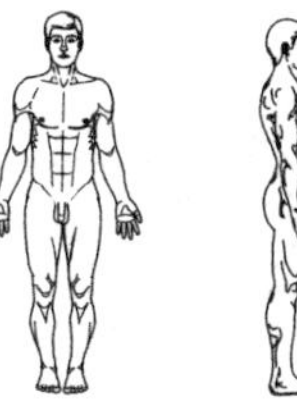

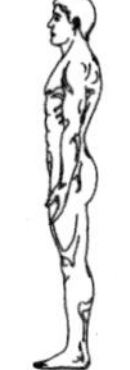

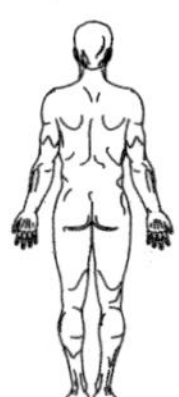

Range of Motion:

Activity	Normal	Active	Passive
Flexion	50		
Extension	0		
Right Rotation	30		
Left Rotation	30		

Neurology

Nerve Supply (Skin):

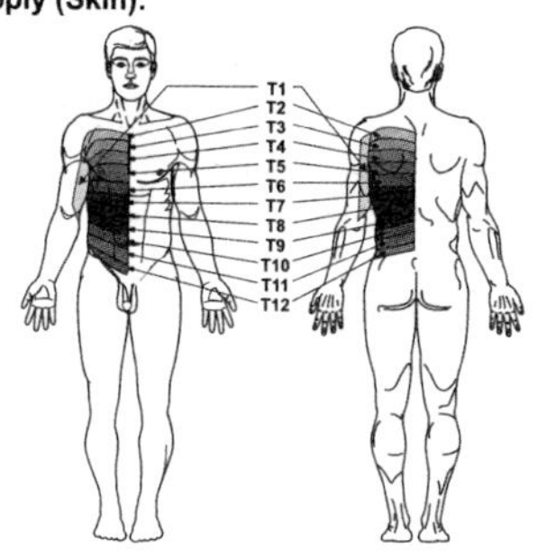

Muscle Testing/Myotomes:

Muscle	Strength L	Strength R
Abdominals (T7-L1)		
Serratus Anterior (C5-7)		

Reflexes:	L	R
Upper Abdominals (T7-10)		
Lower Abdominals (T10-L1)		

Orthopedic: ____________________

Neurological: ____________________

Antalgia: ____________________ **Special:** ____________________

Test Name	Structures	Description of Test	Positive Test
WRIST/HAND			
Allen Test	*Ulnar and radial arteries*	Patient in sitting or lying position. Therapist palpates the radial and ulnar arteries and provides a firm compression while the patient makes a fist and releases 3-4 times, driving blood out of the hand. Therapist releases the arterial compression on one artery while watching for blood refill in the hand.	Reduced blood re-fill from a singular artery may indicate a blockage.
Finkelstein Test	*DeQuervain's Tenosynovitis*	Patient makes a fist with thumb inside the fingers. Therapist stabilizes the forearm and deviates the wrist toward the ulnar side.	Unilateral pain over the abductor pollicis longus and brevis may indicate paratenonitis. Test can produce symptoms in normal populations, so test should be compared to other side. Test is positive only if patient's typical symptoms are produced.
Fromont's Sign	*Adductor Pollicis Brevis/Longus, Ulnar nerve*	Patient grasps a piece of paper between the index finger and the thumb. Therapist pulls paper away while patient attempts to resist this action.	Distal phalanx of thumb flexes when paper is pulled. If, at the same time, the MCP joint hyperextends, the ulnar nerve may be suspected.
Grind Test	*Thumb MCP or metacarpo-trapezial joint*	Therapist holds patient's hand with one hand and grasps the patient's thumb distal to the MCP joint. Therapist then applies an axial compression and rotates the MCP joint. This test may be repeated with any of the MCP joints.	Localized pain and/or grinding may indicate degenerative joint disease.
Phalen's Test	*Carpal Tunnel*	Therapist flexes patient's wrists fully and holds this position for 1 minute by pushing patient's wrists together.	Tingling or numbness in a median nerve distribution (thumb, index and middle finger and radial half of ring finger).
Reverse Phalen's Test	*Carpal Tunnel*	Therapist extends patients hand while asking patient to grip the therapist's hand. Therapist then applies pressure directly over the carpal tunnel for 1 minute. The test may also be performed by placing both hands in a prayer position and pulling back towards the body while keeping the palms in direct contact, although the reliability is reduced using this method.	Tingling or numbness in a median nerve distribution (thumb, index and middle finger and radial half of ring finger).
Supination Lift Test	*TFCC (Triangular fibrocartilage complex)*	Patient in sitting position, forearm supinated, and elbows flexed to 90°. Patient is asked to place hands palms up on the underside of a heavy table, or flat against the therapist's hands (which are palm down). Patient is then asked to lift upward.	Localized pain on the ulnar side of the wrist or difficulty applying the force unilaterally.
Sweater Finger Sign	*Flexor digitorum profundus*	Patient attempts to make a fist.	Distal phalanx of one of the fingers does not flex, may indicate a rupture of the tendon of flexor digitorum profundus.
Tinel's Sign	*Nerve regeneration, Median nerve (in wrist)*	Therapist taps over the carpal tunnel (also can be performed at elbow and shoulder by tapping on various nerve locations).	Tingling or parasthesia distal to the site of pressure.

Wrist & Hand Examination

Patient Name:____________________ **Date:** ________

Diagnosis:____________________ **Examiner:** ________

Vital Signs: Pulse: ____ Blood Pressure:__/__ L R Respiration:____ Temperature: ____

Inspection/Palpation:

P = Pain
X = Trigger Points
B = Bleeding
S = Swelling
C = Contusion
L = Laceration
F = Fracture

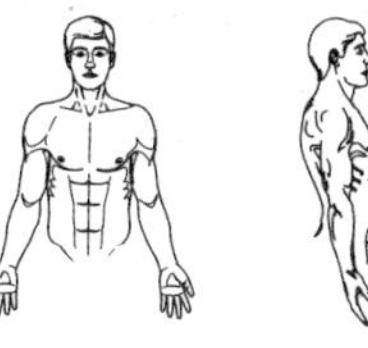

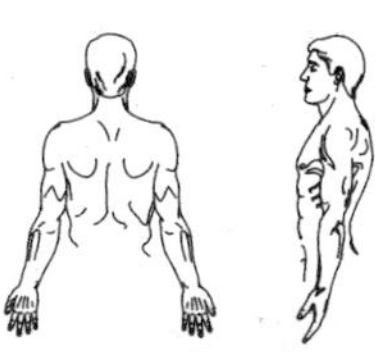

Wrist Range of Motion:

Activity	Normal	Active	Passive
Flexion	80-90		
Extension	70-90		
Radial Deviation	15		
Ulnar Deviation	30-45		

Muscle Testing/Myotomes:

Muscle	Strength L	Strength R
Pronator Quadratus (C8-T1)		
Finger Flexors (C7-T1)		
Finger Extensors (C7-8)		
Thumb Flexors (C8-T1)		

Grip (JAMAR)	L		R	
Trial #1				
Trial #2				
Trial #3				

Nerve Supply (Skin):

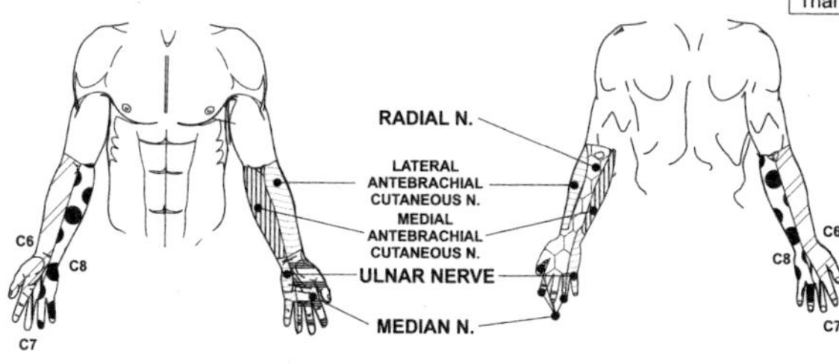

Orthopedic: ____________________

Neurological: ____________________

Antalgia: __________ **Special:** __________

WESTERN

Source: Reproduced with the permission of Lerner Education. Forms can be downloaded at www.lernereducation.com

Pain Patterns & Trigger Points

When treating clients, if you understand the location of pain, it can provide you with a useful map for treating the various muscles associated with client's complaints. A visual map can help massage therapists guide treatment. Treatment can include palpation of trigger points and manual therapy to the associated regions of the muscles. With certain muscles, the referred pain is often exacerbated by simply pressing on a tender trigger point in the region to reproduce a referred pain pattern. If your clients are describing an increase in pain or extreme tenderness coming off the palpated area, you can assume the muscles involved are causing the pain. You can also recommend stretches and exercises to help alleviate pain or perform manual therapy, shiatsu or acupressure to release or alleviate the pain. The following section details common pain patterns and trigger points from different regions of the body.

Recommended reading and resources on trigger point therapy and pain patterns:

Myofascial Pain and Dysfunction: The Trigger Point Manual by Janet G. Travell and David G. Simons
The Trigger Point Therapy Workbook by Clair Davies
Trigger Point Therapy for Myofascial Pain by Donna Finando and Steven Finando
The Concise Book of Trigger Points, Revised Edition by Simeon Niel-Asher

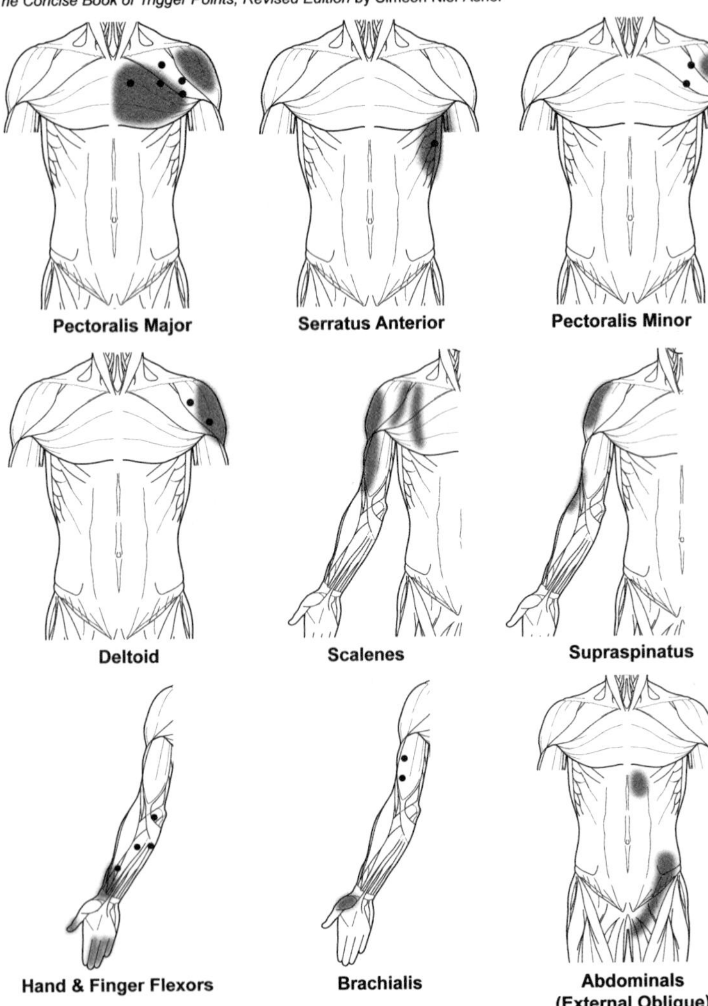

Sources: Simeon Niel-Asher, *The Concise Book of Trigger Points, Revised Edition,* North Atlantic Books, Berkeley, CA 2008. Donna Finando and Steven Finando, *Trigger Point Therapy for Myofascial Pain,* Healing Art Press, Rochester, VT, 2005.

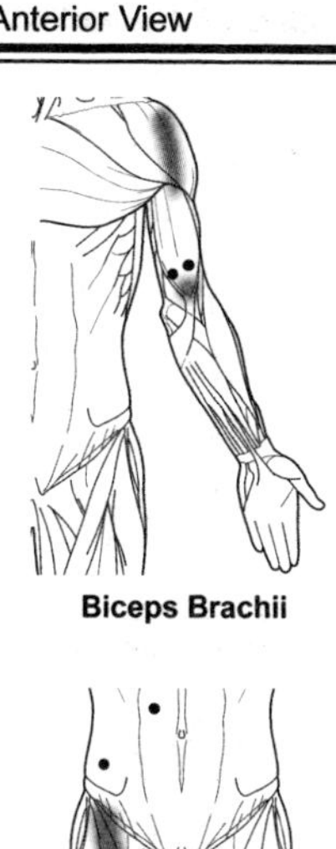
Biceps Brachii

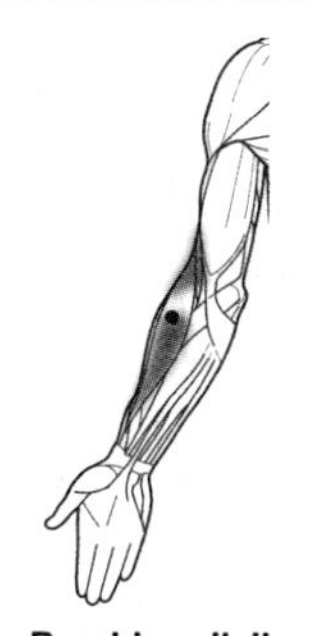
Brachioradialis

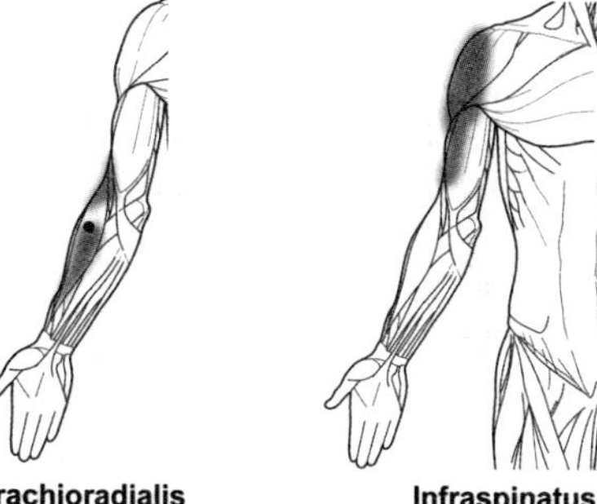
Infraspinatus

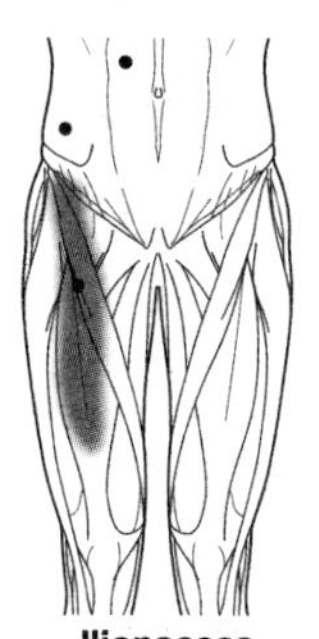
Iliopsosas

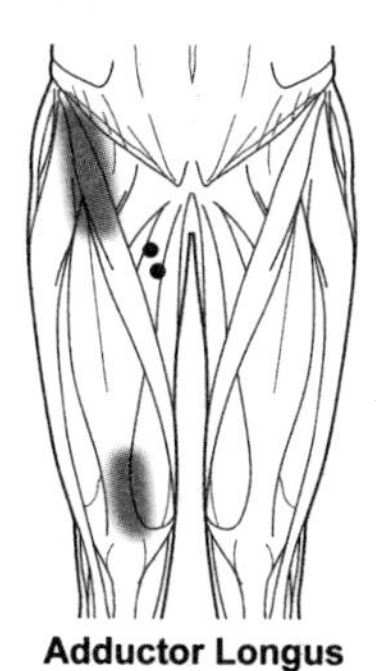
Adductor Longus

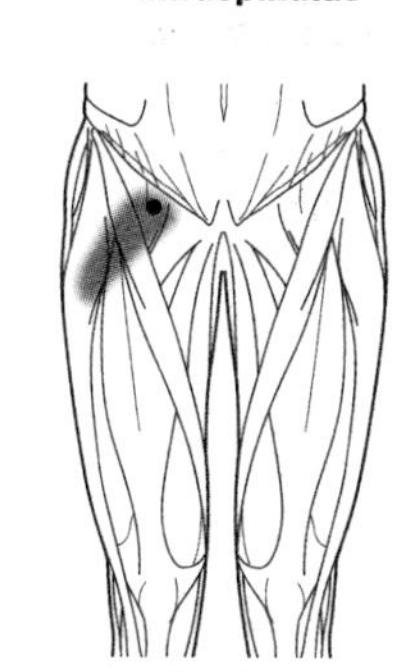
Pectineus

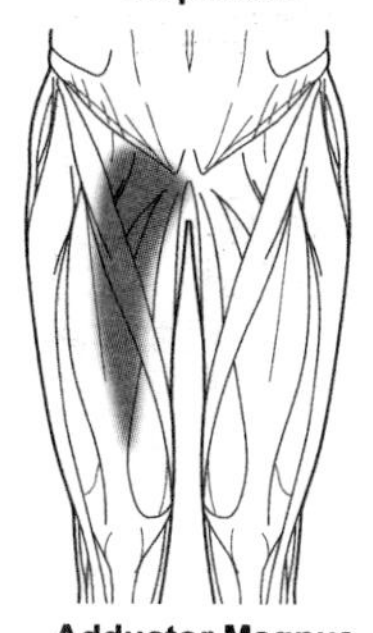
Adductor Magnus

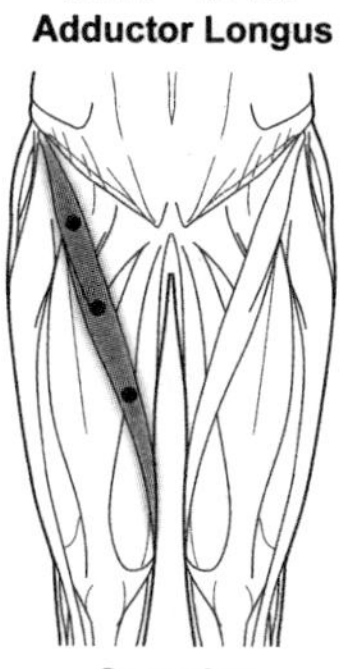
Sartorius

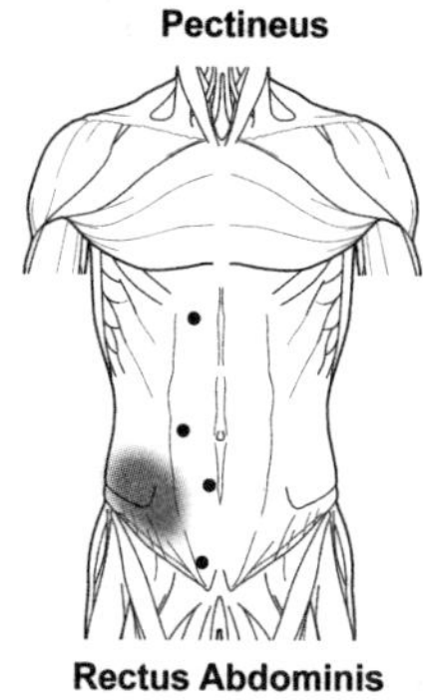
Rectus Abdominis

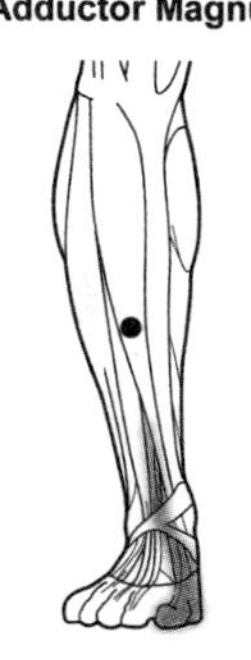
Extensor Hallucis Longus

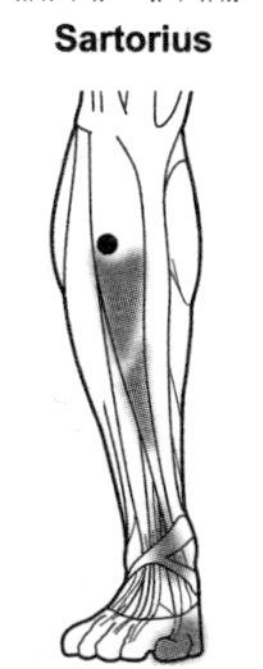
Anterior Tibialis

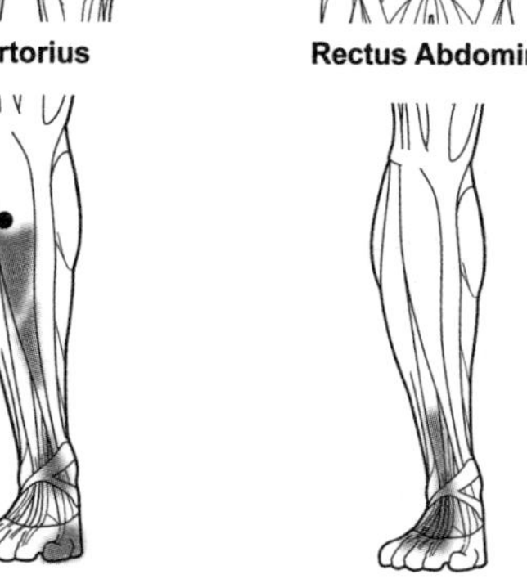
Extensor Digitorum Longus

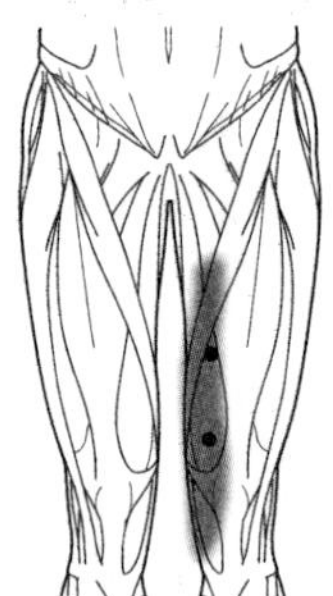
Quadriceps
(Vastus Medialis)

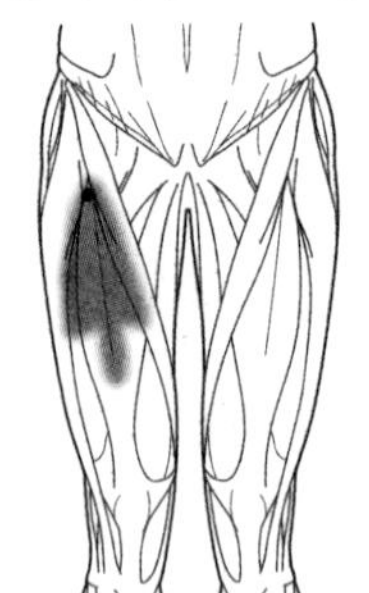
Quadriceps
(Vastus Intermedius)

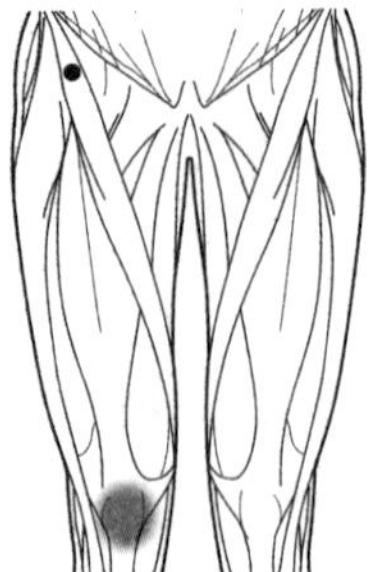
Quadriceps
(Rectus Femoris)

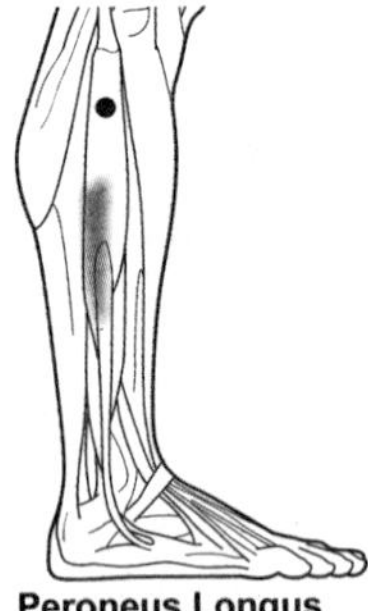
Peroneus Longus

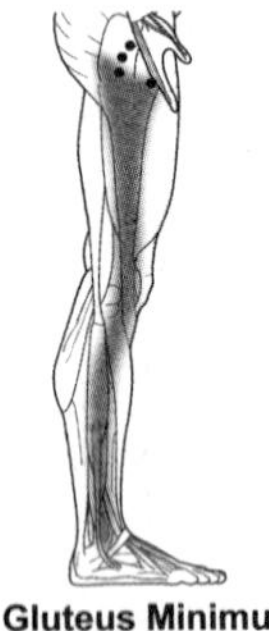
Gluteus Minimus

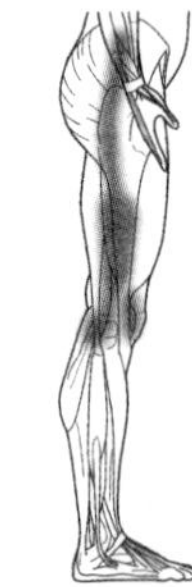
Quadriceps
(Vastus Lateralis)

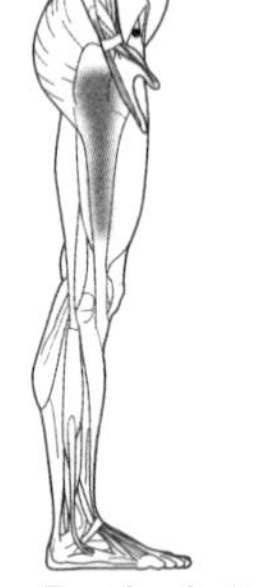
Tensor Fasciae Latae

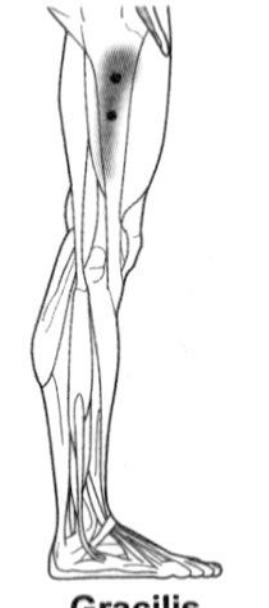
Gracilis

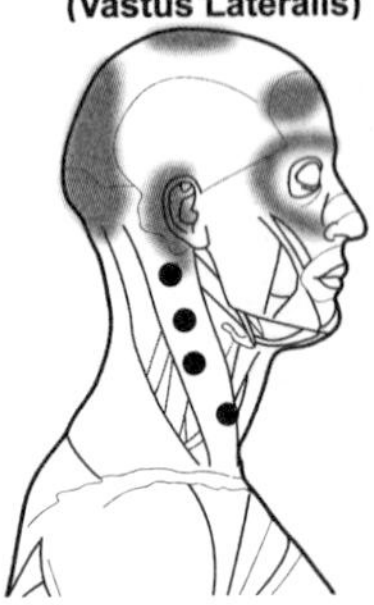
Sternocleidomastoid

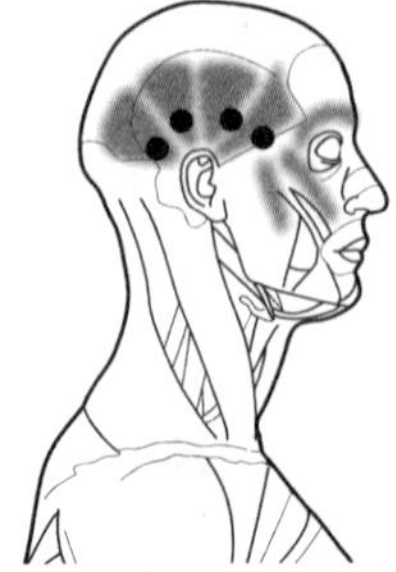
Temporalis

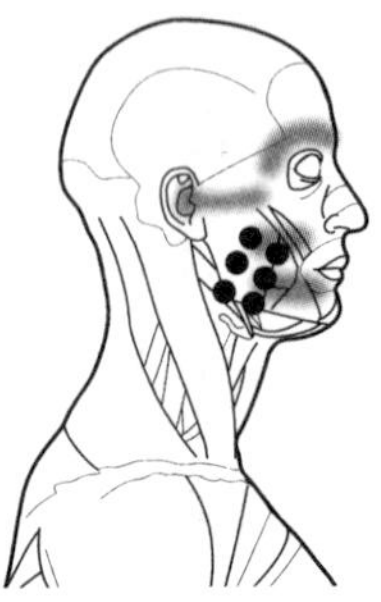
Masseter

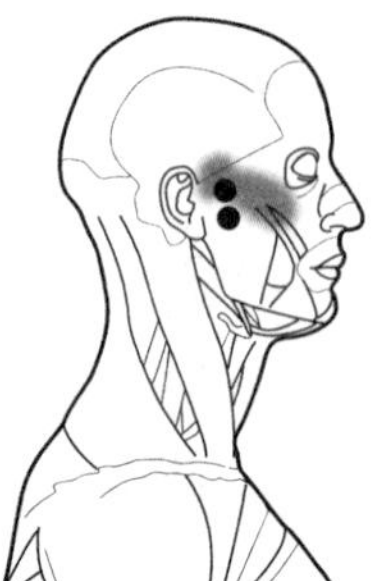
Lateral Pterygoid

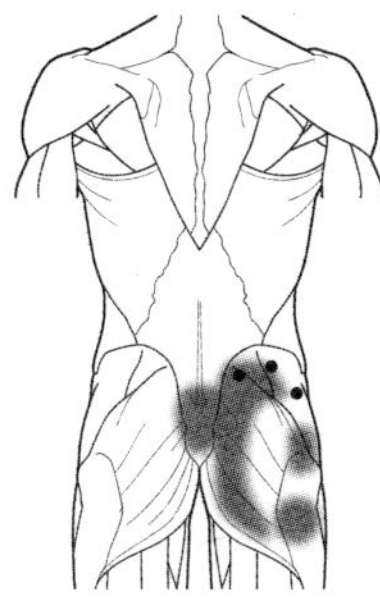
Gluteus Medius

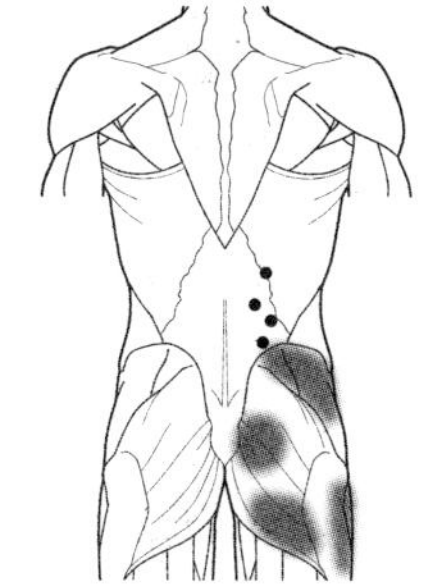
Quadratus Lumborum

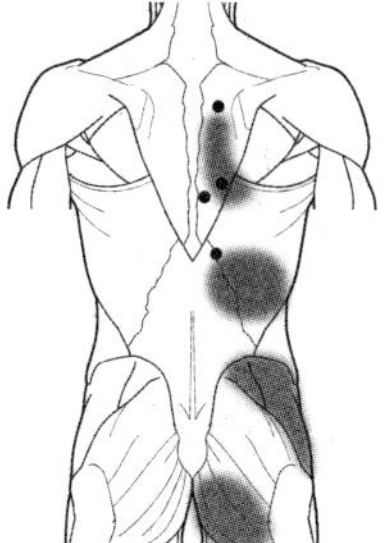
Erector Spinae

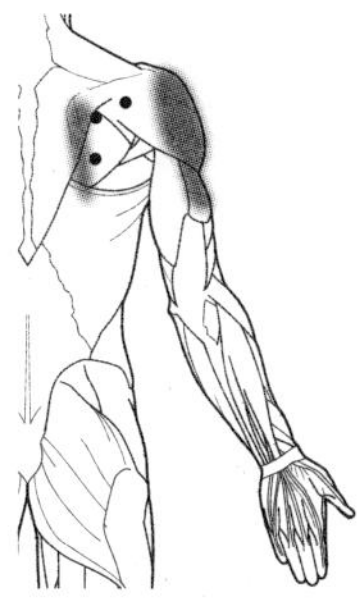
Infraspinatus

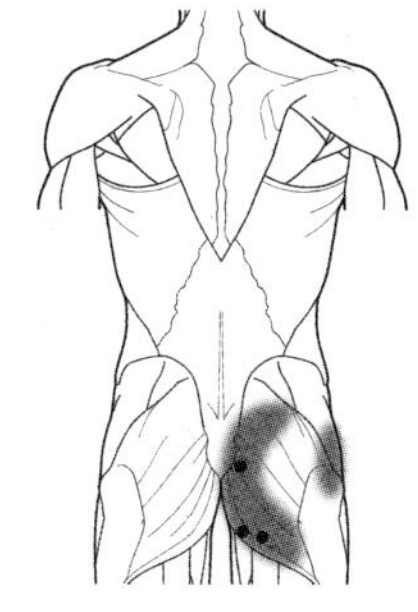
Gluteus Maximus

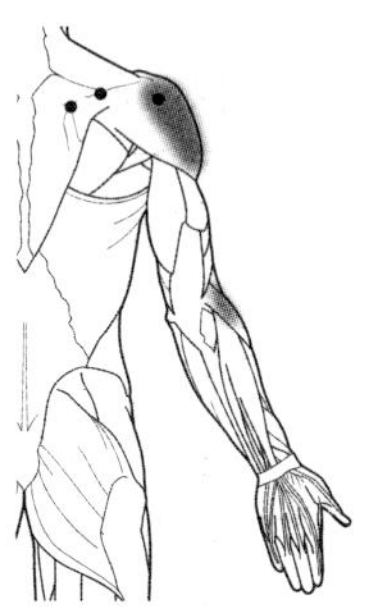
Supraspinatus

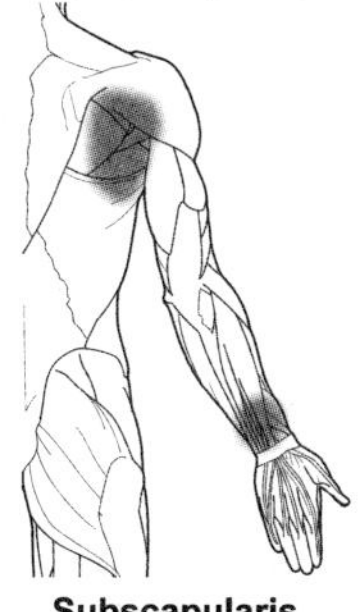
Subscapularis

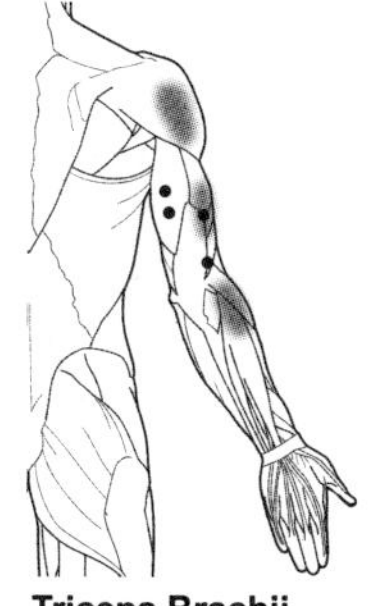
Triceps Brachii

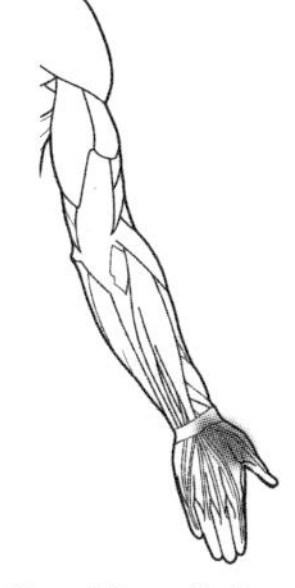
Brachioradialis

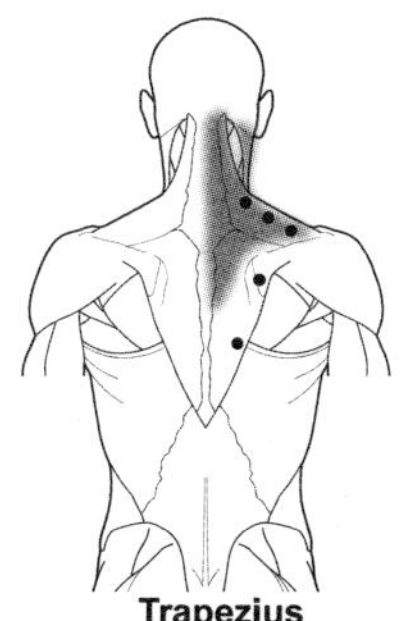
Trapezius

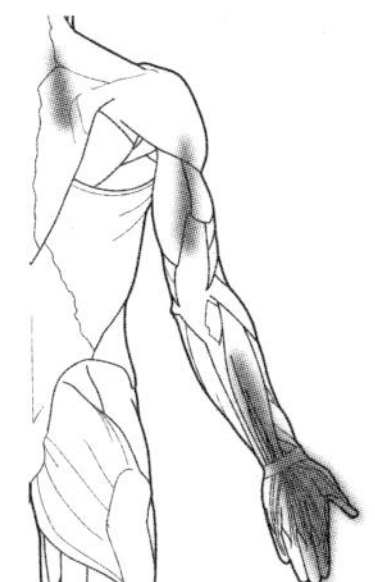
Scalenes

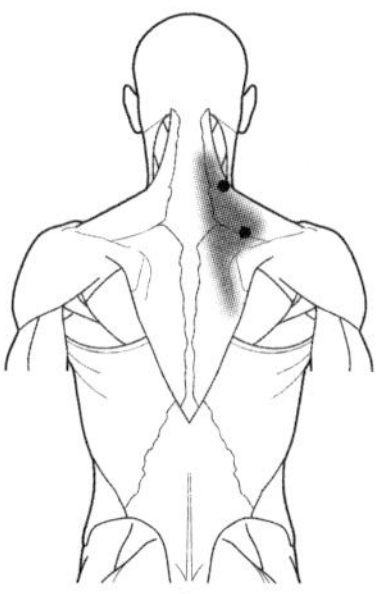
Levator Scapulae

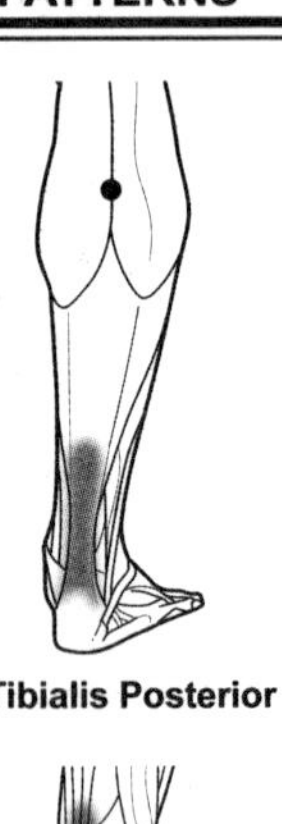
Tibialis Posterior

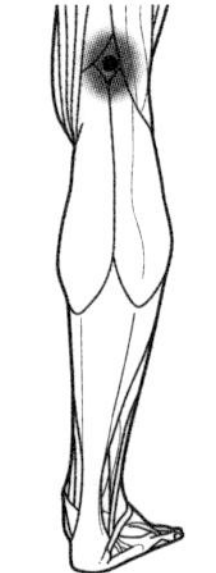
Popliteus

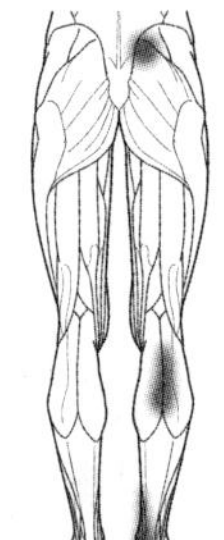
Soleus

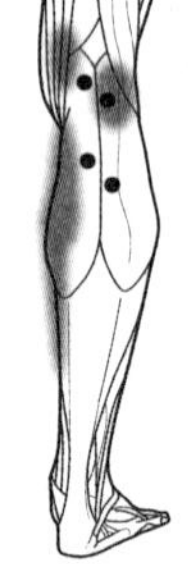
Gastrocnemius

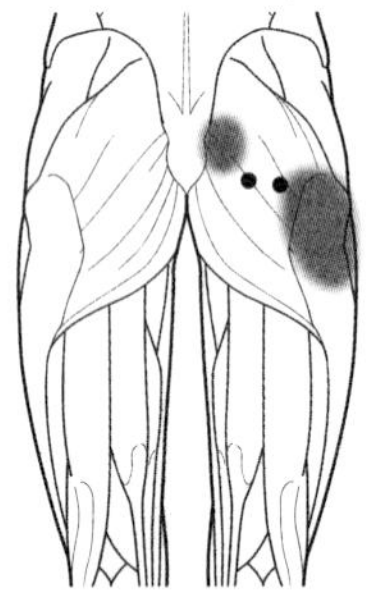
Piriformis

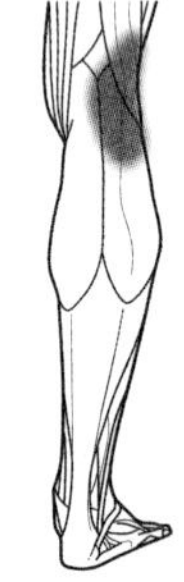
Hamstrings (Biceps Femoris)

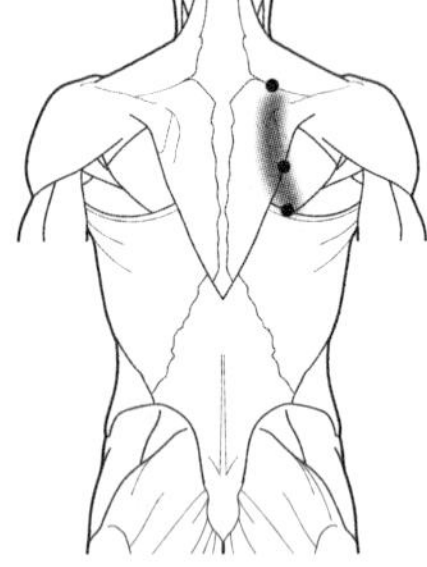
Rhomboids

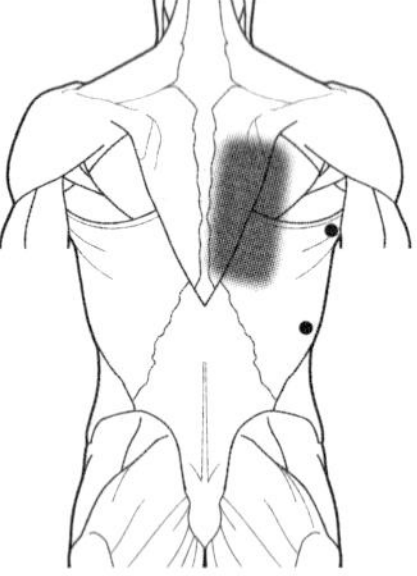
Latissimus Dorsi

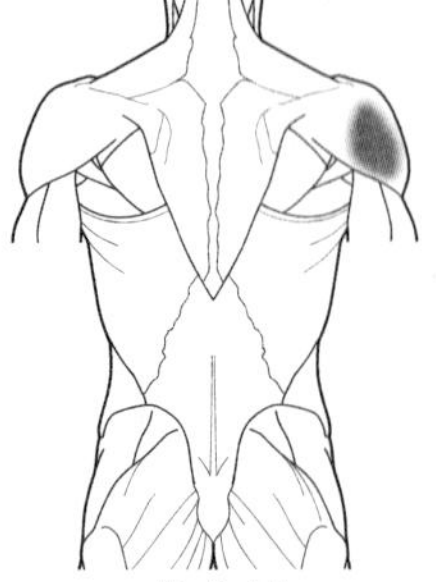
Deltoid

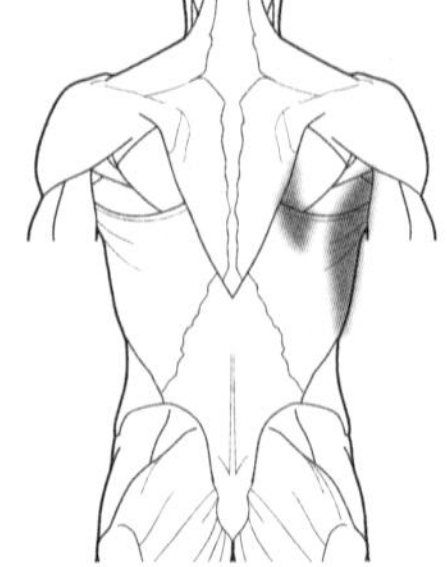
Serratus Anterior

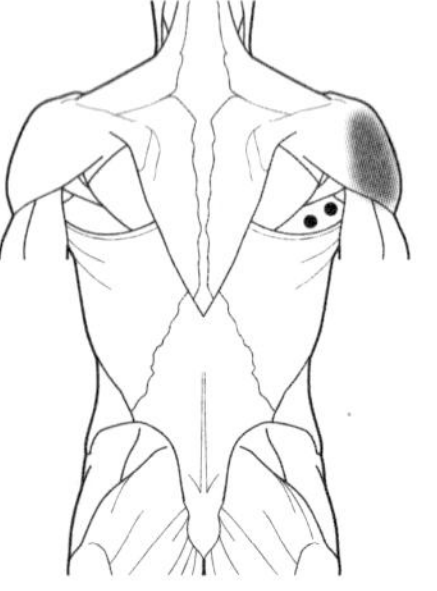
Teres Major

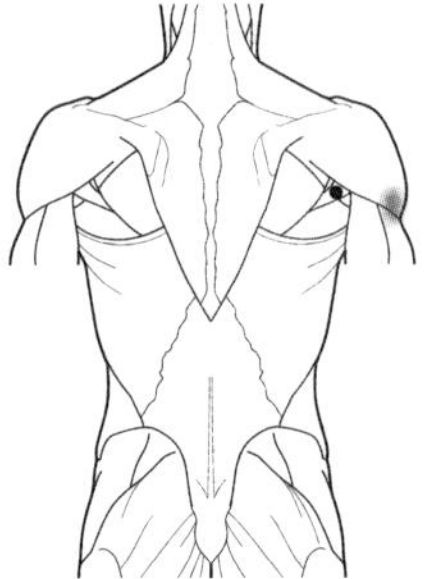
Teres Minor

Chief Complaint History (LOC-Q-SMAT)

1. (L) Location / radiation

- Where? Have client point to the location.
- Write description of location that is as specific as possible (" thoracic or mid-thoracic" is more specific than "low back, "anterior & lateral right shoulder" is preferable to "shoulder")
- Indicate right, left or both sides.
- Does it radiate? If so, where and how far? (ankle, elbow, wrist, hand, fingertips?)
- What surface or aspect? (lateral/medial/anterior/posterior/dorsal)

2. (O) Onset (what happened & when did it occur?)

- When did you first notice this problem? Was it gradual or sudden? What was the cause?
- Look for specific actions, modifications in activities, posture, occupation, exercise.

3. (C) Chronology/Timing (symptom patterns)

- Constant or intermittent patterns (episodic).
- If persistent, is it actually 24 hours a day? Does it affect sleep?
- If irregular, is it associated with specific conditions? (e.g. consuming certain foods? particular activities? time of day?)
- Rate of recurrence & length of the episodes.
- Diurnal patterns (worse in morning or end of day?)
- Is there night pain that wakes you or prevents you from falling asleep?
- Worsening, improving, or staying the same?
- Prior history: Have you ever experienced this type of problem? When? For how long? How did you address it?

4. (Q) Quality

- Have client describe pain or symptoms (sharp, dull, etc.).
- If description is uncommon, use client's words in quotations or open-ended question.

5. (S) Severity/ADL affected (activities daily living)

- Is pain slight, moderate, or intense?
- How would you rate pain on scale from 1 to 10?
- ADL: Can client perform regular daily activity such as work? Is performance affected? Hobbies? Sexual activity? Everyday activities such as putting on a jacket? Get specific actions & how the client is affected (great source of functional outcome markers).

6. (M) Modifying factors

- Does anything make symptoms or pain worse? Be specific.
- Does anything make symptoms better? Avoiding certain things? Changing posture? Rest? Medication (how much relief & how often?)

7. (A) Associated symptoms

- Do you have any other symptoms or problems that you feel are related or relevant to this issue?
- Further detailed questions are asked based on what the client presents with & what the examiner thinks it could be; for example:
  - Is there numbness, tingling, or lack of strength in an extremity?
  - Neck: Any cracking? Headaches? Numbness in the arms?
  - Knees: Any popping, clicking, or snapping? Knees ever lock? Swell? Give way?
  - Low back: Does your back ever catch or get locked? Any changes in bladder or bowel habits? Change in sexual performance?

8. (T) Treatment previous

- Have you been treated by other health care providers? Who did you see? When? What tests were performed?
- What diagnosis? What treatment? Did it help?

9. Relevant injuries

- When? What happened? (Include falls, broken bones, or motor vehicle accidents)
- Were you hospitalized? Did you have any relevant surgeries?
- What was the ultimate outcome? Were there any residual effects?

10. Goal (optional)

- What is the treatment goal of the client?
- If it has been a long-term problem, why is s/he seeking treatment now?

Is there any more information you can provide regarding your condition?

Using appropriate terms, explain why you are inquiring & be compassionate towards client.

Create a differential diagnosis list.

Family & Personal History / Past Health History

Family Health Problems

- Are there any conditions that run in your family, such as cancer, depression, diabetes, high blood pressure, stroke or heart disease?
- I'd like to start with your father. Is he still living? If so, describe any health problems he has
- How about your father's father?
- Your mother? Your siblings?
- If there is a deceased relative, what was their age at time of death? What was the cause of death?
- Are there any other health issues in the family?

1. Living Environment

- How would you describe your living environment? Is it a house/condo/ apartment? What are the relationships of dwellers? Are there children?

2. Occupation

- What is your profession?
- Describe the nature of your work? What is involved? What are the hours you work?
- Do you enjoy your work?

3. Exercise

- Do you partake in regular exercise? (What type? How intense? How often?)

4. Interests/Avocations/ Activities

- Are there any other interests, avocations or activities you enjoy?

5. Diet/Nutrition

- Rate the quality of your overall diet (scale 1 to 10)
- What do you eat for breakfast? Lunch? Dinner? Between meals?
- What do you drink during the day?
- How often do you eat meat? Vegetables? Fruit? Sweets? Fast food?
- How much water a day do you consume?

6. Sleep Pattern

- How much sleep do you get each night?
- Any changes in your sleep lately?
- Do you think you get enough rest?

7. Bowel Habits

- How frequently do you have bowel movements? Any changes recently?
- Any rectal bleeding?

8. Urinary Habits

- Do you have any problems with urinating? Any recent changes? Problems starting or stopping?

9. Habits

- Do you drink alcohol? What type?
- Frequency and amount of alcohol?
- Smoke or use any tobacco products? What kind and how much?
- How long did you smoke? When did you stop?
- Use any recreational drugs? What and for how long? (reiterate client confidentiality if needed)

10. Domestic Violence

- Are you now or have you ever been in a relationship in which you were physically injured or threatened?

11. Stress factors/Depression/Support system

- Any significant stresses in your life lately?
- Noticed a change in your ability to handle stress?
- Feel depressed?
- What resources do you have for support?

Assessing Pain and Symptoms (OPQRST)

O = Onset. When did pain first start? Over days or within hours. Acute vs. chronic.

P = Provoke. What causes the pain? What intensifies or lessens it?

Q = Quality. What does pain feel like? Sharp? Dull? Burning? Stabbing? Crushing? Throbbing?

R = Radiation. Does the pain travel to different places in the body?

S = Severity. Do you think the pain is mild, moderate, or severe?

T = Time. Is pain continuous or sporadic? Has it occurred before? Does it change (get better or worse)? When does it start?

Past Health History

1. Serious Illness
- Ever had one or more serious illnesses?
- Other problems?

2. Hospitalizations/Surgeries
- Ever been hospitalized?
- Ever had surgery of any kind?

3. General Trauma, Accidents, Injury
- Have you experienced any physical trauma that was treated or that you think should have been treated?
- Ever had any accidents? MVA?
- Suffer any residual problems or long-lasting side effects?

4. Menses, Menopause
- What was the first day of your last menstrual period?
- Any problems with your menstrual cycle?
- Any changes in your menstrual cycle? Any abnormal bleeding?

Patients over 50:
- Do you continue to have menstrual periods? If yes, do you remember the first day of your last menstrual period?

Physiologic menopause:
- How old when you first experienced menopause?
- Taken hormone replacements in the past? Currently taking them?
- If yes, which one? How administered?

Surgical menopause:
- Why did you have a hysterectomy? For cancer?
- Were your ovaries removed?
- Taking hormone replacements?
- If yes, which one? How administered?

5. Contraceptives, Pregnancies

Contraceptives:
- Using any type of hormonal contraceptive or an IUD? If yes, have there been any problems?

Pregnancies:
- Ever been pregnant? If is yes, were there any complications?

6. Medications
- Take any prescribed medications?
- Any over-the-counter medications?
- Any vitamins?
- Ever taken any medication such as steroids, antidepressants, NSAIDs, antibiotics, hormones for an extended period of time?

7. Allergies
- Allergic to any foods or medications? If so, are they seasonal?

8. X-rays
- Have you ever had any x-rays? If so, why?
- Any problems identified on the x-ray?

9. Prior Care
- Have you ever received prior care?
- If so, what for? Describe the care. Did it help?
- This will tell what has and hasn't worked prior

10. Last Physical Exam
- When was your last physical exam? Were you experiencing your chief complaint when you had it?
- What was it for?
- Any problems identified?

Females:
- When was your last GYN exam and PAP smear?
- What were the results?

Females over 50:
- Have you had a mammogram? How often?
- Results?

Males 15-35:
- Do you perform self-testicular exams?
- Have you ever been taught how to?

Males over 40:
- Ever had a rectal exam or lab tests to evaluate your prostate?
- If so, do you remember the results?

Review of Findings (ROF)

Review of findings (ROF) is a significant aspect of massage treatment and gives you the chance to determine benefits from your treatment and be an expert in its execution. It also is an excellent outline for massage success by educating client on how you will treat his or her complaints.

Greeting
1. Greet client by name
2. Ask about current status
3. Orient client to ROF
   a. Review of findings and their meanings
   b. Make treatment suggestions
   c. Provide opportunity for questions
   d. Inform client of anticipated duration of each treatment (30 min to 60 min)

Overview
1. Summarize the problem(s)
2. Establish your ability to help
3. Reassure client about his/her condition

Describe condition(s)
1. Explain diagnosis in simple terms
2. The cause (mechanism of injury)
3. Review exam findings how they relate to diagnosis
4. How it manifests
5. How the treatment will address cause

Describe treatment
1. Type of therapy
2. Frequency and duration of treatments

Establish goals
1. Describe goals of massage treatment
2. Relate goals to problem(s) and outcome measures

Describe importance of compliance
1. Relate to cause of problem and complaint
2. Stress client's role in her/his own care
3. Determine and address obstacles to compliance

Describe expectations
1. Outcome measures
2. When to re-evaluate

PAR (Procedures, Alternatives, Risks)
1. Legally required for every new procedure
2. Describe procedures, alternatives to treatment and risks
3. Obtain written informed consent with client's signature to proceed with treatment
4. Address any questions (legally required)

Conclusion
1. Educational materials
2. Answer any of client's questions

Practice Building Tips
1. Be professional, prepared and competent
2. Ensure client's comfort
3. Use appropriate language for client's level of understanding
4. Communication between clinician and client should flow naturally
5. Use clear explanations that make sense
6. Be a good listener
7. Adjust eye contact to client's comfort
8. Have empathy for client's concerns
9. Give client opportunities to ask questions/ verbalize concerns

SOAP NOTES

The purpose of the SOAP note is to be a brief report using abbreviations rather than complete sentences. Keep in mind that abbreviations differ for each specialty. SOAP notes can also be used as documentation on the necessity for continued treatment (especially when dealing with third-party payers or litigation).

S = SUBJECTIVE - Symptoms the client verbally expresses or that are stated by a significant other. Include the client's descriptions of pain or discomfort, the presence of nausea or dizziness and a multitude of other descriptions of dysfunction, discomfort or illness the client describes.

- Record subjective information provided by the client, using quotes if possible
- How has client responded since last treatment
- Address each condition separately
- Keep this section brief unless client has much new information
- If client presents with a new condition, then a new chief complaint history is required

O = OBJECTIVE - Include symptoms that can actually be measured, seen, heard, touched, felt, or smelled. Vital signs such as temperature, pulse, respiration, skin color, swelling and the results of diagnostic tests.

- Record objective information observed about the client
- General observations of the client physical presentation are applicable
- Physical exam parameters are monitored

A = ASSESSMENT - The diagnosis of the client's condition. In some cases the diagnosis may be clear, such as a low back pain, but an assessment might not be clear and could include several diagnosis possibilities.

- Record assessment as to the current status of condition
- Indicate whether improving or not
- For the action, record treatment that was administered during the visit
- Record client response to treatment ask the client how they felt afterwards
- Home care exercises, etc. provided

P = PLAN - May include laboratory and/or radiological tests ordered for the client, medications ordered, treatments performed, client referrals (sending client to a specialist), client disposition (e.g., home care, bed rest, short-term, long-term disability, days excused from work, admission to hospital), client directions and follow-up directions for the client.

- Patient to return (PTR), record the date you want client to return for treatment
- Record any client self-care instructions
- Record any future plans to examine or test

Soap Note Example:
Patient Name: KY DOB: 12/31/1961
Record No. XXX-XXX-XXXX
Date: 09/09/07

S: "Pt. says she has neck pain that cricks upon movement." Had a headache for last 2 weeks, unable to sleep because of pain. PMS symptoms with cramps. Current 7/10 pain.
O: Tight and tender, both sides at occipital ridge, temporal headaches > right side
A: Neck pain, heat to posterior cervical, manual neck stretches.
P: Massage 2x a week, Change habits to lessen workload and avoid being on computer long time. Short Term Goal: Client to begin stretching exercise for every 2 hours of work. Told client to be aware of body and posture while working. Follow-up in one week.

SOAP

Subjective: M / F _____ Age_________

Chief Complaint:
ADLs:
Medications:
Symptoms:
Progress:
Comments:

For Patients with Pain: Pain Scale: None 0 1 2 3 4 5 6 7 8 9 10 Severe

Objective Signs: Visual, palpation, tests and modalities

Physical:
Palpation:
Muscle Testing:
Gait:
Overall:

Other physical/emotional signs and orthopedic examinations:

Assessment/Diagnosis: **with western dx, write "per doctor" or "per patient" or "per records" or "NA" as is applicable**

Western Diagnosis:
Goals:

Plan of Treatment:

Treatment Principle:
Homework & Self care:
Client Comments:
Additional Notes:

Mark the" following" where patient feels pain:

XXX Sharp/stabbing
PPP Pins & Needles
DDD Dull/Aching
NNN Numbness

Swedish ☐ *Heat* ☐
Deep ☐ *Ice* ☐
Reflexology ☐ *Acupressure* ☐
Lymph ☐ *Other* ____

ICD-9 Code:
CPT Code:
Therapist: Signature:
Client Name: Date:

Source: The following general health forms can be downloaded and customized for your usage at www.acupuncturedeskreference.com

PATIENT INFORMATION FORM

Please Note: This is a confidential record of your medical history and will be kept in this office. Information contained here will not be released to any person except when you have authorized us to do so.

Name ____ M.I. ____ Last Name ____

Address ____ City ____ State ____ Zip ____

Home Phone ( ) ____ Cell ( ) ____ Work ( ) ____

SS# ____ Age ____ DOB ____

Drivers License # ____ Male ☐ Female ☐

Employer ____ Occupation ____

Married ☐ Single ☐ Divorced ☐ Name of Spouse ____

Emergency Contact ____ Telephone ( ) ____

Referred by ____ Friend ☐ Relative ☐ Insurance ☐ Other ☐

PRIMARY INSURANCE Cash ☐ Group ☐ Work/Comp ☐ Auto ☐ Other ☐

Name of Insurance Co. ____ ID#. ____ Group# ____

Name of Insured ____ Relationship to Patient: Self ☐ Spouse☐ Parent ☐

Secondary Insurance ____ Name of Insured ____

I understand that this is a quotation of benefits and is NOT a guarantee of payment, and the agreement is between the Insurance Carrier and me. I authorize any and all payment from my insurance carrier directly to this office with the understand that all monies be credit to my account upon receipt. Any denial of payment becomes my responsibility (patient).

____
Patient Name (print) Patient Signature Date

24 HOUR CANCELLATION POLICY & CREDIT AUTHORIZATION RELEASE

__________takes pride in the quality of care he offers his patients. In order to do this he has a strict cancellation policy. Dr. __________ requires a 24-hour cancellation notice prior to your appointment time. If sufficient time is not given, the full fee will be charged to the credit card we have on file.

I, ____________________________________ authorize Dr. ________ to charge the credit card given below, for cancellation fees, insurance co-payments and related charges.

____________-______________-______________-________________ Ex______/_______ Visa ☐ / MC ☐

____
Patient Name (print) Patient Signature Date

Source: The following general health forms can be downloaded and customized for your usage at www.acupuncturedeskreference.com

OUR OFFICE PROTECTS YOUR HEALTH INFORMATION AND PRIVACY

Dear Valued Patient,

This notice describes our office's policy for how medical information about you may be used and disclosed, how you can get access to this information, and how your privacy is being protected.

In order to maintain the level of service that you expect from our office, we may need to share limited personal medical and financial information with your insurance company and with Worker's Compensation (and your employer as well in this instance), or with other medical practitioners. We will obtain your authorization before disclosing any information.

Safeguards in place at our office include:

- Limited access to facilities where information is stored.
- Policies and procedures for handling information.
- Requirements for third parties to contractually comply with privacy laws.
- All medical files and records (including email, regular mail, telephone, and faxes sent) are kept on permanent file.

Types of information that we gather and use:

In administering your health care, we gather and maintain information that may include non-public personal information:

- About your financial transactions with us (billing transactions).
- From your medical history, treatment notes, all test results, and any letters, faxes, emails or telephone conversations to or from other health care practitioners.
- From health care providers, insurance companies, worker's comp and your employer, and other third party administrators (*e.g.* requests for medical records, claim payment information).

In certain states, you may be able to access and correct personal information we have collected about you, (information that can identify you -*e.g.* your name, address, Social Security number, etc.).

We value our relationship with you, and respect your right to privacy. If you have questions about our privacy guidelines, please call us during regular business hours at ________________.

Yours sincerely,

____________________, LMT

Source: The following general health forms can be downloaded and customized for your usage at www.acupuncturedeskreference.com

NAME________________________________ DATE_________________________

I. Goals: What would you most like to achieve through your work at the ABC Massage Center?
1. ____
2. ____
3. ____
4. ____
5. ____

II. Major Symptoms: Please list in order of importance what symptoms are of concern to you.
(most concerning to least, along with the duration of the symptom)
1. ____
2. ____
3. ____
4. ____

Use the following illustration to indicate painful or distressed areas:

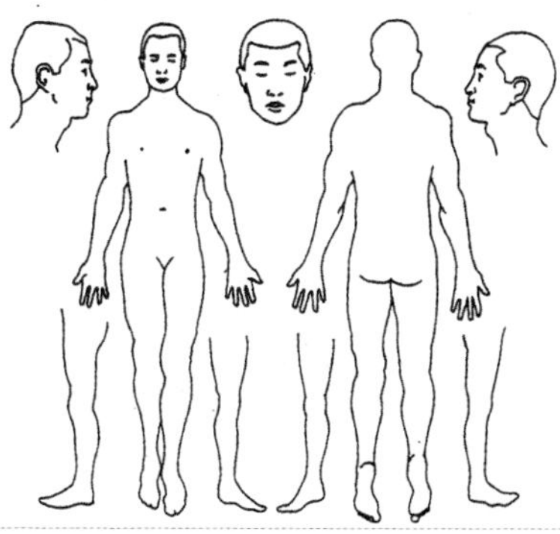

Are you experiencing pain/discomfort in any area of your body? **Y / N**

If yes, using the models to the left, please indicate the location of the discomfort by using the symbol that best describes the feeling:

X X X Sharp/stabbing
P P P Pins & Needles
D D D Dull/Aching
N N N Numbness

For Women:
1. Are you pregnant now? [ ]Yes [ ]No [ ]Unsure

2. Indicate number of occurrences:
Live Births _______ Pregnancies_______ Miscarriages _______ Abortions _______

3. Age: First period _____ Menopause (if applicable) _____

4. Date: Last Pap Smear _____ /_____ Last Mammogram _____ / ______

5. Any History of an Abnormal Pap Smear? [ ] Yes [ ] No If so, what / when? ____________________

Source: The following general health forms can be downloaded and customized for your usage at www.acupuncturedeskreference.com

6. Is your menses cycle regular? [ ] Yes [ ] No
a) Average number of days of flow ______
b) The flow is: [ ] Normal [ ] Heavy [ ] Light
c) The color is: [ ] Normal [ ] Dark [ ] Purple [ ] Light Brown [ ] Brown

7. Do you have the following menstruation related signs/symptoms?

[ ] Difficulty with Orgasm [ ] Cramps [ ] PMS [ ] Heavy Vaginal discharge between periods

[ ] Pain with Intercourse [ ] Nausea [ ] Bleeding between Periods

[ ] Blood Clots [ ] Breast Distention [ ] Vaginal Discharge

For Men:
1. Do you have any bothersome urinary symptoms? [ ] Yes [ ] No

Describe:______________________________

2. Check all that apply:

[ ] Erectile dysfunction [ ] Difficulty with orgasm [ ] Pain or swelling of the testicles [ ] Frequent need to urinate at night

[ ] Impotence/erectile dysfunction [ ] Premature ejaculation [ ] Feeling of coldness or numbness in genitalia

[ ] Pain/Subtly of testicles

3. Do you get up at night to urinate? [ ] Yes [ ] No How often? ______________________

4. To what extent do these conditions interfere with your daily activities (work, sleep, socializing, sex, etc.)?
____

5. Have you sought Medical intervention for these problems? If so, when? ______________________
____

6. What treatments have you tried for these problems and how successful have they been?
____

III. Medical History

Please check all that apply	*Date Diagnosed*		*Date Diagnosed*
Diabetes	___/___/___	High Cholesterol	___/___/___
High Blood Pressure	___/___/___	High Blood Pressure	___/___/___
Thyroid Disease	___/___/___	Seizures	___/___/___
Cancer	___/___/___	Hepatitis	___/___/___
HIV	___/___/___	Others	___/___/___

IV. Surgical History

______________________________ Date __________
______________________________ Date __________
______________________________ Date __________

Source: The following general health forms can be downloaded and customized for your usage at www.acupuncturedeskreference.com

V. Family History

Please check all that apply and state how you are related to the family member with that condition.

Condition	Mother	Father	Sibling	Maternal Grandparent	Paternal Grandparent
Heart disease					
Cancer					
Hypertension					
Stroke					
Asthma					
Allergies					
Migraines					
Depression					
Other mental illness					
Substance abuse					
Osteoporosis					
Diabetes					
Glaucoma					

VI. Medications / Supplements

Medications you are currently taking (please include prescription medicine, supplement, herbal supplements and over the counter medicines you take on a regular basis, along with dosages and brands if known)

Allergies (to medications, chemicals or foods):

VIII. Nutrition

1. Do you follow a special diet? [ ] Yes [ ] No If yes, how would you describe the diet?
   (ie Vegetarian, Vegan, Low Carb, etc.)

2. What do you eat on a "typical" day? ______
a) Breakfast ______
b) Lunch ______
c) Dinner ______
d) Snacks ______
e) Foods you tend to crave: ______
f) Foods you dislike: ______

Source: The following general health forms can be downloaded and customized for your usage at www.acupuncturedeskreference.com

PRACTICE

IX. Social History

1. How much per day do you use of the following?
a) Coffee, tea, soft drinks: ______
b) Alcohol: ______
c) Cigarettes, cigars, other tobacco: ______
d) Other drugs: ______

2. Have you ever had a problem with *alcohol* or *alcoholism*? [ ] Yes [ ] No

3. Have you ever had a problem with *dependency* on other drugs? [ ] Yes [ ] No

4. If yes which and when?
______

5. Do you have a known history of any exposure to *toxic* substances? [ ] Yes [ ] No

6. If so, please list which and when you first noticed symptoms?
______
______

7. In the past year, how many days have been significantly affected by your health? ______

8. How many days did you feel generally poor? ______

9. How many times were you in the hospital? ______

10. Please describe your current exercise regimen:
Hours per week: ______ Activities: ______ [ ] No Exercise

11. How many hours of sleep do you usually get per night during the week? ______

12. Do you awake feeling rested? [ ] Yes [ ] No Do you feel you sleep well at night? [ ] Yes [ ] No

13. Who would you describe as your source of primary social support? (relationship to you)

X. Other Information

Please list and briefly describe the most significant events in your life:
1. ______
2. ______
3. ______
4. ______

Have you been treated for emotional issues? [ ] Yes [ ] No

Have you ever considered or attempted suicide? [ ] Yes [ ] No

Do you have any other neurological or psychological problem? [ ] Yes [ ] No

Please provide us with any other information that you think is relevant for us to know:
______
______
______
______
______
______

Source: The following general health forms can be downloaded and customized for your usage at www.acupuncturedeskreference.com

HEALTH: CHECK ALL THAT APPLY

GENERAL

Past	Current	Condition
[ ]	[ ]	Poor appetite
[ ]	[ ]	Excessive appetite
[ ]	[ ]	Insomnia
[ ]	[ ]	Fatigue
[ ]	[ ]	Fevers
[ ]	[ ]	Night sweats
[ ]	[ ]	Sweat easily
[ ]	[ ]	Chills
[ ]	[ ]	Localized weakness
[ ]	[ ]	Poor coordination
[ ]	[ ]	Bleed or bruise easily
[ ]	[ ]	Catch cold easily
[ ]	[ ]	Change in appetite
[ ]	[ ]	Strong thirst
[ ]	[ ]	Other: ____________

SKIN & HAIR

Past	Current	Condition
[ ]	[ ]	Rashes
[ ]	[ ]	Hives
[ ]	[ ]	Itching
[ ]	[ ]	Eczema
[ ]	[ ]	Pimples
[ ]	[ ]	Dryness
[ ]	[ ]	Tumors, lumps

HECK & NECK

Past	Current	Condition
[ ]	[ ]	Dizziness
[ ]	[ ]	Fainting
[ ]	[ ]	Neck stiffness
[ ]	[ ]	Enlarged lymph glands
[ ]	[ ]	Headaches
[ ]	[ ]	Concussions
[ ]	[ ]	Other: ____________

EARS

Past	Current	Condition
[ ]	[ ]	Infection
[ ]	[ ]	Ringing
[ ]	[ ]	Decreased hearing
[ ]	[ ]	Other: ____________

EYES

Past	Current	Condition
[ ]	[ ]	Blurred vision
[ ]	[ ]	Visual changes
[ ]	[ ]	Poor night vision
[ ]	[ ]	Spots
[ ]	[ ]	Cataracts
[ ]	[ ]	Glasses / contacts
[ ]	[ ]	Eye inflammation
[ ]	[ ]	Other: ____________

NOSE, THROAT, MOUTH

Past	Current	Condition
[ ]	[ ]	Nose bleeds
[ ]	[ ]	Sinus infections
[ ]	[ ]	Hay fever or allergies
[ ]	[ ]	Recurring sore throats
[ ]	[ ]	Grinding teeth
[ ]	[ ]	Difficulty swallowing

CARDIOVASCULAR

Past	Current	Condition
[ ]	[ ]	High blood pressure
[ ]	[ ]	Low blood pressure
[ ]	[ ]	Blood clots
[ ]	[ ]	Palpitations
[ ]	[ ]	Phlebitis
[ ]	[ ]	Chest pain
[ ]	[ ]	Irregular heart beat
[ ]	[ ]	Cold hands / feet
[ ]	[ ]	Fainting
[ ]	[ ]	Difficult breathing
[ ]	[ ]	Swelling of hands / feet
[ ]	[ ]	Other: ____________

RESPIRATORY

Past	Current	Condition
[ ]	[ ]	Asthma
[ ]	[ ]	Bronchitis
[ ]	[ ]	Frequent colds
[ ]	[ ]	Chronic obstructive
[ ]	[ ]	Pulmonary disease
[ ]	[ ]	Pneumonia
[ ]	[ ]	Cough
[ ]	[ ]	Coughing blood
[ ]	[ ]	Production of phlegm
[ ]	[ ]	Other: ____________

GASTRO-INTESTINAL

Past	Current	Condition
[ ]	[ ]	Nausea
[ ]	[ ]	Vomiting
[ ]	[ ]	Diarrhea
[ ]	[ ]	Belching
[ ]	[ ]	Blood in stools/black
[ ]	[ ]	Stools
[ ]	[ ]	Bad breath
[ ]	[ ]	Rectal pain
[ ]	[ ]	Hemorrhoids
[ ]	[ ]	Constipation
[ ]	[ ]	Pain or cramps
[ ]	[ ]	Indigestion
[ ]	[ ]	Gall bladder disorder
[ ]	[ ]	Gas
[ ]	[ ]	Other: ____________

GENITO-URINARY

Past	Current	Condition
[ ]	[ ]	Kidney stones
[ ]	[ ]	Pain or urination
[ ]	[ ]	Frequent urination
[ ]	[ ]	Blood in urine
[ ]	[ ]	Urgency to urinate
[ ]	[ ]	Unable to hold urine
[ ]	[ ]	Other: ____________

MALE

Past	Current	Condition
[ ]	[ ]	Pain / itching genitalia
[ ]	[ ]	Genital lesions/ discharge
[ ]	[ ]	Impotence
[ ]	[ ]	Weak urinary stream
[ ]	[ ]	Lumps in testicles
[ ]	[ ]	Other: ____________

FEMALE

Past	Current	Condition
[ ]	[ ]	Frequent urinary tract infections
[ ]	[ ]	Frequent vaginal infections
[ ]	[ ]	Pain / itching of genitalia
[ ]	[ ]	Genital lesions / discharge
[ ]	[ ]	Pelvic inflammatory disease
[ ]	[ ]	Abnormal pap smear
[ ]	[ ]	Irregular menstrual periods
[ ]	[ ]	Painful menstrual periods
[ ]	[ ]	Premenstrual syndrome
[ ]	[ ]	Abnormal bleeding
[ ]	[ ]	Menopausal syndrome
[ ]	[ ]	Breast lumps
[ ]	[ ]	Hot flashes
[ ]	[ ]	Menopausal syndrome
[ ]	[ ]	Other: ____________

NEUROLOGICAL

Past	Current	Condition
[ ]	[ ]	Seizures
[ ]	[ ]	Tremors
[ ]	[ ]	Numbness/tingling of limbs
[ ]	[ ]	Concussion
[ ]	[ ]	Pain
[ ]	[ ]	Paralysis
[ ]	[ ]	Other: ____________

PSYCHOLOGICAL

Past	Current	Condition
[ ]	[ ]	Depression
[ ]	[ ]	Anxiety / stress
[ ]	[ ]	Irritability
[ ]	[ ]	Treated for emotional or
[ ]	[ ]	Psychological problems
[ ]	[ ]	Other: ____________

INFECTION SCREENING

Past	Current	Condition
[ ]	[ ]	HIV
[ ]	[ ]	TB
[ ]	[ ]	Hepatitis
[ ]	[ ]	Gonorrhea
[ ]	[ ]	Chlamydia
[ ]	[ ]	Syphilis
[ ]	[ ]	Genital warts
[ ]	[ ]	Herpes: oral
[ ]	[ ]	Herpes: genital

MUSCULAR-SKELETAL

Past	Current	Condition
[ ]	[ ]	Stiff neck / shoulders
[ ]	[ ]	Low back pain
[ ]	[ ]	Back pain
[ ]	[ ]	Muscle spasm, twitching, cramps
[ ]	[ ]	Sore, cold or weak knees
[ ]	[ ]	Joint pain

Source: The following general health forms can be downloaded and customized for your usage at www.acupuncturedeskreference.com

COMMON ICD-9 CODES

Condition	Codes
Abdominal pain	789.00
Acid reflux	536.8
Acne	706.1
Adrenal insufficiency	255.5
Alcohol abuse	305.00
Allergic rhinitis	477.9
Allergy, unspecified	995.3
Amenorrhea	626.0
Angina pectoris	413.9
Ankle sprain/strain	845.00
Anxiety disorders	300.00
Arm/leg pain	729.5
Arthritis	716.90
Arthritis - osteoarthritis, hand	715.4
Arthritis - osteoarthritis, lower leg	715.6
Arthritis, gout	274.0
Asthma, unspecified	493.90
Back pain	724.2
Bells palsy	351.0
Bloating	787.3
Brachial radiculitis	723.1
Breast disorders	610.1
Bronchitis, acute	466.0
Bronchitis, chronic	491.9
Carbuncle or furnacle	680.0
Carpal tunnel syndrome	354.0
Chest pain	786.5
Choleycystis, acute	575.0
Chrohn's disease	555.9
Chronic fatigue syndrome	780.71
Colitis, gastroenteritis	558.9
Common cold	460
Constipation	564.00
Cough	786.2
Cystitis, acute	595.0
Depression	311.0
Depressive reaction, prolonged	309.1
Dermatitis, unspecified	564.00
Diabetes	250.0
Diarrhea	787.91
Diarrhea, colitis	558.9
Diverticulitis	562.11
Dizziness/vertigo	780.4
Drug abuse	505.90
Drug dependence	304.00
Dysmenorrhea	625.3
Earache	388.70
Eczema	692.9
Elbow/forearm spr/str	841.9
Endometriosis	617.0
Fatigue, general	780.79
Fatigue/malaise	780.71
Fever	780.6
Fibromyalgia	729.1
Food poisoning	005.9
Foot sprain/strain	845.10
Gastritis, w/ hemorrhage	535.01
Gastritis, w/o hemorrhage	535.00
GERD/reflux	530.81
Gingivitis, acute	523.0
Gout	274.9
Hair loss, alopecia	704.0
Headache	784.0
Headache, migraine	346.90
Headache, tension	707.81
Hearing loss, unspecified	389.9
Hemorrhoids	455.6
Hepatitis	573.3
Herpes zoster	053.9
Herpes, genital	054.10
High blood pressure	796.2
Hip/thigh sprain/stain	843.9
Hypertension	401.9
Hyperthyroidism	424.9
Hypotension	458.1
Hypothyroidism	244.9
Hypothyroidism	244.9
Impotence	302.71
Indigestion, dyspepsia	536.8
Infertility, female	628.9
Infertility, male	606.9
Influenza	487.1
Insomnia	780.52
Insomnia, w/ sleep apnea	780.51
Irregular menstrual cycle	626.4
Irritable bowel syndrome	564.1
Jaundice	782.4
Joint pain	719.4
Knee pain/strain	844.9
Lumbar sprain/strain	847.2
Mastitis	611.0
Menopause	627.2
Menorrhagia, excess	626.2
Migraine	346.1
MS pain/fibromyalgia	729.1
Nausea, no vomiting	787.02
Neck pain	723.1
Neuralgia, neuritis radiculitis	729.2
Night sweats	780.8
Numbness	782.0
Obesity	278.0
Osteoarthritis	715.00
Osteoporosis	733.00
Painful limbs	729.5
Palpitations	785.1
Paresthesias, numbness	782.0
Pelvic pain	625.9
Pharyngitis, chronic	472.1
PMS	625.4
Polycystic ovarian syndrome	256.1
Prostatitis	601.9
Psoriasis	696.1
Radiculopathy	729.2
Respiratory difficulty, SOB	786.05
Rheumatoid arthritis	714.0
Rotator cuff sprain/strain	840.4
Sciatica	724.3
Shingles	053.9
Shoulder pain	719.41
Shoulder strain	840.9
Sinusitis, acute	461.9
Sinusitis, chronic	473.9
Sore throat, acute	462
Sore throat, chronic	472.1
Stress, acute reaction	308.9
Stress, emotions	308.0
Stress, gross	308.9
Tendonitis	726.90
Tennis elbow	726.32
Thoracic outlet syndrome	353.0
Thyroiditis	245.1
Tinnitus	388.30
TMJ	524.60
Tonsillitis, acute	463
Trigeminal neuralgia	3501
Trigger finger	727.03
Ulcerative colitis	556.9
URI	465.9
Urinary incontinence	788.30
Urticaria, allergic	708.0
Uterine fibroid	218.9
UTI	599.0
Vertigo, dizziness	780.4
Voice loss - aphonia	784.41
Vomiting	787.03
Wart, unspecified	078.10
Weakness	780.79
Weight loss	783.2
Wrist sprain/strain	842.00
Yeast infection	112.0
JOINT PAIN	
Ankle, foot	719.47
Cervical, neck	723.1
Coccyx	724.7
Forearm	719.43
Hand	719.44
Knee	719.46
Lower leg	719.46
Lumbar, Low back	724.2
Pelvic, thigh	719.45
Sacrum	724.6
Sciatica	724.3
Shoulder	719.41
Thoracic	724.1
Thoracic or lumbar	724.4
Upper arm	719.42
STRAINS	
Ankle, foot, unspecified	845.00
Bursitis/ankle	726.70
Bursitis/elbow	726.33
Bursitis/knee	726.60
Bursitis/shoulder	726.10
Coccyx	847.4
Elbow, forearm	841.9
Hip, thigh, unspecified	843.9
Knee, leg, unspecified	844.9
Lumbar, Low back	847.2
Neck	547.0
Rotator cuff	840.4
Sacrum	847.3
Shoulder, arm	840.9
Thoracic	847.1
Wrist, carpal (joint)	842.01
Wrist, unspecified	842.00

Massage Insurance & Protection Strategy

It is increasingly clear that massage therapists no longer have the luxury of complacent belief that a malpractice suit "can't happen to me." There are significant financial and legal risks of treating clients without the proper protections and documentation. Unless you can afford to lose your license and/or afford a litigious civil suit, make sure you have proper malpractice insurance coverage, informed consent and policy forms signed and dated by your clients prior to any treatment. It is crucial to protect your business property, personal property, wage earnings, reputation, professional practice and the ability to continue doing massage without the worries of a malpractice suit.

The following is a listing of insurance resources. There are many associations/organizations that provide liability and malpractice insurance at a discount by joining their associations and organizations. (See page 395)

Massage Liability Insurance

American Health Source, Inc
2040 Raybrook SE, Suite 103
Grand Rapids, MI 49546
888-375-7245
http://americanhealthsource.org

AMTA Liability Insurance
500 Davis St.
Evanston, IL 60201
877-905-2700
www.amtamassage.org/InsCoverage.html

International Massage Association
IMA Group Inc
25 South 4th Street
Warrenton, VA 20186
540-351-0800
www.imagroup.com

Associated Bodywork & Massage Professionals (ABMP)
25188 Genesee Trail Road,
Suite 200, Golden, CO 80401
800-458-2267
www.abmp.com

International Association of Animal Massage & Bodywork (IAAMB)
3347 McGregor Lane
Toledo, OH 43623
800-903-9350
www.iaamb.org/insurance-application.php

Hands-On Trade Association
(800) 872-1282
www.handsoninsurance.com

North American Studio Alliance (NAMASTA)
877-626-2782
530-482-2311
www.namasta.com

Cautions and Contraindications

Always use good judgement in massage. If you are in any doubt, ask your client if he/she is under medical supervision or check with client's primary health care provider. Be sure to use an intake form on the first visit that includes a list of contraindications for massage and informed consent, and office policies. This especially applies to cases of cardiovascular conditions, heart disease, cases of thrombosis, phlebitis, and edema. Keep updated on the latest list of new medicines/contraindications that are reasonable for a skilled therapist to know. (See page 31)

Scope of practice

As a licensed massage therapist, it is important to practice within your limits. Only a physician or qualified health care provider has the ability to diagnose clients. Never practice or use techniques that you are not certified or educated to perform. Trust your instincts. If you see red flags, refer them out to the proper health care provider. You alone cannot help everyone that comes through the door. There are different types of therapists, with varying expertise and modalities to meet different types of clients' needs. Build your referral network with other massage therapists and health care providers. Never make false claims or promises to clients regarding treatment. Explain your experiences without making guarantees. Develop and consistently practice your own professional manner. Pay attention to the client's body language. It can reflect whether or not they feel comfortable and secure. And if all else fails, refer them to someone who can help.

Massage Therapy Informed Consent (Example)

I, ______________________________ (client/patient), understand that massage is intended to enhance relaxation, reduce pain caused by muscle tension, increase range of motion, improve circulation and offer a positive experience of touch.

The general benefits of massage, possible massage contraindications and the treatment procedure have been explained to me. I understand that massage therapy is not a substitute for medical treatment or medications, and that it is recommended that I concurrently work with my Primary Health Care Provider for any condition I may have. I am aware that the massage therapist does not diagnose illness or disease, does not prescribe medications, and that spinal manipulations are not part of massage therapy.

I have informed the massage therapist of all my known physical conditions, medical conditions and medications, and I will keep the massage therapist updated on any changes.

Client Signature __________________ Date______________________

Policies and Confidentiality

Respect the limits, outcomes, boundaries, and privacy of your clients. Keep proper SOAPs on each treatment, including what modalities and therapies were effective. Use clear and effective communication with the client about massage policies, outlining cancellations and treatment procedures. Listen to their questions and concerns. Confidentiality is to be maintained in a safe and private manner, with records stored in locked files and out of public sight. Records should be kept for four to seven years after treatment and then disposed of properly. Always practice appropriate and professional boundaries. Respect the therapeutic relationship and avoid any behavior that may violate patient/practitioner trust.

Cancellations (Example)

Your business is valued and your cooperation is appreciated. We are making a commitment to you to guarantee your appointment time and refusing all other requests once you have made the appointment. A 24-hour cancellation notice is required for any scheduled appointments, including gift certificate sessions. Missed or no-show appointments will result in your being charged the full amount of the session booked unless the appointment can be filled. Depending on our booking schedule, late appointments may not receive the full session time allotted for the treatment service booked: Full payment is required. Emergency cancellations are determined at the Massage Therapist's discretion.

Client Signature __________________ Date______________________

Insurance for Massage

Taking clients with medical insurance and filing medical insurance claims with the company for payment can be great for your massage practice if you would like to increase the number of clients you see for massage. More and more policies are now covering medical massage therapy. Always call the health insurance company prior to treatment to see if the policy covers this and what the criteria for payment are.

Before beginning treatment, make sure that you ask your client if this was an accidental injury. If so, it may be covered by auto insurance, Worker's Compensation, or a miscellaneous accident policy. If this is the case, the client's health insurance may not be responsible for any of the payment.

If you are submitting a claim, be sure that you document the client charts, (SOAPs, CPT, ICD-9) as your records can be subpoenaed by attorneys if there is a court case involved. Do not release records to anyone without obtaining a signed release form from the client. Do not send original documents from client charts. Send photocopies.

Many plans will also require a referral from a physician. HMOs require a referral from the patient's primary health care provider. Some require that the therapist be a part of their network of covered providers.

Still other plans will not cover a massage therapist unless the therapist works in the same office as and under the supervision of a covered physician. Other plans do not recognize massage therapists as a covered provider of service, no matter where they practice. Some plans will want a copy of a prescription from a medical doctor stating the diagnosis, the specific types of treatment to be done, the frequency of treatments, and the length of time for the treatments or there is no coverage. Always check with insurance provider prior to treatment for coverage.

When getting ready to send claims in, the address to send the claims to should be on the insurance card. If not, ask the insurance representative while you are on the phone getting coverage information.

Again, to see if medical insurance covers your services, call the insurance company before the treatment and check the plan involved. The insurance company will also let you know if there is a deductible or co-pay. They will state to you that what they tell you is not a guarantee of benefits. Always mention this to the client so the client will understand that he/she is responsible for payment not covered by the health insurance.

One other important note about filing medical insurance claims - if you are a network provider, realize that you will not be reimbursed for your entire fee. You will be paid the network reimbursement amount and you cannot charge the balance to the client as part of the agreement when you sign up to be a part of the network. If you are a non-network provider, then you can bill the balance to the client.

CPT Codes for Massage

97124	**Therapeutic procedure/Medical massage** - Massage including effleurage, petrissage and/or tapotement (stroking, compression, percussion, therapeutic massage) one or more areas, each 15 minutes
97140	**Manual therapy techniques** - Mobilization, manipulation, manual lymphatic drainage, manual traction, one or more regions, each 15 minutes
97122	**Therapeutic procedure** - Neuromuscular re-education of movement, balance, coordination, kinesthetic sense, posture and proprioception. (Includes Proprioceptive Neuromuscular Facilitation (PNF) one or more areas, each 15 minutes

For certain insurance companies, CPT 97124 and 97140 should not be used to bill for activities within the same session.

Other CPT Codes

97010	Hot and cold packs (supervised)
97018	Paraffin bath
97022	Whirlpool
97026	Infrared (supervised)
97530	Therapeutic activities, each 15 minutes
97110	Therapeutic exercise, each 15 minutes
99070	Supplies and materials

Insurance Providers

The following is a listing of some healthcare providers, some of which will provide some form of coverage for varying health plans. This information is provided to enable you to contact healthcare providers directly in order to obtain benefit information for your patients. Be aware that telephone numbers reflect the current numbers at the printing of this book and are subject to change and will vary according to state and regional plans.

In order for insurance companies to reimburse for massage therapy or any medical service, the condition being treated must be medically necessary. The way insurers initially determine medical necessity is by the diagnosis, designated by a code corresponding with the medical condition provided by the treating health care provider. Use sound and ethical judgment. If you use codes to bill insurance companies that are outside your scope of practice of practice, you may find yourself with disciplinary actions taken from your licensing or governing bodies.

Company	Telephone	Notes
Aetna	(800) 624-0756	
Aetna (HMO)	(800) 323-9930	
Aftra	(800) 562-4690	
Anthem / Blue Cross	(800) 333-0912	
Blue Cross (HMO)	(800) 972-4226	
Blue Shield	(800) 351-2465	
Cigna	(800) 832-3211	
Directors Guild	(323) 866-2200	
Empire (Red Bluff)	(800) 676-2583	
Great West / Cigna	(800) 663-8081	
Guardian	(800) 685-4542	
Health Net	(800) 641-7761	
Medicare	(866) 502-9054	
Motion Pictures	(310) 769-0007	
Oxford / United Healthcare	(800) 666-1353	
PacifiCare	(866) 863-9776	
PacifiCare (HMO) / Secure Horizon	(800) 542-8789	
SAG	(818) 954-9400	
United Healthcare	(877) 842-3210	
Writers Guild	(818) 846-1015	

Important Phone Numbers for Emergency, Local, National, and Healthcare Referrals

Local Numbers

Agency	Telephone Number	Notes
Emergency	*911*	
Police		
Fire		
Poison Control		
Hospital 1		
Hospital 2		
Hospital 3		
County Health Department		
Mental Health Referral		
Domestic Abuse Hotline		
Alcoholic Anonymous		
Rape and Battering Hotline		
Alcoholic Anonymous		
Elder Abuse		
Child Abuse		
Suicide Prevention		
Other		

Many of the numbers can be found in your local telephone directory. We have also listed national directory information in this section that will provide you the number.

Other Massage Therapists & Their Specialties

The best practice management is to know when to refer out. Regardless of your specialty, building a referral network with other healthcare professionals can be a great resource for your patients and complement your practice. The following section offers a location where you refer your patients or specialties. Check with your colleagues or other physicians in the area.

Acupuncturist	Specialty/Area	Telephone	Address
John Doe, LMT	*Rolfing*	*555-1212*	*123 ABC Street, Los Angeles*
Pat White, CMT	*Pregnancy*	*555-1213*	*456 D Street, Santa Monica*

Referral to other Healthcare Professionals

Massage therapists who successfully work with other healthcare professionals have found that one of the key ingredients in development of such relationships is the quality of referrals. MDs are more likely to work with LMTs and CMTs who demonstrate a high level of professionalism with referrals. The following section provides a list of other healthcare professionals that are essential to client care. Talk to your client as well as with your colleagues to find the out which MDs are open to building a referral network in your area.

Healthcare Professional Referral Numbers

Specialty	Physician	Telephone	Address
Allergy			
Acupuncturist			
Acupuncturist			
Cardiologist			
Chiropractor			
Chiropractor			
Chiropractor			
Emergency Medicine			
Endocrinology			
Family Practice			
Family Practice			
Family Practice			
Family Practice			
Gastroenterology			
General Surgery			
General Surgery			
Infectious Diseases			
Internal Medicine			
Midwife			
Neurology			
OB/GYN			
OB/GYN			
Oncology			
Optometry			
Orthopaedic Surgery			
Orthopaedic Surgery			
Pediatrics			
Podiatry			
Psychiatry			
Psychologist			
Radiology			
Rheumatology			
Urology			

Massage-Related Numbers

Massage Agency	Telephone	Notes
National Massage Regulatory		
State Regulatory Agency		
National OSHA	(800) 356-4674	
State OSHA		
U.S. Food and Drug Administration	(888) 463-6332	
CDC	(800) 311-3435	
National Organizations		
State Massage Organizations		

Many of the addresses and phone numbers can be found on the following pages. It is advisable to have them on hand in case of emergencies or questions regarding your practice.

National Numbers

You can contact the following agencies to get more information on local or regional offices, and many provide a wealth of information on their websites. The numbers are subject to change.

	Agency	Telephone
Aging	National Council on Aging	(800) 424-9046
Aging	National Institute on Aging Information Center	(800) 222-2225
AIDS / HIV	AIDS Hotline	(800) 367-2437
AIDS / HIV	National AIDS Hotline	(800) 342-2437
AIDS / HIV	Sexually Transmitted Disease National Hotline	(800) 227-8922
AIDS/HIV	HIV/AIDS Treatment Hotline	(800) 822-7422
Alcohol	A1-Anon/Alateen Family Group Headquarters, Inc	(800) 344-2666
Alcohol	Alcohol and Drug Addictions/Trauma hotline	(800) 544-1177
Alcohol	Alcohol and Drug Information	(800) 729-6686
Alcohol	Alcohol Hotline	(800) 331-2900
Alcohol	Alcoholism and Drug Dependence Hopeline	(800) 622-2255
Alcohol	Children of Alcoholics Foundation, Inc	(800) 359-2623
Alcohol	National Drug and Alcohol Treatment Referral Service	(800) 662-HELP
Child Abuse	Child Abuse Hotline	(800) 4-A-CHILD
Child Abuse	Child Abuse Hotline	(800) 792-5200
Child Abuse	Child Abuse prevention	(800) 257-3223
Child Abuse	Information Services for Child Support	(800) 537-7072
Child Abuse	National Child Abuse Hotline	(800) 422-4453
Depression	National Depressive & Manic-Depressive Association	(800) 826-3632
Disease	Center for Disease Control	(800) 277-8922
Domestic Abuse	Domestic Abuse Hotline	(800) 978-3600
Drug Abuse	Alcohol and Drag Abuse Hotline	(800) 237-6237
Drug Abuse	American Council for Drug Education	(800) 488-3784

Drug Abuse	Center for Substance Abuse Treatment	(800) 662-HELP
Drug Abuse	Cocaine Hotline	(800) COCAINE
Drug Abuse	Drug and Alcohol Treatment Routing Service	(800) 662-4357
Drug Abuse	Marijuana Anonymous	(800) 766-6779
Eating Disorder	Eating Disorders - Bulimia, Anorexia Self Help	(800) 762-3334
Eating Disorder	Eating Disorders Hotline	(800) 445-1900
Elder Abuse	Abuse Registry (Elderly & Disabled)	(800) 962-2873
Elder Abuse	Elder Abuse Hotline	(800) 922-1660
Family Violence	National Domestic Violence/Abuse Hotline	(800) 7997233
Family Violence	Parent Helpline	(800) 942-4357
Family Violence	Parents' Stress Hotline	(800) 632-8188
Grief	Grief Recovery Institute	(800) 445-4808
Health - Alzheimer's	Alzheimer's Association	(800) 272-3900
Health - Cancer	Cancer Information Service	(800) 422-6237
Health - Cystic	Cystic Fibrosis Foundation	(800) 344-4823
Health - Diabetes	Juvenile Diabetes Foundation	(800) 223-1138
Health - Donor	Organ Donor Hotline	(800) 243-6667
Health - Down	National Down Syndrome Congress	(800) 232-6372
Health - Dyslexia	Dyslexia Society	(800) 222-3123
Health - Epilepsy	Epilepsy Foundation	(800) 332-1000
Health - Hearing	Better Hearing Institute	(800) 327-9355
Health - Heart	American Heart Association	(800) 242-8721
Health - Info	National Health Information Center	(800) 336-4797
Health - Info	National OCD Information Hotline	(800) NEWS-4-OCD
Health - Kidney	American Kidney Fund	(800) 638-8299
Health - Liver	American Liver Foundation	(800) 223-0179
Health - Lupus	Lupus Foundation of America	(800) 800-4532
Health - MS	National Multiple Sclerosis Society	(800) 532-7667
Health - Nutrition	National Center for Nutrition	(800) 366-1655
Health - Panic	Panic Disorder Information Hotline	(800) 64-PANIC
Health - Parkinson	National Parkinson Foundation	(800) 327-4545
Health - Reyes	National Reyes Syndrome Foundation	(800) 233-7393
Health - SID	Sudden Infant Death Syndrome Alliance	(800) 221-7437
Health - Spina	Spina Bifida Association	(800) 621-3141
Health - Spine	Spinal Cord Injury	(800) 526-3456
Health - STD	Center for Disease Control-National STD Hotline	(800) 227-8922
Mental Health	Anxiety and Panic	(800) 64-PANIC
Mental Health	Depression Awareness	(800) 421-4211
Mental Health	Mental Health Clearing House	(800) 654-1247
Mental Health	Mental Health Referral	(800) 843-7274
Mental Health	National Council on Compulsive Gambling	(800) 522-4700
Mental Health	National Foundation for Depressive Illness	(800) 248-4344
Mental Health	National Mental Health Association	(800) 969-6642
Poison	Poison Information Center	(800) 777-6476

Pregnancy	Planned Parenthood	(800) 230-7526
Pregnancy	Pregnancy Hotline	(800) 848-5683
Rape	Crisis Help Line -For Any Kind of Crisis	(800) 233-4357
Rape	Crisis Hotlines Abuse/Assault	(800) 962-2873
Rape	Crisis Line	(800) 866-9600
Rape	Crisis Line for the Handicapped	(800) 426-4263
Rape	National Victims Center (for rape or assault)	(800) FYI-CALL
Rape	Rape, Abuse, Incest National Network (RAINN)	(800) 656-HOPE
Rape	Sexual Assault Crisis Line -Hotlines & Information	(800) 643-6250
Rape	Victims of Crime Resources Center	(800) 842-8467
Rape	VOICES, Victims Of Incest Can Emerge Survivors	(800) 7-VOICE-8
Runaways	Boys Town National Hotline	(800) 448-3000
Runaways	Center For Missing and Exploited Children	(800) 843-5678
Runaways	Help Now Hotline	(800) 435-7609
Runaways	Missing and Exploited Children Hotline	(800) 843-5678
Runaways	Missing Children	(888) 356-4774
Runaways	Missing Children Hotline	(800) THE-LOST
Runaways	National Child Safety Council	(800) 327-5107
Runaways	National Hotline for Missing & Exploited Children	(800) 843-5678
Runaways	National Runaway Hotline	(800) 231-6946
Runaways	National Runaway Hotline	(800) 621-4000
Runaways	National Runaway Switchboard	(800) 462-6642
Runaways	National Youth Crisis Hotline	(800) 442-HOPE
Runaways	National Youth Crisis Hotline, Help for Kids	(800) 448-4663
Runaways	Youth Crisis Hot Line	(800) 448-4663
Runaways	Youth Development International	(800) HIT-HOME
Spousal Abuse	National Domestic Violence/Abuse Hotline	(800) 799-7233
Substance Abuse	Cocaine Anonymous (CA)	(800) 347-8998
Substance Abuse	National Treatment Hotline	(800) 662-HELP
Suicide	National Adolescent Suicide Hotline	(800) 621-4000
Suicide	National Cocaine and Suicide Prevention Hotline	(800) 288-1022
Suicide	National Suicide Referral	(202) 237-2280
Suicide	Suicide Crisis Intervention Center	(800) 784-2433

Manufacturer and Distributor Information

Below is a resource listing of massage equipment suppliers and manufacturers/distributors of massage tables. This information is provided to enable you to contact these companies to order or to obtain further information about their products. None of the manufacturers or distributors mentioned has had any connection with the production of this book. Rather, we list these companies because we believe their products to be effective and of high quality. Be aware that addresses, numbers, and URLs are subject to change.

Massage Equipment & Supplies

Advanced Health Products
2257 Old Middlefield Way
Mountain View, CA 94043
800-676-7976
www.massageproducts.com

Banner Therapy Products, Inc.
891 Broadway St.
Asheville, NC 28804
828-277-1189
www.bannertherapy.com

BestMassage.com
1419 W. Howard St.
Chicago, IL 60626
773-764-6542
www.bestmassage.com

BML Basic
501 West Kingshighway
Paragould, AK 72450
800-643-4751
www.bmlbasic.com

Bodywork Central
1522 Shattuck Ave.
Berkeley, CA 94709
888-226-8500
www.bodyworkcentral.com

Bodyworkmall.com
200 E. South Temple, Suite 190
Salt Lake City, UT 84111
866-717-6753
www.bodyworkmall.com

Buymassage.com
Core Institute, FL
866.830.0108
www.coreinstitute.com

Ebodylogic.com
4887 Alpha Rd #210
Farmers Branch, TX 75244
800-662-3306
www.ebodylogic.com

Edcat Enterprise
733 North Beach Street
Daytona Beach, FL 32114
386-253-2385

Gotyourback.com
521 E. Hector Street
Conshohocken, PA 19428
800-677-9830
www.gotyourback.com

Hands-on-supply
800-842-9874
www.handsonsupply.com

Here's The Rub
66 Evergreen Ave.
Warminster, PA 18974
877-484-3782
www.herestherub.net

Masageleader.com
www.massageleader.com

Massage Central
12235 Santa Monica Blvd.
West Los Angeles, CA 90025
310-826-2209
www.mcla.com

Massage King
800-290-3932
www.massageking.com

Massage Supplies and Such
10748 Reading Rd
Cincinnati, OH 45241
800-650-3178
www.massagesuppliesandsuch.com

MHP International
7520 N. St. Louis Avenue
Skokie, IL 60076
888-710-7206
www.mastermassagetables.com

Perfect Touch
110 Broadway
Costa Mesa, CA 92627
949-515-8825
www.perfecttouch1.com

Spa & Bodywork Market
10 River St.
Red Bank, NJ 07701
800-228-6457
www.bestofnature.com

Sunset Park Massage Supplies
4344 S. Manhattan Ave.
Tampa, FL 33611
800-344-7677
www.massagesupplies.com

Yan Jing Supply
1441 York St # 200
Denver, CO 80206
866-837-1346
www.yanjingsupply.com

Massage Table Manufacturers

Astralite
120 Manfre Road
Watsonville, CA 95076
800-368-5483
www.astra-lite.com

Colorado Healing Arts
4635 Broadway
Boulder, CO 80304
800-728-2426
www.greatmassagetables.com

Creative Touch
P.O. Box 912
Lotus, California 95651
530-295-3769
www.massageresources.com

Custom Craftworks
760 Bailey Hill Road
Eugene, OR 97402
800-627-2387
www.customcraftworks.com

Earthlite
3210 Executive Ridge Dr.
Vista, CA 92081
800-872-0560
www.earthlite.com

Galaxy Enteripses Inc
5411 Sheila Street
City of Commerce, CA 90040
323-728-3980
www.galaxymfg.com

Golden Ratio Woodworks
PO Box 440
Emigrant, MT 59027
406-222-5928
www.goldenratio.com

Living Earth Crafts
3210 Executive Ridge Dr.
Vista, CA 92081
800-358-8292
www.livingearthcrafts.com

Oakworks
923 E. Wellspring Rd.
New Freedom, PA 17349
800-558-8850
www.oakworks.com

Pisces Productions
380A Morris Street
Sebastapol, CA 95472
800-822-5333
http://piscespro.com

Stronglite
369 S. Orange St. #7
Salt Lake City, UT 84104
800-289-5487
www.stronglite.com

Touch America
437 Dimmocks Mill Road
Hillsborough, NC 27278
800-678-6824
www.touchamerica.com

Massage Supports

Body Support Systems, Inc
1040 Benson Way
Ashland, OR 97520
800-448-2400
www.bodysupport.com

Massage Linens

Body Linen
9713 South 600 West
Sandy, UT 84070
877-215-9004
www.bodylinen.com

Inner Peace
PO Box 940
Walpole, NH 03608
800-949-7650
www.innerpeace.com

Professional Organizations

There are a number of professional organizations that promote massage/bodywork professions which are needed at this time with all of the issues surrounding licensing and legislation. Many of these organizations are defining professional standards of practice, training, and the ability to bill insurance companies for massage services. We encourage you to support these organizations. You can also contact many of these organizations for information on CEUs, schools, and obtain professional liability insurance and legal requirements in your area.

Organizations and Associations

American Massage Therapy Association (AMTA)
500 Davis St.
Evanston, IL 60201.
877-905-2700
www.amtamassage.org

American Medical Massage Association
2040 Raybrook SE, Suite 103
Grand Rapids, MI 49546
888-375-7245
www.americanmedicalmassage.com

Associated Bodywork & Massage Professionals (ABMP)
25188 Genesee Trail Road,
Suite 200, Golden, CO 80401
800-458-2267
www.abmp.com

National Association for Holistic Aromatherapy (NAHA)
3327 W. Indian Trail Road PMB 144
Spokane, WA 99208
509-325-3419

International Massage Association (IMA)
25 South 4th Street
Warrenton, VA 20186
540-351-0800
www.imagroup.com

International Institute of Reflexology
5650 First Avenue North
PO Box 12642
St Petersburg FL 33733
727-343-4811
www.reflexology-usa.net

International SPA Association (ISPA)
2365 Harrodsburg Road, Suite A325
Lexington, KY 40504
859-226-4326
www.experienceispa.com

Alexander Technique International (ATI)
1692 Massachusetts Ave, 3rd floor
Cambridge, MA 2138
888-668-8996
www.ati-net.com

American Society for the Alexander Technique
P.O. Box 60008
Florence, MA 01062
800-473-0620
www.alexandertech.org

National Association for Holistic Aromatherapy
3327 W. Indian Trail Road PMB 144
Spokane, WA 99208
509-325-3419
www.naha.org

International Association of Animal Massage & Bodywork
3347 McGregor Lane
Toledo, OH 43623
800-903-9350
www.iaamb.org

Worldwide Aquatic Bodywork Association
P.O. Box 889
Middletown, CA 95461
707-987-3801
www.waba.edu

American Organization for Bodywork Therapies of Asia
1010 Haddonfield-Berlin Road Suite 408
Voorhees, NJ 08043
856-782-1616
www.aobta.org

International Myotherapy Association
P.O. Box 65240
Tucson, AR 85728
800-221-4634
www.myotherapy.org

International Association of Healthcare Practitioners
(IAHP) /The Upledger Institute, Inc.
11211 Prosperity Farms Road, Suite D-325
Palm Beach Gardens, FL 33410
800-311-9204
www.iahp.com
www.upledger.com

Esalen Massage and Bodywork Association
55000 Highway 1
Big Sur, CA 93920
831-667-3018
www.esalenmassage.org

The Feldenkrais Guild of North America
3611 SW Hood Avenue Ste100
Portland, OR 97201
800-775-2118
www.feldenkrais.com

Day-Break Geriatric Massage Institute
5760 Northdale Lake Court #C
Indianapolis, IN 46220
317-722-9896
www.daybreak-massage.com/

Healing Touch International
445 Union Blvd., Suite 105
Lakewood, CO 80228
303-989-7982
www.healingtouch.net

Hellerwork® International
406 Berry St.
Mt. Shasta, CA 96067
530-926-2500
www.hellerwork.com

Association for Holotropic Breathwork™ International
P.O Box 400267
Cambridge, MA 02140
617-674-2474
www.breathwork.com

Hospital-Based Massage Network
612 S College Avenue Ste 1
Fort Collins, CO 80524
970-407-9232
www.info4people.com

National Association of Nurse Masage Therapist (NANMT)
28 Lowry Drive
P.O. Box 232
West Milton, OH 45383
800-262-4017
www.nanmt.org

International Association of Infant Massage
1891 Goodyear Avenue, Suite 622
Ventura, CA 93003
805-644-8524
www.iaim-us.com

Hawaiian Lomilomi Association
15-156 Puni Kahakai Loop
Pahoa, HI 96778
808-965-8917
www.lomilomi.org

United States Medical Massage Association
PO Box 2394
Surf City, NC 28445
910-328 3323
www.usmedicalmassage.org

Ancient Healing Arts Association
P.O. Box 1785
Bensalem, PA 19020
1-866-843-2422
www.ancienthealingarts.org

Society of Ortho-Bionomy International®
5335 North Tacoma Street, Suite 21G
Indianapolis, IN 46220
www.ortho-bionomy.org

International Association of Pfrimmer Deep Muscle Therapists
2107 East, 1250 North
Alexandria, IN 46001
877-484-7773
www.pfrimmer.com

American Polarity Therapy Association
PO Box 19858
Boulder, CO. 80308
303-545-2080
www.polaritytherapy.org

International Association of Rubenfeld Synergists (INARS)
19 Thrush Lane
Harpers Ferry, WV 25425
877-RSM-2468
www.rubenfeldsynergy.com

United States Association for Body Psychotherapy (USABP)
8639 B 16th St., Suite 119
Silver Spring, MD 20910
202-466-4619
www.usabp.org

The Day Spa Association
310 17th Street
Union City, NJ 07087
201-865-206
www.dayspaassociation.com/

International Spa Association
2365 Harrodsburg Rd Ste A325
Lexington, KY 40504
888-651-ISPA
www.experienceispa.com

The Spa Association (SPAA)
PO Box 273283
Fort Collins, CO 80527
602-540-4696

National Association of Bodyworkers in Religious Service
5 Big Stone Court
Baltimore, MD 21228-1018
410-455-0277

U.S. Sports Massage Federation/
International Sports Massage Federation
2156 Newport Blvd
Costa Mesa, CA 92627
949-642-0735

Guild for Structural Integration
3197 28th Street
Boulder, CO 80301
800-447-0122
www.rolfguild.org

Rolf Institute® of Structural Integration
5055 Chaparral Court, Suite 103
Boulder, CO 80301
303-449-5903
www.rolf.org

International Thai Therapists Association
P.O. Box 1048
Palm Springs, CA 92263
773-792-4121
www.thaimassage.com

Nurse Healers-Professional Assoc., Inc.
Box 419
Craryville, NY 12521
518-325-1185
www.therapeutic-touch.org

Trager International
3800 Park East Drive
Ste 100 Rm 1
www.trager.com

US Trager Association
13801 W Center St Suite C
Burton OH 44021
440-834-0308
www.tragerus.org

Zero Balancing Health Association
Kings Contrivance Village Center
8640 Guilford Road, Suite 240
Columbia MD 21046
410-381-8956
www.zerobalancing.com/

New York State Society of Medical Massage Therapist
P.O. Box 442
Bellmore, NY 11710
877-697-7668
www.nysmassage.org

Continuing Education (CEU) / Massage Training

Massage therapy license requirements vary from state to state, region to region, city to city, and the laws are constantly changing. It certain states you are required to complete continuing education courses on specific subjects including, professional ethics, HIV, CPR, and prevention of medical errors. There are also specific CEU requirements in certain cities for license renewal in your area. We recommend that you contact the police department in the city and your state licensing board (see page 400) to confirm practice and hours of requirements for license renewal and massage therapy continuing education acceptance. The following is a list of specific instructors/institutes/schools/practitioners that offer CEUs and advanced training in massage therapy.

Acupressure

Acupressure Institute
1533 Shattuck Avenue
Berkeley, CA 94709
800-442-2232
www.acupressureinstitute.com

Acupressure Therapy Institute
One Billings Road
Quincy, MA 02171
617-697-1477
www.acupressuretherapy.com

Aston Pattering

Aston Kinetics
P.O. Box 3568
Incline Village, NV 89450
775-831-8228
www.astonkinetics.com

Body Rolling

Yamuna Body Rolling
132 Perry St.
New York, NY 10014
212-633-2143
www.yamunabodyrolling.com

Bowen Therapy

Bowenwork Academy USA
337 North Rush Street
Prescott, AR 86301
866-862-6936
www.bowtech.com

Breema

Breema Center
6076 Claremont Avenue
Oakland, CA 94618
510-428-0937
www.breema.com

Business Practices

Success Beyond Work
P.O. Box 398238
Miami Beach, FL 33239
www.successbeyondwork.com

Cancer Massage

Tracy Walton
617- 661-5800
www.tracywalton.com

Chair Massage

Touch Pro Institute
584 Castro Street #555
San Francisco, CA 94114
415-621-6817
www.touchpro.com

Connective Tissue Massage

John Latz
7700 Center Bay Drive
North Bay Village, FL 33141
305 754-0983
www.johnlatz.com

Tom Myers
318 Clarks Cove Road
Walpole, ME 04573
207 563-7121
www.anatomytrains.com

Cranialsacral Therapy

G. Dallas Hancock
7827 N. Armenia Avenue
Tampa, FL 33604
813-933-6335
www.dallashancock.com

Milne Institute Inc.
P.O. Box 220
Big Sur, CA 93920
831-667-2323
www.milneinstitute.com

Energywork

California Academy for the Healing Arts
2488 Newport Blvd. Ste D
Costa Mesa, CA 92627
949-574-9480
www.cahaschool.com

Equine Massage

Equi-Myo
800-523-2876
www.equimyo.com

Wilson Meagher Sports therapy
Box 1155
Concord, MA 01742
978-772-9702
www.sportsmassageinc.com

Esalen Massage

Esalen Institute
55000 Highway 1
Big Sur, CA 93920
831-667-3000
www.esalen.org

Feldenkrais

Feldenkrais Method
5436 N. Albina Ave
Portland, OR 97217
800-775-2118
www.feldenkrais.com

Geriatric Massage

Daybreak
7434 - A King George Dr,
Indianapolis, IN 46260
317-722-9896
www.daybreak-massage.com

Hellerwork®

Hellerwork® International
PO Box 17373
Anaheim, CA 92817
714-873-6131
www.hellerwork.com

Hellerwork® International
406 Berry St.
Mt. Shasta, CA 96067
530-926-250
www.hellerwork.com

Hot Stone

LaStone
8110 S. Houghton Road Suite
158-154
Tucson, AR 85747
520-319-6414
www.lastonetherapy.com

Lymphatic Masage

Bruno Chikly
28607 N 152nd St
Scottsdale, AR 85262
561 622-4334
www.iahp.com

Vodder School International
PO Box 5121
Victoria BC V8R 6N4
250-598-9862
www.vodderschool.com

Massage All

International Alliance of Healthcare
Educators (IAHE)
11211 Prosperity Farms Rd. D-325
Palm Beach Gardens, FL 33410
561-622-4334
www.uiahe.com

Medical Massage

Ralph Stephens
PO Box 8267
Cedar Rapids, IA 52408
888-570-9040
www.ralphstephens.com

Muscle Alignment

Erik Dalton
5801 N. Ann Arbor Avenue
Oklahoma City, OK 73122
800-709-505
http://erikdalton.com

Myofascial Release

Bonnie Prudden Myotherapy
P.O. Box 65240
Tucson, AR 85728
520-529-3979
www.bonnieprudden.com

John Barnes
222 West Lancaster Avenue, Suite 100
Paoli, PA 19301
610-644-0136
www.myofascialrelease.com

NMT

CORE Institute
223 West Carolina Street
Tallahassee, FL 32301
850-222-8673
http://coreinstitute.com

Judith Delany
900 14th Avenue North
St. Petersburg, FL 33705
727-821-7167
www.nmtcenter.com

St. John Neuromuscular Therapy Seminars
6565 Park Blvd.
Pinellas Park, FL 33781
http://stjohnseminars.com

Ortho-Bionomy

Society of Ortho-Bionomy International
5335 North Tacoma Street, Suite 21G
Indianapolis, IN 46220
317-536-0064
www.ortho-bionomy.org

Orthopedic Massage

James Waslaski
PO Box 822141
N. Richland Hills, TX 76182
800-643-5543
www.orthomassage.net

OMERI
PO Box 3500, PMB #409
Sisters, OR 97759
888-340-1614
www.omeri.com

Polarity

American Polarity Therapy
122 N. Elm Street, Suite 512
Greensboro, NC 27401
336-574-1121
www.polaritytherapy.org

Fritz Smith
8640 Guilford Road, Suite 240
Columbia, MD 21046
www.zerobalancing.com

Randolph Stone
122 N Elm Street, #512
Greensboro, NC 27401
336-574-1121
www.polaritytherapy.org

Pregnancy Massage

Carole Osborne-Sheets
9449 Balboa Ave. Suite 310
San Diego, CA 92123
858-277-8827
www.bodytherapyassociates

Claire Marie Miller
8703 Rollingwood Road
Chapel Hill, NC 27516
919-967-9015
www.nurturingthemother.com

Elaine Stillerman
P O Box 150337
Brooklyn, NY 11215
212-533-3188
www.mothermassage.net

Kate Jordan Seminars
8950 Villa La Jolla Dr. #A217
La Jolla, CA 92037
760-436-0418
www.katejordanseminars.com

Kelly Lott
P.O. 40444
Ft. Worth, TX 76140
817-516-7037
www.kellylott.com

Reflexology

American Academy of Reflexology
725 E. Santa Anita Avenue, # B
Burbank, CA 91501
818-841-7741
www.americanacademyofreflexology.com

Connecticut Center for Universal Reflexology
102 Wolcott Road
Wolcott, CT 06716
203-879-5551
www.universalreflexology.net

International Institute of Reflexology
5650 First Avenue North
St Petersburg, FL 33733
727-343-4811
www.reflexology-usa.net

Rolfing® Structural Integration

Guild for Structural Integration
P.O. Box 1559
Boulder, CO 80306
303-447-0122
www.rolfguild.org

The Rolf Institute of Structural Integration
5055 Chaparral Ct. Suite 103
Boulder, CO 80301
303-449-5903
www.rolf.org

Hellerwork® International
406 Berry St.
Mt. Shasta, CA 96067
530-926-250
www.hellerwork.com

Shiatsu

Namasté Institute
328 Main Street, Studio 201
Rockland, ME 04841
207-593-7455
www.namasteinstitute.com

Ohashi Institute
147 West 25th Street
New York, NY 10001
800-810-4190
www.ohashiatsu.org

Shiatsu Massage School
2309 Main Street
Santa Monica, CA 90405
310-581-0097
www.smsconline.com/

Zen Shiatsu Chicago
825A Chicago Ave
Evanston, IL 60202
847-864-1130
www.zenshiatsuchicago.org

Soft Tissue Release

Stuart Taws
P.B.BOX 2252
Garden Grove, CA 92842
714-539-9351
www.softtissuerelease.com

Somatics

Lawrence Gold
1574 Coburg Road, #300
Eugene, OR 97401
505 699-8284
www.somatics.com

Sound Therapy

Kairos Institute of Sound Healing
157 Pacheco Rd., Box 8
Llano de San Juan, NM 87543
575-587-2689
www.acutonics.com

Sports Massage

James Malley
7525 Auburn Blvd., Suite 9
Citrus Heights, CA 95610

www.abundanthealth.com

Stretching

Aaron Mattes (Active Isolated Stretching)
P.O. Box 17217
Sarasota, FL 34276
800-809-3747
http://stretchingusa.com

Spiri Physical Inc.
P.O. Box 370761
Miami, FL 33137
305-438-9649
www.spiriphysical.com

Thai Massage

ITM international Training Massage
17/6-7 Morakot Road
Chiang Mai 50300 Thailand
(66 53) 218632
www.itmthaimassage.com

Universal Touch
406 Republic Court
Deerfield Beach, FL. 33442
954-429-9213
www.universaltouchinc.com

Trager

Milton Trager
13801 West Center Street, Suite C
Burton, OH 44021
440-834-0308
www.tragerus.org

Watsu / Water Massage

Harold Dull
P.O. Box 1817
Middletown, CA 95461
707-987-3801
www.waba.edu

Resources You Can Use

There are many reliable resources and information in alternative remedies. We have listed the following professional associations and health organizations. Besides brochures, booklets and hotlines, many provide reliable on-line information.

Acupuncture & Oriental Medicine

Accreditation Commission for Acupuncture and Oriental Medicine (ACAOM)
Maryland Trade Center #3, 7501 Greenway Center Drive,
Suite 760, Greenbelt, MD 20770
301-313-0855
www.acaom.org

American Association of Acupuncture & Oriental Medicine (AAAOM) AKA AOM Alliance
PO Box 162340
Sacramento, CA 95816
916-443-4770
www.aaom.org or www.aaaomonline.org

Council of Acupuncture and Oriental Medicine Associations
1217 Washington Street
Calistoga, CA 94515
707-942-9380
www.acucouncil.org

National Acupuncture Detoxification Association (NADA)
PO Box 1927
Vancouver WA 98668-1927
360-254-0186
http://acudetox.com

National Certification Commission for Acupuncture and Oriental Medicine (NCCAOM)
76 South Laura Street, Suite 1290
Jacksonville, FL 32202
904-598-1005
www.nccaom.org

Aromatherapy

The National Association for Holistic Aromatherapy
3327 W. Indian Trail Road PMB 144
Spokane, WA 99208
509-325-3419
www.naha.org

Ayurvedic Medicine

American Academy of Ayurvedic Medicine, Inc.
100 Jersey Avenue
Building B, Suite 300
New Brunswick, N.J. 08901
732-247-3301
www.ayurvedicacademy.com

National Institute of Ayurvedic Medicine
584 Milltown Road Brewster,
New York 10509
845-278-8700
www.niam.com

Biofeedback

Association for Applied Psychophysiology and Biofeedback
10200 W 44th Ave #304
Wheat Ridge, CO 80033
303-422-8436
www.aapb.org

Chelation Therapy

American Association of Naturopathic Physicians
4435 Wisconsin Ave NW Ste 403
Washington DC 20016
866-538-2267
www.naturopathic.org

Chiropractic

American Chiropractic Association
1701 Clarendon Boulevard
Arlington, VA 22209
703-276-8800
www.amerchiro.org

Craniosacral Therapy
(see massage organization)

Herbal Medicine

American Botanical Council
6200 Manor Road
Austin, TX 78723
512-926-4900
www.herbalgram.org

Herb Research Foundation
4140 15th St.
Boulder, CO 80304
303-449-2265
www.herbs.org

Homeopathy

National Center for Homeopathy
801 North Fairfax Street Suite 306
Alexandria, VA 22314
703-548-7790
http://nationalcenterforhomeopathy.org

North American Society of Homeopaths
PO BOX 450039
Sunrise, FL 33345-0039
206-720-7000
www.homeopathy.org

Naturopathic Medicine

American Association of Naturopathic Physicians
4435 Wisconsin Ave NW Ste 403
Washington DC 20016
866-538-2267
www.naturopathic.org

Nutrition

National Association of Nutrition Professionals
P.O. Box 1172
Danville, CA 94526
800-342-8037
www.nanp.org

American Dietetic Association
120 South Riverside Plaza, Suite 2000
Chicago, Illinois 60606-6995
800-877-1600
www.eatright.org

Council for Responsible Nutrition
1828 L Street, NW, Suite 900
Washington, DC, 20036-5114
202-776-7929
www.crnusa.org

Osteopathic Medicine

American Osteopathic Association
142 East Ontario Street
Chicago, IL 60611
800-621-1773
www.osteopathic.org

Reflexology
(see massage organization)

Yoga

American Yoga Association
P.O. Box 19986
Sarasota, FL 34276
941-927-4977
www.americanyogaassociation.org

Massage Regulatory State Agencies

We have listed the following state regulatory agencies on massage licensing, laws, and regulation. Codes and laws can be found through their respective agencies. Due to the changing nature of laws, the information, regulations, and regulatory agencies are subject to change.

Alabama	
State of Alabama Board of Massage Therapy 610 S McDonough St. Montgomery, AL 36104 334-269-9990, 866-873-4664 334-263-6115 (fax) **Required Education & Exams** 650 Hours, Written **Exam** NCETMB	**Fees & Interval** Application: $25.00 Licensing: $100.00 (every 2 years) Renewal: $100.00 **Title & Credential Type** Massage Therapist/License (LMT) **CEUs, Interval** 16 every 2 years
Alaska	Does not have state licensing requirements

Arizona	
Arizona Board of Massage Therapy 1400 West Washington, Suite 230 Phoenix, AZ 85007 602-542-8604 334-263-6115 (fax) **Required Education & Exams** 700 Hr., Written **Exam** NCETMB	**Fees & Interval** Application & Initial License: $165.00 Fingerprint: $24.00 Duplicate license: $40.00 Renewal: $75.00 every 2 years **Title & Credential Type** Massage Therapist/License (LMT) **CEUs, Interval** 25 every 2 years

Arkansas	
Akansas State Board of Massage Therapy PO Box 20739 Hot Springs, AR 71903 501-520-0555 501-623-4130 (fax) **Required Education & Exams** 500 Hours, Written **Exam** MBLEx	**Fees & Interval** Application & Initial License: $130.00 Annual Renewal: $30.00 (LMT) every 2 years Annual Renewal: $40.00 (Master) Annual Renewal: $45.00 (Instructor) **Title & Credential Type** Massage Therapist/License (LMT) Master Massage/Therapist/ Instructor **CEUs, Interval** 6 per year

California	
California Massage Therapy Council One Capitol Mall, Suite 320 Sacramento, CA 95814 916-669-5336 916-444-7462 (fax) **Required Education & Exams** Contact State/Local Office 500 Hours, Written 250 Hours, Written **Exam** Contact State/Local Office	**Fees & Interval** Contact State/Local Office **Title & Credential Type** Voluntary Certification Massage Therapist/License (LMT) or Practitioner (CMP) **CEUs, Interval** Contact State/Local Office

Colorado	
Colorado Department of Regulatory Agencies 1560 Broadway, Suite 1550 Denver, CO 80202 303-894-7855 ext. 7800 303-894-7693 (fax) **Required Education & Exams** 500 Hours **Exam** NCETMB or MBLEx	**Fees & Interval** Application & Initial License: $90 CBI Fingerprint: $39.50 Renewal: Contact State/ Local Office **Title & Credential Type** Massage Therapist/ Certification (RMT) **CEUs, Interval** 16 every 2 years

Connecticut	
Connecticut Department of Public Health - Massage Therapy Licensure 410 Capitol Avenue Hartford, CT 06134 860-509-7603 860-509-8457 (fax) **Required Education & Exams** 500 Hours **Exam** NCETMB	**Fees & Interval** Application: $300.00 Renewal: $200.00 every 2 years **Title & Credential Type** Massage Therapist/License (LMT) **CEUs, Interval** 24 every 4 years

Delaware	
Delaware Board of Massage and Bodywork Cannon Building 861 Silver Lake Blvd., Suite 203 Dover, DE 19904 302-744-4500 302-739-2711 (fax) **Required Education & Exams** 300 Hr., CMT 200 Hr., Temp. CMT 500 Hr., LMT, Written or Practical **Exam** NCETMB	**Fees & Interval** Application: $104 (CMT and LMT) Upgrade from Active CMT to LMT: $32 Temporary Massage Technician: $52 Renewal: $104 every 2 years **Title & Credential Type** Massage Technician Massage Therapist/License (LMT) **CEUs, Interval** 12, 2 Yr., CMT 24, 2 Yr., LMT

Florida	
Florida Board of Massage Therapy 4052 Bald Cypress Way, Bin# C06 Tallahassee, FL 32399 850-245-4161 850-921-6184 (fax) **Required Education & Exams** 500 Hr., Written **Exam** NCETMB	**Fees & Interval** Application: $205.00 Renewal: $155.00 every 2 years **Title & Credential Type** Massage Therapist/License (LMT) **CEUs, Interval** 25 every 2 years Course HIV/Aids

Georgia	
Georgia Board of Massage Therapy 237 Coliseum Drive Macon, GA 31217 478-207-2440 478-207-1663 (fax) **Required Education & Exams** 500 Hr., Written & Practical **Exam** NCETMB or MBLEx	**Fees & Interval** Application: $125 Renewal: $75 every 2 years **Title & Credential Type** Massage Therapist/License (LMT) **CEUs, Interval** 24 every 2 years

Hawaii	
Hawaii Board of Massage Therapy P.O. Box 3469 Honolulu, HI 96801 808-587-3222 **Required Education & Exams** 570 Hr., Written **Exam** State Exam	**Fees & Interval** Application: $50.00 License: $25.00 Renewal: $25.00 MT Apprentice: $50 **Title & Credential Type** Massage Therapist/License (LMT) Massage Apprentice/Permit **CEUs, Interval** None
Idaho	Does not have state licensing requirements

Illinois	
Illinois Division of Professional Regulation 320 West Washington Street, 3rd Floor Springfield, IL 62786 217-785-0800 217-782-7645 (fax) **Required Education & Exams** 500 Hr., Written **Exam** NCETMB	**Fees & Interval** License: $175.00 Renewal: $175.00 every 2 years **Title & Credential Type** Massage Therapist/License (LMT) **CEUs, Interval** 24 every 2 years

Indiana	
Indiana State Board of Massage Therapy 402 W Washington St, Room W072 Indianapolis, Indiana 46204 317-234-2051 **Required Education & Exams** 500 Hr., Written **Exam** NCETMB	**Fees & Interval** Application: $100.00 Renewal: $100 every 4 years **Title & Credential Type** Massage Therapist/ Certification (CMT) **CEUs and Interval** Contact State/Local Office

Iowa	
Iowa Bureau of Professional Licensure 321 E. 12th Street Des Moines, IA 50319 515-281-6959 515-281-3121 (fax) **Required Education & Exams** 500 Hr., Written **Exam** NCETMB or MBLEx	**Fees & Interval** Application: $120.00 Renewal: $120.00 every 2 years **Title & Credential Type** Massage Therapist/License (LMT) **CEUs and Interval** 24 every 2 years

Kansas	Does not have state licensing requirements

Kentucky	
Kentucky Board of Licensure for Massage Therapy P.O. Box 1360 Frankfort, KY 40602 502-564-3296 502-564-4818 (fax) **Required Education & Exams** 600 Hr., Written **Exam** NCETMB	**Fees & Interval** Application: $50.00 Initial License: $75.00 Renewal: $100.00 every 2 years **Title & Credential Type** Massage Therapist/License (LMT) **CEUs and Interval** 24 every 2 years

Louisiana	
Louisiana Board of Massage Therapy 12022 Plank Road Baton Rouge, LA 70811 225-771-4090 225-771-4021 (fax) **Required Education & Exams** 500 Hr., Written & Oral **Exam** NCETMB or MBLEx	**Fees & Interval** Application: $75.00 Renewal: $125.00 every 2 years **Title & Credential Type** Massage Therapist/License (LMT) **CEUs and Interval** 12 per year

Maine	
Maine Massage Therapy Licensure 35 State House Station Augusta, ME 04333 207-624-8624 207-624-8637 (fax) **Required Education & Exams** 500 Hr. or Exam **Exam** NCETMB or MBLEx	**Fees & Interval** Application & Initial License: $71.00 Renewal: $25.00 per year **Title & Credential Type** Massage Therapist/License (LMT) **CEUs and Interval** Contact State/Local Office

Maryland	
Maryland Board of Chiropractic and Massage Therapy Examiners 4201 Patterson Avenue Baltimore, Maryland 21215 410-764-4726 410-358-1879 (fax) **Required Education & Exams** 500 Hr., RMP, Written 500 Hr. & 60 College Credits, LMT, Written **Exam** NCETMB or NCCAOM	**Fees & Interval** Application & Initial License: $350.00 State Jurisprudence Exam: $200.00 Renewal: $250.00 every 2 years **Title & Credential Type** Massage Practitioner/ Registration Massage Therapist/License (CMT) **CEUs and Interval** 24 every 2 years

Massachusetts	
Massachusetts Board of Registration of Massage Therapy 239 Causeway Street, Suite 500 Boston, MA 02114 617-727-1747 617-727-0139 (fax) **Required Education & Exams** 500 Hr., Written **Exam** Contact State/Local Office	**Fees & Interval** App & License: $225.00 Annual Renewal: $150.00 **Title & Credential Type** Massage Therapist/License (LMT) **CEUs and Interval** Contact State/Local Office

Michigan	
Michigan Department of Community Health Capitol View Building 201 Townsend Street Lansing, MI 48913 517-373-3740 **Required Education & Exams** 500 Hr., Written **Exam** NCETMB	**Fees & Interval** Renewal: $75 per year **Title & Credential Type** Massage Therapist/License **CEUs and Interval** 18 every 3 years

Minnesota	Does not have state licensing requirements

Mississippi	
Mississippi State Board of Massage Therapy PO Box 20 Morton, MS 39117 601-732-6038 **Required Education & Exams** 700 Hr., Written **Exam** NCETMB or MBLEx	**Fees & Interval** Initial Application: $50.00 Renewal: $192 every 2 years **Title & Credential Type** Massage Therapist/License (LMT) CEUs and Interval 24 every 2 years

Missouri	
Missouri Board of Therapeutic Massage P.O. Box 1335 Jefferson City, MO 65102 573-522-6277 573-751-0735 (fax) **Required Education & Exams** 500 Hr., Written **Exam** NCETMB, MBLEx, NCCAOM or AMMA	**Fees & Interval** Student License: $25.00 Provisional License: $50.00 Permanent License: $100.00 Renewal: $200.00 every 2 years **Title & Credential Type** Massage Therapist/License (LMT) **CEUs, Interval** 12 every 2 years

Montana	
Montana Board of Massage Therapists PO Box 200513 Helena, MT 59620 406-841-2380 406-841-2305 (fax)	

RESOURCE

Nebraska	
Nebraska Department of Health and Human Services PO Box 94986 Lincoln, NE 68509 402-471-2115 402-471-3577 (fax) **Required Education & Exams** 1,000 Hr., Written **Exam** NCETMB	**Fees & Interval** Initial License: $110.00 Temporary License: $25.00 Renewal: $110.00 every 2 years **Title & Credential Type** Massage Therapist/License (LMT) **CEUs, Interval** 24 every 2 years

Nevada	
State of Nevada Board of Massage Therapy 1755 E. Plumb Lane Suite 252 Reno, NV 89502 775-688-1888 775-786-4264 (fax) **Required Education & Exams** 500 Hr., Written **Exam** NCETMB	**Fees & Interval** Application: $100.00 License: $150.00 Background Check: $125.00 Fingerprint: check with local authorities Renewal: $150.00 per year **Title & Credential Type** Massage Therapist/License (LMT) **CEUs, Interval** 12 every year

New Hampshire	
New Hampshire Department of Health and Human Services 129 Pleasant St. Concord, NH 03301 603-271-0853 603-271-5590 (fax) **Required Education & Exams** 750 Hr., Written & Practical **Exam** NCETMB	**Fees & Interval** Application: $125.00 Renewal: $100.00 every 2 years **Title & Credential Type** Massage Therapist/License (LMT) **CEUs, Interval** 12 every 2 years

New Jersey	
Massage, Bodywork and Therapy Examining Committee PO Box 45010 Newark, NJ 07101 973-504-6430 **Required Education & Exams** 500 Hr. or Written **Exam** NCETMB or NCCAOM	**Fees & Interval** Application: $75.00 Certification: $120.00 Criminal Background Check: $78.00 Renewal: $120 every 2 years **Title & Credential Type** Massage Therapist/ Certification (CMT) **CEUs, Interval** 20 every 2 years

New Mexico	
New Mexico Massage Therapy Board 2550 Cerrillos Road Santa Fe, NM 87505 505-476-4870 505-476-4645 (fax) **Required Education & Exams** 650 Hr., Written **Exam** NCETMB	**Fees & Interval** Application: $75.00 Initial License: Pro-rated at $5.00 per month Renewal: $125.00 every 2 years **Title & Credential Type** Massage Therapist/License (LMT) **CEUs, Interval** 16 every 2 years

New York	
Office of the Professions Massage Therapy Unit 89 Washington Avenue Albany, NY 12234 518-474-3817 ext. 150 518-486-2981 (fax) **Required Education & Exams** 1,000 Hr., Written **Exam** State Exam	**Fees & Interval** Application: $150.00 Limited Permit: $35.00 Renewal: $50.00 every 3 years **Title & Credential Type** Massage Therapist/License (LMT)/Registration **CEUs, Interval** Contact State/Local Office

North Carolina	
North Carolina Board of Massage and Bodywork Therapy PO Box 2539 Raleigh, NC 27602 919-546-0050 919-833-1059 (fax) **Required Education & Exams** 500 Hr., Written **Exam** ABTE, NCETM or MBLEx	**Fees & Interval** Licensure: $150.00 Renewal: $100.00 every 2 years **Title & Credential Type** Massage and Bodywork/ License (LMT) **CEUs, Interval** 24 every 2 years

North Dakota	
North Dakota Board of Massage PO Box 218 Beach, ND 58621 701-872-4895 **Required Education & Exams** 750 Hr., Written **Exam** State Exam, NCETM	**Fees & Interval** Licensure: $150.00 Renewal: $100.00 every year **Title & Credential Type** Massage Therapist/License (LMT) **CEUs, Interval** 18 every year

Oklahoma	Does not have state licensing requirements

Oregon	
Oregon Board of Massage Therapists 748 Hawthorne Avenue NE Salem, OR 97301 503-365-8657 503-385-4465 **Required Education & Exams** 500 Hr., Written & Practical **Exam** MBLEx	**Fees & Interval** Application & Initial License: $150.00 Practical Exam: $150.00 Renewal: $100.00 every 2 years **Title & Credential Type** Massage Therapist/License (LMT) **CEUs, Interval** 25 every 2 years

Pennsylvania	Does not have state licensing requirements

Rhode Island	
Office of Health Professionals Regulation 3 Capitol Hill - Room 105 Providence, RI 02908 401-222-2827 401-222-1272 (fax) **Required Education & Exams** 500 Hr., Written & Practical **Exam** NCETMB or NCETM	**Fees & Interval** Licensing: $50.00 Renewal: $50.00 every year **Title & Credential Type** Massage Therapist/License (LMT) **CEUs, Interval** Call State/Local Office

South Carolina	
South Carolina Massage/ Bodywork Panel PO Box 11329 Columbia, S.C. 29211 803-896-4501 803-896-4525 (fax) **Required Education & Exams** 500 Hr., Written **Exam** NCETMB or MBLEx	**Fees & Interval** Application: $50.00 Initial License: $100.00 Renewal: $160.00 every 2 years Late Renewal: $210.00 **Title & Credential Type** Massage/Bodywork License (LMT) **CEUs, Interval** 12 every 2 years

South Dakota	
South Carolina Board of Massage Therapy P.O. Box 1062 Sioux Falls, SD 57101 605-271-7103 605-331-2043 (fax) **Required Education & Exams** 500 Hr., Written **Exam** NCETMB or NBCA exam from AMMA	**Fees & Interval** Application Fee: $100.00 Initial License: $65.00 Renewal Fee: $65.00 every year **Title & Credential Type** Massage Therapist/License (LMT) **CEUs, Interval** 8 every 2 years

RESOURCE

Tennessee	
Tennessee Board of Massage Licensure 227 French Landing, Suite 300 Nashville, TN 37243 615-532-3202 **Required Education & Exams** 500 Hr., Written **Exam** NCETMB or MBLEx	**Fees & Interval** Application: $60.00 FBI Fingerprint: $48.00 **Title & Credential Type** Massage Therapist/License (LMT) **CEUs, Interval** 25 every 2 years

Texas	
Texas Massage Therapy Licensing Program P.O. Box 149347, Mail Code 1982 Austin , Texas 78714 512-834-6616 512-834-6677 (fax) **Required Education & Exams** 500 Hr., Written **Exam** NCETMB or MBLEx	**Fees & Interval** Application: $117.00 Renewal: $106.00 every 2 years **Title & Credential Type** Massage Therapist/License (LMT) **CEUs, Interval** 12 every 2 years

Utah	
Utah Division of Occupation and Professional Licensing 160 East 300 South Salt Lake City, Utah 84111 801-530-6628 801-530-6511 (fax) **Required Education & Exams** 600 Hr., LMT 1,000 Hr. Apprenticeship, AMT **Exam** NCETMB or MBLEx	**Fees & Interval** Application: $60.00 BCI Fingerprint: $15.00 FBI Fingerprint: $20.00 Renewal: $52.00 every 2 years **Title & Credential Type** Massage Therapist/License (LMT) Massage Therapist/ Apprentice **CEUs, Interval** Call State/Local Office

Vermont	Does not have state licensing requirements

Virginia	
Virginia Board of Nursing Perimeter Center 9960 Mayland Drive, Suite 300 Henrico, Virginia 23233 804-367-4515 804-527-4455 (fax) **Required Education & Exams** 500 Hr., Written **Exam** NCETMB	**Fees & Interval** Application and Initial Certification: $105.00 Renewal: $70.00 every 2 year **Title & Credential Type** Massage Therapist/ Certification (CMT) **CEUs, Interval** 25 every 2 years

Washington	
Board of Massage P.O. Box 47865 Olympia, WA 98504 804-367-4403 804-527-4466 (fax) **Required Education & Exams** 500 Hr., Written **Exam** MBLEx, NCE or NESL	**Fees & Interval** Initial License: $115.00 Renewal: $90.00 **Title & Credential Type** Massage Practitioner/License **CEUs, Interval** 16 every 2 years

West Virginia	
West Virginia Massage Licensure Board 179 Summers Street, Suite 711 Charleston, WV 25301 304-558-1060 304-558-1061 (fax) **Required Education & Exams** 500 Hr., Written **Exam** NCETMB or MBLEx	**Fees & Interval** Initial Application: $25.00 Biennial License: $200.00 Renewal: $100.00 every 2 years **Title & Credential Type** Massage Therapist/License (LMT) **CEUs, Interval** 24 every 2 years

Wisconsin	
State of Wisconsin Department of Regulation and Licensing 1400 E. Washington Ave. Madison, WI 53703 608-266-2112 608-261-7083 (fax) **Required Education & Exams** 600 Hr., Written **Exam** NCETMB, NCETM, NCCAOM	**Fees & Interval** Exam: $57.00 Certification: $53.00 Renewal: $53.00 every 2 years **Title & Credential Type** Massage Therapist/License (CMT) **CEUs, Interval** Contact State/Local Office

Wyoming	Does not have state licensing requirements

MBLEx: licensing offered by Federation of State Massage Therapy Boards
CEU: Continuing education hours required for renewal of license
NCBTMB: Offers 2 exams, the **NCETMB** & **NCETM**; check with your state to determine which it accepts

Diagnostic Laboratories

The following diagnostic laboratories offer innovative tests for integrative health professionals, including female and male hormone screenings, adrenal stress hormone tests, thyroid panels, platelet or urine catecholamine panels, digestive stool analysis, candida antibody tests, Chronic Fatigue Immune Dysfunction Syndrome evaluation, ELISA food allergy testing, hair analysis for toxic and essential elements, nutritional assays, amino acid assays, essential fatty acids profile, vitamin and mineral analysis. Many of the laboratories are physician-friendly and can be obtained by blood, saliva or urine. The range of tests will vary according to specialties and will require massage practitioner to setup an account. We have listed some specialties, however many labs offer a broad spectrum of tests.

Aeron Lifecycles Clinical Laboratory
1933 Davis St., Suite 310
San Leandro, CA 94577
800-631-7900
www.aeron.com

Aeron LifeCycles is a clinical laboratory with research interests in linking hormonal changes with many of the diseases and symptoms of aging including osteoporosis, cardiovascular disease and cancer. Accurate salivary hormone tests are currently available for: estradiol, progesterone, testosterone, DHEA, and melatonin.

Alletess
216 Pleasant Street
Rockland, MA 02370
800-225-5404
www.foodallergy.com

Alletess specializes in food and inhalant allergy testing, food sensitivities and other tests to assess the immune system.

Biochemical Laboratories
P.O.Box 157
Edgewood, NM 87015
505-832-4100

Specializes in hair trace mineral analysis tests.

Doctors Choice
P.O.Box 337
Washington Depot, CT 06794
888-852-2723
www.doctorschoice.net

Turnkey services setup for all organized testing results from various laboratories.

Doctors Data, Inc.
3755 Illinois Avenue
St. Charles, IL 60174-2420
800-323-2784
708-231-3649
www.doctorsdata.com

Doctor's Data, Inc. is an independent reference laboratory that provides tests in the following area: toxic and hair analysis, amino acids, and metabolites in blood and urine tests.

ELISA/ACT Biotechnologies
14 Pidgeon Hill #300
Sterling, VA 22181
800-553-5472
703-450.2980
www.elisaact.com

Provides a range of comprehensive allergy and hypersensitivity tests.

Genova Diagnostics
63 Zillicoa Street
Asheville, N.C. 28801
800-522-4762
www.genovadiagnostics.com

Specializes in tests of physiological function. All tests use samples of stool, urine, saliva, blood, and hair. Results focus on how well the body is doing its job in six important areas: digestion, nutrition, detoxification/ oxidative stress, immunology/allergy, production and regulation of hormones, and heart and cardiovascular systems.

Immuno Laboratories, Inc.
1620 W. Oakland Park Blvd.
Ft. Lauderdale, FL 33311
954-691-2500
800-231-9197
www.immunolabs.com

Offers ELISA delayed food allergy testing, a highly sensitive candida assay, as well as an ELISA gluten/ gliadin assay.

Immunosciences Lab, Inc.
8730 Wilshire Blvd., Suite 305
Beverly Hills, CA 90211
310-657-1077
800-950-4686
www.immuno-sci-lab.com

A diagnostic and research facility that specializes in innovative microbiology and immunology laboratory testing. Tests in the following categories: allergy, autoimmune diseases, cancer and its early diagnosis, chronic fatigue syndrome, immunology and serology, immunotoxicology and intestinal health.

King James Medical Laboratory/Omegatech
24700 Center Ridge Rd., #113
Cleveland, OH 44145
216-835-2150
800-437-1404
www.kingjamesomegatech-lab.com

The King James Medical Laboratory, Inc. provides the analysis of metals in hair and water samples to both the general public and healthcare practitioners.

Medtox
1238 Anthony Road
Burlington, NC 27215
336-226-6311
www.medtox.com

Medtox laboratories offer full range clinical tests and toxicology reports,

Meridian Valley Lab
801 SW 16th Street Suite 126
Renton, WA 98055
425-271.8689
www.meridianvalleylab.com

A clinical reference lab and nutritional testing for practitioners. The lab offers the following tests: allergy (ELISA), amino acids, bone density, complete stool and digestive analysis, essential fatty acids profile, mineral analysis, steroid, hormone panels, thyroid panels.

Metametrix Clinical Laboratory
3425 Corporate Way
Duluth, GA 30096
770-446-5483
800-221-4640
www.metametrix.com

Metametrix Clinical Laboratory provides a wide range of test in nutritional insufficiencies, metabolic dysfunction, and toxicity and detoxification.

Optimum Health Resource Laboratories, Inc.
419 South Federal Highway
Dania Beach, FL 33004
954-926-8020
www.optimumhealthresource.com

Optimum Health Resource provides food intolerance testing.

Quest Diagnostics
3 Giralda Farms
Madison, NJ 07940
800-222-0446
www.questdiagnostics.com

Quest Diagnostics offer full range of routine and specialty laboratory tests and services in laboratories throughout the USA.

Spectracell Laboratories, Inc.
10401 Town Park Drive
Houston, TX 77027
800-227-5227
713-621-3101
www.spectracell.com

SpectraCell Laboratories Inc. specializes in functional intracellular testing. Their tests offer application for assessing many clinical conditions including cardiovascular risk, immunological disorders, metabolism measurements and nutritional analysis.

U.S. BioTek Laboratories
13500 Linden Ave North
Seattle, WA 98125
877-318-8728
206-365-1256
www.usbiotek.com

US BioTek Laboratories provides a range of tests including: antibody, amino acids, bone density, complete stool and digestive analysis, urinary metabolic tests, hormone panels, thyroid panels.

Vitamin Diagnostics
2 Industrial Dr # A
Keyport, NJ 07735
732-583-7773

Offers specialized nutritional testing for nutrient status.

RESOURCES FOR THE STUDY OF MASSAGE

The following pages detail resources for the study of massage, providing for each the name of the book and its author(s), publisher, and principal city and publication date for the publisher's distribution.

Clearly, there will be substantial differences in opinion about the quality of each book; in fact, it was not always easy to place the books within one of the categories based on the criteria established here since many books overlap categories and many provide broad discussions on wide-ranging topics of massage modalities and treatments. Emphasis is placed on such features as: inclusion of quality of work; comprehensiveness in dealing with the subject at hand; apparent reliability of the information presented; and readability.

A massage therapist with an extensive library would have books from each category (at least from those that correspond to his or her scope of practice). A minimum library of about 15-30 such books in these categories would likely provide the resource information that is essential to conduct a successful massage practice.

MASSAGE

Barbara Ann Brennan, *Hands of Light: A Guide to Healing Through the Human Energy Field*, Bantam Doubleday Dell Pub, 1993.

Ben E. Benjamin & Gale Borden, *Listen to Your Pain: The Active Person's Guide to Understanding, Identifying, and Treating Pain and Injury*, Viking Press, New York, NY, 1984.

Carla-Krystin Andrade & Paul Clifford, *Outcome-Based Massage: From Evidence to Practice (2nd Edition)*, Lippincott Williams & Wilkins, Philadelphia, PA, 2008.

Carole Osborne-Sheets, *Pre and Perinatal Massage Therapy: A Comprehensive Practioners' Guide to Pregnancy, Labor, Postpartum*, Body Therapy Associates, 1988.

Clair Davies, *The Frozen Shoulder Workbook: Trigger Point Therapy for Overcoming Pain & Regaining Range of Motion*, New Harbinger Publications, Oakland, CA, 2006.

David Hoffmann, *Healthy Bones & Joints: A Natural Approach to Treating Arthritis, Osteoporosis, Tendinitis, Myalgia & Bursitis*, Storey Books, New York, NY, 2000.

Eilean Bentley, *Head, Neck and Shoulders Massage: A Step-by-Step*, St. Martins Press, New York, NY, 2000.

Frances Tappan & Patricia Benjamin, *Tappan's Handbook Of Healing Massage Techniques: Classic, Holistic, And Emerging Methods (3rd Edition)*, Prentice Hall, Saddle River, NJ, 1998.

Jack W. Painter, *Technical Manual of Deep Wholistic Bodywork: Postural Integration*, Bodymind Books, 1987.

James Clay & David Pounds, *Basic Clinical Massage Therapy: Integrating Anatomy and Treatment (2nd Edition)*, Lippincott Williams & Wilkins, Philadelphia, PA, 2003.

John Hamwee & Fritz Smith, *Zero Balancing: Touching the Energy*, North Atlantic Books, Berkeley, CA, 2000.

Joseph Ashton & Duke Cassel, *Review for Therapeutic Massage and Bodywork Certification*, Lippincott Williams & Wilkins, Philadelphia, PA, 2006.

Kalyani Pemkumar, *The Massage Connection: Anatomy and Physiology*, Lippincott Williams & Wilkins, Philadelphia, PA, 2003.

Lawrence Jones, Randall Kusunose & Edward Goering, *Strain CounterStrain*, Jones Strain-CounterStrain, Inc, Carlsbad, CA, 1995.

Mark F. Beck, *Milady's Theory and Practice of Therapeutic Massage (3rd Edition)*, Delmar Publishers, Florence, KY, 1999.

R. Louis Schultz, Rosemary Feitis, Diana Salles & Ronald Thompson, *The Endless Web: Fascial Anatomy and Physical Reality*, North Atlantic Books, Berkeley, CA, 1996.

Rene Cailliet, *Soft Tissue Pain and Disability (3rd Edition)*, F A Davis Co, Philadelphia, PA, 1996.

Ron Kurtz, *Body-Centered Psychotherapy: The Hakomi Method: The Integrated Use of Mindfulness, Nonviolence and the Body*, Liferhythm, Medocino, CA, 1997.

Rosie Spiegel, *Bodies, Health and Consciousness: A Guide to Living Successfully in Your Body Through Rolfing and Yoga*, Srg Pub, 1994.

Ruth Werner, *A Massage Therapist's Guide to Pathology (Lww Massage Therapy & Bodywork*, Lippincott Williams & Wilkins, Philadelphia, PA, 2008.

Susan Salvo, *Massage Therapy: Principles and Practice*, Saunders Comapany, New York, NY, 2007.

Thomas Hendrickson, *Massage for Orthopedic Conditions*, Lippincott Williams & Wilkins, Philadelphia, PA, 2002.

Thomas W. Myers, *Anatomy Trains: Myofascial Meridians for Manual and Movement Therapists (2nd Edition)*, Churchill Livingstone, London, England, 2008.

Tom Valentine & Carole Valentine, *Applied Kinesiology: Muscle Response in Diagnosis, Therapy and Preventive Medicine*, Amer Intl Distribution Corp, 1989.

ACUPRESSURE

Alon Lotan, *Acupoint Location Guide*, Estem, Yodfat, Isreal, 2000.

Andrew Ellis, Nigel Wiseman, & Ken Boss, *Fundamentals of Chinese Acupuncture*, Paradigm Publications, Brookline, MA, 1988.

Chris Jarmey, *A Practical Guide to Acu-points*, North Atlantic Books, Berkeley, CA, 2008.

F. M. Houston, *The Healing Benefits of Acupressure: Acupuncture Without Needles*, Keats Pub, Lincolnwood, IL, 1993.

Giovanni Maciocia, *Diagnosis in Chinese Medicine, A Comprehensive Guide*, Churchill Livingstone, London, England, 2004.

Giovanni Maciocia, *Foundations of Chinesel Medicine*, Churchill Livingstone, London, England, 1989.

Giovanni Maciocia, *The Practice of Chinese Medicine*, Churchill Livingstone, London, England, 1994.

Iona Marsaa Teeguarden, *Acupressure Way of Health: Jin Shin Do*, Japan Publications, Japan, 1978.

Jack Forem, *Healing with Pressure Point Therapy: Simple, Effective Techniques for Massaging Away More Than 100 Common Ailments*, Prentice Hall Press, Saddle River, NJ, 1999.

John & Dan Bensky, *Acupuncture: A Comprehensive Text*, Eastland Press, Seattle, WA, 1981.

Julian Kenyon M.D., *Acupressure Techniques: A Self-Help Guide*, Healing Arts Press, Rochester, VT, 1996.

Maoliang Qiu, *Chinese Acupuncture and Moxibustion*, Churchill Livingstone, London, England, 1993.

Michael Reed Gach, *Acupressure's Potent Points: a Guide to Self-Care for Common Ailments*, Bantam, New York, NY, 1990.

Paul Lundberg, *The New Book of Shiatsu: Vitality and Health Through the Art of Touch*, Gaia Books Ltd, London, England, 2005.

Peter Deadmean & Mazin Al-Khafaji, *A Manual of Acupuncture*, Journal of Chinese Medicine Publications, East Sussex, England, 1998.

Sun Peilin, *The Treatment of Pain with Chinese Herbs and Acupuncture*, Churchill Livingstone, London, England, 2002.

Ted Kaptchuk, *The Web That Has No Weaver: Understanding Chinese Medicine*, McGraw-Hill, New York, NY, 2000.

Zhang Enquin, *Chinese Acupuncture and Moxibustion*, Publishing House of Shanghai College of Traditional Chinese Medicine, Shanghai, China, 1990.

Zhu Ming Ching, *Handbook for Treatment of Acute Syndromes by Using Acupuncture and Moxibustion*, Eight Dragons Publishing, Hong Kong, 1992.

ALTERNATIVE MEDICINE

Bill Gottlieb, *Alternative Cures: The Most Effective Natural Home Remedies for 160 Health Problems*, Da Capo Press, Cambridge, MA, 1998.

Charles Fetrow, *The Complete Guide to Herbal Medicines*, Pocketbooks, New York, NY, 2000.

Daniel Krinsky & James LaValle, *Lexi-Comp's Natural Therapeutics Pocket Guide, 2nd Edition*, Lexi-Comp, Inc, Hudson, OH, 2003.

Earl Mindell & Virginia Hopkins, *Prescription Alternatives, Third Edition: Hundreds of Safe, Natural Prescription-Free Remedies to Restore and Maintain Your Health*, McGraw Hill, Random House, 2003.

Gary Null, *The Complete Encyclopedia of Natural Healing*, Kensington Books, New York, NY, 2005.

Hazel Courtney, *500 of the Most Important Health Tips You'll Ever Need*, Cico Books, London, England, 2001.

James Balch & Mark Stengler, *Prescription for Natural Cures: A Self-Care Guide for Treating Health Problems with Natural Remedies Including Diet and Nutrition, Nutritional Supplements, Bodywork, and More*, John Wiley & Sons, Hoboken, NJ, 2004.

Larry Trivieri & John Anderson, *Alternative Medicine: The Definitive Guide (2nd Edition)*, Celestial Arts, Berkeley, CA, 2002.

Linda Page, *Healthy Healing: A Guide to Self-Healing for Everyone, 12th Edition*, Traditional Wisdom, Inc., New York, NY, 2004.

Linda Skidmore-Roth, *Mosby's Handbook of Herbs & Natural Supplements*, Mosby, St. Louis, MO, 2001.

Michael Murray & Joseph E. Pizzorno, *Encyclopedia of Natural Medicine*, Prima Publishing, Rocklin, CA, 1998.

Michael Murray & Joseph Pizzorno, *Encyclopedia of Natural Medicine, Revised Second Edition*, Three Rivers Press, New York, NY, 1997.

Michael Murray & Joseph Pizzorno, *Encyclopedia of Nutritional Supplements: The Essential Guide for Improving Your Health Naturally*, Three Rivers Press, New York, NY, 1996.

Michael Van Straten, *Organic Super Foods*, Octopus Publishing, London, England, 2003.

Phyllis Balch, *Prescription for Herbal Healing: An Easy-to-Use A-Z Reference to Hundreds of Common Disorders and Their Herbal Remedies*, Penguin Putnam, New York, NY, 2002.

Phyllis Balch, *Prescription for Nutritional Healing, 4th Edition: A Practical A-to-Z Reference to Drug-Free Remedies Using Vitamins, Minerals, Herbs & Food Supplements ... A-To-Z Reference to Drug-Free Remedies)*,, Penguin Putnam, New York, NY, 2004.

Phyllis Balch, *Prescription for Nutritional Healing: The A-to-Z Guide to Supplements: The A-to-Z Guide to Supplements*, Penguin Putnam, New York, NY, 2002.

Ralph Golan, *Optimal Wellness*, Wellspring/Ballantine, New York, NY, 1995.

Steven Brantman & Andrea Girman, *Mosby's Handbook of Herbs and Supplements and Their Therapeutic Use*, Mosby, St. Louis, MO, 2003.

Vance Ferrell & Edgar Archbold, *Natural Remedies Encyclopedia*, Harvestime Books, Altamount, TN, 2002.

ANATOMY

Andrew Biel, *Trail Guide to the Body*, Books of Discovery, 2005.

Blandine Germain, *Anatomy of Movement*, Eastland Press, Seattle, WA, 1993.

Carmine Clemente, *Anatomy: A Regional Atlas of the Human body (4th Edition)*, Lippincott Williams & Wilkins, Philadelphia, PA, 1997.

Deane Juhan, *Job's Body: A Handbook for Bodywork (Third Edition)*, Station Hill Press, Barrytown, NY, 1998.

Frank Netter, *Atlas of Anatomy*, Rittenhouse Book Distributors Inc, King of Prussia, PA, 1997.

Gerald Tortura, *Principles of Human Anatomy*, John Wiley & Sons, Hoboken, NJ, 1999.

Kay Sieg & Sandra Adams, *Illustrated Essentials of Musculoskeletal Anantomy*, Megabooks, Gainesville, FL, 1996.

Paul Blakey, *The Muscle Book*, Himalayan Institute Press, Honesdale, PA, 1992.

Stanley Hoppenfeld, *Physical Examination of the Spine Extremities*, Prentice Hall, Saddle River, NJ, 1976.

AROMATHERAPY

Kurt Schnaubelt Ph.D., *Advanced Aromatherapy: The Science of Essential Oil Therapy*, Healing Arts Press, Rochester, VT, 1998.

Len Price & Shirley Price, *Aromatherapy for Health Professionals*, Churchill Livingstone, London, England, 2006.

BOWEN THERAPY

Frank Navratil, *Bowen Therapy: Tom Bowen's Gift to the World*, Return to Health Books, 2003.

Julian Bakeer, *The Bowen Technique*, Human Kinetics, Champaign, IL, 2002.

BREEMA

Jon Schreiber, *Breema and the Nine Principles of Harmony*, Breema Center Publishing. Oakland, CA 2007.

Jon Schreiber, *Every Moment Is Eternal*, Breema Center Publishing. Oakland, CA 2007.

Jon Schreiber, *Self-Breema: Exercises for Harmonious Life*, Breema Center Publishing. Oakland, CA 2004.

Jon Schreiber, *Freedom Is in this Moment*, Breema Center Publishing. Oakland, CA 2004.

NUTRITION

E.N. Anderson, *The Food of China*, Yale University Press, New Haven, CT, 1988.

Henry Lu, *Chinese System of Food Cures*, Sterling, New York, NY, 1986.

Maoshing Ni & Cathy NcNease, *The Tao of Nutrition*, College of Tao & Traditional Chinese Healing, Los Angeles, CA, 1987.

Paul Pitchford, *Healing with Whole Foods*, North Atlantic Books, Berkeley, CA, 2002.

Rosa LoSan & Suzanne LeVert, *Chinese Healing Foods*, Pocket Books, New York, NY, 1998.

Zhang Enquin, *Chinese Medicated Diet*, Publishing House of Shanghai College of Traditional Chinese Medicine, Shanghai, China, 1988.

CRANIOSACRAL THERAPY

Don Cohen & John E. Upledger, *An Introduction to Craniosacral Therapy: Anatomy, Function, and Treatment*, North Atlantic Books, Berkeley, CA, 1983.

Hugh Milne, *The Heart of Listening: A Visionary Approach to Craniosacral Work VOL. 1*, North Atlantic Books, Berkeley, CA, 1998.

John E. Upledger, *Your Inner Physician and You: Craniosacral Therapy and Somatoemotional Release, 2nd Ed*, North Atlantic Books, Berkeley, CA, 1997.

John E. Upledger & Jon Vredevoogd, *Craniosacral Therapy*, Eastland Press, Seattle, WA, 1983.

DEEP TISSUE

Art Riggs, *Deep Tissue Massage: A Visual Guide to Techniques*, North Atlantic Books, Berkeley, CA, 2002.

Don Scheumann, *The Balanced Body: A Guide to Deep Tissue and Neuromuscular Therapy*, Lippincott Williams & Wilkins, Philadelphia, PA, 2002.

ENERGYWORK

Robert O Becker & Gary Selden, *The Body Electric, Electromagnetism and the Foundation of Life*, Quill, William Morrow, New York, 1985.

Barbara Brennan, *Hands of Light and Light Emerging, The Journey of Personal Healing*, Bantam Books, New York, 1991 and 1993.

Donna Eden, *Energy Medicine*, Tarcher/Putnam, New York, 1999.

Ariel, F Hubbard, *Come From the Heart: A Practical Guidebook to Healing with Divine Energy, Part One and Part Two*, California Academy for the Healing Arts, Costa Mesa, CA 2000.

Michael Gerber, *Vibrational Medicine for the 21st Century: A Complete Guide to Healing with Energy and Vibrational Medicine*, Eagle Brook/Harper Collins, New York, 2000.

HELLERWORK®

Joseph Heller & William Henkin, *Bodywise: An Introduction to Hellerwork for Regaining Flexibility and Well-Being*, North Atlantic Books, Berkeley, CA, 2004.

Joseph Heller, *Bodywise*. Wingbow Press, Berkely, CA, 1991.

LOMI LOMI

Makana Risser Chai, *Na Mo'olelo Lomilomi: The Traditions of Hawaiian Massage and Healing*, Bishop Museum Press, Honolulu, HI, 2005.

Nancy, S Kahalewai, *Hawaiian Lomilomi: Big Island Massage*, IM Publishing, 2005.

LYMPHATIC MASSAGE

Michael Foldi & Roman Strossenreuther, *Foundations of Manual Lymph Drainage*, Mosby, St. Louis, MO, 2004.

Ramona Moody French, *Milady's Guide to Lymph Drainage Massage*, Milady, Albany, NY, 2003.

Roger Uren, John Thompson & Robert Howman-Giles, *Lymphatic Drainage of the Skin and Breast: Locating the Sentinel Nodes*, Harwood Academic Publisher, 1999.

William N. Brown, *The Touch that Heals, The Art of Lymphatic Massage*, Self-published, 2008.

MYOFASCIAL

Donna Finando & Steven Finando, *Trigger Point Therapy for Myofascial Pain: The Practice of Informed Touch*, Healing Arts Press, Rochester, VT, 2005.

Leon Chaitow & Sandy Fritz, *A Massage Therapist's Guide to Understanding, Locating and Treating Myofascial Trigger Points*, Churchill Livingstone, London, England, 2006.

Marian Wolfe-Dixon, *Myofascial Massage (Lww Massage Therapy & Bodywork Educational*, Lippincott Williams & Wilkins, Philadelphia, PA, 2006.

Robert King, *Myofascial Massage Therapy*, Bobkat, 1996.

ROLFING® STRUCTURAL INTEGRATION

Hans Georg Brecklinghaus, *Balancing Your Body: A Self-Help Approach to Rolfing Movement*, Lebenshaus Verlag, 2002.

Ida Rolf, *Rolfing: Reestablishing the Natural Alignment and Structural Integration of the Human Body for Vitality and Well-Being*, Healing Arts Press, Rochester, VT, 1989.

Ida Rolf, *Rolfing and Physical Reality*, Inner Traditions Intl Ltd, Rochester, VT, 1990.

Betsy Sise, *The Rolfing Experience, Integration in the Field of Gravity*, Hohm Press, Prescott, AZ, 2005.

Rosemary Feitis & Louis Schultz, *Remembering Ida Rolf*, North Atlantic Books, Berkeley, CA, May 1997.

Briah Anson, *Rolfing Stories of Personal Empowerment*, North Atlantic Books, Berkeley, CA, July 1998.

SHIATSU

Chris Jarmey, *The Foundations of Shiatsu*, North Atlantic Books, Berkeley, CA, 2007.

Chris Jarmey, *Shiatsu, Revised Edition*, Thorsons, New York, NY, 2000.

DoAnn T. Kaneko, *Oriental Healing Arts: Doann's Long Form (Spiral-bound)*, Shiatsu Massage School of California, Santa Monica, CA, 1994.

Paul Lundberg, *The Book of Shiatsu: A Complete Guide to Using Hand Pressure and Gentle Manipulation to Improve Your Health, Vitality and Stamina*, Fireside, 2003.

Shizuto Masunaga, *Zen Shiatsu: How to Harmonize Yin and Yang for Better Health*, Japan Publications, Japan, 1977.

Toru Namikoshi, *The Complete Book of Shiatsu Therapy*, Japan Publications, Japan, 2001.

Wataru Ohashi, *Reading the Body: Ohashi's Book of Oriental Diagnosis*, Penguin, New York, NY, 1991.

SPORTS MASSAGE

Joan Watt, *Massage for Sport*, Crowood Press, Marlborough, England, 1999.

Lars Peterson & Per Renström, *Sports Injuries: Their Prevention and Treatment - 3rd Edition*, Human Kinetics, Champaign, IL, 2000.

Mel Cash, *Sport & Remedial Massage Therapy*, Ebury Press, London, England, 1996.

Pat Archer, *Therapeutic Massage in Athletics*, Lippincott Williams & Wilkins, Philadelphia, PA, 2006.

Patricia Benjamin & Scott Lamp, *Understanding Sports Massage*, Human Kinetics Pub, Champaign, IL, 1996.

Sandy Fritz, *Sports & Exercise Massage: Comprehensive Care in Athletics, Fitness, & Rehabilitation*, Mosby, St. Louis, MO, 2005.

Simeno Niel-Asher, *The Concise Book of Trigger Points, Revised Edition*, North Atlantic Books, Berkeley, CA, 2006.

William Weintraub, *Tendon and Ligament Healing: A New Approach Through Manual Therapy*, North Atlantic Books, Berkeley, CA, 1999.

THAI MASSAGE

C. Pierce Salguero, *Thai Massage Workbook: Basic and Advanced Courses*, Findhorn Press, Findhorn, Scotland, 2007.

Harald Brust, *Art of Traditional Thai Massage*, Unknown, 1997.

Howard Derek Evans, *A Myofascial Approach to Thai Massage: East meets West*, Churchill Livingstone, London, England, 2009.

Kam Thye Chow, *Thai Yoga Massage: A Dynamic Therapy for Physical Well-Being and Spiritual Energy*, Healing Arts Press, Rochester, VT, 2004.

Kay Rynerson, *The Thai Massage Workbook*, Crow's Wing Studio, Seattle, WA, 2009.

Maneewan Chia; Max Chia, *Nuad Thai: Traditional Thai Massage*, Healing Tao Books, Los Angeles, CA, 2005.

Maria Mercati, *Thai Massage Manual: Natural Therapy for Flexibility, Relaxation, and Energy Balance*, Sterling, New York, NY, 2005.

TRIGGER POINT

Bonnie Prudden, *Myotherapy: Bonnie Prudden's Complete Guide to Pain-Free Living*, Ballantine Books, 1985.

Clair Davies, Amber Davies & David G. Simons, *The Trigger Point Therapy Workbook: Your Self-Treatment Guide for Pain Relief, Second Edition*, New Harbinger Publications, Oakland, CA, 2004.

Dimitrios Kostopoulos & Konstantine Rizopoulos, *The Manual of Trigger Point and Myofascial Therapy*, Slack Incorporated, 2001.

John Sharkey, *The Concise Book of Neuromuscular Therapy: A Trigger Point Manual*, North Atlantic Books, Berkeley, CA, 2008.

Leon Chaitow, *Soft-Tissue Manipulation: A Practitioner's Guide to the Diagnosis and Treatment of Soft-Tissue Dysfunction and Reflex Activity*, Healing Arts Press, Rochester, VT, 1987.

TUINA THERAPY

Jinxue Li, *Chinese Manipulation and Massage: Chinese Manipulative Therapy*, Elsevier Science, London, England, 1990.

Maria Mercati, *The Handbook of Chinese Massage: Tui Na Techniques to Awaken Body and Mind*, Healing Arts Press, Rochester, VT, 1997.

Sarah Pritchard, *Chinese Massage Manual: The Healing Art of Tui Na*, Sterling, New York, NY, 1999.

Shen Guoquan & Yan Juntao, *Illustrations of Tuina Manipulations*, Shanghai Scientific & Technical Publisher, Shanghai, China, 2004.

Sun Chengnan, *Chinese Bodywork: A Complete Manual of Chinese Therapeutic Massage*, Pacific View Press, Shanghai, China, 2000.

Sun Shuchun, *Atlas of Therapeutic Motion for Treatment and Health: A Guide to Traditional Chinese Massage and Exercise Therapy*, Foreign Languages Press, Beijing, China, 1989.

Wang Fu, *Chinese Tuina Therapy*, Foreign Languages Press, Beijing, China, 1994.

Xu Xiangcai, *Chinese Tui Na Massage: The Essential Guide to Treating Injuries, Improving Health & Balancing Qi*, YMAA Publication Center, Jamaica Plains, MA, 2002.

Wei Guikang, *Illustrated Therapeutic Manipulation in TCM Orthopedics and Traumatology*, Shanghai Scientific and Technical Publishers, Shanghai, China 2003.

Zhang Enqin, *Chinese Massage: A Practical English-Chinese Library of Traditional Chinese Medicine*, Publishing House of Shanghai College of Traditional Chinese Medicine, Shanghai, China, 1992.

WESTERN MEDICINE

AMA, *AMA Encyclopedia of Medicine*, Random House, New York, NY, 2003.

Fred Ferri, *Guide to the Care of Medical Patient, 4th Edition*, Mosby, St. Louis, MO, 1998.

James J. Rybacki, *The Essential Guide to Prescription Drugs*, Harper Perennial, New York, NY, 2006.

Kathleen Mahan and Sylvia Escott-Stump, *Krause's Food, Nutrition, & Diet Therapy, 10th Edition*, Saunders Company, New York, NY, 2000.

Mark Beers & Robert Porter, *The Merck Manual (18th ed.)*, Merck & Co., Rahway, NJ, 2007.

John Boik, *Natural Compounds in Cancer Therapy*, Oregon Medical Press, Princeton, MN, 2001.

Winter Griffith and Stephen Moore, *Complete Guide to Prescription and Nonprescription Drugs 2007 (Complete Guide to Prescription and Nonprescription Drugs)*, Harper Collins, New York, NY, 2007.

James J. Rybacki, *The Essential Guide to Prescription Drugs*, Harper Perennial, New York, 2006.

Melvyn R. Werbach, *Foundations of Nutritional Medicine,* Third Line Press, Tarzana, CA, 1997.

Melvyn R. Werbach, *Healing Through Nutrition*, 1993, Harper Collins, New York, NY, 1993.

Melvyn R. Werbach, *Nutritional Influences on Illness, Second Edition*, Third Line Press, Tarzana, CA, 1993.

Melvyn R. Werbach, *Nutritional Influences on Mental Illness, Second Edition*, Third Line Press, Tarzana, CA, 1999.

Lawrence M. Tierney, *Current Medical Diagnosis & Treatment, 2006*, McGraw Hill, New York, NY, 2006.

ALASKA

Alaska Learning Institute
Anchorage, AK
907-242-6369

CB Healing Institute
Anchorage, AK
907-248-8961

Oriental Healing Arts School of Massage Therapy
Anchorage, AK
907-279-0135

ALABAMA

Birmingham School of Massage.
Birmingham, AL
205-414-1477

Virginia College at Birmingham
Birmingham, AL
205-943-2110

Calhoun Community College
Decatur, AL
256-306-2555

Massage Therapy Institute
Decatur, AL
256-306-0444

North Alabama Wellness School of Massage
Florence, AL
256-767-1890

Gadsden State Community College
Gadsden, AL
256-549-8320

Red Mountain Institute, Inc.
Homewood, AL
205-933-0702

Virginia College at Huntsville
Huntsville, AL
256-533-7837

International School of Structural Integration
Madison, AL
256-772-0669

Madison School of Massage Therapy
Madison, AL
256-430-9756

Blue Cliff Career College
Mobile, AL
251-473-2220

Capps College
Mobile, AL
251-344-1203

Capps College Massage Therapy School
Mobile, AL
251-344-1203

H. Councill Trenholm State Technical College
Montgomery, AL
334-420-4397

Montgomery School of Bodywork & Massage
Montgomery, AL
334-270-9340

Virginia College at Montgomery
Montgomery, AL
334-277-3390

Southern Union State Community College
Opelika, AL
334-745-6437

Aromatherapy Institute
Theodore, AL
251-653-9900

ARKANSAS

Lurleen B. Wallace Community College
Opp, AL
334-493-5375

White River School of Massage
Fayetteville, AR
479-521-2550

ARIZONA

Arizona School of Integrative Studies
Clarkdale, AZ
928-639-3455

East Valley Institute of Technology
Mesa, AZ
480-461-4000

Desert Wind Healing Arts
Oro Valley, AZ
520-360-7469

Arizona School of Massage Therapy - Phoenix
Phoenix, AZ
602-331-4325

Bryman School
Phoenix, AZ
602-274-4300

Denver School of Massage
Phoenix, AZ
602-331-4325

Phoenix College
Phoenix, AZ
602-285-7800

WestWind Massage Academy
Phoenix, AZ
602-265-4466

Cortiva Institute
Scottsdale, AZ
480-945-9461

RainStar University of Complementary and Alternative Medicine
Scottsdale, AZ
480-423-0375

Northern Arizona Massage Therapy Institute (NAMTI)
Sedona, AZ
928-282-7737

Sedona School of Massage
Sedona, AZ
928-284-3693

Arizona School of Massage Therapy -Tempe
Tempe, AZ
480-784-9461

Southwest Institute of Healing Arts
Tempe, AZ
480-994-9244

Cortiva Institute
Tucson, AZ
520-792-1191

Providence Institute
Tucson, AZ
520-881-4765

CALIFORNIA

Hellerwork International
Anaheim, CA
714-873-6131

American Institute of Natural Healings
Antioch, CA
925-777-9995

Arcata School of Massage
Arcata, CA
707-822-5223

Vitality College of Healing Arts
Carlsbad, CA
760-931-0704

School of Healing Touch
Castro Valley, CA
510-886-0893

Fremont College
Cerritos, CA
562-809-5100

Massage Center
Chatsworth, CA
818-773-0140

Healing Arts Institute
Citrus Heights, CA
916-725-3999

Institute of Conscious Bodywork
Corte Madera, CA
415-945-9945

California Academy for the Healing Arts
Costa Mesa, CA
949-574-9480

Institute of Psycho-Structural Balancing
Culver City, CA
310-342-7130

De Anza College
Cupertino, CA
408-864-8814

Massage Therapy Institute
Davis, CA
530-753-4428

National Holistic Institute College of Massage Therapy
Emeryville, CA
510-547-6442

Natural Healing Institute of Naturopathy
Encinitas, CA
760-943-8485

Touch Therapy Institute
Encino, CA
818-788-0824

Healing Hands School of Holistic Health
Escondido, CA
760-746-9364

Fair Oaks Massage Institute
Fair Oaks, CA
916-965-4063

Trinity College
Fairfield, CA
707-424-6027

Dahn Healing Institute of Massage Therapy
Fullerton, CA
714-992-5126

Fullerton College
Fullerton, CA
714-992-7000

Heartwood Institute
Garberville, CA
707-923-5000

Bryan College
Gold River, CA
800-878-5515

CalCopa Massage School
Huntington Beach, CA
714-964-7744

United Education Institute - Huntington Park Campus
Huntington Park, CA
213-427-3700

Konocti College of Holistic Studies
Kelseyville, CA
707-279-2539

Hendrickson Method Institute
Kensington, CA
510-524-3107

Western Institute of Neuromuscular Therapy
Laguna Hills, CA
949-830-6151

California Professional College
Los Angeles, CA
213-387-5900

LA Vocational Institute
Los Angeles, CA
213-480-4882

Watsu Institute School of Shiatsu & Massage
Middletown, CA
707-987-3801

School of Traditional Medical Thai Massage
Mill Valley, CA
415-384-0242

Abrams College
Modesto, CA
209-527-7777

Lifestream Massage School
Napa, CA
707-226-2090

Napa Valley School of Massage
Napa, CA
707-253-0627

Phillips School of Massage
Nevada City, CA
530-265-4645

Institute of Professional Practical Therapy
North Hollywood, CA
818-980-8990

Kingston University
Norwalk, CA
562-868-6488

McKinnon Institute of Massage
Oakland, CA
510-465-3488

Ojai School of Massage
Ojai, CA
805-640-9798

West Coast College - Ontario
Ontario, CA
909-986-3200

Career Networks Institute
Orange, CA
714-568-1566

Lincoln Institute of Body Therapy
Orange, CA
714-998-4943

SCHOOLS

As of printing of this book and changing nature of businesses the information is subect to change.

Desert Resorts School of Somatherapy
Palm Springs, CA
760-323-5806

Body Therapy Center
Palo Alto, CA
650-328-9400

McKinnon Body Therapy Center
Palo Alto, CA
510-465-3488

Sky Hill Institute School of Wholistic Healing Arts
Petaluma, CA
707-778-9445

Mesa Academy of Massage
Placentia, CA
714-579-3330

Poway Academy of Hair Design
Poway, CA
858-748-1490

New Life Institute of Massage Therapy
Redding, CA
530-222-1467

Hands-on Medical Massage School
Redlands, CA
909-793-4263

Mendocino School of Holistic Massage and Advanced Healing Arts
Redwood Valley, CA
707-485-8197

Touching For Health Center
Salida, CA
209-543-9170

Diamond Light School of Massage & Healing Arts
San Anselmo, CA
415-454-6651

Body Mind College
San Diego, CA
858-453-3295

International Professional School of Bodywork
San Diego, CA
858-490-1154

Meridian International School of Health Sciences
San Diego, CA
619-275-2345

Mueller College of Holistic Studies
San Diego, CA
619-291-9811

Pacific College of Oriental Medicine
San Diego, CA
619-574-6909

American College of Traditional Chinese Medicine
San Francisco, CA
415-282-7600

California Pacific Medical Center
San Francisco, CA
415-600-6000

San Francisco School of Massage
San Francisco, CA
415-474-4600

Sonoma College - San Francisco
San Francisco, CA
415-543-1833

World School of Massage and Holistic Healing Arts
San Francisco, CA
415-221-2533

Five Branches Institute College
San Jose, CA
408-260-0208

Just for Your Health
San Jose, CA
408-723-2131

Trinity College
San Jose, CA
408-287-5100

American Institute of Massage Therapy
Santa Ana, CA
714-432-7879

Santa Barbara Body Therapy Institute
Santa Barbara, CA
805-966-5802

Santa Barbara Bodyworks
Santa Barbara, CA
805-569-3230

Midline School of Integrated Bodywork
Santa Cruz, CA
831-421-9222

Mind in Motion
Santa Cruz, CA
831-459-8173

Twin Lakes College of the Healing Arts
Santa Cruz, CA
831-476-2152

Shiatsu Massage School of California
Santa Monica, CA
310-581-0097

Sebastopol Massage Center
Sebastopol, CA
707-823-3550

California Institute of Massage & Spa Services
Sonoma, CA
707-939-9431

Body TuneUp School of Massage Therapy
Stockton, CA
209-473-4993

University of East-West Medicine
Sunnyvale, CA
408-733-1878

Bryman College
Torrance, CA
310-320-3200

Hands On Healing Institute
Tujunga, CA
818-951-5811

Massage School of Santa Monica
Valley Glen, CA
818-763-4912

Kali Institute for Massage & Somatic Therapies
Ventura, CA
805-648-6204

West Coast College - Victorville
Victorville, CA
760-241-7332

Milan Institute
Visalia, CA
559-733-4040

California Healing Arts College
West Los Angeles, CA
310-826-7622

Center For Natural Healing
Westlake Village, CA
818-879-0411

Makoto Kai Healing Arts
Woodland, CA
530-662-5662

COLORADO

Denver School of Massage
Aurora, CO
303-366-4325

Boulder College of Massage Therapy
Boulder, CO
303-530-2100

Healing Spirits
Boulder, CO
303-443-5396

Rolf Institute
Boulder, CO
303-449-5903

Colorado Institute of Massage Therapy
Colorado Springs, CO
719-634-7347

Mountain Heart School
Crested Butte, CO
970-349-0473

Heritage College
Denver, CO
303-872-0609

Massage Therapy Institute of Colorado
Denver, CO
303-329-3670

Rocky Mountain Institute of Healing Arts
Durango, CO
970-385-5142

Academy of Natural Therapy
Greeley, CO
970-454-2628

Colorado School of Healing Arts
Lakewood, CO
303-986-2320

Denver School of Massage
Westminster, CO
303-426-5621

CONNECTICUT

Connecticut Center for Massage Therapy
Groton, CT
860-446-2299

Connecticut Center for Massage Therapy
Newington, CT
860-667-1886

Connecticut Center for Massage Therapy
Westport, CT
203-221-7325

Branford Hall Career Institute - Windsor Campus
Windsor, CT
860-683-4900

DISTRICT OF COLUMBIA

Potomac Massage Training Institute
Washington, DC
202-686-7046

DELAWARE

Academy of Massage and Bodywork
Bear, DE
302-392-6768

Delaware Learning Institute - Millsboro Campus
Millsboro, DE
302-732-6704

National Massage Therapy Institute
Wilmington, DE
302-656-2328

FLORIDA

Boca Beauty Academy
Boca Raton, FL
561-487-1191

Florida College of Natural Health
Bradenton, FL
941-744-1244

Manatee Technical Institute
Bradenton, FL
941-751-7900

Broward College - North Campus
Coconut Creek, FL
954-201-2074

Daytona State College
Daytona Beach, FL
386-506-3185

Keiser University
Daytona Beach, FL
386-274-5060

Lee County High Tech Center Central
Ft. Meyers, FL
239-334-4544

Southwest Florida College - Ft. Meyers
Ft. Meyers, FL
239-939-4766

Florida Academy of Massage & Skin Care
Ft. Myers, FL
239-489-2282

Heritage Institute
Ft. Myers, FL
239-936-5822

Florida School of Massage
Gainesville, FL
352-378-7891

Hollywood Institute of Beauty Careers
Hollywood, FL
954-922-5505

Sheridan Technical Center
Hollywood, FL
754-321-5400

Withlacoochee Technical Institute
Inverness, Fl
352-726-2430

Everest University - Jacksonville
Jacksonville, FL
904-731-4949

Heritage College
Jacksonville, FL
904-332-0910

Florida College of Natural Health
Maitland, FL
407-261-0319

Academy of Cosmetology
Merritt Island, FL
321-452-8490

Educating Hands School of Massage
Miami, FL
305-285-6991

Florida College of Natural Health
Miami, FL
305-597-9599

Praxis Institute
Miami, FL
305-642-4104

Soothing Arts - Healing Therapies School of Massage
Miramar Beach, Fl
850-269-0820

Florida Health Academy
Naples, FL
239-263-9391

Lorenzo Walker Institute of Technology
Naples, FL
239-377-0918

High Tech Institute
Orlando, FL
407-673-9900

Daytona College
Ormond Beach, FL
386-267-0565

Humanities Center Institute of Allied Health
Pinellas Park, FL
727-541-5200

American Institute of Massage Therapy
Pompano Beach, FL
954-781-2468

Florida College of Natural Health
Pompano Beach, FL
954-975-6400

Alpha Institute of the Treasure Coast
Port St. Lucie, FL
772-337-5533

Sarasota School of Massage Therapy
Sarasota, FL
941-957-0577

International Academy
South Daytona, FL
386-767-4600

CORE Institute School of Massage Therapy
Tallahassee, FL
850-222-8673

Southwest Florida College - Tampa
Tampa, FL
813-630-4401

Space Coast Health Institute
West Melbourne, FL
321-308-8000

Palm Beach Academy of Health & Beauty
West Palm Beach, FL
561-845-1400

Ridge Career Center
Winter Haven, FL
863-419-3060

Central Florida School of Massage Therapy
Winter Park, FL
407-673-6776

GEORGIA

Atlanta Polarity Center
Atlanta, GA
404-231-9481

Atlanta School of Massage
Atlanta, GA
770-454-7167

Gwinnett College - Sandy Springs
Atlanta, GA
770-457-2021

Rising Spirit Institute of Natural Health
Atlanta, GA
770-457-2021

Georgia Career Institute
Conyers, GA
770-922-7653

Gwinnett College
Lilburn, GA
770-381-7200

American Professional Institute
Macon, GA
478-314-4444

Lincoln College of Technology
Marietta, GA
770-226-0056

Georgia Academy of Massage
Martinez, GA
706-869-7575

Academy of Somatic Healing Arts ASHA
Norcross, GA
770-368-2661

Coosa Valley Technical College
Rome, GA
706-295-6963

Savannah School of Massage Therapy
Savannah, GA
912-355-3011

Georgia Massage School
Suwanee, GA
678-482-1100

Georgia Massage Institute
Winder, GA
770-307-0873

HAWAII

Spa Luna ~ Holistic School of Massage Therapy
Haiku, Maui, HI
808-575-9267

Hawaiian Massage School of Kauai
Hanalei, HI
808-828-6418

Big Island Academy of Massage
Hilo, HI
808 935-1405

Hawaii Massage Academy
Honolulu, HI
808-955-4555

International School of Beauty & Esthetique
Honolulu, HI
808-942-0088

Aloha School of Massage Therapy
Kahului, Maui, HI
808-871-9966

Aloha Institute of Massage & Healing Arts
Kailua, HI
808-263-2468

Hawaii Healing Arts College
Kailua, HI
808-266-2462

Hawaiian Islands School of Massage
Kealakekua, HI
808-323-3800

Maui Academy of the Healing Arts
Kihei, HI
808-879-4266

Maui School of Therapeutic Massage
Makawao, Maui, HI
808-572-2277

Kalani Oceanside Retreat
Pahoa, HI
808-965-0468

West Oahu Wellness and Massage Education Center
Waipahu, HI
808-393-1404

IOWA

Salon Professional Academy
Ames, IA
515-232-7250

Carlson College of Massage Therapy
Anamosa, IA
319-462-3402

Iowa College of Natural Health
Ankeny, IA
515-965-3991

La' James International College - Cedar Falls
Cedar Falls, IA
319-277-2150

Ancient Wisdom College of Healing Arts & Wellness Center
Council Bluffs, IA
712-256-3600

Windemere Institute of Healing Arts
Decorah, IA
563-382-8495

Iowa Massage Institute
Des Moines, IA
515-280-7611

IDAHO

College of Massage Therapy at Bingham Memorial Hospital
Blackfoot, ID
208-785-3823

Wellspring School for Healing Arts
Boise, ID
208-388-0206

Twin Falls Institute of Holistic Studies
Filer, ID
208-326-4870

Idaho School of Massage Therapy
Meridian, ID
208-343-1847

Moscow School of Massage
Moscow, ID
208-882-7867

Idaho State University Massage Therapy Program
Pocatello, ID
208-282-2622

American Institute of Clinical Massage
Post Falls, ID
208-773-5890

ILLINOIS

Chicago College of Healing Arts
Chicago, IL
773-596-5012

Hired Hands International University
Chicago, IL
773-296-0129

National College of Naprapathic Medicine
Chicago, IL
773-282-2686

Pacific College of Oriental Medicine, School of Massage, Inc
Chicago, IL
773-477-4822

Soma Institute
Chicago, Il
312-939-2723

Thai Bodywork School of Thai Massage
Evanston, IL
847-440-7525

SoderWorld Healing Arts Center & Spa
Hinsdale, IL
630-455-5885

National University of Health Sciences
Lombard, IL
630-889-6566

Kishwaukee College
Malta, IL
815-825-2086

Alive & Wellness, Inc. School of Massage Therapy
Moline, IL
309-764-2442

Black Hawk College - Quad-Cities
Moline, IL
309-796-5000

Northwestern College - Massage Therapy Program
Naperville, IL
888-205-2283

Harper College
Palatine, IL
847-925-6000

European Massage Therapy School
Skokie, IL
847-673-7595

Halsa Hem School of Massage
Springfield, IL
217-546-9011

Solex Massage Academy
Wheeling, IL
847-229-9595

Wellness and Massage Training Institute
Woodridge, IL
630-739-9684

INDIANA

Alexandria School of Scientific Therapeutics
Alexandria, IN
765-724-9152

Midwest Academy of Healing Arts
Brownsburg, IN
317-293-8076

American Certified Massage School
Crown Point, IN
219-661-9099

American Certified Massage School - Elkhart
Elkhart, IN
574-522-9095

Bodyworks School of Massage
Evansville, IN
812-490-9009

Center For Vital Living School of Therapeutic Massage and Bodywork
Fort Wayne, IN
260-436-8807

Aquarian Age Alternatives
Indianapolis, IN
317-843-1138

Indiana College of Massage
Indianapolis, IN
317-850-1994

Teresa's School of Therapeutic Massage
Kokomo, IN
765-455-0570

KANSAS

Colby Community College
Colby, KS
785-462-3984

American Academy of Massage Therapy - Manhattan
Manhattan, KS
785-539-1837

BMSI Institute, LLC
Overland Park, KS
913-649-3322

Johnson County Community College
Overland Park, KS
913-469-8500

American Academy of Massage Therapy - Topeka
Topeka, KS
785-539-1837

Heritage College
Wichita, KS
316-681-1615

Kansas College of Chinese Medicine
Wichita, KS
316-691-8822

Total Health Works Massage Clinic & School
Wichita, KS
316-262-8401

KENTUCKY

Natural Health Institute
Bowling Green, KY
270-783-8001

Southwestern College
Florence, KY
859 282-9999

Bluegrass Professional School of Massage Therapy
Lexington, KY
859-264-1450

Louisville School of Massage
Louisville, KY
502-429-5765

Sun Touch
Mayfield, KY
270-247-8923

LOUISIANA

Medical Training College
Baton Rouge, LA
225-926-5820

South Louisiana Institute of Massage
Gretna, LA
504-368-4263

Louisiana Institute of Massage Therapy
Lake Charles, LA
337-474-3737

MASSACHUSETTS

NE Inst Reflexology & Universal Studies
E. Wareham, MA
508-317-3044

Salter School - Fall River
Fall River, MA
508-730-2740

MassBay Community College
Framingham, MA
781-239-3000

Mildred Elley School of Massage
Pittsfield, MA
413-442-0333

Palmer Institute of Massage & Bodywork
Salem, MA
978-740-0044

Central Mass School of Massage and Therapy
Spencer, MA
508-885-0306

Kripalu School of Massage
Stockbridge, MA
413-448-3152

Healing Touch Institute
Stoneham, MA
978-846-3521

Salter School - Tewksbury
Tewksbury, MA
978-934-9300

Cortiva Institute - Muscular Therapy Institute
Watertown, MA
617-668-1000

Bancroft School of Massage Therapy
Worcester, MA
508-757-7923

Salter School - Worchester
Worcester, MA
781-324-5454

MARYLAND

Anne Arundel Community College
Arnold, MD
410-777-2222

Holistic Massage Training Institute
Baltimore, MD
410-243-4688

Massage Institute of Maryland
Catonsville, MD
410-744-9130

Zero Balancing Health Association
Columbia, MD
410-381-8956

Allegany College of Maryland
Cumberland, MD
301-724-7700

Baltimore School of Massage
Linthicum, MD
410-636-7929

MAINE

Acadia School of Massage
Bar Harbor, ME
207 288-8222

Fuller Circles School for Therapeutic Massage
Oakland, ME
207-877-5650

Pierre's School of Cosmetology
Portland, ME
207-774-1913

Namaste Institute
Rockport, ME
207-236-2744

Downeast School of Massage
Waldoboro, ME
207-832-5531

MICHIGAN

Ann Arbor Institute of Massage Therapy
Ann Arbor, MI
734-677-4430

Mary Light
Ann Arbor, MI
734-769-7794

School of Orthopedic Massage & Bodywork
Ann Arbor, MI
734-222-3300

Michigan School Myomassology
Berkley, MI
248-542-7228

Flint School of Therapeutic Massage
Flint, MI
810-767-1000

Schoolcraft College Radcliff Center
Garden City, MI
734-462-4770

Institute of Sanative Arts
Grand Rapids, MI
616-791-0472

Institute of Natural Therapies
Hancock, MI
906-482-2222

Michigan Institute of Therapeutic Massage
Holland, MI
616-494-9055

Kalamazoo Center for the Healing Arts
Kalamazoo, MI
269-373-1000

Lansing Community College
Lansing, MI
517-483-1957

Health Enrichment Center, Inc.
Lapeer, MI
810-667-9453

Marquette School of Therapeutic Massage
Marquette, MI
906-225-1700

Naturopathic Institute of Therapies and Education
Mt. Pleasant, MI
989-773-1714

American Medical Massage Association
Muskegon, MI
231-733-0717

Lakewood School of Therapeutic Massage
Port Huron, MI
810-987-3959

St. Clair County Community College
Port Huron, MI
810-989-5500

Kirtland Community College
Roscommon, MI
989-275-5000

Spring Renewal Professional Massage Training Program
Saugatuck, MI
269-857-2602

Irene's Myomassology Institute
Southfield, MI
248-350-1400

MINNESOTA

National American University - Bloomington
Bloomington, MN
952-356-3600

Northwestern Health Sciences University
Bloomington, MN
952-888-4777

National American University - Brooklyn Center
Brooklyn Center, MN
763-852-7500

Aveda Institute - Minneapolis
Minneapolis, MN
612-378-7401

Center Point Massage & Shiatsu Therapy School & Clinic
Minneapolis, MN
612-617-9090

Healing Touch School of Massage Therapy
Rochester, MN
507-536-4076

American Academy of Acupuncture and Oriental Medicine
Roseville, MN
651-631-0204

National American University - Roseville
Roseville, MN
651-855-6300

Saint Paul College
Saint Paul, MN
651-846-1600

Tao Institute Inc.
St. Cloud, MN
320-253-8028

Sister Rosalind Schools & Clinics of Massage
West St. Paul, MN
651-554-3010

MISSOURI

Massage Therapy Institute of Missouri
Columbia, MO
573-875-7905

Orler School of Massage Therapy Technology
Joplin, MO
417-623-7359

Heritage College
Kansas City, MO
816-942-5474

Massage Therapy Training Institute
Kansas City, MO
816-523-9140

Midwest Institute of Natural Healing
Kansas City, MO
816-453-3577

A Gathering Place Wellness Education Center, LLC
Maryland Heights, MO
314-739-5559

SOMA Massage Therapy School of Massage Arts
Nixa, MO
417-725-0800

Missouri College
Saint Louis, MO
314-821-7700

Professional Massage Training Center Inc.
Springfield, MO
417-863-7682

St. Charles School of Massage Therapy
St. Charles, MO
636-498-0777

Elements of Wellness
University City, MO
314-727-1778

MISSISSIPPI

Virginia College - Biloxi
Biloxi, MS
228-546-9100

Antonelli College - Hattiesburg
Hattiesburg, MS
601-583-4100

Healing Touch School of Massage Therapy and Spa
Hattiesburg, MS
601-261-0147

Antonelli College - Jackson
Jackson, MS
601-362-9991

Virginia College - Jackson
Jackson, MS
601-977-0960

Natural Healing Arts School of Massage Therapy
Oxford, MS
662-234-1037

Delta Technical College
Southaven, MS
662-280-1443

MONTANA

Health Works Institute
Bozeman, MT
406-582-1555

Big Sky Somatic Institute
Helena, MT
406-442-8998

Montana Institute of Massage Therapy
Kalispell, MT
406-257-6468

Montana School of Massage
Missoula, MT
406-549-9244

Serenity Center
Whitefish, MT
406-862-3808

NORTH CAROLINA

Asheville School of Massage & Yoga
Asheville, NC
828-252-7377

Gaston College - East
Belmont, NC
704-825-3737

Southeastern School of Neuromuscular Massage
Charlotte, NC
704-527-4979

Therapeutic Massage Training Institute
Charlotte, NC
704-338-9660

Blue Ridge Healing Arts Academy
Concord, NC
704-795-7478

Edmund Morgan School Of Neuromuscular & Massage Therapy
Cornelius, NC
704-896-2636

Gaston College - Dallas
Dallas, NC
704-922-6200

Natural Touch School of Massage Therapy
Greensboro, NC
336-808-0178

Natural Touch School of Massage
Hickory, NC
828-267-1901

Gaston College - Lincoln
Lincolnton, NC
704-748-1040

Sandhills Community College - Main Campus
Pinehurst, NC
910-692-6185

American & European Massage Center
Raleigh, NC
919-790-9750

Healing Arts and Massage School
Raleigh, NC
919-821-1444

Medical Arts School
Raleigh, NC
919-872-6386

Wake Technical Community College
Raleigh, NC
919-662-3400

The Whole You School of Massage & Bodywork
Rutherfordton, NC
828-287-0955

Body Therapy Institute
Siler City, NC
919-663-3111

Johnston Community College
Smithfield, NC
919-934-3051

Southwestern Community College
Sylva, NC
828-586-4091

Center for Massage & Natural Health
Weaverville, NC
828-658-0814

NORTH DAKOTA

Josef's School of Hair Design Skin & Bodywork Institute
Grand Forks, ND
701-795-1312

NEBRASKA

Midwest School of Massage
Omaha, NE
402-331-8383

Universal College of Healing Arts
Omaha, NE
402-556-4456

NEW HAMPSHIRE

Earth Heart Farm
Belmont, NH
603-520-5445

Vital Kneads Institute for Massage Therapy
Belmont, NH
603-267-1208

New Hampshire Institute for Therapeutic Arts
Bridgton, NH
603-882-3022

New England Academy of Therapeutic Sciences
Dublin, NH
603-563-7760

DoveStar Schools of Holistic Technology
Hooksett, NH
603-669-5104

North Eastern Institute of Whole Health
Manchester, NH
603-623-5018

NEW JERSEY

Dover Business College - Clifton
Clifton, NJ
973-546-0123

Lourdes Institute of Wholistic Studies
Collingswood, NJ
856-869-3125

Gentle Healing School of Massage
Cranbury, NJ
609-409-2700

Body Concepts wellness Institute
East Rutherford, NJ
201-635-1099

National Massage Therapy Institute
Egg Harbor Township, NJ
800-509-5058

Academy of Massage Therapy
Hackensack, NJ
201-568-3220

Health-Choices Holistic Massage School
Hillsborough, NJ
908-359-3995

School of Integrative Therapies
Holmdel, NJ
732-332-1500

Rizzieri Institute for Massage Therapy
Marlton, NJ
856-988-8600

JSG School of Massage Therapy
Midland Park, NJ
845-351-5444

Lincoln Technical Institute
Mt. Laurel, NJ
856 722-9333

Somerset School of Massage Therapy
Piscataway, NJ
732-885-3400

Institute for Therapeutic Massage, Inc.
Pompton Lakes, NJ
973-839-6131

Gloucester County School of Massage
Sewell, NJ
856-582-3500

Seashore Healing Arts Center
Somers Point, NJ
609-601-9272

Body, Mind, and Spirit Learning Alliance
Toms River, NJ
732-349-7153

Mercer County Technical Schools
Trenton, NJ
609-587-7640

National Massage Therapy Institute
Turnersville, NJ
800-509-5058

Essex Group Institute for Massage and Bodywork
Verona, NJ
973-571-9801

Academy of Therapeutic Massage & Healing Arts
Vineland, NJ
856-692-8111

Warren County Community College
Washington, NJ
908-835-9222

Berdan Institute
Wayne, NJ
973-837-1818

Center for Therapeutic Massage and School
West Long Branch, NJ
732-571-9111

Therapeutic Massage Training Center
Westfield, NJ
908-789-2288

Healing Hands Institute for Massage Therapy
Westwood, NJ
201-722-0099

Academy of Natural Health Sciences
Woodbridge, NJ
732-634-2155

NEW MEXICO

Body Dynamics School of Massage Therapy
Albuquerque, NM
505-881-1314

Crystal Mountain School of Therapeutic Massage
Albuquerque, NM
505-872-2030

Taos School of Massage
El Prado, NM
575-758-2725

Northern New Mexico College
Espanola, NM
505-747-2100

Massage Therapy Training Institute
Las Cruces, NM
505-523-6811

New Mexico Academy of Healing Arts
Santa Fe, NM
505-982-6271

Scherer Institute of Natural Healing
Santa Fe, NM
505-982-8398

NEVADA

Baum Healing Arts Center
Carson City, NV
775-884-1145

Ki-Atsu Institute for Healing Arts
Henderson, NV
702-263-9000

European Massage Therapy School - Las Vegas
Las Vegas, NV
702-202-2455

Northwest Health Careers
Las Vegas, NV
702-254-7577

Nevada School of Massage Therapy
Las Vegas, NV
702-456-4325

NEW YORK

Center for Natural Wellness School of Massage Therapy
Albany, NY
518-489-4026

Mildred Elley School of Massage
Albany, NY
518-786-3171

Nayada Institute of Thai Massage
Amherst, NY
716-833-8031

One Light Healing Touch
Brewster, NY
845-876-0259

Brooklyn Institute of Massage Therapy
Brooklyn, NY
718-853-8606

New York Institute of Massage
Buffalo, NY
716-633-0355

Trocaire College
Buffalo, NY
716-826-1200

Finger Lakes Community College
Canandaigua, NY
585- 394-3500

Hudson Valley School of Massage Therapy
Highland, NY
845-691-2547

Finger Lakes School of Massage
Ithaca, NY
607-272-9024

New York Open Center
New York, NY
212-219-2527

Ohashi Institute
New York, NY
646-486-1137

Pacific College of Oriental Medicine - New York
New York, NY
212-982-3456

Swedish Institute
New York, NY
212-924-5900

Onondaga School of Therapeutic Massage
Rochester, NY
585-241-0070

North Country Community College
Saranac Lake, NY
518-891-2915

New York College of Health Professions
Syosset, NY
516-364-0808

Onondaga School of Therapeutic Massage
Syracuse, NY
315-424-1159

OHIO

Stautzenberger College
Brecksville, OH
440-838-1999

United States Trager Association
Burton, OH
440-834-0308

Antonelli College - Cincinnati
Cincinnati, OH
513-241-4338

Cincinnati School of Medical Massage
Cincinnati, OH
513-469-6300

Integrated Touch Therapy
Circleville, OH
740-474-6436

Cuyahoga Community College
Cleveland, OH
866-806-2677

American Institute of Alternative Medicine
Columbus, OH
614-825-6278

Dayton School of Medical Massage
Dayton, OH
937-294-6994

Blanchard Valley Academy of Massage Therapy
Findlay, OH
419-423-2628

Owens Community College - Findlay
Findlay, OH
567-429-3500

Southwestern College
Florence, OH
513-874-0432

Lakeland Community College
Kirtland, OH
440-525-7000

Lima School of Medical Massage
Lima, OH
419-998-3000

Oakes School of Massage Therapy
Massillon, OH
330-832-2002

Northwest Academy of Massotherapy
Maumee, OH
419-893-6464

Cleveland Institute of Medical Massage
Middleburg Heights, OH
440-243-8650

EHOVE Career Center
Milan, OH
419-499-4663

Stark State College of Technology
North Canton, OH
330-494-6170

Institute of Therapeutic Massage
Ottawa, OH
419-523-9580

Healing Arts Institute
Perrysburg, OH
419-874-4496

Owens Community College - Toledo
Perrysburg, OH
567-661-7000

Harmony Path School of Massage Therapy
Rocky River, OH
440-333-6633

Carnegie Institute of Integrative Medicine
Suffield, OH
330-630-1132

OKLAHOMA

Body Business School of Massage Therapy
Durant, OK
580-931-9093

AcuCollege of America
Oklahoma City, OK
405-524-4000

Heritage College
Oklahoma City, OK
405-631-3399

Praxis College of Health Arts & Sciences
Oklahoma City, OK
405-879-0224

Community Care College
Tulsa, OK
918-610-0027

OREGON

Ashland Institute of Massage
Ashland, OR
541-482-5134

Sage School of Massage & Healing Arts
Bend, OR
541-419-5659

East West College
Portland, OR
503-233-6500

Oregon School of Massage
Portland, OR
503-244-3420

Portland Beauty School
Portland, OR
503-255-6303

Western States Chiropractic College
Portland, OR
503-256-3180

Silverton School of Massage
Silverton, OR
503-873-6131

PENNSYLVANIA

Pennsylvania Myotherapy Institute
Abbottstown, PA
717-259-7000

Lincoln Tech Institute
Alentown, PA
610-398-5300

Lehigh Valley Healing Arts Academy
Allentown, PA
610-398-9642

HunaMua Wellness Center
Ardmore, PA
610-360-2427

Health Options Institute
Bethlehem, PA
610-419-3535

Institute for Therapeutic Massage and Bodywork
Chaddsford, PA
610-358-5800

International School of Shiatsu
Doylestown, PA
215-340-9918

Great Lakes Institute of Technology
Erie, PA
814-864-6666

National Massage Therapy Institute
Falls Church, PA
800-509-5058

MBO Massage School
Feasterville Trevose, PA
215-355-9955

Cortiva Institute - Pennsylvania School of Muscle Therapy
King of Prussia, PA
610-666-9060

National Academy of Massage Therapy & Healing Sciences
Kulpsville, PA
215-412-4121

Omega Healing Arts School Massage and Bodywork Therapies
Lafayette Hill, PA
484-994-6086

Lancaster School of Massage
Lancaster, PA
717-293-9698

Professional School of Massage
Langhorne, PA
215-750-0700

Alternative Conjunction Clinic and School of Massage Therapy
Lemoyne, PA
717-737-6001

Community College of Allegheny County - Boyce
Monroeville, PA
724-325-6614

Massage Therapy Institute of Western Pennsylvania
Murrysville, PA
724-327-1194

Pennsylvania School of Muscle Therapy
Oaks, PA
610-666-9060

Center for Human Integration School of Integrative Body/Mind Therapies
Philadelphia, PA
215-742-3505

Lincoln Tech Institute
Philadelphia, PA
215-969-0869

Massage Arts Center of Philadelphia
Philadelphia, PA
267-321-0200

National Massage Therapy Institute
Philadelphia, PA
800-509-5058

Community College of Allegheny County - Pittsburg
Pittsburgh, PA
412-237-2709

Pittsburgh School of Massage Therapy
Pittsburgh, PA
412-241-5155

Valley School of Healing Arts
Port Trevorton, PA
570-374-2222

Academy of Massage & Bodyworks
Pottstown, PA
610-705-4401

Pennsylvania Institute of Massage Therapy
Quakertown, PA
215-538-5339

Central Pennsylvania School of Massage
State College, PA
814-234-4900

Mt. Nittany Institute of Natural Health
State College, PA
814-238-1121

Laurel Business Institute
Uniontown, PA
724-439-4900

Pfrimmer Institute for Corrective Muscle Therapy
Valley Forge, PA
610-666-9553

East West School of Massage Therapy
Wyomissing, PA
610-375-7520

Baltimore School of Massage - York
York, PA
717-268-1881

RHODE ISLAND

Lincoln Tech Institute
Lincoln, RI
401-334-2430

Community College of Rhode Island
Warwick, RI
401-825-1000

SOUTH CAROLINA

South Carolina Massage Therapy Institute
Bluffton, SC
803-939-9600

Charleston School of Massage
Charleston, SC
843-762-7727

Trident Technical College
Charleston, SC
843-722-5542

Southeastern Institute
Columbia, SC
803-798-8800

Carolina Bodywork Institute, Inc.
Greenville, SC
864-421-9481

Virginia College
Greenville, SC
864-679-4900

South Carolina Massage Therapy Institute
Myrtle Beach, SC
843-293-2225

Southeastern School of Neuromuscular & Massage Therapy of Charleston
North Charleston, SC
843-747-1279

South Carolina Massage & Esthetics Institute
West Columbia, SC
803-939-9600

SOUTH DAKOTA

Black Hills Health & Education Center School of Massage
Hermosa, SD
605-255-4101

Springs Bath House School of Massage Therapy
Hot Springs, SD
605-745-4424

Headlines Academy
Rapid City, SD
605-348-4247

National American University - Sioux Falls
Sioux Falls, SD
605-336-4600

Sioux Falls Therapeutic Massage and Education
Sioux Falls, SD
605-338-9266

South Dakota School of Massage Therapy
Sioux Falls, SD
605-334-4422

TENNESSEE

Virginia College
Chattanooga, TN
888-232-7887

Massage Institute of Cleveland
Cleveland, TN
423-559-0380

Southern Massage Institute
Collierville, TN
901-854-9095

Holston Institute of Healing Arts
Johnson City, TN
423-239-5043

Reflection of Health School of Massage
Johnson City, TN
423-929-3331

Tennessee School of Therapeutic Massage
Knoxville, TN
865-588-2324

Massage Institute of Memphis
Memphis, TN
901-324-4411

Tennessee School of Massage
Memphis, TN
901-843-2706

High-Tech Institute
Nashville, TN
901-432-3800

Natural Health Institute
Nashville, TN
615-242-6811

Southeastern Institute
Nashville, TN
615-889-9388

Roane State Community College
Oak Ridge, TN
865-481-2017

TEXAS

Abilene Institute of Massage
Abilene, TX
325-672-3444

Ace School for Massage
Amarillo, TX
806-359-8888

Amarillo Massage Therapy Institute
Amarillo, TX
806-331-0795

Massage Therapy Training Centre
Amarillo, TX
806-331-1665

West Texas Massage Institute
Amarillo, TX
806-354-8840

North Texas School of Massage
Arlington, TX
817-446-6629

Lauterstein-Conway Massage School
Austin, TX
512-374-9222

Texas Healing Arts Institute
Austin, TX
512-323-6042

Hands On School of Massage
Beaumont, TX
409-866-8911

Healing Handz Massage Academy
Bryan, TX
979-823-2989

Carrollton Massage Institute
Carrollton, TX
972-394-9700

Institute of Natural Healing Sciences
Colleyville, TX
817-498-0716

Aveda Institute
Conroe, TX
936-271-7700

ATI Career Training Center
Dallas, TX
214-306-8390

ATI Career Training Center
Dallas, TX
214-989-3001

Hands On Approach
Dallas, TX
972-484-8180

Sterling Health Center
Dallas, TX
972-991-9293

El Paso Community College
El Paso, TX
915-831-2000

Training Academy 4 U
Ferris, TX
972-842-2999

Texas Massage Institute - Fort Worth
Fort Worth, TX
817-838-3800

ATI Career Training Center
Houston, TX
713-581-8001

Avalon School of Massage
Houston, TX
713-333-5250

European Institute for Massage Therapy
Houston, TX
713-783-1446

Fountain Massage School
Houston, TX
713-771-5399

Houston Community College
Houston, TX
713-718-7389

Houston School of Massage
Houston, TX
713-681-5275

Memorial Hermann Massage & Spa Therapy School
Houston, TX
713-456-4304

Texas School of Massage
Houston, TX
281-488-3903

Relax Station
Kingwood, TX
281-358-0600

Laredo Massage Therapy Institute
Laredo, TX
956-717-2838

Institute of Bodywork Studies
Lewisville, TX
972-353-8989

ATI Career Training Center
Lewisville, TX
469-293-2880

Power of Touch Massage Therapy Institute
Longview, TX
903-295-8090

Oceans Massage Therapy School
Lubbock, TX
806-722-3300

Rub Me The Right Way
Massage School
Lubbock, TX
806-866-0089

Hands On Therapy Massage
School - Mesquite
Mesquite, TX
972-285-6133

ATI Career Training Center
North Richland Hills, TX
817-284-1141

Massage Masters School
Pharr, TX
956-787-9100

Ke Kino Massage Academy
Plano, TX
972-509-5588

Texas Massage Institute - Plano
Plano, TX
972-881-1496

Academy for Massage Therapy
Training
San Antonio, TX
210-375-2688

Mind Body Naturopathic Institute
San Antonio, TX
210-308-8888

River City Massage School
San Antonio, TX
210-798-7988

Therapeutic Body Concepts
San Antonio, TX
210-684-6563

Caring Hands Massage
School of Texas
Spring, TX
936-273-6055

McLennan Community College
Waco, TX
254-299-8000

UTAH

Vista College
Clearfield, UT
801-774-9900

Utah Career College
Layton, UT
801-660-6000

Utah College of Massage - Provo
Lindon, UT
801-796-0300

Ogden Institute of
Massage Therapy
Ogden, UT
801-627-8227

Utah Career College
Orem, UT
801-822-5800

Eagle Gate College
Salt Lake City, UT
801-287-9640

Healing Mountain Massage School
Salt Lake City, UT
801-355-6300

Utah College of Massage - Provo
Salt Lake City, UT
801-521-3330

Sensory Development Institute
School of Massage Therapy
St. George, UT
435-652-9003

Utah Career College
West Jordan, UT
801-304-4224

Renaissance School of
Therapeutic Massage
Woods Cross, UT
801-292-8515

VIRGINIA

Appalachian Institute of
Healing Arts
Abingdon, VA
276-698-3160

Applied Career Training -
The Allied Health School
Alexandria, VA
703-527-6660

Centura College
Alexandria, VA
703-778-4444

Blue Ridge School of
Massage and Yoga
Blacksburg, VA
540-552-2177

Natural Touch School of
Massage Therapy
Blairs, VA
434-836-6640

Virginia School of Massage
Charlottesville, VA
434-293-4031

Centura College
Chesapeake, VA
757-549-2121

Everest Institute
Chesapeake, VA
757-361-3900

Associates of Integrative Health
Damascus, VA
812-330-0053

Shenandoah Valley School of
Therapeutic Massage
Edinburg, VA
888-836-0400

Columbia College
Fairfax, VA
877-307- 2232

Greater Washington
Institute of Massage
Fairfax, VA
703-425-8692

Northern Virginia School of
Therapeutic Massage
Falls Church, VA
703-533-3113

Career Training Solutions
Fredericksburg, VA
540-373-2200

American Spirit Institute
Glen Allen, VA
804-822-1558

AKS Massage School, Inc
Herndon, VA
703-476-9095

Heritage Institute - Manassas
Manassas, VA
703-334-2501

Everest College
Mc Lean, VA
703-288-3131

Centura College
Newport News, VA
757-874-2121

Everest Institute
Newport News, VA
757-873-1111

Fordes College
Norfolk, VA
757-499-5447

Pate School
Neuromuscular Therapy
Norfolk, VA
757-303-4636

American Institute of Massage
Richmond, VA
804-290-0980

Centura College
Richmond, VA
804-330-0111

Richmond Academy of Massage
Richmond, VA
804-282-5003

Virginia Career Institute
Richmond, VA
804-323-1020

Advanced Fuller School of
Massage Therapy, Inc
Virginia Beach, VA
757-340-3080

American Spirit Institute
Virginia Beach, VA
757-220-8000

Cayce/Reilly School
of Massotherapy
Virginia Beach, VA
757-428-3588

Centura College
Virginia Beach, VA
757-340-2121

American Spirit Institute
Williamsburg, VA
757-220-8000

Piedmont School of
Professional Massage
Woodbridge, VA
703-499-9909

VERMONT

Community College of Vermont
Bennington, VT
802-524-6541

Community College of Vermont
Burlington, VT
802-865-4422

Touchstone Healing Arts
School of Massage
Burlington, VT
802-658-7715

Vermont Institute of Massage
Milton, VT
802-893-2760

Community College of Vermont
Morrisville, VT
802-888-4258

Green Mountain Institute for
Integrative Therapy
North Bennington, VT
802-442-3886

Wellness Massage Center
Saint Albans, VT
802-527-1601

O'Briens Training Center
South Burlington, VT
802-658-9591

Community College of Vermont
Springfield, VT
802-885-8360

WASHINGTON

Denton Massage School
Arlington, WA
360-435-8490

Bellevue Massage School/
Center for Healing Arts
Bellevue, WA
425-641-3409

Body Mind Academy
Bellevue, WA
206-367-9060

Whatcom Community College
Bellingham, WA
360-383-3726

Everest College
Bremerton, WA
360-473-1120

Soma Institute of
Neuromuscular Integration
Buckley, WA
360-829-1025

Barlen Institute of Massage
Ellensburg, WA
509-962-3535

Tri-City School of Massage
Kennewick, WA
509-586-6434

Northwest School of Massage
East Side
Kirkland, WA
866-713-1212

Spectrum Center School
of Massage
Lake Steven, WA
425-334-5409

Clover Park Technical College
Lakewood, WA
253-589-5536

Bodymechanics School of
Myotherapy and Massage
Olympia, WA
800-615-5594

Peninsula College Massage
Port Angeles, WA
360-417-6569

Port Townsend School of Massage
Port Townsend, WA
360-379-4066

Renton Technical College
Renton, WA
425-235-2352

Ancient Arts Massage School
Richland, WA
509-943-9589

Cortiva Institute Seattle School
of Massage Therapy
Seattle, WA
206-282-1233

Everest College
Seattle, WA
206-440-3090

Inland Massage Institute
Spokane, WA
509-465-3033

NW Noetic School of Massage & Education Center
Spokane, WA
509-835-4000

Spokane Community College
Spokane, WA
509-533-7000

Wellness Education Center
Spokane, WA
509-624-8608

Apollo College
Spokane Valley, WA
509-532-8888

Alexander School of Natural Therapeutics, Inc.
Tacoma, WA
253-473-1142

Everest Institute
Tacoma, WA
253-926-1435

Massage Connection School of Natural Healing
Tacoma, WA
253-444-3381

Northwest Academy of Healing Arts
Tacoma, WA
800-929-9441

Institute of Structural Medicine
Twisp, WA
509-997-9392

Everest Institute
Vancouver, WA
360-885-3152

Evergreen Center for the Healing Arts
Vancouver, WA
360-750-7272

WISCONSIN

Fox Valley School Of Massage
Appleton, WI
920-993-8660

Wisconsin Indianhead Technical College
Ashland, WI
715-682-4591

Blue Sky Educational Foundation
De Pere, WI
920-338-9500

Professional Hair Design Academy
Eau Claire, WI
715-835-2345

Blue Sky School of Professional Massage and Therapeutic Bodywork
Fredonia, WI
262-692-9500

Wisconsin School of Massage Therapy
Germantown, WI
262-250-1276

Blue Sky School of Professional Massage and Therapeutic Bodywork
Madison, WI
608-270-5241

East-West Healing Arts Institute
Madison, WI
608-236-9000

TIBIA Massage School
Madison, WI
608-238-7378

Institute of Beauty & Wellness
Milwaukee, WI
414-227-2889

Lakeside School of Massage Therapy, Milwaukee
Milwaukee, WI
414-372-4345

Wisconsin Indianhead Technical College
New Richmond, WI
715-246-6561

Wisconsin Indianhead Technical College
Rice Lake, WI
800-243-9482

Wisconsin Indianhead Technical College
Superior, WI
715-394-6677

WEST VIRGINIA

Everest Institute
Charleston, WV
304-776-6290

Mountain State School of Massage
Charleston, WV
304-926-8822

Clarksburg Beauty School & School of Massage Therapy
Clarksburg, WV
304-624-6475

Art & Science Institute of Cosmetology & Massage Therapy
Fairmont, WV
304-363-2015

I-N Touch School of Massage Therapy Inc.
Huntington, WV
304-523-1234

Morgantown Beauty College
Morgantown, WV
304-292-8475

WYOMING

Eastern WY College
Douglas, WY
307-433-8363

Sheridan College
Sheridan, WY
307-674-6446

Terms	Definitions
Abduction	Movement of a limb or any other part away from the midline of the body.
Abrasion	A superficial skin wound as a result of scraping skin against a hard or rough surface.
Accessory Joint Motion	The range of motion within synovial and secondary cartilaginous joints that is not under voluntary control and can therefore only be obtained passively by the clinician. These motions, also known as joint play movements, are essential for full and pain-free active range of motion.
Achilles Tendonitis	Inflammation of the Achilles tendon.
Acromion Clavicular (AC) Separation	Stretching or tearing injury to the ligament that attaches the collarbone to the shoulder blade forming the shoulder joint. Slight deformity and extreme tenderness at the end of the collarbone are typical. The injury is often seen with athletes as a result of a fall to the shoulder. Commonly known as shoulder separation.
Active Assisted Movement	Movement of a joint in which both the client and the therapist produce the motion.
Active Assisted Range of Motion (AAROM)	The range of movement at a particular joint achieved with some assistance. Assistance may include another person aiding in the movement or using opposite hand to move the involved arm.
Active Joint Movement	Movement of a joint through its range of motion by the client.
Active Range of Motion (AROM)	The amount of joint motion that can be achieved by the client during the performance of unassisted voluntary joint motion.
Active Resistive Movement	Movement of a joint by the client against resistance provided by the therapist.
Active Rest	Continuance of movement after the cessation of activity, opposite of stopping abruptly.
Active Trigger Point	A trigger point which refers pain in a characteristic pattern whether the muscle in which it is located is working or at rest.
Acupressure	A type of massage which uses specific compression to stimulate acupoints and meridians to achieve complex effects on physiological function that are usually manifested in areas that are remote to the point of application.
Acute	Describes a condition in which the signs and symptoms develop quickly, last a short time, and then disappear.
Acute Illness	A short-term illness that resolves by means of the normal healing process and, if necessary, supportive medical care.
Acute Pain	A symptom of a disease condition or a temporary aspect of medical treatment. Acute pain acts as a warning signal because it can activate the sympathetic nervous system. It usually is temporary, of sudden onset, and localized. The client frequently can describe the pain, which often subsides without treatment.
Acute Traumatic Injury	Describing a condition of rapid onset with severe symptoms and brief duration. Also describing any intense symptom, such a severe pain. An acute injury is characterized by a rapid onset and results from a traumatic event.
Adaptation	A response to a continual or constant sensory stimulation in which nerve signaling is reduced or ceases.
Adaptive Shortening	Shortening of muscle fibers and decrease of range of motion, secondary to inactivity. The muscles will become progressively tighter unless optimal muscle length is maintained with stretching and physical activity.
Adduction	Movement of a limb or any other part towards the midline of the body.
Adhesion	A binding together with dense connective tissue that normally glide or move in relation to each other, with resultant loss of mobility. Like scars, adhesions may result from the replacement of normal tissue that has been destroyed by burn, wound, surgery, radiation, or disease with connective tissue.
Adhesive Capsulitis	Adhesive inflammation between the joint capsule and the peripheral articular cartilage of the shoulder. Causes pain, stiffness, and limitation of movement. Also called frozen shoulder.
Aerobic	Means "in the presence of oxygen." Aerobic exercise is sustained rhythmical movement using the large muscle groups of the body during activities such as walking, jogging, cycling and swimming.
Agonist Muscle (Prime Mover)	A muscle whose active contraction causes movement of a body part. Contraction of an agonist results in relaxation of its antagonist. For example, in bending of the elbow, the biceps muscle is the agonist and the triceps the antagonist.
Alcoholic Hepatitis	An acute or chronic inflammation of the liver caused by alcohol ingestion. This disease can sometimes improve if alcohol is avoided. It can be serious, however, and is a risk factor for developing cirrhosis and liver cancer.
Alignment	The arrangement of body parts forming a straight line. Proper alignment involves positioning the head, neck, back, and knees in proper posture with all activities to prevent injury.
Allied Health	Occupations of medical personnel who are not physicians, and are qualified by special training and, frequently, by licensure to work in supporting roles in the health care field. These occupations include, but are not limited to, medical technology, physical therapy, physician assistant, etc.
Amino Acid	A protein which performs a specific role in a particular biochemical process in the body.
Anaerobic	Exercise performed without oxygen or too intense to utilize fat as an energy source. Anaerobic activities are typically performed at high intensity for a short duration. (e.g. sprinting, weight training).
Anatomic Barriers	Anatomic structures determined by the shape and fit of the bones at the joint.
Aneurysm	A blood-filled sac formed in a weakened area of the wall of an artery or vein; usually will protrude from the vessel.

Terms	Definitions
Angina	Name for the chest pain that occurs when the muscular wall of the heart becomes temporarily short of oxygen. When the oxygen requirement falls, the pain usually improves and disappears.
Ankylosing Spondylitis	Form of degenerative joint disease that affects the spine. Systemic illness, producing pain and stiffness as a result of inflammation of the sacroiliac, intervertebral, and costovertebral joints.
Anorexia Nervosa	An eating disorder characterized by a distorted body image, an extreme fear of obesity, refusal to maintain a minimally normal weight and, in women, the absence of menstrual periods. Anorexics often maintain a body weight at least 15% or more below the normal for their gender and height.
Antagonism	An interaction between chemicals in which one partially or completely inhibits the effect of the other (for example, a drug that blocks a hormone's receptor site would be a hormone antagonist).
Antagonist Muscle	A muscle whose contraction opposes that of another muscle, the agonist or prime mover. The antagonist muscle relaxes and provides smooth movement by balancing opposing forces to allow the agonist to effect movement. For example, in bending the elbow, the triceps muscle is the antagonist and the biceps the agonist.
Antagonists	The muscles that oppose the movement of the prime movers.
Anterior	Refers to before, towards, or in front of the body. Pertains to the abdominal side of the body. Anterior is the opposite of posterior and synonymous with ventral. (e.g. the tip of the nose is anterior to the ears)
Anterior Tibial Compartment Syndrome	Rapid swelling, increased tension, and pain of the anterior tibial compartment of the leg. Usually a history of excessive exertion.
Antibiotics	Natural or synthetic substances used in the treatment of infectious diseases.
Antioxidants	Compounds that protect your body from the cell damage that causes health problems, such as cancer, heart disease, cataracts, and arthritis. Popular antioxidant vitamins are vitamin E, vitamin C, selenium and beta-carotene.
Antirheumatics	Drugs used to reduce inflammation in many chronic, non-infective diseases, such as rheumatoid arthritis and gout.
Aortic Aneurism	Sac formed by the dilation of the wall of the aorta, which is filled with fluid or clotted blood.
Apley's Scratch Test	Determines range of motion: internal rotation and adduction; internal rotation, extension, and adduction; abduction, flexion, and external rotation.
Applied Kinesiology	Methods of evaluation and bodywork that use a specialized type of muscle testing and various forms of massage and bodywork for corrective procedures.
Approximation	The technique of pushing muscle fibers together in the belly of the muscle.
Armoring	Myofascial hardness associated with chronically elevated resting level of muscle tone.
Arousal	Cortical vigilance or readiness of tone, presumed to be in response to sensory stimulation via the reticular activating system.
Arterial Circulation	Movement of oxygenated blood under pressure from the heart to the body through the arteries.
Arteries	Blood vessels that carry blood away from the heart.
Arteriosclerosis	The sclerosis or narrowing and thickening of the walls of the smaller arteries. This term is most often used in referring to diseases of the smaller arteries.
Arthritis	An inflammatory condition involving the joints. A general term for a number of different conditions that involve swollen, painful or stiff joints. Common causes are infection, autoimmune diseases, or trauma.
Arthropathy	Any joint disease.
Articular Dysfunction	Disturbance, impairment, or abnormality of a joint.
Aseptic Technique	Procedures that kill or disable pathogens on surfaces to prevent transmission.
Assessment	The collection and interpretation of information provided by the client, the client's family and friends, the massage practitioner, and referring medical professionals.
Asymmetry	Lacks symmetry. The opposite sides of the body, right and left, are not equal in size, shape, and relative position.
Atherosclerosis	Hardening of the arteries in which cholesterol and fat build up in the walls of arteries, and can lead to a heart attack or stroke. Often used interchangeably with "arteriosclerosis".
Atrophy	Wasting away of a normally developed organ or tissue due to degeneration of cells. This may occur through undernourishment, disease, disuse such as inactivity or casting, or aging. For example, reduction of muscle size indicates muscle atrophy. Atrophy is the opposite of hypertrophy.
Attention	The clinician's capacity to focus on the sensory information that she receives primarily, but not exclusively, through her hands.
Autoimmune Disease	A disease that occurs when the body produces antibodies that attack its own tissues.
Autonomic Nervous System	The body system that regulates involuntary body function using the sympathetic "fight/flight/fear" response and the restorative parasympathetic "relaxation response." The sympathetic and parasympathetic systems work together to maintain homeostasis through a feedback loop system.
Autoregulation	Any of several physiological processes in which an inhibitory feedback system counteracts change. For examples, the process that maintains a constant flow of blood to an organ despite changes in arterial pressure.
Avulsion Fracture	Indirect fracture caused by compressive forces from direct trauma or excessive tensile forces.
Axis of Rotation	An imaginary line or point that an object, such as a body or lever, rotates around (e.g. the knee joint is the axis of rotation in a leg extension exercise).

GLOSSARY

Terms	Definitions
Ayurveda	A system of health and medicine that grew from East Indian roots.
Bacteria	Primitive cells that have no nuclei. Bacteria cause disease by secreting toxic substances that damage human tissues, by becoming parasites inside human cells, or by forming colonies in the body that disrupt normal function.
Bad Body Mechanics	Applying pressure with hyperextension of the wrists and abduction of thumb or crouched over the client.
Baker's Cyst	Swelling behind the knee caused by leakage of synovial fluid which has become enclosed in a sac of membrane.
Balance Point	The point of contact between the practitioner and client.
Ballistic Stretch	Characterized by momentum, relatively high force, and rapid bouncing at the end range of a stretch, activating the stretch reflex opposing the desired stretch. This stretch is short in duration. Exercise caution due to increased risk of injury.
Barrett's Syndrome	Peptic ulcer of the lower esophagus, sometimes containing functional mucous cells, instead of the normal squamous cell epithelium.
Barrier-Release Phenomenon	The clinician engages the tissue barrier at the point at which the clinician palpates a resistance to tissue motion. If the clinician sustains the pressure on the tissue barrier, a "release" may occur after a latency period that will vary with the nature and state of health of the tissue. This release results in a reduction of the resistance that will enable the clinician to move the tissue beyond the location of the original barrier without increasing the pressure of palpation.
Basal Cell Carcinoma	An epidermal tumor with the potential for local invasion and destruction. It is the most common type of skin cancer. Cells just below the surface of the skin become cancerous, and a tumor develops and becomes ulcerated.
Basic Daily Calorie Needs	The number of calories you need every day to sustain life. This includes calories required to maintain breathing, heart rate, and bodily functions. It does not include calories required for activity.
Beating	A percussion massage technique applied with a lightly closed fist using the hypothenar eminence and small finger as the striking surface, used for stimulation.
Beats Per Minute (BPM)	The number of times the heart beats in a minute.
Benign	A term that describes an abnormal growth that will neither spread to surrounding tissue nor recur after complete removal. The opposite of malignant.
Benign Prostate Hyperplasia	A non-cancerous enlargement of the prostate gland.
Biochemical	Having to do with the chemistry of the substances involved in the life processes of any living organism.
Blockage	Obstruction of a vessel or physiological process that may cause disease.
Body Armor	Patterns in the musculoskeletal system which are reflections of emotional patterns.
Body Mechanics	The utilization of correct muscles to complete a task safely and efficiently, without undue strain on any muscle or joint.
Body Segment	The area of the body between joints that provides movement during walking and balance.
Body Supports	Pillows, folded blankets, foam forms, or commercial products that help contour the flat surface of a massage table or mat.
Body/Mind	The interaction between thought and physiology that is connected to the limbic system, hypothalamic influence on the autonomic nervous system, and the endocrine system.
Bodywork	A term that encompasses all the various forms of massage, movement, and other touch therapies.
Boundary	Personal space that exists within an arm length's perimeter. Personal emotional space is designated by morals, values, and experience.
Breathing Pattern Disorders	A complex set of behaviors that lead to overbreathing in the absence of a pathologic condition. These disorders are considered a functional syndrome because all the parts are working effectively; therefore a specific pathologic condition does not exist.
Bruxism	Involuntary spasmodic gnashing, grinding, and clenching of teeth. Related to repressed aggression, emotional tension, etc.
Bunion	Abnormal prominence of the inner aspect of the first metatarsal head, resulting in displacement of the great toe (hallux valgus).
Burnout	A condition that occurs when a person uses up energy faster than it can be restored.
Bursa	A small connective tissue-lined sac filled with synovial fluid, found at the joints and acting as cushions.
Calcaneus	Bone of the heel.
Calcific Tendonitis	Inflammation and calcification of the subacromial or subdeltoid bursa. This results in pain and limitation of movement of the shoulder.
Calcium	A mineral found in many foods that is essential for many body functions, including the regulation of the heartbeat, conduction of nerve impulses, clotting of blood, and the building and maintaining of a healthy skeleton.
Callus	Development of thick skin where there is excess friction or pressure.
Capsular Laxity	Anatomical or pathological lengthening of the joint capsule.
Capsular Restrictions	Anatomical or pathological shortening of the joint capsule.
Capsulitis and Synovitis	Inflammation of the joint capsule and associated internal ligaments, and of the synovium.
Carbohydrates	A nutrient in food, which is your body's main source of fuel, and includes both sugars and starches. Each gram of carbohydrate has 4 calories.
Carcinogen	A cancer causing substance.

Terms	Definitions
Cardiovascular System	Transport system carrying oxygen, carbon dioxide, nutrients, and wastes.
Carpal Tunnel Syndrome	Compression of the median nerve as it passes through the carpal tunnel, leading to pain and tingling in the hand.
Cartilage	Hard, connective tissue found at the ends of bones which absorbs shock and prevents direct wearing of the bones.
Centering	The ability to focus the mind by screening out sensation.
Centripetal	Directed towards the heart or proximally.
Chakra	Energy fields or centers of consciousness within the body.
Charley Horse	A cramp of the quadriceps muscle group characterized by muscle cramping and pain usually caused by a strain or injury.
Chronic	Long-standing or recurring.
Chronic Illness	A disease, injury, or syndrome that shows little change or slow progression.
Chronic Liver Disease	Caused by some forms of hepatitis and may persist for a lifetime. It can be mild or severe and have episodes of remission. Signs and symptoms include: upper abdominal pain, low-grade fever, nausea, vomiting, and diarrhea, lack of appetite, muscle aches, and headache.
Chronic Obstructive Pulmonary Disease	Pulmonary disorders that are characterized by the presence of increased airway resistance.
Chronic Pain	Pain that persists or recurs for indefinite periods, usually for longer than 6 months. It frequently has an insidious onset, and the character and quality of the pain change over time. It frequently involves deep somatic and visceral structures. Chronic pain usually is diffuse and poorly localized.
Chronic Spasm	Alternating involuntary contraction and relaxation of a muscle.
Chronic Stress	A prolonged and heightened state of arousal that has negative physiological and psychological consequences.
Circuit Training	A strength-training program during which one moves through a circuit of exercises, with minimal rest, until the entire major muscle groups are covered.
Circular Friction	A friction massage technique applied in a circular motion covering no more than 1 square inch at a time; used to break adhesions and for specific warming.
Circulatory	Systems such as the arterial, venous and respiratory that depend on the pumping action of the skeletal muscle.
Circulatory System	The heart, arteries, veins and capillaries that function to move blood, oxygen and nutrients through the body.
Circumduction	Movement of a part, e.g., an extremity, in a circular direction.
Cirrhosis	A liver disease marked by progressive destruction of liver cells, most commonly caused by alcohol. The liver shrinks, becomes hard and nodular, and eventually malfunctions. This can lead to total liver failure. (See hepatitis)
Clapping	A form of percussion which uses the fingers and palms to mechanically loosen secretions in the lungs and to facilitate airway clearance.
Claw Toe	Toe deformity, particularly in clients with rheumatoid arthritis, consisting of dorsal subluxation of toes 2-5; painful condition during walking. The client develops a shuffling gait.
Client Information Form	A document used to obtain information from the client about health, preexisting conditions, and expectations for the massage.
Client Outcome	The results desired from the massage and the massage therapist.
Clinical Breast Exam	Inspection by a clinician for breast abnormalities usually performed during an annual PAP or pelvic exam.
Clinical Decision-Making	The process by which clinicians synthesize and analyze information on their clients' conditions and use the results of their analysis to formulate and progress a therapeutic regimen for their clients. Also known as clinical reasoning and clinical problem-solving.
Clinical Hypothesis	The clinician's hypothesis about the client's key clinical problems.
Clinical Indication	A sign, symptom, evaluation or diagnosis which directs the clinician to apply a certain procedure.
Clonus	A cyclical, spasmodic hyperactivity of antagonistic muscles that occurs at a regular frequency in response to a quick stretch stimulus.
Closed Fracture	A fracture in which skin is intact at site of fracture.
Coalition	A group formed for a particular purpose.
Coccydynia	Pain in the coccyx and neighboring region. Also known as coccygodynia.
Cognition	Conscious awareness and perception, reasoning, judgment, intuition, and memory.
Cognitive Transactional Model of Stress	Lazarus and Folkman's model of stress as the condition that results when a person's interactions with his environment leads him to perceive a discrepancy between the demands of the situation and the resources of the person's biological, psychological, or social systems.
Cogwheel Rigidity	A ratchet-like response to passive movement, alternating between giving way and resistance.
Coherence	Consistent order and structure of a massage sequence or intervention that results from clear and consistent intention(s) on the part of the clinician.
Collagen	The protein substance of the white fibers (collagenous fibers) of skin, tendon, bone, cartilage and all other connective tissue.
Colon Cancer	A malignancy that arises from the lining of either the colon or the rectum (large intestine). The second most common form of cancer found in males and females.
Comfort Barrier	The first point of resistance short of the client perceiving any discomfort at the physiologic or pathologic barrier.
Comminuted Fracture	A fracture in which the bone is broken into several pieces.

Terms	Definitions
Commitment	The ability and willingness to be involved in what is happening around us so as to have a purpose for being.
Communicable Disease	A disease caused by pathogens that are easily spread; a contagious disease.
Compartment Syndrome	Condition in which increased intramuscular pressure impedes blood flow and function of tissues within that compartment.
Compensation	The process of counterbalancing a defect in body structure or function.
Complex Carbohydrate	A type of carbohydrate that is high in starch such as bread, cereals, fruits, and vegetables. These foods generally contain more fiber, which increases satiety to help in weight control, blood sugar control, and regular bowel movements.
Complex Regional Pain Syndrome	Syndrome of vascular changes secondary to autonomic nervous system dysfunction (vaso nervorum / vaso vasorum).
Compound Fracture	Complete break in bone with protrusion from skin.
Compression	A massage technique that employs a gradual compressing of tissue followed by a gradual reduction of pressure; used to increase circulation.
Compressive Force	The amount of pressure exerted against the surface of the body in order to apply pressure to the deeper body structures; pressure directed in a particular direction.
Concave	Having a rounded, somewhat depressed surface, resembling the hollow inner segment of a sphere. Concave is the opposite of convex.
Concentric Contraction	Shortening of muscle fibers during a muscle contraction, or when the opposite ends of the muscle come close together. Concentric is the opposite of eccentric. (e.g. the biceps muscles concentrically contract during the curling phase of a biceps curl).
Concentric Isotonic Contraction	Application of a counterforce by the massage therapist while allowing the client to move, which brings the origin and insertion of the target muscle together against the pressure.
Conceptual Framework	A set of empirical generalizations that provides a means of organizing and integrating observations about a specific set of behaviors that one observes in a particular setting.
Conceptual Model	A diagram that shows the proposed causal linkages among a set of concepts that the individual believes to be related to a particular health problem.
Condition Management	The use of massage methods to support clients who are unable to undergo a therapeutic change but who wish to function as effectively as possible under a set of circumstances.
Confidentiality	Respect for the privacy of information obtained during therapeutic sessions and all other time spent with clients.
Conflict	An expressed struggle between at least two interdependent parties who perceive incompatible goals, scarce resources, and/or interference from the other party in achieving their goals.
Congenital	A condition that is present at birth and usually exists before birth.
Congenital Nevi	Moles that form before birth.
Congestive Heart Failure (CHF)	A condition in which the heart fails to pump out blood efficiently. As a result, blood that would normally enter the heart backs up in the veins depriving body tissues of oxygen. The backup of blood causes fluid to collect in the lungs, lower legs, ankles, arms, and liver.
Connective Tissue	Tissues that consist of several different types of cells, such as fibroblasts and fat cells, and elastin and collagen fibers embedded in a matrix of gelatinous material, the consistency of which varies in response to many factors. Nerves, blood vessels, lymph vessels, myofibrils, and organs are found within connective tissue.
Connective Tissue Massage	A system of massage developed by Elizabeth Dicke and popular in Europe in which connective tissue techniques are applied in precise sequences to the skin and superficial fascial layers to elicit specific physiological reflex effects.
Connective Tissue Techniques	Massage techniques that palpate, lengthen, and promote remodeling of connective tissue.
Conservation Withdrawal	A basic survival mechanism marked by adaptation or surrender to overwhelming circumstances (instead of fight or flight in manageable circumstances). Marked by weakness, tiredness, fatigue, hypotonia, emptiness, and depressive type symptoms.
Constipation	Describes the infrequent or difficult passing of hard bowel movements.
Contact Surface	The portion of the clinician's hand or arm that is used to execute the stroke.
Context	A brief description of how a massage technique is conventionally sequenced in relation to other techniques.
Contract (Muscle Contraction)	To develop tension within a muscle. There are three basic types of muscle contractions - isometric, concentric or eccentric.
Contract / Relax	An active movement used to promote muscular relaxation through consciously tensing and then relaxing a specific muscle or muscle group.
Contracture	A permanent muscular shortening due to a variety of physiological changes in muscle, such as fibrosis or loss of muscular balance.
Contraindicated	Not advisable, as use may cause problems.
Contraindication	Any condition that renders a particular treatment improper or undesirable.
Control	The belief that we can influence events by the way we feel, think, and act.
Control center (Homeostatic control mechanisms)	Analyzes information from receptors and determines the appropriate response. Works through feedback mechanisms. In most feedback loops, the control center is the brain.
Controlled Lean Posture	An inclined, aligned posture used to efficiently transfer the clinician's body weight to the client in a controlled manner.
Contusion	A bruising of body tissue without a break in the skin.
Convex	Having a rounded, evenly curved, somewhat elevated surface, resembling the external surface of a sphere. Convex is the opposite of concave.

Terms	Definitions
Cool Down	The time at the end of a workout allowing the body to return to near resting levels. Cool down includes an active aerobic cool down and a final cool down consisting of stretching exercises.
Coordination	The act of various muscles working together to produce a specific movement.
Core Muscles	The muscles that support the spine and pelvis and control movement through a "braking" action to produce quality movement and prevent injury to the spine. They provide a stable base of support for the muscles to power the arms and legs and center of gravity is in the core area leading to balanced skillful movements.
Coronary Arteries	Arteries that deliver oxygenated blood to the heart muscle (myocardium).
Coronary Artery Disease (CAD)	A form of heart disease caused by obstructions in the arteries that supply the heart with blood.
Coronary Heart Disease (CHD)	When myocardial tissue goes without oxygen resulting in damage (ischemia) or death (infarction).
Cortisol	A stress hormone produced by the adrenal glands that is released during long-term stress. An elevated level indicates increased sympathetic arousal.
Counseling	The giving of advice and assistance to individuals with educational or personal needs.
Counter Pressure	Force applied to an area that is designated to match exactly (isometric contraction) or partly (isotonic contraction) the effort or force produced by the muscles of that area.
Counter Transference	The personalization of the professional relationship by the therapist in which the practitioner is unable to separate the therapeutic relationship from personal feelings and expectations for the client.
Counterirritant	A substance applied to the skin which produces an analgesic effect.
Cramp	A painful contraction or spasm of a muscle.
Cream	A type of lubricate that is in a semisolid or solid state.
Credential	A designation earned by completing a process that verifies a certain level of expertise in a given skill.
Creep	Visco-elastic stretch of connective tissue that occurs when it is subjected to sustained tension, and which is palpable.
Crepitus	A rubbing, grinding, or cracking sensation experienced with joint movement; it is usually associated with arthritis or tendonitis and may be associated with pain.
Cross Directional Stretching	Tissue stretching that pulls and twists connective tissue against its fiber direction.
Cross Gender Massage	Client and therapist are of different sex or gender.
Cross Training	A method of adding active recovery to a training program. For example, for a regular runner, substituting swimming or cycling instead of running is cross training. The benefits include decreased injury incidence, reduced boredom through variety, and increased physical challenge for the body.
Cross-Directional Stretching	Tissue stretching that pulls and twists connective tissue against its fiber direction.
Cryotherapy	Therapeutic use of ice.
Cryptorchidism	A condition in which one or both testes (testicles) fail to descend through the abdominal wall into the scrotum by birth. An operation (orchidopexy) is performed to lower the testicle into the correct position within the scrotum.
CSF	Cerebrospinal fluid
Culture	The arts, beliefs, customs, institutions, and all other products of human work and thought created by a specific group of people at a particular time.
Cupping	A percussion technique applied with cupped hands used for stimulation.
De Quervain's Tenosynovitis	Inflammatory narrowing tenosynovitis of the abductor pollicis longus and extensor pollicis brevis tendons.
Decerebrate Rigidity	Rigidity that occurs as a result of brainstem lesions. It presents clinically as sustained contraction and posturing of the trunk and lower limbs in extension.
Decorticate Rigidity	Rigidity that occurs as a result of brainstem lesions. It presents clinically as sustained contraction and posturing of the trunk and lower limbs in extension and the upper limbs in flexion.
Deep Effleurage	A general gliding manipulation performed with moderate-to-heavy centripetal pressure that deforms superficial or deep layers of muscle.
Deep Fascia	Connective tissue layer that lies immediately superficial to, or between, muscle fibers. The primary functions of the deep fascia are to allow muscles to move freely, to carry nerve and blood vessels, to fill the space between muscles, and to provide an origin for muscles.
Deep Inspiration	Movement of air into the body by hard breathing to meet an increased demand for oxygen. Any muscles that can pull the ribs up are called into action.
Deep Transverse Friction	A specific rehabilitation technique that creates therapeutic inflammation by creating a specific controlled reinjury of tissues by applying concentrated therapeutic movement that moves the tissue against its grain over only a very small area.
Deep Vein Thrombosis (DVT)	The formation of a stationary blood clot in the wall of one or more of the deep veins of the lower leg.
Defensive Measures	The means by which our bodies defend against stressors (e.g., production of antibodies and white blood cells or through behavioral or emotional means).
Deformation	The change in shape of a tissue or structure when it is subjected to pressure.
Denial	The ability to retreat and to ignore stressors.
Dependent Edema	An increase in extracellular fluid volume that is localized in a dependent area, such as a limb.

Terms	Definitions
Depression	A condition characterized by a decrease in vital functional activity and by mood disturbances of exaggerated emptiness, hopelessness, and melancholy or of unbridled high energy with no purpose or outcome.
Dermatomal Pain	Pain in the pattern of a dermatome. A dermatome is an area of skin supplied by one dorsal nerve root. Injury of a dorsal root may result in sensory loss in the skin or may be felt as a burning or electric pain.
Dermatome	Cutaneous (skin) distribution of spinal nerve sensation.
Dermatomyositis	Chronic, progressive inflammatory disease of skeletal muscle, occurring in association with characteristic inflammatory skin changes.
Dermis	The first layer of connective tissue.
Dermomyotome	Zone of undifferentiated embryological tissue - pre-cursor of skin cells and muscle cells.
Diagnosis	The process and result of analyzing and organizing the findings from the client examination into clusters or syndromes.
Diaphragm	A broad sheet of muscle with attachments at the lower ribs, lumbar vertebrae and sternum, having its action influenced by breathing.
Direct Fascial Technique	A slow, gliding connective tissue technique that applies a moderate, sustained tensional force to the superficial fascia or to the deep fascia and associated muscle. It results in palpable visco-elastic lengthening and plastic deformation of the fascia.
Direct Inhibitory Pressure	Specific compression applied to a tendon as a means of inhibiting the tone of the related muscle for a short period of time.
Direction of Ease	The position the body assumes with postural changes and muscle shortening or weakening, depending on how it has balanced against gravity.
Direction of Technique	The direction of the applied force. The direction given in the description of techniques is the direction in which the greatest force is applied during the pressure phase of the stroke.
Disability	When an individual is unable to perform his socially defined tasks, activities, or roles to the expected level.
Disc	A pad of cartilage located between each vertebra.
Disclosure	Acknowledging and informing the client of any situation that interferes with or affects the professional relationship.
Discogenic Pain	Pain caused by derangement of an intervertebral disc.
Discopathy	Disease of an intervertebral cartilage (disc).
Discrimination	The clinician's ability to distinguish fine gradations of sensory information.
Disinfection	The process by which pathogens are destroyed.
Dislocation	The movement of a bone from its normal position.
Dissociation	A defense mechanism (detachment, discontentedness, separation, isolation) in which a group of mental processes are segregated from the rest of a person's mental activity in order to avoid emotional distress, or in which an idea or object is segregated from its emotional significance.
Diverticular Disease	Symptomatic congenital or acquired diverticula (a small sac-like structure that sometimes forms in the walls of the intestines) of any portion of the gastrointestinal tract.
Drag	The amount of pull (stretch) on the tissue (tensile stress).
Draping	The process by which the clinician covers and uncovers portions of the client's body during treatment, while maintaining modesty and respecting appropriate client-clinician boundaries.
Dual Role	Overlap in the scope of practice, with one professional providing support in more than one area of expertise.
Dupuytren's Contracture	Shortening, thickening, and fibrosis of the palmar fascia, producing a flexion deformity of a finger / toe.
Duration	The length of time a method lasts or stays in the same location.
Duration of Technique	An estimate of a reasonable length of time for which a single technique may have to be applied by a competent clinician to begin to achieve the specified impairment-level outcomes of care.
Dysfunction	An in-between state in which one is "not healthy" but also "not sick" (i.e., experiencing disease).
Dysmenorrhea	Difficult or painful menstruation.
Dyspareunia	Difficult or painful sexual intercourse.
Dyspnea	Shortness of breath, labored or difficult breathing or uncomfortable awareness of one's breathing.
Eccentric Isotonic Contraction	Application of a counterforce while the client moves the jointed area, which allows the origin and insertion to separate. The muscle lengthens against the pressure.
Edema	An accumulation of fluid in cells, tissues, or serous cavities. Edema has four main causes: increased permeability of capillaries, decreased plasma protein osmotic pressure, increased pressure in capillaries and venules, and lymphatic flow obstruction.
Effleurage	A group of general gliding manipulations performed with centripetal pressure and varying pressures.
Effusion	Excessive fluid in the joint capsule, indicating irritation or inflammation of the synovium.
Elastic Barrier in Soft Tissue	The resistance that the clinician feels at the end of the passive range of motion of the tissue when she is taking the "slack" out of the tissue.
Elastic Deformation	Deformation in response to applied force that disappears after the force is removed; spring-like behavior.
End Feel	The qualities of motion or resistance to motion that the clinician palpates in the joint at the end of passive range of motion.

Terms	Definitions
Endangerment Site	Any area of the body where nerves and blood vessels surface close to the skin and are not well protected by muscle or connective tissue; therefore deep, sustained pressure into these areas could damage these vessels and nerves. The kidney area is included because the kidneys are loosely suspended in fat and connective tissue, and heavy pounding is contraindicated in that area.
Endogenous	Made in the body.
Endurance	A measure of fitness. The ability to work for prolonged periods and the ability to resist fatigue.
Energetic Approaches	Methods of bodywork that work with subtle body responses.
Energy Fields	Vibrational or electromagnetic pathways.
Enkephalins And Endorphins	Neurochemicals that elevate mood, support satiety (reduce hunger and cravings), and modulate pain.
Entrapment	Pathologic pressure placed on a nerve or vessel by soft tissue.
Epicondylitis	Inflammation and micro rupturing of the soft tissues on the epicondyles of the distal humerus.
Epinephrine/Adrenaline	A neurochemical that activates arousal mechanisms in the body; the activation, arousal, alertness, and alarm chemical of the fight-or-flight response and all sympathetic arousal functions and behaviors.
Episode of Care	A single period of treatment (initial visit to discharge) that a client receives for a specific condition.
Epithelium	A layer of closely packed columnar or squamous cells that have little intercellular material between them.
Equilibrium	A state of balance or harmony.
Erythema	Redness of the skin produced by congestion of the capillaries.
Esoteric	Intended for or understood by a small group of people, often applied in mysticism.
Essential Touch	Vital, fundamental, and primary touch that is crucial to well-being.
Ethical Behavior	Right and good conduct that is based on moral and cultural standards as defined by the society in which we live.
Ethics	The science or study of morals, values, or principles, including ideals of autonomy, beneficence, and justice; principles of right and good conduct.
Evaluation	The synthesis of the information from the client examination.
Eversion	Turning outward, away from the body midline.
Examination	The collection of information on the client's health status and clinical condition through history-taking, a general systems review, and tests and measures.
Exemption	A situation in which a professional is not required to comply with an existing law because of educational or professional standing.
Experiment	A method of testing a hypothesis.
External Sensory Information	Stimulation from an origin exterior to the surface of the skin that is detected by the body.
Facilitation	The state of a nerve in which it is stimulated but not to the point of threshold, the point at which it transmits a nerve signal.
Fascia	A sheet or band of fibrous connective tissue that covers, supports, or separates muscles. It also binds skin with underlying tissues.
Fascial Restrictions	The loss of mobility of one fascial layer with respect to another because of the loss of fluid consistency of ground substance and development of collagenous cross-links. Fascial restrictions can result from repair of tissue damage and from prolonged immobility.
Fascial Sheath	A flat sheet of connective tissue used for separation, stability, and muscular attachment points.
Fasciculations	Localized, subconscious muscle contractions that result from the contraction of the muscle cells innervated by a single motor axon and thus do not involve the entire muscle.
Fasciitis	Inflammation of the fascia surrounding portions of a muscle.
Fast Twitch	A type of muscle fiber designed for quick speed of contraction, rapid movements, and high capacity for sudden bursts of energy. Recruited primarily for high intensity and short duration activities such as sprinting, jumping, and throwing.
Fasting Blood Sugar (FBS)	The level of sugar in the bloodstream after a period of fasting.
Fat	A nutrient in food that supplies energy and is used by the body to make cell membranes and regulating chemicals. A gram of fat has 9 calories.
Fat Soluble Vitamins	Vitamins (A, D, E, and K) which can dissolve in fat or fat-based solvents; they will not dissolve well in water.
Fatigue fracture	A hairline or microscopic break in the bone that is not demonstrable with conventional X-rays.
Feedback	A noninvasive, continual exchange of information between the client and the professional. Verbal or nonverbal communication from client regarding effectiveness of techniques.
Fetal Alcohol Syndrome	Birth defects in infants born to mothers whose chronic alcoholism continued during pregnancy.
Fiber	A substance found in foods that come from plants (fruits and vegetables) and typically cannot be digested. Also called bulk or roughage, it is thought to lower cholesterol and help control blood glucose.
Fibromyalgia	Pain and stiffness in the muscles and joints that is either diffuse or has multiple trigger points.
Fine Vibration	A superficial reflex technique in which a fast, oscillating or trembling movement is produced on the client's skin that result in minimal deformation of subcutaneous tissues.
First Degree Sprain or Strain	Stretched fibers, minimal swelling, and minimal limitations.
Flaccid	Lacking firmness or tone.

GLOSSARY

Terms	Definitions
Flexibility	The capacity of a muscle to lengthen or stretch; the range of motion at a specific joint. Synonymous with pliability.
Flexion	Movement about a joint in which the bones on either side of the joint are brought closer together, or decrease the angle of the bones forming a joint. Flexion is the opposite of extension. (e.g. bending the elbow or a biceps curl).
Flight phase	The stage of jogging or running when both feet is off the ground. Increased risk of injury with added body weight during flight phase activities.
Fracture	A broken bone.
Fremitus	A pulmonary vibration that a clinician can palpate over the rib cage as the client speaks or vocalizes.
Frequency	The number of times a method repeats itself in a time period.
Friction	A repetitive, specific, non-gliding, connective tissue technique that produces movement between the fibers of dense connective tissue, increasing tissue extensibility.
Frozen Shoulder Syndrome	See Adhesive Capsulitis.
Functional Limitation	A restriction of the individual's ability to perform actions or activities within the range considered normal for the organ or organ system.
Functional Outcome of Care	The outcome of care that is related to the client's functional limitation.
Gait	Walking pattern.
Gall Bladder Disease	Infection or inflammation in the pear-shaped sac located on the visceral surface of the right lobe of the liver.
General Relaxation	Physiological state characterized by decreases in heart rate, oxygen consumption, respiration, and skeletal muscular activity and by increases in skin resistance and alpha brain waves; sometimes called relaxation response.
General Technique	A technique that is applied to an entire region or a larger portion of the body, or applied using a broad surface such as the palm, or both.
Genetics	The scientific study of the process of biological inheritance. Its findings explain how and why certain traits such as hair color or blood types run in families.
Genital Warts	A viral skin tumor found on moist skin of the reproductive organs. The warts are caused by viruses belonging to the family of human papilloma viruses and transmitted through sexual contact.
Genu	Refers to the knee.
Genu Recurvatum	Hyperextension of the knee joint.
Genu Valgus	A condition where the knees are close together and the feet are apart, knock-knee.
Genu Varus	A condition where the knees are apart and the feet are close together, bow-legged.
Gestational Diabetes Mellitus (GDM)	Diabetes that develops during pregnancy, usually noticed between weeks 24-28 of pregnancy.
Glide	Movement of the clinician's hand across the client's skin.
Glucose	A simple sugar; the form in which all carbohydrates are used as the body's principal energy source.
Glucose Tolerance Test (GTT)	A test used for diagnosing diabetes. Glucose (blood sugar) is measured in intervals after a glucose-rich meal is ingested.
Glycogen	The storage form of glucose found in the liver and muscles.
Goiter	An enlargement of the thyroid gland usually visible as a swelling in the anterior portion of the neck.
Golfer's Elbow	Inflammation of the medical epicondyle of the humerus caused by activities (e.g. golf) that involve gripping and twisting, especially when there is a forceful grip.
Golgi Tendon	Receptors in the tendon that sense tension.
Golgi Tendon Organ (GTO)	A sensory receptor that responds to the tension or stretching of the tendon and relays impulses to the central nervous system. When stimulated, the GTO inhibits or relaxes the entire muscle group to protect against excessive force and injury.
Golgi Tendon Receptors	Receptors in the tendons that sense tension.
Gout	A metabolic disease that is a form of acute arthritis, marked by joint inflammation and an abnormally increased level of uric acid in the blood. It can be genetic or caused by a high intake of foods with purines (e.g. organ meats, alcohol).
Gross Anatomy	Large easily observed organs and organ systems.
Growth Hormone	A hormone that promotes cell division; in adults it is implicated in the repair and regeneration of tissue.
Guarding	Contraction of muscles in a splinting action, surrounding an injured area.
Hacking	A type of tapotement that alternately strikes to the surface of the body with quick, snapping movements.
Hallux Rigidus	Painful flexion deformity of the great toe, in which there is limitation of motion at the metatarsophalangeal joint.
Hallux Valgus	Angulation of the great toe away from the midline of the body, or toward the other toes.
Hammer Toe	A condition in which the big toe points upward and the second and third toes point downward.
HBIG	(Hepatitis B Immune Globulin) An injection that contains antibodies to hepatitis B virus and offers prompt but short lived protection against Hepatitis B.

Terms	Definitions
HBSAG	(Hepatitis B Surface Antigen) A serologic marker on the surface of the hepatitis B virus. The body will normally produce antibodies to hepatitis B surface antigen as part of the normal immune response to infection. The presence of antibodies to the hepatitis B surface antigen that are detected in a positive hepatitis blood test.
Headache	Pain felt in the head or upper neck.
Healing	The restoration of wellness or health.
Health	Optimal functioning with freedom from disease or abnormal processes; being free from physical and/or psychological disease or ailment.
Health-Related Quality of Life	The objective and subjective dimensions of an individual's ability to function in, and derive satisfaction from, a variety of social roles in the presence of impaired health status.
Healthy Weight	A weight range that correlates with a less than average risk for weight-related health problems.
Heart	A muscular organ that pumps blood throughout the body.
Heart Disease	An abnormal condition of the heart and/or circulation. See also "Cardiovascular Disease."
Heart Rate Reserve (HRR)	Also called Maximum HRR is defined as the difference between the maximum Heart Rate and the resting Heart Rate.
Heat Exhaustion	Heat disorders, resulting from the body's inability to efficiently dissipate heat through the sweating mechanism. Characterized by elevated body temperature, breathlessness, extreme tiredness, dizziness, and rapid pulse.
Heat Stress	The first stage of heat related illnesses from exercise in the heat. Heat stress begins when the body cannot sufficiently cool itself. A major factor is the percent relative humidity.
Heavy Pressure	Compressive force that extends to the bone under the tissue.
Heberden's Node	Small hard nodule(s), formed at the distal interphalangeal articulations of the fingers. Associated with interphalangeal osteoarthritis.
Heel Spur	A bone projection on the lower surface of the calcaneus (heel bone) that causes pain when walking.
Heel Strike	The phase during locomotion when the heel contacts the ground following the swing through of the leg and before the entire foot contacts the ground for push off.
Hemarthrosis	Joint pain and swelling caused by bleeding into a joint.
Hematoma	An accumulation of blood, released from a broken blood vessel, into the surrounding tissues resulting in a clot formation (solid mass) and swelling.
Hemiplegia	Paralysis of one side of the body.
Hemochromatosis	A rare disease of iron metabolism in which iron accumulates in body tissues. It can lead to sexual dysfunction, heart failure, joint pains, liver cirrhosis, diabetes mellitus, fatigue, and darkening of skin.
Hemorrhage	An escape of blood or bleeding through ruptured or un-ruptured vessels.
Hemorrhagic Stroke	(Cerebral Hemorrhage) Occurs when an artery bursts and blood seeps from the rupture into surrounding brain tissue and continues to do so until the seepage is blocked or the blood clots.
Hepatitis	Inflammation caused by viruses and chemicals (alcohol and some medications). New forms of hepatitis have been identified and the etiology and treatments are different for each. Hepatitis B is the most common type.
Hepatitis Type A	A form of viral hepatitis also called infectious hepatitis. It can spread through personal contact with oral secretions and bowel movements, and is also transmitted sexually. There is no specific treatment for hepatitis A.
Hepatitis Type B	(HepB) Inflammation caused by a virus that infects the liver. This form of viral hepatitis is known as serum hepatitis, because it is commonly spread through contact with infected blood products (transfusions or contaminated needles). Hepatitis B may also be spread sexually or from mother to child during pregnancy.
Hepatitis Type C	A chronic viral form of hepatitis primarily caused through transfusions or contaminated needles. Sexual transmission is rare. There is no specific treatment yet, although interferon may be successful in some people.
Hepatitis Type D	A rare form of hepatitis that occurs in some individuals with hepatitis B. Treatment is the same as for hepatitis B and individuals who develop this type of hepatitis are more likely to suffer more severe illness.
Hernia	Protrusion of abdominal viscera through a weakened portion of the abdominal wall.
Herniated Disc	Refers to a protrusion of a vertebral disc, a disorder involving displacement of the internal components of the vertebral disc beyond the outer wall of the disc. A herniated disc may occur either in the cervical or lumbar spine. Symptoms vary in degree and severity, but radiating pain, numbness or tingling, and weakness in the arms or legs, is common.
Herpes Zoster	Acute infectious, usually self-limited, disease believed to represent activation of latent human herpes virus 3 in those who have been made partially immune after a previous attack of chickenpox.
High Density Lipoproteins (HDL)	Known as good cholesterol; it helps carry bad cholesterol away from the artery walls, thus preventing build-up of cholesterol in the artery walls.
High Impact Activities	An activity or exercise in which both feet leave the ground simultaneously (aerobics, jogging, running).
Hip Flexors	The muscles located on the front aspect of the hip, joining the hip and the femur (thighbone). These muscles contract to decrease the angle between the legs and torso. (e.g. walking, sit-up, knee lift).
HIPAA	Health Insurance Portability and Accountability Act. Requires health care provider to inform clients about privacy rights and how their information can be used.
Histamine	A chemical produced by the body that dilates the blood vessels.

GLOSSARY

Terms	Definitions
HLA	A genetic fingerprint on white blood cells and platelets, composed of proteins that play a critical role in activating the body's immune system to respond to foreign organisms.
Homeostasis	Dynamic equilibrium of the internal environment of the body through processes of feedback and regulation.
Hormonal stimulus	Stimulus by chemical messengers that travel through the bloodstream to stimulate other organs.
Hormone	A chemical messenger in the bloodstream.
Horner's Syndrome	A nerve condition causing sinking in of the eyeball, ptosis of the upper eyelid, slight elevation of the lower lid, flushing of the affected side of the face, and constriction of the pupil.
HR Max	Maximum Heart Rate. The highest heart rate value attainable during an all-out effort to the point of exhaustion.
Human Immunodeficiency Virus (HIV)	A type of retrovirus that is responsible for the fatal illness AIDS (Acquired Immune Deficiency Syndrome). It weakens the body's immune system, decreasing its ability to fight lethal infections and cancers. (See AIDS).
Human Papilloma Virus (HPV)	A disease caused by the human papilloma virus, characterized by a soft, wart-like growth on the genitalia, called genital warts.
Humeral Head	Top portion of the upper arm bone, humerus, which moves at the shoulder joint to allow motion at the joint.
Humerus	Upper arm bone extending from the shoulder to the elbow.
Hyperextension	Overextension, excessive extension of a body part.
Hypersensitivity	An exaggerated response to a stimulus or foreign property.
Hyperstimulation Analgesia	Diminishing the perception of a sensation by stimulating large-diameter nerve fibers. Some methods used are application of ice or heat, counterirritation, acupressure, acupuncture, rocking, music, and repetitive massage strokes.
Hyperstimulation Analgesia	The relief of pain through the stimulation of large-diameter nerves using a variety of techniques, such as acupuncture, acupressure, ice packs, etc.
Hypertension	(High Blood Pressure) A disease in which the heart pumps blood through the circulatory system with much greater force than necessary, eventually damaging the arteries. Diagnosed with a systolic (top) blood pressure reading of >140mm/hg or a diastolic (bottom) of >90mm/hg on 2 separate readings.
Hyperthyroidism	Excessive secretion by the thyroid gland, which increases basal metabolic rate.
Hypertonia	A general term used to refer to muscle tone that is above normal resting levels, regardless of the mechanism for the increase in tone.
Hypertonic	The existence of a greater level of tension. Also: Of a fluid, sufficiently concentrated to cause osmotic shrinkage of cells immersed in it.
Hypertonicity	Increase in muscle tone resulting in muscle tension. Also: An increased effective osmotic pressure of body fluids.
Hypertrophy	Increase in the size of a tissue or organ brought about by the enlargement of its cells rather than by cell multiplication. Muscles undergo this change in response to increased stimulus/ demands/work. For example, muscle hypertrophy occurs with strength training.
Hypo	Used in prefix form; meaning below normal or deficient.
Hypomobility	Deficient or abnormally decreased range of motion in a joint; movement is within the normal plane of motion, but limited. The opposite of hypomobility is hypermobility.
Hypothalamus	A portion of the brain which lies beneath the thalamus and secretes substances which control metabolism by exerting an influence on pituitary gland function. The hypothalamus is also involved in the regulation of body temperature, water balance, blood sugar and fat metabolism. The hypothalamus also regulates other glands such as the ovaries, parathyroid and thyroid.
Hypothermia	Low core body temperature.
Hypothyroidism	Deficiency of thyroid secretion, which decreases basal metabolic rate.
Hypotonia	A general term used to refer to muscle tone that is below normal resting levels, regardless of the mechanism for the decrease in tone.
Hypotonic	A tissue that possesses a lesser degree of tension. Also: Having a lesser osmotic pressure than a reference solution, which is ordinarily assumed to be blood plasma or interstitial fluid; more specifically, refers to a fluid in which cells would swell.
Hypoxia	Below normal levels of oxygen; insufficient amount of oxygen.
Ideal Body Weight (IBW)	An ideal weight based on height and weight charts.
Identification	The clinician's ability to distinguish between healthy and dysfunctional tissue states and to identify tissues and structures and their responses to applied force.
Iliotibial Band (IT Band)	A wide band of thick fibrous tissue that runs along the outside of the thigh from the hip to the knee.
Iliotibial Band Syndrome	A condition characterized by irritation and tenderness on the outside of the knee where the band crosses the knee. Local swelling and/or snapping of the band may occur with bending and straightening of the knee. Overuse, excessive running, and poor running mechanics are the primary causes of this condition.
Immunosuppressive Therapy	Use of a substance or procedure that lessens or prevents an immune response.
Impacted Fracture	One end of broken bone is pushed into the other end of the broken bone.
Impairment	A loss or abnormality of the affected individual's physiological, anatomical, cognitive, or emotional structure or function that occurs as a result of the initial or subsequent pathophysiology.

Terms	Definitions
Impairment-Level Outcome of Care	The outcome of care that is related to the client's impairment.
Impingement Syndrome	A condition characterized by a painful shoulder with motion, particularly overhead activities. Usually caused by a combination of several conditions occurring at the same time (e.g. bursitis and tendinitis of the rotator cuff and/or biceps tendinitis). May occur secondary to trauma or overuse.
Indication	A therapeutic application that promotes health or assists in the healing process. When there is justification to work an existing condition with a positive outcome.
Indigestion	Abnormal digestion, which usually includes one or more symptoms: pain, nausea and vomiting, heartburn, acid regurgitation, and gas or belching.
Inferior	Indicates the undersurface of a structure or a structure lower in relation to another structure (e.g. - away from the head). For example, the mouth is inferior to the eyes. The opposite is superior.
Inflammation	The reaction of tissues to injury or disease, characterized by redness, pain and swelling often seen at the site of infection or trauma.
Inflammatory Response	A normal mechanism characterized by pain, heat, redness, and swelling, that usually speeds recovery from an infection or injury.
Influenza (flu)	A viral illness with the following symptoms: fever, inflammation of the nose, larynx and bronchi, cough, fatigue, muscular pain, gastrointestinal disorders and nervous disturbances (headaches, dizziness). Influenza primarily affects the respiratory tract; however it can involve other body systems.
Informed Consent	Explains what therapist is going to do, tells what the client can expect and asks permission to work on the client; the client is informed that he/she can say no at any time.
Inguinal Hernia	A bulge or protrusion of soft tissue that forces its way through or between muscles in the groin area.
Inhibition	A decrease in or the cessation of a response or function.
Injury	Trauma or damage inflicted to a body part by an external force.
Inquiring Touch	Intelligent touch is inquiring touch. A good clinician is constantly asking questions, and the use of massage is no exception to this requirement. The use of inquiring touch does not imply that the clinician's touch feels tentative to the client or that it lacks firmness when required.
Insertion	The muscle attachment point that is closest to the moving joint.
Insulin Sensitivity	An allergic reaction to insulin rarely manifests urticaria, angioedema, or anaphylaxis. Also: the body system's responsiveness to glucose.
Integrated Approaches	Combined methods of various forms of massage and bodywork styles.
Integration	The process of remembering an event while being able to remain in the present moment, with an awareness of the difference between then and now, to bring some sort of resolution to the event.
Integumentary System	Forms the external body covering (mainly, skin) protecting deeper tissue from injury.
Intelligent Touch	The learned skills essential for successful clinical use of massage: attention and concentration, discrimination, identification, inquiry, and intention.
Intensity	How much exertion or how hard the exercise is performed.
Interferon	A family of glycoproteins derived from human cells, which normally has a role in fighting viral infections by preventing virus multiplication in cells. Is currently being used to treat some forms of hepatitis.
Internal Rotation	Turning around the axis of a joint toward the midline of the body. Opposite of external or lateral rotation, but synonymous with medial rotation (e.g. turning the shoulder inward internally rotates the shoulder, or turning the toes inward internally rotates the lower leg).
Intervals	Alternating short, fairly intense spurts of exercise with periods of relatively easy exercise. Vary distance and speed; allow sufficient recovery time between training days. Perform sets with specific numbers of repetitions.
Intervention	A single purposeful and skilled interaction between the clinician and the client.
Intervention Model	Seven step system to address a client-situation that has become inappropriate.
Intimacy	A tender, familiar, and understanding experience between beings.
Intra-abdominal	Within the abdominal cavity.
Intra-thoracic	Within the thoracic (chest) cavity.
Intrinsic	Situated on the inside, or pertaining exclusively to a certain body part; due to causes or elements internal to the body, organ, or part. Intrinsic is synonymous with internal. Opposite is extrinsic.
Intuition	Knowing something by using subconscious information.
Inversion	A turning inward, toward the body midline.
Ischemia	Insufficient blood flow to tissue that results in a decreased oxygen supply (hypoxia), increased carbon dioxide and an insufficient supply of nutrients. Can cause pain, stiffness, and soreness in the affected area.
Ischemic Compression	See trigger point pressure release.
Isolation	Exercises involving motion at one joint, targeting one specific muscle. In a properly performed biceps curl, the joint motion occurs only at the elbow and targets only the biceps muscle.
Isometric	A type of muscle contraction where the joint does not move and the muscle fiber neither lengthens nor shortens, but still produces a force. (e.g. pushing against a wall isometrically contracts the muscles of the arm)

Terms	Definitions
Isometric Contraction	A contraction in which the effort of the muscle or group of muscles is exactly matched by a counter pressure, so that no movement occurs, only effort.
Isoniazid (INH)	An antibacterial, used principally in treating tuberculosis.
Isotonic	A type of muscle contraction where the resistance remains constant throughout the exercise. (e.g. both raising and lowering a weight create an isotonic contraction). Also: denoting a solution having the same tonicity as some other solution with which it is compared, such as physiologic salt solution and the blood serum.
Joint End Feel	The sensation felt when a normal joint is taken to its physiological limit.
Joint Inflammation	Localized redness, swelling, and pain in a joint (the hinge-like structure between neighboring bones) that occurs as a result of overuse, injury, or infection.
Joint Instability	A condition in which a joint is unstable or loose. The individual may experience "giving way" of the joint.
Joint Integrity	The extent to which a joint conforms to the expected anatomical and biomechanical norms.
Joint Kinesthetic Receptors	Receptors in the capsules of joints that respond to pressure and to acceleration and deceleration of joint movement.
Joint Movement	The movement of the joint through its normal range of motion.
Joint Range of Motion	The capacity of the joint to move within the anatomic or physiological range of motion that is available at that joint based upon its arthrokinematics and the ability of the periarticular connective tissue to deform. Range of motion reflects the function of the contractile, nervous, inert, and bony tissues and the client's willingness to perform a movement.
Jojoba	Oil-like substance made from jojoba seeds used in massage therapy; it is hypoallergenic and healthy for skin and easily washes out of sheets and towels.
Jostling	A massage technique in which the soft tissues are shaken back and forth with short, quick, loose movements; may be accompanied by mobilization of surrounding joints; used to loosed up an area.
Karvonen Formula	The calculation of determining training heart rate by adding a given percentage of the maximal heart rate reserve to the resting heart rate.
Ketones	Compounds produced in the body from the breakdown of fat. This occurs when there aren't sufficient carbohydrate stores for energy. Ketones can cause weakness, nausea, dehydration, and extra stress on kidneys.
Kidney Failure	The inability of the kidneys to adequately remove wastes from the bloodstream, which can result in severe metabolic imbalances.
Kinesiology	The study of body motion and its relationship to the brain, nerves and muscles.
Kinesthetic Awareness	The ability to sense the extent, direction, or weight of movement. An individual's ability to feel where his/her body is in relation to space.
Klinefelter's Syndrome	An inherited abnormality of the sex chromosomes occurring in males.
Kneading	A massage movement, in which the hands alternately and rhythmically lift squeeze, and release the soft tissues; used for muscular relaxation and increasing circulation in the tissues.
Kyphosis	An exaggerated convex curvature in the thoracic region of the spine, causing a hunching of the back. Sometimes called a humpback.
Kyphotic curve	Outward curve of the spine.
Laceration	A wound made by tearing. Usually a jagged or irregular cut to the soft tissue.
Lactic Acid	A substance formed in the breakdown of glycogen in the muscles and found in fatigued muscles.
Lactose	A carbohydrate composed of the 2 sugars, glucose and galactose, commonly known as milk sugar.
Lactose intolerant	Unable to tolerate lactose found in dairy products; symptoms include nausea, bloating, gas and loose stools.
Latent Trigger Points	Trigger points which are not painful in and of themselves unless they are being palpated.
Lateral	Outer side, away from the body midline.
Lateral Flexion	Flexion toward the side of the body (e.g. bending the neck to the side so that the ear meets the shoulder is lateral flexion).
Lateral Rotation	Turning the axis of a joint away from the midline of the body. Opposite of internal or medial rotation, but synonymous with external rotation (e.g. turning the shoulder outward laterally rotates the shoulder, or turning the toes outward laterally rotates the lower leg).
Law of Similars	The concept that certain parts and organs of the body are related to other parts by virtue of their similar shape (e.g. the sacrum and the calcaneus, the buttocks and the calf muscles).
Laxative	A food or chemical substance that acts to loosen the bowels and prevent/relieve constipation.
Laxity (joint)	Looseness in the muscles and soft tissues surrounding a joint, resulting in an inability to maintain the integrity of the joint.
Lead-Pipe Rigidity	Constant resistance to passive movement.
Lengthening	The process in which the muscle assumes a normal resting length by means of the neuromuscular mechanism.
Lesion	Any pathological or traumatic discontinuity of tissue or loss of function of a part.
Leucine	An essential amino acid which is the most abundant amino acid found in protein.
Leukemia	A fatal disease of the blood-forming organs, characterized by a marked increase in the number of white blood cells, together with enlargement and proliferation of the lymphoid tissue of the spleen, lymphatic glands, and bone marrow.
Leukoplakia	A disease characterized by the development of white, thickened patches that sometimes fissure (crack). It develops in the cheeks, gums or tongue and is common in smokers and users of tobacco products.

Terms	Definitions
Leverage	Leaning with the body weight to provide pressure.
Life Events Model of Stress	Holmes and Rahe's model of stress that examined the nature and consequences of negative life events and proposed that interpersonal stressors are predictive of increases in disease activity.
Ligament	A strong band of fibrous connective tissue that connects bone to bone and supports and strengthens joints. Ligaments are flexible but inelastic.
Ligament Insufficiency	Anatomical or pathological shortening of the capsular ligament.
Ligament Laxity	Anatomical or pathological lengthening of the capsular ligament.
Liniment	Topical liquid or semi-liquid used for therapeutic purposes.
Lipoproteins	Lipid means fat. Proteins are the transport system for fats that allows them to travel throughout the body. A lipoprotein is therefore, a fat particle produced in the liver that travels in the body.
Liver Cancer	(Hepatocellular Carcinoma) A tumor of the liver. Risk factors include chronic active hepatitis B and cirrhosis of the liver.
Locking	Term used for straightening an arm or leg, to the point where the joint is locked in place, such as the elbow and knee joints. This typically involves hyperextension of the joint placing undue stress on the joint.
Long Term Goals	Objectives met within a year to a lifetime. (e.g. maintaining muscular strength and endurance by regular aerobic exercise and strength training).
Longitudinal Stretching	A stretch applied along the fiber direction of the connective tissues and muscles.
Lordosis	Excessive convex curve in the lumbar region of the spine.
Lordotic Curve	Inward curve of the spine.
Lotions	Semi-liquid substance containing agents for moisturizing the skin or for therapeutic proposes.
Lou Gehrig's Disease	This disease causes the motor nerve cells of the spinal cord to degenerate.
Low Density Lipoproteins (LDL)	Known as bad cholesterol; responsible for depositing cholesterol in the artery walls, which increases one's risk for heart disease.
Low Impact Activities	An activity or exercise in which both feet do not leave the ground simultaneously (water aerobics, walking).
Lubricant	A substance that reduces friction on the skin during massage movements.
Lumbar Spine	The area of the spinal column located directly below the last vertebra of the thoracic spine to the sacrum (tail bone), labeled L1-L5. Often referred to as the "low back," it provides mobility for the back, support for the upper portion of the body, and transmits weight to the pelvis and lower extremities.
Lumbar Vertebral Disc	Cartilage situated between each of the vertebrae in the low back or lumbar spine to reduce friction and provide shock absorption for the spine.
Lumbodorsal Fascia	A deep membrane or fibrous band of connective tissue that covers, supports, or separates muscles of the trunk and back. It also binds skin with underlying tissues. Synonymous with thoracolumbar fascia.
Lung Cancer	A cancerous growth in lung tissue; lung cancer may be metastatic from another source (e.g. the colon) or may be primary (originating in the lung).
Lymph Glands	Small bean-shaped organ made up of a loose meshwork of reticular tissue in which are enmeshed large numbers of lymphocytes, macrophages and accessory cells located along the lymphatic system.
Lymph Nodes	Molecules found throughout the body that act as filters, especially to keep bacteria from entering the bloodstream.
Lymphadenopathy	Disease of the lymph nodes.
Lymphatic Drainage	A specific type of massage that enhances lymphatic flow.
Lymphatic System	Open system of vessels distribution intra-cellular fluids.
Lymphedema	Accumulation of abnormal amounts of lymph fluid and associated swelling of subcutaneous tissues that result from the obstruction, destruction, or hypoplasia of lymph vessels.
Lymphoma	A general term applied to any neoplastic (abnormal growth of cells, such as cancer) disorder of the lymphoid tissue. Lymphoma can be a malignant or life-threatening tumor of the lymph glands.
Maintenance	An all-purpose application of sports massage that is scheduled between competitions. It aims at recovery, normalizing stressed tissues, and treating minor injuries and complaints.
Malignant	A term applied to a cancerous growth to indicate that it is likely to penetrate the tissues in which it originated to spread further (metastasize). The opposite of benign.
Malignant Melanoma (MM)	The most serious of the 3 types of skin cancer, often metastasizing, or spreading, throughout the body. Changes in the underlying skin cells that produce skin-coloring pigment (melanin) cause a malignant tumor to develop. This cancerous lump can develop from a mole.
Malleolus	A protruding bone found at the ankle joint.
Malocclusion	Malposition of the maxillary and mandibular teeth, affecting movements of the jaw that are essential for mastication.
Malunion	Faulty or poor union of the two fractured ends of a bone.
Mammogram	A special kind of breast x-ray that can detect malignant tumors and other breast abnormalities.
Manipulation	Skillful use of the hands in a therapeutic manner. Massage manipulations focus on the soft tissues of the body and are not to be confused with joint manipulation using a high-velocity thrust.
Manual Lymph Drainage	Methods of bodywork that influence lymphatic movement.
Massage Routine	The step-by-step protocol and sequence used to give a massage.

GLOSSARY

Terms	Definitions
Matrix	The intercellular substance of a tissue.
McBurney's Point	Sits one-third the distance between the anterior superior iliac spine (ASIS) and umbilicus that, with deep palpation, produces rebound tenderness, indicating appendicitis.
Mechanical Methods	Techniques that directly affect the soft tissue by normalizing the connective tissue or moving body fluids and intestinal contents.
Mechanical Response	A response that is based on a structure change in the tissue. The tissue change is caused directly by application of the technique.
Medial	Inner side, toward the body midline.
Medial Rotation	Turning around the axis of a joint toward the midline of the body. Opposite of external or lateral rotation, but synonymous with internal rotation (e.g. turning the shoulder inward medially rotates the shoulder, or turning the toes inward medially rotates the lower leg).
Medications	Substances prescribed to stimulate or inhibit a body process or replace a chemical in the body.
Mega-doses	Extremely high intake of vitamins, minerals, or other supplements that may lead to health problems and toxicity. At high doses, nutrients act as drugs rather than supplements.
Membrane	A thin, pliable layer of tissue covering or separating body structures and organs.
Meningoencephalitis	Infection that involves both meninges and brain.
Meniscus	A crescent-shaped cartilage located in the knee joint.
Menopause	A term that refers to the event that signifies the cessation of menstruation in the human female, usually occurring between the age of 46 and 50.
Menstrual Period	The cyclic (usually 4-week intervals), physiologic uterine bleeding which normally recurs in the absence of pregnancy during the reproductive period of the female.
Mentoring	Career support by someone with more experience.
Meralgia Paresthetica	Entrapment of the lateral femoral cutaneous nerve at the inguinal ligament, causing pain and numbness of the outer surface of the thigh in the region supplied by the nerve.
Meridian	In Traditional Chinese Medicine, a conduit or channel through which energy (qi, chi) circulates through the body in well-defined cycles.
Metabolic Disorder	Disorder in which a mutation of a single gene or a small number of related genes causes a metabolic disorder, such as diabetes.
Metabolism	All physical, chemical and energy changes that take place within the body.
Metabolite	A substance essential to the metabolism of a particular organism or to a particular metabolic process; a product of metabolism. Amino acids are metabolites of protein metabolism.
Metastasis	Migration of cancer cells.
Metastasize	A term applied to a malignant growth that develops in one part of the body as a result of the spread of abnormal cells from another part. The term also refers to the process of spreading (i.e., cancers that spread (metastasize) show up in other parts of the body and are called metastasis).
Metatarsal	The 5 bones of the forefoot that array with the toes. The metatarsal heads are located at the ball of the foot. The first metatarsal arrays with the great (big) toe and the fifth arrays with the little toe and so on.
Metatarsalgia	Condition involving general discomfort around the metatarsal's heads.
Microscopic Anatomy	Cells and tissues that can only be observed with magnifying instruments.
Migraine	Vascular headache usually temporal and unilateral in onset, with symptoms including lack of tolerance for sound and/or light.
Minerals	One of a group of nutrients essential for life. They help release energy from foods and play a vital role in all the processes that take place throughout the body.
MmHg	Unit used to measure pressure (millimeters of mercury).
Mobility	The amount of joint motion that occurs before being limited by surrounding tissues.
Mode of Exercise	The particular type of exercise being done (e.g. running, walking, cycling, swimming, water aerobics, aerobics, water polo, etc).
Moderate Pressure	Compressive pressure that extends to the muscle layer but does not press the tissue against the underlying bone.
Modifiable (Controllable) Risk Factors	Those risk factors that can be altered or changed by the individual through behavior changes. Examples include smoking, weight loss, and exercise.
Mole	A pigmented fleshy growth that can occur anywhere on the body. They are small, roughly circular areas of skin that are much darker than the surrounding skin.
Monounsaturated Fats	Fats associated with a decreased risk of heart disease and are generally liquid at room temperature (e.g. olive oil, canola oil, peanut oil).
Morbid Obesity	30% over ideal body weight, which places individual at risk for life-threatening weight-related medical conditions.
Mortality	Death rate; the ratio of the number of deaths to a given population.
Morton's Neuralgia	Form of foot pain, metatarsalgia caused by compression of a branch of the plantar nerve by the metatarsal heads.
Morton's Neuroma	Tumor growing from a nerve or made up largely of nerve cells and nerve fibres, resulting from Morton's neuralgia.
Motor Control	The ability to physically perform skillful movements involving agility, balance, and coordination.
Motor Point	The point where a motor nerve enters the muscle it innervates and causes a muscle to twitch if stimulated.
Multiple Sclerosis	A degenerative disease of the central nervous system characterized by the gradual accumulation of plaques of demyelization in the brain.

Terms	Definitions
Mumps	A contagious, feverish disease caused by a virus, and marked by inflammation and swelling of the parotid (saliva-making) gland (near the ear). The infection may also affect other organs, especially in adults.
Muscle Endurance	A muscle's ability to contract, or maintain torque, over a number of contractions or a period of time. Conversely, fatigue is inability to maintain torque, or the loss of power, over time.
Muscle Extensibility	The ability of a muscle and its associated fascia to undergo lengthening deformation during the movement of a joint through its anatomic range.
Muscle Fatigue	A state in which a muscle has lost its power to contract.
Muscle Integrity	The extent to which a muscle conforms to the expected anatomical and biomechanical norms.
Muscle Performance	A muscle's capacity to do work based on its length, tension, and velocity. Neurological stimulus, fuel storage, fuel delivery, and balance, timing and sequencing of muscle contraction influence integrated muscle performance.
Muscle Power	Work produced by a muscle per unit of time (strength x speed).
Muscle Resting Tension	The firmness to palpation at rest observed in muscles with normal innervation. Traditionally, resting muscle tension has been described as resulting from the physiological properties of muscle, such as viscosity, elasticity, and plasticity rather than from motor unit firing.
Muscle Soreness	Tenderness/soreness felt in the muscles as a result of a buildup of the end products of exercise. It usually disappears within a few minutes or several hours after exercise.
Muscle Spasm	Involuntary contraction of a muscle that results in increased muscular tension and shortness that cannot be released voluntarily.
Muscle Spindles	Structures located primarily in the belly of the muscle that respond to both sudden and prolonged stretches.
Muscle Squeezing	A petrissage technique in which one or both hands are used to grasp, lift, and squeeze a muscle, muscle group, or body segment without glide.
Muscle Strain or Tear	Lesion or inflammation of muscle fibers that can occur in response to trauma.
Muscle Strength	The force or torque produced by a muscle or group of muscles to overcome a resistance during a maximum voluntary contraction.
Muscle Tear	The separation of muscle tissue. A muscle tear may involve a partial tear or a complete tear. Complete tears typically require surgical intervention.
Muscle Testing Procedures	An assessment process that uses muscle contraction. Strength testing is done to determine whether a muscle responds with sufficient strength to perform the required body functions. Neurologic muscle testing is designed to determine whether the neurologic interaction of the muscles is working smoothly. The third type, applied kinesiology, uses muscle strength or weakness as an indicator of body function.
Muscular Balance	Opposing muscles groups have comparable strength, endurance, and flexibility.
Muscular System	Allows locomotion and facial expression while producing internal body heat.
Musculoskeletal	Refers to the muscles, bones, and supporting structures such as ligaments, tendons and fascia.
Musculotendinous Junction	The point where muscle fibers end and the connective tissue continues to form the tendon; a major site of injury.
Mutate	To change in form, quality or some other characteristic. To change the genetic material (DNA) inside the cell.
Myalgia	Muscle pain.
Myocardial Infarction (MI)	The medical term for a heart attack. The most common type is caused by a thrombosis, or blockage, of one of the coronary arteries by a blood clot. This cuts off the blood supply to one region of the heart muscle. Lack of an adequate blood supply damages the deprived tissue.
Myofascial Pain Syndrome	The sensory, motor, and autonomic symptoms caused by myofascial trigger points.
Myofascial Release	A system of bodywork that affects the connective tissue of the body through various methods that elongate and alter the plastic component and ground matrix of the connective tissue.
Myofascial Trigger Point	A hyperirritable spot in skeletal muscle that is associated with a hypersensitive palpable nodule in a taut band. The area is painful on compression and can give rise to a variety of symptoms, such as referred pain, referred tenderness, motor dysfunction, and autonomic phenomena.
Myofibril	A very small longitudinal fiber found in skeletal or cardiac muscle fiber.
Myotatic Stretch Reflex	Reflex contraction of a muscle in response to it being stretched. The muscle will try to contract to oppose the attempt to elongate it.
Myotomal Pain	Pain in a myotome, or a group of muscles that are supplied by one nerve root.
Nephropathy	Any disease of the kidneys.
Nerve Impingement	Pressure against a nerve by skin, fascia, muscles, ligaments, or joints.
Nervous System	Control system of the body, responding to internal and external stimuli.
Neural Stimulus	Endocrine organs are stimulated by nerve impulses.
Neuralgia	Nerve pain
Neuritis	Inflammation of a nerve, with pain and tenderness.
Neurogenic	Forming nervous tissue, or originating in the nervous system.
Neurogenic Pain	Pain that result from noninflammatory dysfunction of the peripheral or central nervous system that does not involve nociceptor stimulation or trauma.
Neurologic Muscle Testing	Testing designed to determine whether the neurologic interaction of the muscles is proceeding smoothly.
Neurological	Pertaining to the nervous system.

GLOSSARY

Terms	Definitions
Neuromuscular	The interaction between nervous system control of the muscles and the response of the muscles to the nerve signals.
Neuromuscular Approaches	Methods of bodywork that influence the reflexive responses of the nervous system and its connection to muscular function.
Neuromuscular Mechanism	The interplay and reflex connection between sensory and motor neurons and muscle function.
Neuromuscular or Muscle Tone	Muscle resting tension and responsiveness of muscles to passive elongation or stretch.
Neuromuscular Technique	As defined by Chaitow and others, complex massage system that includes specific finger and thumb techniques that resemble stripping and direct fascial technique.
Neuropathy	A term describing functional and/or pathological changes in the peripheral nervous system, usually causing abnormal sensation (such as numbness, tingling, burning, or feelings of coldness) in the hands and feet; weakness in distal area of a peripheral nerve as a result of trauma or degeneration.
Neurotransmitter	A chemical messenger in the synapse of a nerve.
Neutral Position	Neither flexion nor extension.
Neutral Position (Neutral Spine/Neutral Trunk Posture)	Position the spine in such a way to avoid extreme stress on any part of the spine. Maintain natural curvature of the spine.
Nicotine	The addictive substance found in tobacco products.
Nociceptive Pain	Sensitization of peripheral nociceptors as a result of injury to a muscle or a joint that causes increased release of neurotransmitters in the dorsal horn of the spinal cord. The sensitized dorsal horn neurons demonstrate increased background activity, increased receptive field size, and increased responses to peripherally applied stimuli.
Nodule	A small lump, swelling or collection of tissue.
Non Myofascial Trigger Points	A hyperirritable spot in scar tissue, fascia, periosteum, ligament, or joint capsule that is associated with a hypersensitive palpable nodule in a taut band.
Non-Impact Activities	Activities such as swimming.
Nonunion	Failure of fractured ends of a bone to unite.
Norepinephrine	A neurochemical that functions in a manner similar to epinephrine but that is more concentrated in the brain.
NSAIDs	~Nonsteroidal Anti-Inflammatory Drugs ~ Medications designed to reduce pain and inflammation of chronic conditions. Many available over-the-counter. Some common generic names: aspirin, ibuprofen, and naproxen. Avoid use within the first few days of an injury as they may retard the healing process.
Obesity	A condition where surplus fat is stored by the body. A person may be considered obese if he/she exceeds the "desirable" weight for his/her height, build, and age by more than 20%.
Object Being Palpated	The chosen portion of the sensory field on which the clinician focuses attention during palpation. The object being palpated is not necessarily a physical object; instead, it may be a characteristic, such as temperature, or a phenomenon, such as resistance to movement.
Occlusion	A blockage; an obstruction to the flow of blood through an artery resulting from a spasm of the vessel or the presence of a clot.
Odynophagia	Pain during swallowing.
Omega-3 Fatty Acids	Types of polyunsaturated fat that may help lower the risk of heart attack or stroke. Found in seafood, especially higher fat fish, such as albacore tuna, mackerel, sardines, lake trout, herring, and salmon.
Omega-6 Fatty Acids	Types of polyunsaturated fat found in vegetable oils, such as sunflower, safflower, corn & vegetable oils.
Oncologist	A doctor who specializes in the diagnosis, treatment, and rehabilitation of individuals suffering with cancer.
One Repetition Maximal (1RM)	The maximal amount of weight lifted or moved in one effort. Bench press is typically used for upper body, leg press for lower body.
Open Fracture	Compound fracture in which the skin is perforated and there is an open wound down to the fracture.
Opposing Muscles	The muscles on the opposite side of a joint that perform the opposite movement of the muscles that are contracting [e.g. the hamstrings (knee flexors) and the quadriceps (knee extensors)].
Oral	Pertaining to the mouth. Also refers to ingestion through the mouth.
Oral Cancer	Cancer affecting the mouth.
Orchitis	Inflammation (swelling) of a testis (testicle), usually caused by bacteria. It causes pain, swelling, and a feeling of testicle heaviness.
Organ Systems	Composed of two or more organs working together to perform a higher function.
Organism	Living thing composed of many organ systems.
Organs	Composed of different tissue that works together to form a structure that performs a specific function.
Origin	The attachment point of a muscle at the fixed point during movement.
Orthopedist	A physician treating disorders of the skeletal system.
Orthotics	A material usually made of plastic or rubber, individually fitted and inserted into everyday footwear to correct foot problems such as flat feet (e.g. arch supports).
Osteitis	Inflammation of a bone, causing enlargement of the bone, tenderness, and a dull, aching pain.

Terms	Definitions
Osteo kinematic Movements	The movements of flexion, extension, abduction, adduction, and rotation; also known as physiological movements.
Osteoarthritis	Noninflammatory degenerative joint disease, characterized by degeneration of the particular cartilage, hypertrophy of bone at the margins, and changes in the synovial membrane. Seen particularly in older persons.
Osteopath	A physician using therapeutic bone manipulation in addition to other medical procedures.
Osteoporosis	A condition characterized by the loss of calcium from and porosity of the bones, common to the elderly.
Outcome of Care	The results of an intervention or the treatment regimen as a whole.
Ovarian Cancer	Cancer of the ovaries. It is the leading cause of death from gynecologic malignancies.
Overload	To place a greater workload on the body than what it is normally accustomed; also known as stimulus.
Overload Principle	A stress on an organism that is greater than the one regularly encountered during everyday life.
Over-training	The attempt to do more work than can be physically tolerated. Over-training results from performing activities at an unnecessarily high training volume, training intensity, or both.
Overuse (Injury)	Any injury that has been caused by small, repetitive overloaded forces on the structural and force generating parts of the body. Too much activity that places excessive stress on the body or body part (e.g. tennis elbow, shin splints, stress fractures, tendinitis).
Oxytocin	A hormone that is implicated in pair or couple bonding, parental bonding, feelings of attachment, and care taking, along with its more commonly known functions in pregnancy, delivery, and lactation.
Pacing	Refers to the speed of performing techniques.
Paget's Disease	Rare disease where bone is replaced by fibrous tissue that then becomes hard and brittle, with much pain. Particularly affecting the skull, spine, and leg bones.
Pain	An unpleasant sensation associated with actual or potential tissue damage that is mediated by specific nerve fibers to the brain where its conscious appreciation may be modified by various factors.
Painful Arc Syndrome	Pain located within a limited number of degrees in the range of motion.
Palliative Care	Care intended to relieve or reduce the intensity of uncomfortable symptoms but that cannot affect a cure.
Palmar	Pertaining to the palm.
Pancreatitis	Inflammation of the pancreas. It can be an acute or chronic condition, and is caused by auto-digestion of a pancreatic tissue by its own enzymes.
PAP Test	(Named after Dr. Papanicolaou) A cervical cancer-screening test. Cells are scraped from the outside of the cervix and just inside the cervical canal, then tested to identify the presence of abnormal cervical and other reproductive tract cells.
Paralysis	Loss or impairment of motor or sensory function.
Parasympathetic Autonomic Nervous System	The restorative part of the autonomic nervous system. The parasympathetic response often is called the relaxation response or the "rest and digest" response.
Parkinsonian Rigidity	Rigidity that occurs as a result of basal ganglia lesions. It presents clinically as a tight contraction of both agonist and antagonist muscles throughout the movement (lead-pipe rigidity).
Passive	Not produced by active efforts, does not require energy.
Passive Joint Movement	Movement of a joint by the massage practitioner without the assistance of the client.
Passive Movement	Client is relaxed while the practitioner moves his/her body.
Passive Movement Techniques	Massage techniques that primarily palpate the movement of tissues and structures, and result in the repetitive movement of soft tissue masses over the underlying structure(s) with varying degrees of joint motion.
Passive Range of Motion	The amount of joint motion available when an examiner moves a joint through its anatomic or physiological range, without assistance from the client, while the client is relaxed.
Passive Rest	Cessation of all movements after exercise.
Patella	Pertaining to the kneecap.
Patellar Tendinitis	Inflammation of the patellar tendon, the tendon that attaches the muscles of the leg (quadriceps) to the patella (kneecap) and tibia (lower leg).
Patellofemoral	Pertaining to the patella (kneecap) and the femur (thighbone).
Pathogenic Animals	Large, multicellular organisms sometimes called metazoa. Most metazoa are worms that feed off human tissue or cause other disease processes.
Pathologic Barrier	An adaptation of the physiologic barrier that allows the protective function to limit rather than support optimal functioning.
Pathology	The study of disease.
Pelvis	The bony structure formed by the innominate (hip) bones, sacrum and coccyx (tailbone) and the surrounding ligaments. The structure supports the vertebral column and movement of the legs.
Percussion, or Percussive Techniques	Massage techniques that deform and release tissues quickly through controlled, repeated, rhythmical, light striking.
Perimysium	Wraps bundles of fibers within a muscle.
Periosteum	Wraps bone and connects to tendons.

GLOSSARY

Terms	Definitions
Peripheral Artery Disease	Progressive occlusive disease of the arteries that supply the extremities. Risk factors include atherosclerosis and diabetes. Symptoms often occur in the hands and feet.
Peripheral Muscles	Muscles surrounding the moving joint, but not involved in the action of the joint (e.g. the supinator is a peripheral muscle in elbow flexion).
Peripheral Neuropathy	A condition in which injury to the peripheral (surface) nerves causes abnormal sensation to the tissues in the periphery. It most commonly involves the arms, legs, hands, and feet. See neuropathy.
Peripheral Vascular Disease (PVD)	A broad term used to describe a disease of the arteries and veins of the extremities; i.e. atherosclerosis, which is accompanied by narrowing of the arteries.
Pes	Refers to the foot.
Pes Cavus	Abnormal concavity of the sole or arch of the foot. Possessing high arched feet.
Pes Planus	Abnormal flattening of the sole or arch of the foot. Possessing flat feet.
Petrissage	Kneading, rhythmic rolling, lifting, squeezing, and wringing of soft tissue.
Phasic Muscles	The muscles that move the body.
Phlebitis	Inflammation of a vein, usually caused by blockage of the vein.
Physical Assessment	Evaluation of body balance, efficient function, basic symmetry, range of motion, and ability to function.
Physiologic Barriers	The result of the limits in range of motion imposed by protective nerve and sensory function to support optimal performance.
Physiological Adaptations	The body's ability to adjust and adapt body functions to physical activity.
Physiological Model of Stress	Hans Selye's model of stress that is based on the interaction of the adrenal cortex and the neuroendocrine and immune systems during stress. Stress in this model is defined as the body's automatic response ("fight or flight") to a demand that is placed on it.
Physiotherapy	The treatment of disease through the use of water, air, heat, massage, exercise or other physical forms of therapy.
Phytochemicals	Plant chemicals found in fruits, vegetables, dry beans and whole grains that help protect against some cancers, heart disease, and other chronic health conditions.
Picking Up	A one-handed or two-handed gliding petrissage technique in which muscle is lifted and squeezed between the fingers and the abducted thumb.
Piezoelectricity	The production of an electrical current by application of pressure to certain crystals such as mica, quartz, Rochelle salt, and connective tissue.
Pitting Edema	Edema that retains the indentation produced by the pressure of palpation.
Placebo	A medicinal preparation having no specific pharmacological activity against the client's illness or complaint given solely for the psycho physiological effects of the treatment.
Plantar	Having to do with the sole of the foot.
Plantar Fascia	A broad band of connective tissue located on the bottom of the foot and extending the length of the foot, heel to toes. It supports the arch of the foot.
Plantar Fasciitis	Irritation and inflammation of the plantar fascia, usually due to stretching and tearing of the tissue as a result of overuse. The pain is most severe at the heel bone and particularly with weight bearing. A heel spur may develop as the condition worsens. Maintaining proper flexibility in the plantar fascia and Achilles tendon will minimize the chance of developing this problem.
Plantar Flexion	The act of extending of the foot to increase the angle between the top of the foot and the front of the leg (e.g. pointing the toes). Dorsiflexion is the opposite of plantarflexion.
Plaque	A mass of fatty tissue (cholesterol, other fat particles, and debris from the blood) that builds up on the walls of an artery and can cause a blockage to the flow of blood.
Pliability	The inherent quality of tissue that refers to the ease with which it is bent, twisted, sheared, elongated, or compressed.
Pneumonia	A disease marked by inflammation and/or infection of the lungs. Symptoms can include a chill, followed by sudden elevation of temperature, difficult and rapid breathing, pain in the chest and side, and cough. Viruses and bacteria most commonly cause pneumonia.
Polarity	A holistic health practice that encompasses some of the theory base of Asian medicine and Ayurveda. Polarity is an eclectic, multifaceted system.
Poliomyelitis	An infectious disease, causing paralysis of the muscles.
Polymyalgia Rheumatica	Syndrome characterized by proximal joint and muscle pain; often affects the elderly.
Polyp	A small, benign growth in the large intestine that develops as an outgrowth of tissue from the skin or mucous membrane. They appear as a short stalk with a knob on the end.
Polyunsaturated Fats	Fats associated with a decreased risk of heart disease, which are generally liquid at room temperature (e.g. safflower, sunflower, soybean, corn, and vegetable oils).
Positional Release	Methods of moving the body into the direction of ease (the way the body wants to move out of the position that causes pain); the positioning places the painful area in a state of safety and may cause it to stop signaling for protective spasm.
Positioning	Placing the body in such a way that specific joints of muscles are isolated.
Post Isometric Relaxation (PIR)	The state that occurs after isometric contraction of a muscle; it results from the activity of minute neural reporting stations called the Golgi tendon bodies.
Posterior Tibial Compartment Syndrome	Pain in the posterior compartment of the lower leg, including soleus, gastrocnemius, tibialis posterior, flexor digitorum longus, and flexor hallucis longus. Site of pain varies depending on muscles affected.

Terms	Definitions
Postpartum	After childbirth or delivery.
Postural Drainage	The use of positioning to promote the movement of bronchial secretions through the lungs; conventionally used in conjunction with percussion.
Postural Malalignment	Abnormal joint alignment caused by soft-tissue imbalance or deformity within a bone.
Postural Muscles	Muscles that support the body against gravity.
Postural Tone	The development of muscular tension in skeletal muscles that participate in maintaining the positions of different parts of the skeleton. The cerebellum regulates postural tone. Unlike muscle resting tension, constant muscle activation is required for the maintenance of postural tone, and the self-sustained firing of motoneurons may reduce the need for prolonged synaptic input in this situation.
Posture	The positioning and alignment of the skeleton and associated soft tissues in relation to gravity, the center of mass, and the base of support of the body.
Powder	A type of lubricant that consists of a finely ground substance.
Pressure of Technique	The amount of force per unit area of contact surface that the clinician applies.
Process of Care	The manner in which care is delivered; the activities that take place within and between the clinician and the client. This encompasses the interpersonal aspects of the client-clinician interaction and the technical aspects of how the clinician provides care.
Prognosis	The process of predicting the client's level and timing of improvement.
Prone	Lying face down.
Proprioceptive Neuromuscular Facilitation (PNF)	Specific application of muscle energy techniques that uses strong contraction combined with stretching and muscular pattern retraining.
Proprioceptive Palpation	A form of palpation in which the clinician uses proprioceptive sense to gauge how the client's compressed tissues are deforming under the application of the clinician's body weight.
Proprioceptor	Sensory receptors that detect joint and muscle activity.
Psychogenic Stress	Stress which is triggered by the autonomic nervous system and is psychologically oriented.
Ptosis	Downward displacement.
Pulse	Throbbing or beat caused by expansion and contraction of the arterial walls.
Quadriceps	The muscle group located in the front of the thigh.
R.I.C.E. First Aid	First aid treatment for acute muscle injuries (rest, ice, compression, elevation).
Radiation	Electromagnetic waves.
Radicular Pain	Pain that is felt in a dermatome, myotome, or sclerotome because of direct involvement of a spinal nerve or nerve root. Also known as nerve root pain.
Radiculopathy	Disease of the nerve roots.
Radioactive iodine	Iodine that gives off radiation, often used for thyroid testing.
Range of Motion	Movement of joints. The degree of motion allowed at a specific joint.
Rapport	The development of a relationship based on mutual trust and harmony.
Rate of Technique	An indication of how fast the force is applied. The rate may describe the speed of the movement of the clinician's hand over the client's skin (distance per second), or the frequency of repetitions of a described technique (repetitions per second), or both.
Receptor (homeostatic control mechanism)	Monitors and responds to changes in the environment.
Reciprocal Inhibition (RI)	The effect that occurs when a muscle contracts, obliging its antagonist to relax in order to allow normal movement to take place.
Reciprocity	The exchange of privileges between governing bodies.
Reclining	Face up with a back-rest to prop up torso.
Recommended Dietary Allowance (RDA)	The levels of intake of essential nutrients that, on the basis of scientific knowledge, are judged by the Food and Nutrition Board to be adequate to meet the known nutrient needs of practically all healthy persons.
Recovery Heart Rate	The heart rate response at the cessation of exercise. An indication of fitness levels; higher fitness levels will produce a rapid drop in heart rate post exercise due to heart and lung efficiency.
Recovery Massage	Massage structured primarily for the uninjured athlete who wants to recover from a strenuous workout or competition.
Recurrent	Returning at intervals or happening time after time.
Reenactment	Reliving an event as though it were happening at the moment.
Referral	Sending a client to a health care professional for specific diagnosis and treatment of a disease.
Referred Pain	Pain felt in a region of the body distant from site of tissue damage or injury.
Reflex	An involuntary response to a stimulus, a pressure point which affects another area in the body.
Reflexive Methods	Massage techniques that stimulate the nervous system, the endocrine system, and the chemicals of the body. Reflexive methods work by stimulating the nervous system (sensory neurons), and tissue changes occur in response to the body's adaptation to the neural stimulation.
Reflexology	A system of manual treatment which applies specific compression to reflex points in the foot or hand to normalize function in distant body segments or organs.
Refractory Period	The period after a muscle contraction during which the muscle is unable to contract again.
Rehabilitation	The treatment and education process to restore maximum function resulting from a disease or injury.
Rehabilitation Massage	Massage used for severe injury or as part of intervention after surgery.

Terms	Definitions
Relaxation Phase	The stage of exercise when the muscles are no longer contracting.
Renal	Pertaining to the kidney.
Repetitive strain injury (RSI)	Refers to any overuse condition, such as strain, or tendonitis in any part of the body.
Reproductive System	Responsible for the production of offspring.
Resilience	The inherent quality of tissue which restores original form after deformation by applied force.
Resistance	That inherent quality of tissue which counteracts the tendency of applied force to produce movement of the tissue.
Resisted Movement	Client attempts to move while the practitioner resists the movement.
Resourceful Compensation	Adjustments made by the body to manage a permanent or chronic dysfunction.
Respiratory System	Keeps the blood constantly supplied with oxygen and removes carbon dioxide.
Resting Heart Rate (RHR)	The number of times the heart beats each minute while the body is at rest.
Resting Position	The first stroke of the massage; the simple laying on of hands.
Restrictive or Pathological Barriers In Soft Tissue	Barriers that are observed when soft tissue dysfunction is present. They can be located anywhere between the normal physiological barriers, can limit the available range of motion within the tissues, and can alter the position of the midrange. A restrictive barrier will change the quality of the movement and the "feel" at the end of the tissue range of motion. This is analogous to the abnormal end feels observed in joints.
Retinopathy	Disease of the structure of the eye called the retina, the light-sensitive layer of the eye.
Retraction	The act or condition of drawing back (e.g. squeezing the shoulder blades together). Opposite of protraction.
Retropatellar Pain Syndrome	Pain behind the patella (kneecap) caused by overuse or trauma. The condition may progress to Chondromalacia Patella.
Rheumatoid Arthritis	An autoimmune disease causing inflammation of the connective tissue, particularly the membranes that line the joints. The inflamed joints are painful, swollen and warm to the touch. The wrists and knuckles are most commonly affected.
Rhythm	The regularity of application of a technique. If the method is applied at regular intervals, it is considered even or rhythmic. If it is choppy or irregular, it is considered uneven or not rhythmic.
Rhythmical Mobilization	A technique in which entire structures are repetitively moved, resulting in the movement of soft tissue over bone and the movement of related joints and internal organs.
Right Of Refusal	The entitlement of both the client and the professional to stop the session.
Rigidity	Increased muscular tone that results from brainstem or basal ganglia lesions. Rigidity involves a uniformly increased resistance in both agonist and antagonist muscles, resulting in stiff, immovable body parts, independent of the velocity of the stretch stimulus.
Risk Factor	A clearly defined occurrence or characteristic that has been associated with the increased rate of a subsequently occurring disease.
Rocking	A technique in which gentle, repetitive oscillation of the body is produced by repeatedly pushing the pelvis or torso from a midline resting position into lateral deviation and then allowing it to return.
Rolling	A condition in which the inner border of the foot falls inward.
Rotation	Movement of a joint around its own axis.
S.O.A.P.	A problem-oriented method of medical record keeping; the acronym soap stands for subjective, objective, assessment, and plan.
Sacroiliitis	Inflammation (arthritis) in the sacroiliac joint.
Safe Touch	Secure, respectful, considerate, sensitive, responsive, sympathetic, understanding, supportive, and empathetic contact.
Salicylates	A group of chemical substances with anti-inflammatory properties. These drug compounds are similar to and include aspirin.
Same Gender Massage	Client and therapist are of same sex or gender.
Sanitation	The formulation and application of measures to promote and establish conditions favorable to health, specifically public health.
Saturated Fats	Fats associated with an increased risk of heart disease and are generally solid at room temperature. (e.g. butter, bacon grease, fats in meats and cheese, and the tropical oils: coconut, palm kernel and palm)
Scalene Syndrome	Thoracic outlet syndrome caused by compression of nerves and vessels between a cervical rib and scalenus anterior.
Scapulocostal Syndrome	Pain in the superior or posterior aspect of the shoulder girdle, as a result of long-standing alteration of the relationship of the scapula and the posterior thoracic wall.
Scar	The fibrous tissue that replaces normal tissues that have been destroyed by a burn, wound, surgery, radiation or disease.
Sciatica	Compression of a spinal nerve due to a herniated disc, a muscle-related or facet joint disease, or compression between the two parts of the piriformis.
Scleroderma	Chronic hardening and thickening of the skin, occurring in a localized or focal form as well as a systemic disease.
Sclerotomal Pain	Pain in a sclerotome, an area of bone or fascia innervated by one segmental nerve root.
Scoliosis	An abnormal lateral curvature of the spine.
Scope of Practice	The knowledge base and practice parameters of a profession.

Terms	Definitions
Screening Tests	Examination of people with no symptoms, to detect unsuspected diseases.
Second Degree Sprain or Strain	Partially torn tendon or muscle fibers, moderate swelling, and moderate limitations.
Sedation	The process of calming or allaying nervous excitement.
Sedentary	(Referring to lifestyle) Engaging in no regular exercise, performing minimal walking and movement, 75% of the day spent sitting or lying down.
Self Testicular Exam (STE)	A self-examination in which an individual performs a manual inspection of the testes (testicles), palpating (feeling) for lumps.
Semi-Supine	Face up with a back-rest to prop up torso (as used in pregnancy massage).
Sequence	A structured, outcome-based series or succession of massage techniques that comprise an intervention or a part of an intervention.
Seronegative Spondyloarthropathy	A general term comprising a number of degenerative joint diseases having common features, e.g. synovitis of the peripheral joints.
Serotonin	The neurochemical that regulates mood in terms of appropriate emotions, attention to thoughts, calming, quieting, and comforting effects; it also subdues irritability and regulates drive states.
Set	A number of repetitions performed without any rest (e.g. one set of ten repetitions or 1 X 10).
Sever's Disease	A traction-type injury, or osteochondrosis, of the calcaneal apophysis, seen in young adolescents.
Sexual Misconduct	Any behavior that is sexually oriented in the professional setting.
Shaking	A technique in which the body area is grasped and shaken in a quick, loose movement; sometimes classified as rhythmic mobilization.
Shattered	Comminuted fracture in which the bone is broken into pieces.
Shiatsu	A complex Japanese system of massage, based on the meridian system, which makes extensive use of specific compression.
Shin Splints	A straining of the muscles of the lower leg, causing pain.
Short Term Goals	Objectives usually to be met within a year (e.g. losing 1-2 lbs. each week for the next month).
Shoulder Girdle	Consists of shoulder blades (scapula), collarbones (clavicles) and supportive structures that attach the bones of the upper extremities (arms) to the spine.
Side Lying	Lying on side with pillows under head, arm and knee.
Skin	A layer of epithelium, the epidermis, and the dermis.
Skin Rolling	A gliding connective tissue technique in which tissue superficial to the investing layer of deep fascia is grasped, continuously lifted, and rolled over underlying tissues in a wave-like motion.
Social Skills Learning Theory	A behavioral theory that postulates that persons with unhealthy social skills (e.g. distorted views on eating) can adapt healthy social skills through behavioral training.
Societal Limitations	Those limitations to an individual's level of function that can be attributed to physical or attitudinal barriers in society.
Sodium	A mineral needed by the body to regulate fluid balance, help muscles relax, transmit nerve impulses and regulate blood pressure. Table salt (sodium chloride) is made up of 40% sodium and 60% chlorine.
Sodium Intake	The amount of sodium consumed in an individual's diet. American Heart Association recommends consumption of no more than 3,000 milligrams of sodium chloride per day.
Soft Tissue	The skin, fascia, muscles, tendons, joint capsules, and ligaments of the body; tissue that is not bone.
Soft Tissue Injury	Injury to a muscle, tendon or ligament; NOT injury to a bone. Ligament sprains and muscle strains are examples of soft tissue injuries.
Soft Tissue Range of Motion	Available range of motion of soft tissue that is analogous to the range of motion available in joints. Within this range of motion, normal soft tissue has three barriers or resistances that can limit movement.
Somatic	Pertaining to the body.
Somatic Pain	Pain that arises from stimulation of receptors in the skin (superficial somatic pain) or in skeletal muscles, joints, tendons, and fascia (deep somatic pain).
Spasm	An involuntary and sudden muscular contraction.
Spasticity	A state of increased muscle tone with exaggerated muscle tendon reflexes.
Specific Compression	A non-gliding neuromuscular technique in which pressure is applied to the target tissue with a specific contact surface in a direction that is perpendicular to the target tissue.
Specific Kneading	A gliding petrissage technique performed in circles or ellipses and delivered with a small contact surface such as the thumb.
Specific Technique	A technique that is applied to a localized area or applied with a small contact surface, or both.
Specificity	Focusing massage techniques on a specific condition and in a small area.
Specificity of Training	Training should be relevant to the demands of the activity and work the muscles involved in a manner resembling the movements performed during the activity (e.g. if training to improve a softball pitch, concentrate on the muscles of the upper arm and shoulder; also training should imitate the throwing motion).
Speed of Movement	The speed that repetitions are performed.
Spindle Cells	Sensory receptors in the belly of the muscle that detect stretch.
Spondyloarthropathy	Disease of the joints of the spine.
Spondylolisthesis	Forward displacement of one vertebra over another.
Spondylolysis	Dissolution of a vertebra.

GLOSSARY

Terms	Definitions
Spondylosis	Degenerative spinal changes due to osteoarthritis.
Sports Massage	Massage performed on athletes for the purpose of preparation, recovery, maintenance, or rehabilitation.
Sprain	The tearing of supporting ligaments.
Spur	A bony projection.
SSE (skin self exam)	A self-examination in which an individual performs a visual inspection of the skin, looking for new skin lesions and changes to existing lesions such as moles.
Stabilization	Holding the body in a fixed position during joint movement, lengthening, and stretching.
Stabilize	To maintain firm or steady.
Stabilizer Muscles	Muscles designed to protect the integrity of a joint and responsible for stabilizing one joint, so a specific movement can occur at another (e.g. the intrinsic muscles of the foot protect the ankle and the hip abductor on one side stabilizes the pelvis and trunk while the opposite leg abducts).
Stacking the joints	Pressure applied along the line of the bones and through the joints.
Staging	A system used to determine how far a type of cancer has spread. Health providers select appropriate treatment based on the stage.
Static Contact	A superficial reflex technique in which the clinician's hands contact the client's body without motion and with minimal force.
Static Stabilizers	Synonymous with stabilizer muscles. Muscles designed to protect the integrity of a joint. They function to maintain equilibrium without movement.
Static Stretch	Stretching muscle tissue to a comfortable position, and then holding this position for a period of time, usually 10-30 seconds. This stretch is low force, long duration, and is the safest stretch to perform if performed properly.
STD	Sexually transmitted disease such as genital herpes, gonorrhea, HIV or chlamydia, whose usual means of transmission is by sexual contact.
Stenosis	Abnormal narrowing of a duct or canal, e.g. spinal stenosis, a narrowing of the vertebral canal, caused by encroachment of the bone upon the space.
Sterilization	The process by which all microorganisms are destroyed on a particular object or area .
Sternum (breast bone)	A flat, narrow bone, situated in the median line of the front of the chest.
Steroid Medications	Hormonal preparations that are used primarily for anti-inflammatory purposes in arthritis or asthma; however they are also useful for treating malignancies or compensating for a deficiency of natural hormones (i.e. synthroid is a synthetic hormone taken by persons with hypothyroidism).
Steroids	Name given to some hormones produced by the body that act as chemical transmitters.
Stimulation	Excitation that activates the sensory nerves.
Stool	Fecal discharge of the bowels.
Stored Fat	Approximately 98-99% of body fat is composed of white fat cells, also called storage fat. Commonly seen on hips and buttocks in women; upper torso or abdominal area for men. Excessive caloric intake combined with inactivity will promote production of white fat cells, increasing total body fat weight.
Strain	A traumatic injury causing overstretching or tearing of a muscle or tendon beyond its normal limits.
Strain-Counterstrain	Using tender points to guide the positioning of the body into a space where the muscle tension can release on its own.
Strength	The force or tension that a muscle or muscle group can exert against a resistance.
Strength Testing	Testing intended to determine whether a muscle is responding with sufficient strength to perform the required body functions. Strength testing determines a muscle's force of contraction.
Streptococcus Pneumonia	A type of pneumonia caused by streptococcal bacteria.
Stress	Any substantial change in routine or any activity that forces the body to adapt.
Stress Fracture	A micro fracture or incomplete fracture caused by frequent, excessive, or repeated stresses or overuse to a bone (such as in running or marching long distances). The rate of bone breakdown exceeds the rate of bone repair.
Stress Response	The individual's cognitive, physiological, affective or behavioral response to the stressor, or stress causing agent.
Stressors	Any internal perceptions or external stimuli that demand a change in the body.
Stretch Receptor	A cell or group of cells found between muscle fibers responding to stretch of the muscle by transmitting impulses to the central nervous system. Stretch receptors are part of the proprioceptive system necessary for the performance of coordinated muscular activity. The golgi tendon organ is an example of a sensory receptor.
Stretch Reflex	Involuntary reflex contraction of a muscle in response to it being stretched. The muscle will try to contract to oppose the stretch. The muscle spindle is the sensory organ responsible for initiating the contraction. The stretch reflex occurs with ballistic stretching and inhibits the desired stretch.
Stretching	The act of elongating (making long) muscle and connective tissues to improve range of motion around a joint; mechanical tension applied to lengthen the myofascial unit (muscles and fascia).
Stripping	A slow, specific, gliding, neuromuscular technique that is applied from the origin of a muscle to its insertion for the purpose of reducing the activity of trigger points.

Terms	Definitions
Stroke	A technique of therapeutic massage that is applied with a movement on the surface of the body, whether superficial or deep.
Structural Integration	Methods of bodywork derived from biomechanics, postural alignment, and the importance of the connective tissue structures.
Structure of Care	The human, physical, and financial resources that is available for the delivery of care.
Subacute	Describing a condition, illness, or disease that progresses more rapidly than a chronic condition but does not become acute. Improvement from an acute condition.
Subluxation	Partial or incomplete dislocation of a joint so that the bone ends are misaligned, but still in contact; usually a subluxation is self-reducing (returns to normal position on its own).
Subtle Energies	Weak electrical fields that surround and run through the body.
Suffering	An overall impairment of a person's quality of life.
Suicide	The taking of one's own life.
Superficial Effleurage	A gliding manipulation performed with light centripetal pressure that deforms subcutaneous tissue down to the investing layer of the deep fascia.
Superficial Fascia	The connective tissue layer just under the skin.
Superficial Fluid Techniques	Massage techniques that are applied to tissues superficial to muscle that increase the return flow of lymph and possibly venous blood.
Superficial Lymph Drainage Technique	A non-gliding technique performed in the direction of lymphatic flow using short, rhythmical stokes with light pressure, which deforms subcutaneous tissue without engaging muscle.
Superficial Pressure	Pressure that remains on the skin.
Superficial Reflex Techniques	Massage techniques that palpate the skin and primarily affect level of arousal, autonomic balance, or the perception of pain.
Superficial Stroking	A superficial reflex technique that involves unidirectional pressureless gliding over the client's skin with minimal deformation of subcutaneous tissues; usually applied over large areas.
Superior	Situated higher in the body in relation to another structure or surface (e.g. towards the head). For example, the eyes are superior to the mouth. The opposite of inferior.
Supination	The act of assuming a supine position, or lying on the back face up. The act of turning the palm up or shifting the body weight to the outside of the foot. The opposite of supination is pronation.
Supine	The position in which the client is lying face up.
Supports	Objects such as pillows and bolsters that are used to make the client more comfortable, stable, or accessible during massage.
Swedish Massage	A system of massage, consolidated by Per Henrik Ling (1776-1839), which includes effleurage, petrissage, friction, tapotement, and shaking (or vibration), and which constitutes one of the technical foundations for outcome-based massage.
Swelling	An abnormal enlargement of a segment of the body.
Symmetry	The opposite sides of the body, right and left, are equal in size, shape and relative position. The right and left sides of the superficial body are mirror images of each other.
Sympathetic Autonomic Nervous System	The energy-using part of the autonomic nervous system, the division in which the fight-or-flight response is activated.
Symptomatic	Referring to the indication, sensation or appearance of a disorder or disease.
Symptoms	The subjective abnormalities felt only by the client.
Syndrome	A group of different signs and symptoms that usually arise from a common cause.
Synergistic	The interaction of medication and massage by combining two things to create an outcome greater than each would create on its own.
Synergy	Coordination of muscles or organs by the nervous system so that a specific action can be performed.
Synovial Fluid	A thick colorless lubricating fluid that surrounds a joint or bursa and fills a tendon sheath that nourishes and lubricates the cartilage of a joint.
Synovial Joint	A joint lined with synovial membrane that secretes synovial fluid.
Synovitis	Inflammation of the synovial membrane. A swollen and painful joint, especially with motion, characterizes the condition.
System	A group of interacting elements that function as a complex whole.
Systemic Disease	Pertaining to or affecting the body as a whole.
Systemic Massage	Massage structured to affect one body system primarily. This approach usually is used for lymphatic and circulation enhancement massage.
Systolic	The maximum pressure in the arteries, which occurs when the heart is contracting. Represented by the top number in the fraction of the blood pressure reading.
Tapotement	Springy blows to the body at a fast rate to create rhythmic compression of the tissue; also called percussion.
Tapping	A type of tapotement that uses the fingertips.
Target Heart Rate Range (THRR)	The Karvonen method takes into account an individual's resting HR as well as HR during activity.
Target Muscle	The muscle or groups of muscles on which the response of the methods is specifically focused.
Techniques	Methods of therapeutic massage that provide sensory stimulation or mechanical change of the soft tissue of the body.
Temporomandibular Joint	The joint at the junction of the temporal bone and the mandible (jaw), commonly called the TMJ.

Terms	Definitions
Tendinitis	Continuous low-grade inflammation of a tendon with pain on movement, usually caused by injury or overuse. Can progress to a partial or complete tendon rupture if not treated properly.
Tendinopathy	Disease of a tendon.
Tendinosis	Unlike tendinitis, which is an inflammatory condition, tendinosis refers to common overuse conditions of tendon that have a histopathology that is consistent with a noninflammatory, degenerative process of unclear etiology.
Tendon	Strong, fibrous tissue which connects muscle to bone.
Tendon Organs	Structures found in the tendon and musculotendinous junction that responds to tension at the tendon.
Tendon Rupture	A complete tear or breaking apart of the tendon. A common injury is the Achilles tendon rupture.
Tennis Elbow	Tendinitis of the muscles of the back of the forearm at their insertion and is caused by excessive hammering or sawing type movements, or a tense, awkward grip on a tennis racquet.
Tenosynovitis	Inflammation of the synovial sheath around the tendons.
Tension, or Tensile Force	Any force that is so oriented that its effect is to lengthen a tissue or structure.
Tenting	Technique that allows client to turn conveniently while maintaining boundaries.
Theory	An organized set of facts that explains the relationships between a groups of observed phenomenon.
Therapeutic	Having healing or curative powers.
Therapeutic Change	Beneficial change produced by a bodywork process that resulted in a modification of physical form or function that can affect a client's physical, mental, and/or spiritual state.
Thiamin Deficiency	A nutritional condition produced by a deficiency of thiamin in the diet, characterized by loss of appetite, irritability, and weight loss. In addition to being caused by a poor diet, thiamin deficiency in the United States most commonly occurs as a result of alcoholism.
Thixotropy	The property of some colloids by which they become more fluid when subjected to movement or heat, and less fluid when subjected to stasis or cold.
Thoracic Outlet Syndrome	Compression of the brachial plexus rather than the nerve roots; combination of pain in the neck and shoulder, numbness and tingling of the fingers, and a weak grip.
Thoracolumbar Fascia	A deep membrane or fibrous band of connective tissue that covers, supports, or separates muscles of the thoracic (trunk) and lumbar (low back) regions of the spine. It also binds skin with underlying tissues.
Thrombosis	The formation or presence of a blood clot.
Thrombus	Stationary blood clot along the wall of a blood vessel, frequently causing vascular obstruction.
Thyroid Gland	A butterfly shaped endocrine gland in the neck that is found on both sides of the trachea (windpipe).
Tibia	The larger of the two bones in the lower leg located on the inside between the knee and ankle.
Tic Douloureux	See Trigeminal Neuralgia.
Tietze's Syndrome	Swellings of one or more costal cartilages, especially the second rib. The anterior chest pain may mimic that of coronary artery disease.
Tissue	Composed of cells with similar form and function.
Tissues Engaged By Technique	The target tissues or layers of tissue to which the clinician directs the pressure of the stroke and that are mechanically deformed by application of the technique.
TMJ (Temporomandibular Joint) Syndrome	Complex of symptoms including tinnitus, dizziness, headache, and clicking of the TMJ. Causes suggested include mandibular overclosure, and stress.
Tonic Vibration Reflex	Reflex that tones a muscle with stimulation through vibration methods at the tendon.
Total Daily Caloric Needs	The total amount of calories your body needs every day, including for physical activity.
Total Joint Replacement	A surgical procedure in which the connection point between 2 bones (joint) is removed and replaced with an artificial device.
Total Skin Examination (TSE)	Examination of skin from head to toe.
Touch	Primary mode of personal interaction during massage; to come into contact with.
Touch Technique	The basis of soft tissue forms of bodywork methods.
Toughening/Hardening	The reaction to repeated exposure to stimuli that elicit arousal responses.
Trachea	Also called windpipe; a cylinder-shaped tube about 41/2" long that extends from the larynx to the bronchial tubes.
Traction	Gentle pull on the joint capsule to increase the joint space.
Training Stimulus Threshold	The stimulus that elicits a training response.
Trans Fatty Acid	Unsaturated fats that are chemically changed to become more like saturated fats. This makes them more stable and solid at room temperature (e.g. shortening, some margarines, crackers, cookies, and desserts). Also found naturally in beef, pork, lamb, butter, and milk.
Transference	When a client responds to practitioners as they might have responded to an important person from their childhood; the personalization of the professional relationship by the client.

Terms	Definitions
Transient Ischemic Attack (TIA)	A process caused by brain blood flow interruption causing symptoms of a stroke for up to 24 hours. They are often caused by blood cells blocking off a small artery in the brain. Blood flow is restored quickly, when the blood cells break up and are swept away. Recurrent attacks often warn of an impending stroke.
Trauma	Physical injury caused by violent or disruptive action, toxic substances, or psychic injury resulting from a severe long- or short-term emotional shock.
Traumatic	Caused by or pertaining to an injury.
Treatment	A series of interventions that make up an episode of care.
Treatment Plan	The plan used to achieve therapeutic goals. It outlines the agreed objectives; the frequency, duration, and number of visits; progress measurements; the date of reassessment; and massage methods to be used.
Tremors	Rhythmic movements of a joint that result from involuntary contractions of antagonist and agonist muscle groups.
Trigeminal Neuralgia	Excruciating episodic pain in the area supplied by the trigeminal nerve, often precipitated by stimulation of well-defined trigger points.
Trigger Point	An area of local nerve facilitation; pressure on the trigger point results in hypertonicity of a muscle bundle and referred pain patterns. Muscle fibers in this area have gone through injury and have not completely healed and when touched present moderate to severe pain.
Triglycerides	A type of lipoprotein made up of mostly fat and sugar, which is primarily stored in fat tissue.
Trismus	Motor disturbance of the trigeminal nerve, especially spasm of the masticatory muscles, with difficulty in opening the mouth.
Tuberculosis (TB)	A highly infectious disease characterized by the formation of rounded nodules in the tissues that spread in all directions, primarily through the respiratory system, but also through the lymph vessels and blood vessels disseminating through the body. Most common symptoms are cough, fever, and fatigue.
Tumor	A mass of new tissue which persists and grows independently of its surrounding structures, and which has no physiologic use.
Types of fascia	Superficial (on the surface) and deep.
Ulcerative colitis	A long term, inflammatory disease of the colon, in which raw, inflamed areas called ulcers, and small abscesses, develop in the lining of the large intestine.
Ulcers	Holes (wounds) that develop in the lining of the esophagus, stomach, or a part of the small intestine closest to the stomach caused by digestive secretions that irritate the lining of the gastrointestinal tract.
Ultrasound	A diagnostic procedure in which high-frequency sound waves are bounced off certain internal structures of the body. The reflections and echoes of these waves create a picture for the clinician to use to assess health of an organ, body part, or fetus.
Unilateral	Relating to or affecting one side of the body or one side of an organ or other part.
Urethra	The tube that carries urine from the bladder out of the body.
Urethritis	Inflammation of the urethra.
Uric Acid Crystallization	The deposit of uric acid, a waste product, in a part of the body.
Urinary	Pertaining to the urine, or the urinary system.
Urinary system	Eliminates nitrogenous wastes while maintaining a balance of electrolytes in the blood; includes the kidneys, ureter, bladder, and urethra.
Utero (in utero)	Refers to events that occur within the uterus.
Vaccination	The injection of vaccine for the purpose of inducing immunity.
Vaccine	A suspension of attenuated or killed microorganisms administered for the prevention or treatment of infectious diseases.
Valsalva Maneuver	A force created within the thoracic cavity as a result of holding breath and extreme exertion. *Particularly dangerous for hypertensive individuals.
Valsalva's Man Oeuvre	Forcible exhalation effort against a closed glottis, or occluded nostrils and a closed mouth.
Varicocele	Condition in males characterized by varicosity of the veins in the skin of the scrotum. Accompanied by a constant dull pain.
Varicose Veins	Abnormal stretching and swelling of the walls of the veins usually occurring in the legs and caused by excessive standing, obesity or pregnancy.
Vascular	Pertaining to the blood vessels.
Veins	Blood vessels that carry blood towards the heart.
Ventral	Pertaining to the belly, or indicating a position more toward the belly surface than some other object of reference. The opposite of dorsal. Synonymous with anterior in reference to human anatomy.
Vertebrae	Any one of the 33 bones of the spinal column, comprising the 7 cervical, 12 thoracic, 5 lumbar, 5 sacral, and 4 coccygeal vertebrae. Bony or cartilaginous segments, separated by discs to form the spinal column.
Vertebral Artery Syndrome	Vascular insufficiency involving compression of the vertebral artery in the cervical spine.
Vertebral Disc	Cartilage situated between each of the vertebrae to reduce friction and provide shock absorption for the spine.
Vibration	Fine or coarse tremulous movement that creates reflexive responses.
Viral	A virus is an ultramicroscopic infectious agent that replicates itself only within cells of living hosts
Visceral Pain	Pain resulting from injury or disease to an organ in the thoracic or abdominal cavity.

GLOSSARY

Terms	Definitions
Visco-Elastic Deformation	Deformation in response to applied force, which partially remains after the force is removed; visco-elastic deformation combines spring-like and putty-like behavior.
Viscosity, or Fluid Viscosity	The property of fluids and semi fluids that offers resistance to flow, i.e., stickiness.
Vital Force	Sum total of the body's energy or life force.
Warm up	A slow, rhythmic activity of larger muscle groups designed to help the body adapt from rest to exercise and should imitate the activity. Should last a minimum of 10-15 minutes.
Weight Bearing Exercise	Any exercise that requires the body to work against a resistance. Weight training/lifting, walking and jogging are weight-bearing exercises.
Wellness	The efficient balance of body, mind, and spirit, all working in a harmonious way to provide quality of life; the state of being whole in body, mind, and soul.
Wellness Massage	General massage in which the main outcomes of care are the reduction of anxiety, stress response, and muscle resting tension.
Wholistic/Holistic	A state in which, in nature, the individual (entity) or other completely organism cannot be reduced to the sum of its parts, but functions as a complete unit.
Wick	Term used to facilitate evaporation of sweat in cold temperatures, while still maintaining body heat. Refers to a function of clothing.
Wringing	A petrissage technique in which muscle is lifted and sheared between contact surfaces that are moving in opposite directions.
Yang	The portion of the whole realm of function of the body, mind, and spirit in Eastern thought that corresponds with sympathetic autonomic nervous system functions.
Yin	The portion of the whole realm of function of the body, mind, and spirit in Eastern thought that corresponds with parasympathetic autonomic nervous system functions.

Alon Lotan, *Acupoint Location Guide*, Estem, Yodfat, Isreal, 2000.

AMA, *AMA Encyclopedia of Medicine*, Random House, New York, NY, 2003.

Andrew Biel, *Trail Guide to the Body*, Books of Discovery, 2005.

Andrew Ellis, Nigel Wiseman, & Ken Boss, *Fundamentals of Chinese Acupuncture*, Paradigm Publications, Brookline, MA, 1988.

Art Riggs, *Deep Tissue Massage: A Visual Guide to Techniques*, North Atlantic Books, Berkeley, CA, 2002.

Barbara Ann Brennan, *Hands of Light: A Guide to Healing Through the Human Energy Field*, Bantam Doubleday Dell Pub, 1993.

Ben E. Benjamin & Gale Borden, *Listen to Your Pain: The Active Person's Guide to Understanding, Identifying, and Treating Pain and Injury*, Viking Press, New York, NY, 1984.

Bill Gottlieb, *Alternative Cures: The Most Effective Natural Home Remedies for 160 Health Problems*, Da Capo Press, Cambridge, MA, 1998.

Blandine Germain, *Anatomy of Movement*, Eastland Press, Seattle, WA, 1993.

Bonnie Prudden, *Myotherapy: Bonnie Prudden's Complete Guide to Pain-Free Living*, Ballantine Books, 1985.

C. Pierce Salguero, *Thai Massage Workbook: Basic and Advanced Courses*, Findhorn Press, Findhorn, Scotland, 2007.

Carla-Krystin Andrade & Paul Clifford, *Outcome-Based Massage: From Evidence to Practice (2nd Edition)*, Lippincott Williams & Wilkins, Philadelphia, PA, 2008.

Carmine Clemente, *Anatomy: A Regional Atlas of the Human body (4th Edition)*, Lippincott Williams & Wilkins, Philadelphia, PA, 1997.

Carole Osborne-Sheets, *Pre and Perinatal Massage Therapy: A Comprehensive Practioners' Guide to Pregnancy, Labor, Postpartum*, Body Therapy Associates, 1988.

Charles Fetrow, *The Complete Guide to Herbal Medicines*, Pocketbooks, New York, NY, 2000.

Chris Jarmey, *A Practical Guide to Acu-points*, North Atlantic Books, Berkeley, CA, 2008.

Chris Jarmey, *The Foundations of Shiatsu*, North Atlantic Books, Berkeley, CA, 2007.

Chris Jarmey, *Shiatsu, Revised Edition*, Thorsons, New York, NY, 2000.

Clair Davies, *The Frozen Shoulder Workbook: Trigger Point Therapy for Overcoming Pain & Regaining Range of Motion*, New Harbinger Publications, Oakland, CA, 2006.

Clair Davies, Amber Davies & David G. Simons, *The Trigger Point Therapy Workbook: Your Self-Treatment Guide for Pain Relief, Second Edition*, New Harbinger Publications, Oakland, CA, 2004.

Daniel Krinsky & James LaValle, *Lexi-Comp's Natural Therapeutics Pocket Guide, 2nd Edition*, Lexi-Comp, Inc, Hudson, OH, 2003.

David Hoffmann, *Healthy Bones & Joints: A Natural Approach to Treating Arthritis, Osteoporosis, Tendinitis, Myalgia & Bursitis*, Storey Books, New York, NY, 2000.

Deane Juhan, *Job's Body: A Handbook for Bodywork (Third Edition)*, Station Hill Press, Barrytown, NY, 1998.

Dimitrios Kostopoulos & Konstantine Rizopoulos, *The Manual of Trigger Point and Myofascial Therapy*, Slack Incorporated, 2001.

DoAnn T. Kaneko, *Oriental Healing Arts: Doann's Long Form (Spiral-bound)*, Shiatsu Massage School of California, Santa Monica, CA, 1994.

Don Cohen & John E. Upledger, *An Introduction to Craniosacral Therapy: Anatomy, Function, and Treatment*, North Atlantic Books, Berkeley, CA, 1983.

Don Scheumann, *The Balanced Body: A Guide to Deep Tissue and Neuromuscular Therapy*, Lippincott Williams & Wilkins, Philadelphia, PA, 2002.

Donna Finando & Steven Finando, *Trigger Point Therapy for Myofascial Pain: The Practice of Informed Touch*, Healing Arts Press, Rochester, VT, 2005.

E.N. Anderson, *The Food of China*, Yale University Press, New Haven, CT, 1988.

Earl Mindell & Virginia Hopkins, *Prescription Alternatives, Third Edition: Hundreds of Safe, Natural Prescription-Free Remedies to Restore and Maintain Your Health*, McGraw Hill, Random House, 2003.

Eilean Bentley, *Head, Neck and Shoulders Massage: A Step-by-Step*, St. Martins Press, New York, NY, 2000.

F. M. Houston, *The Healing Benefits of Acupressure: Acupuncture Without Needles*, Keats Pub, Lincolnwood, IL, 1993.

Frances Tappan & Patricia Benjamin, *Tappan's Handbook Of Healing Massage Techniques: Classic, Holistic, And Emerging Methods (3rd Edition)*, Prentice Hall, Saddle River, NJ, 1998.

Frank Navratil, *Bowen Therapy: Tom Bowen's Gift to the World*, Return to Health Books, 2003.

Frank Netter, *Atlas of Anatomy*, Rittenhouse Book Distributors Inc, King of Prussia, PA, 1997.

Fred Ferri, *Guide to the Care of Medical Patient, 4th Edition*, Mosby, St. Louis, MO, 1998.

Gary Null, *The Complete Encyclopedia of Natural Healing*, Kensington Books, New York, NY, 2005.

Gerald Tortura, *Principles of Human Anatomy*, John Wiley & Sons, Hoboken, NJ, 1999.

Giovanni Maciocia, *Diagnosis in Chinese Medicine, A Comprehensive Guide*, Churchill Livingstone, London, England, 2004.

Giovanni Maciocia, *Foundations of Chinesel Medicine*, Churchill Livingstone, London, England, 1989.

Giovanni Maciocia, *The Practice of Chinese Medicine*, Churchill Livingstone, London, England, 1994.

Hans Georg Brecklinghaus, *Balancing Your Body: A Self-Help Approach to Rolfing Movement*, Lebenshaus Verlag, 2002.

Harald Brust, *Art of Traditional Thai Massage*, Unknown, 1997.

Hazel Courtney, *500 of the Most Important Health Tips You'll Ever Need*, Cico Books, London, England, 2001.

Henry Lu, *Chinese System of Food Cures*, Sterling, New York, NY, 1986.

Howard Derek Evans, *A Myofascial Approach to Thai Massage: East meets West*, Churchill Livingstone, London, England, 2009.

Hugh Milne, *The Heart of Listening: A Visionary Approach to Craniosacral Work VOL. 1*, North Atlantic Books, Berkeley, CA, 1998.

Ida Rolf, *Rolfing: Reestablishing the Natural Alignment and Structural Integration of the Human Body for Vitality and Well-Being*, Healing Arts Press, Rochester, VT, 1989.

Ida Rolf, *Rolfing and Physical Reality*, Inner Traditions Intl Ltd, Rochester, VT, 1990.

Iona Marsaa Teeguarden, *Acupressure Way of Health: Jin Shin Do*, Japan Publications, Japan, 1978.

Jack Forem, *Healing with Pressure Point Therapy: Simple, Effective Techniques for Massaging Away More Than 100 Common Ailments*, Prentice Hall Press, Saddle River, NJ, 1999.

Jack W. Painter, *Technical Manual of Deep Wholistic Bodywork: Postural Integration*, Bodymind Books, 1987.

James Balch & Mark Stengler, *Prescription for Natural Cures: A Self-Care Guide for Treating Health Problems with Natural Remedies Including Diet and Nutrition, Nutritional Supplements, Bodywork, and More*, John Wiley & Sons, Hoboken, NJ, 2004.

James Clay & David Pounds, *Basic Clinical Massage Therapy: Integrating Anatomy and Treatment (2nd Edition)*, Lippincott Williams & Wilkins, Philadelphia, PA, 2003.

James J. Rybacki, *The Essential Guide to Prescription Drugs*, Harper Perennial, New York, NY, 2006.

Jinxue Li, *Chinese Manipulation and Massage: Chinese Manipulative Therapy*, Elsevier Science, London, England, 1990.

Joan Watt, *Massage for Sport*, Crowood Press, Marlborough, England, 1999.

John & Dan Bensky, *Acupuncture: A Comprehensive Text*, Eastland Press, Seattle, WA, 1981.

John E. Upledger, *Your Inner Physician and You: Craniosacral Therapy and Somatoemotional Release, 2nd Ed*, North Atlantic Books, Berkeley, CA, 1997.

John E. Upledger & Jon Vredevoogd, *Craniosacral Therapy*, Eastland Press, Seattle, WA, 1983.

John Hamwee & Fritz Smith, *Zero Balancing: Touching the Energy*, North Atlantic Books, Berkeley, CA, 2000.

John Sharkey, *The Concise Book of Neuromuscular Therapy: A Trigger Point Manual*, North Atlantic Books, Berkeley, CA, 2008.

Joseph Ashton & Duke Cassel, *Review for Therapeutic Massage and Bodywork Certification*, Lippincott Williams & Wilkins, Philadelphia, PA, 2006.

Joseph Heller & William Henkin, *Bodywise: An Introduction to Hellerwork for Regaining Flexibility and Well-Being*, North Atlantic Books, Berkeley, CA, 2004.

Julian Bakeer, *The Bowen Technique*, Human Kinetics, Champaign, IL, 2002.

Julian Kenyon M.D., *Acupressure Techniques: A Self-Help Guide*, Healing Arts Press, Rochester, VT, 1996.

Kalyani Pemkumar, *The Massage Connection: Anatomy and Physiology*, Lippincott Williams & Wilkins, Philadelphia, PA, 2003.

Kam Thye Chow, *Thai Yoga Massage: A Dynamic Therapy for Physical Well-Being and Spiritual Energy*, Healing Arts Press, Rochester, VT, 2004.

Kathleen Mahan and Sylvia Escott-Stump, *Krause's Food, Nutrition, & Diet Therapy, 10th Edition*, Saunders Company, New York, NY, 2000.

Kay Rynerson, *The Thai Massage Workbook*, Crow's Wing Studio, Seattle, WA, 2009.

Kay Sieg & Sandra Adams, *Illustrated Essentials of Musculoskeletal Anantomy*, Megabooks, Gainesville, FL, 1996.

Kurt Schnaubelt Ph.D., *Advanced Aromatherapy: The Science of Essential Oil Therapy*, Healing Arts Press, Rochester, VT, 1998.

Larry Trivieri & John Anderson, *Alternative Medicine: The Definitive Guide (2nd Edition)*, Celestial Arts, Berkeley, CA, 2002.

Lars Peterson & Per Renström, *Sports Injuries: Their Prevention and Treatment - 3rd Edition*, Human Kinetics, Champaign, IL, 2000.

Lawrence Jones, Randall Kusunose & Edward Goering, *Strain CounterStrain*, Jones Strain-CounterStrain, Inc, Carlsbad, CA, 1995.

Lawrence M. Tierney, *Current Medical Diagnosis & Treatment, 2006*, McGraw Hill, New York, NY, 2006.

Len Price & Shirley Price, *Aromatherapy for Health Professionals*, Churchill Livingstone, London, England, 2006.

Leon Chaitow, *Soft-Tissue Manipulation: A Practitioner's Guide to the Diagnosis and Treatment of Soft-Tissue Dysfunction and Reflex Activity*, Healing Arts Press, Rochester, VT, 1987.

Linda Page, *Healthy Healing: A Guide to Self-Healing for Everyone, 12th Edition*, Traditional Wisdom, Inc., New York, NY, 2004.

Linda Skidmore-Roth, *Mosby's Handbook of Herbs & Natural Supplements*, Mosby, St. Louis, MO, 2001.

Makana Risser Chai, *Na Mo'olelo Lomilomi: The Traditions of Hawaiian Massage and Healing*, Bishop Museum Press, Honolulu, HI, 2005.

Maneewan Chia; Max Chia, *Nuad Thai: Traditional Thai Massage*, Healing Tao Books, Los Angeles, CA, 2005.

Maoliang Qiu, *Chinese Acupuncture and Moxibustion*, Churchill Livingstone, London, England, 1993.

Maoshing Ni & Cathy NcNease, *The Tao of Nutrition*, College of Tao & Traditional Chinese Healing, Los Angeles, CA, 1987.

Maria Mercati, *The Handbook of Chinese Massage: Tui Na Techniques to Awaken Body and Mind*, Healing Arts Press, Rochester, VT, 1997.

Maria Mercati, *Thai Massage Manual: Natural Therapy for Flexibility, Relaxation, and Energy Balance*, Sterling, New York, NY, 2005.

Mark Beers & Robert Porter, *The Merck Manual (18th ed.)*, Merck & Co., Rahway, NJ, 2007.

Mark F. Beck, *Milady's Theory and Practice of Therapeutic Massage (3rd Edition)*, Delmar Publishers, Florence, KY, 1999.

Mel Cash, *Sport & Remedial Massage Therapy*, Ebury Press, London, England, 1996.

Melvyn R. Werbach, *Foundations of Nutritional Medicine*, Third Line Press, Tarzana, CA, 1997.

Melvyn R. Werbach, *Nutritional Influences on Mental Illness, Second Edition*, Third Line Press, Tarzana, CA, 1999.

Michael Foldi & Roman Strossenreuther, *Foundations of Manual Lymph Drainage (3rd Edition)*, Mosby, St. Louis, MO, 2004.

Michael Foldi & Roman Strossenreuther, *Foundations of Manual Lymph Drainage*, Mosby, St. Louis, MO, 2004.

Michael Murray & Joseph E. Pizzorno, *Encyclopedia of Natural Medicine*, Prima Publishing, Rocklin, CA, 1998.

Michael Murray & Joseph Pizzorno, *Encyclopedia of Natural Medicine, Revised Second Edition*, Three Rivers Press, New York, NY, 1997.

Michael Murray & Joseph Pizzorno, *Encyclopedia of Nutritional Supplements: The Essential Guide for Improving Your Health Naturally*, Three Rivers Press, New York, NY, 1996.

Michael Reed Gach, *Acupressure's Potent Points: a Guide to Self-Care for Common Ailments*, Bantam, New York, NY, 1990.

Michael Van Straten, *Organic Super Foods*, Octopus Publishing, London, England, 2003.

Nancy, S Kahalewai, *Hawaiian Lomilomi: Big Island Massage*, IM Publishing, 2005.

Nikita Vizniak, *Quick Reference Clinical Consultant Physical Assessment*, Professional Health Systems, Canada, 2006.

Pat Archer, *Therapeutic Massage in Athletics*, Lippincott Williams & Wilkins, Philadelphia, PA, 2006.

Patricia Benjamin & Scott Lamp, *Understanding Sports Massage*, Human Kinetics Pub, Champaign, IL, 1996.

Paul Blakey, *The Muscle Book*, Himalayan Institute Press, Honesdale, PA, 1992.

Paul Lundberg, *The Book of Shiatsu: A Complete Guide to Using Hand Pressure and Gentle Manipulation to Improve Your Health, Vitality and Stamina*, Fireside, 2003.

Paul Lundberg, *The New Book of Shiatsu: Vitality and Health Through the Art of Touch*, Gaia Books Ltd, London, England, 2005.

Paul Pitchford, *Healing with Whole Foods*, North Atlantic Books, Berkeley, CA, 2002.

Peter Deadmean & Mazin Al-Khafaji, *A Manual of Acupuncture*, Journal of Chinese Medicine Publications, East Sussex, England, 1998.

Phyllis Balch, *Prescription for Herbal Healing: An Easy-to-Use A-Z Reference to Hundreds of Common Disorders and Their Herbal Remedies*, Penguin Putnam, New York, NY, 2002.

Phyllis Balch, *Prescription for Nutritional Healing, 4th Edition: A Practical A-to-Z Reference to Drug-Free Remedies Using Vitamins, Minerals, Herbs & Food Supplements ... A-To-Z Reference to Drug-Free Remedies)*,, Penguin Putnam, New York, NY, 2004.

Phyllis Balch, *Prescription for Nutritional Healing: The A-to-Z Guide to Supplements: The A-to-Z Guide to Supplements*, Penguin Putnam, New York, NY, 2002.

R. Louis Schultz, Rosemary Feitis, Diana Salles & Ronald Thompson, *The Endless Web: Fascial Anatomy and Physical Reality*, North Atlantic Books, Berkeley, CA, 1996.

Rudolph Ballentine, *Radical Healing: Integrating the World's Great Therapeutic Traditions to Create a New Transformative Medicine*, Three Rivers Pr, Princeton, MN, 2000.

Ralph Golan, *Optimal Wellness*, Wellspring/ Ballantine, New York, NY, 1995.

Ramona Moody French, *Introduction to Lymph Drainage Massage*, Empire Pub, Desert Hot Springs, CA, 2001.

Ramona Moody French, *Milady's Guide to Lymph Drainage Massage*, Milady, Albany, NY, 2003.

Rene Cailliet, *Soft Tissue Pain and Disability (3rd Edition)*, F A Davis Co, Philadelphia, PA, 1996.

Roger Uren, John Thompson & Robert Howman-Giles, *Lymphatic Drainage of the Skin and Breast: Locating the Sentinel Nodes*, Harwood Academic Publisher, 1999.

Ron Kurtz, *Body-Centered Psychotherapy: The Hakomi Method: The Integrated Use of Mindfulness, Nonviolence and the Body*, Liferhythm, Medocino, CA, 1997.

Rosa LoSan & Suzanne LeVert, *Chinese Healing Foods*, Pocket Books, New York, NY, 1998.

Rosie Spiegel, *Bodies, Health and Consciousness: A Guide to Living Successfully in Your Body Through Rolfing and Yoga*, Srg Pub, 1994.

Ruth Werner, *A Massage Therapist's Guide to Pathology (Lww Massage Therapy & Bodywork*, Lippincott Williams & Wilkins, Philadelphia, PA, 2008.

Sandy Fritz, *Sports & Exercise Massage: Comprehensive Care in Athletics, Fitness, & Rehabilitation*, Mosby, St. Louis, MO, 2005.

Sarah Pritchard, *Chinese Massage Manual: The Healing Art of Tui Na*, Sterling, New York, NY, 1999.

Shen Guoquan & Yan Juntao, *Illustrations of Tuina Manipulations*, Shanghai Scientific & Technical Publisher, Shanghai, China, 2004.

Shizuto Masunaga, *Zen Shiatsu: How to Harmonize Yin and Yang for Better Health*, Japan Publications, Japan, 1977.

Simeno Niel-Asher, *The Concise Book of Trigger Points, Revised Edition*, North Atlantic Books, Berkeley, CA, 2006.

Stanley Hoppenfeld, *Physical Examination of the Spine Extremities*, Prentice Hall, Saddle River, NJ, 1976.

Steven Brantman & Andrea Girman, *Mosby's Handbook of Herbs and Supplements and Their Therapeutic Use*, Mosby, St. Louis, MO, 2003.

Sun Chengnan, *Chinese Bodywork: A Complete Manual of Chinese Therapeutic Massage*, Pacific View Press, Shanghai, China, 2000.

Sun Peilin, *The Treatment of Pain with Chinese Herbs and Acupuncture*, Churchill Livingstone, London, England, 2002.

Sun Shuchun, *Atlas of Therapeutic Motion for Treatment and Health: A Guide to Traditional Chinese Massage and Exercise Therapy*, Foreign Languages Press, Beijing, China, 1989.

Susan Salvo, *Massage Therapy: Principles and Practice*, Saunders Comapany, New York, NY, 2007.

Ted Kaptchuk, *The Web That Has No Weaver: Understanding Chinese Medicine*, McGraw-Hill, New York, NY, 2000.

Thomas Hendrickson, *Massage for Orthopedic Conditions*, Lippincott Williams & Wilkins, Philadelphia, PA, 2002.

Thomas W. Myers, *Anatomy Trains: Myofascial Meridians for Manual and Movement Therapists (2nd Edition)*, Churchill Livingstone, London, England, 2008.

Tom Valentine & Carole Valentine, *Applied Kinesiology: Muscle Response in Diagnosis, Therapy and Preventive Medicine*, Amer Intl Distribution Corp, 1989.

Toru Namikoshi, *The Complete Book of Shiatsu Therapy*, Japan Publications, Japan, 2001.

Vance Ferrell & Edgar Archbold, *Natural Remedies Encyclopedia*, Harvestime Books, Altamount, TN, 2002.

Wang Fu, *Chinese Tuina Therapy*, Foreign Languages Press, Beijing, China, 1994.

Wataru Ohashi, *Reading the Body: Ohashi's Book of Oriental Diagnosis*, Penguin, New York, NY, 1991.

William N. Brown, *The Touch that Heals, The Art of Lymphatic Massage*, Self-published, 2008.

William Weintraub, *Tendon and Ligament Healing: A New Approach Through Manual Therapy*, North Atlantic Books, Berkeley, CA, 1999.

Winter Griffith and Stephen Moore, *Complete Guide to Prescription and Nonprescription Drugs 2007 (Complete Guide to Prescription and Nonprescription Drugs)*, Harper Collins, New York, NY, 2007.

Wolfgang Luckmann, *Lomi Lomi Hawaiian Therapeutic Massage Deep Tissue*, Self-published.

Xu Xiangcai, *Chinese Tui Na Massage: The Essential Guide to Treating Injuries, Improving Health & Balancing Qi*, YMAA Publication Center, Jamaica Plains, MA, 2002.

Tell the Editors

The information is constantly evolving. We view MDR similar to a clearing house of information for the massage community. Our research and editorial team analyzes information periodically. If you spot information that needs to be changed or updated, you can use this form, or a copy of it, to communicate directly with the editors. You can email or snail-mail the information. We appreciate your help!

We are constantly looking for feedback to improve future versions of Massage Desk Reference.

1. What part of MDR are you commenting about?	Page Number
2. What wording should be added?	
(Please be specific about exact wording that you propose adding)	
3. What wording should be deleted?	
4. What reference citations support this change?	
(Please give us specific reference citations). We base on reliable studies published in peer-reviewed professional literature. Please give us enough information so that we can find the reference.	
5. What would you like to see in future versions of MDR?	

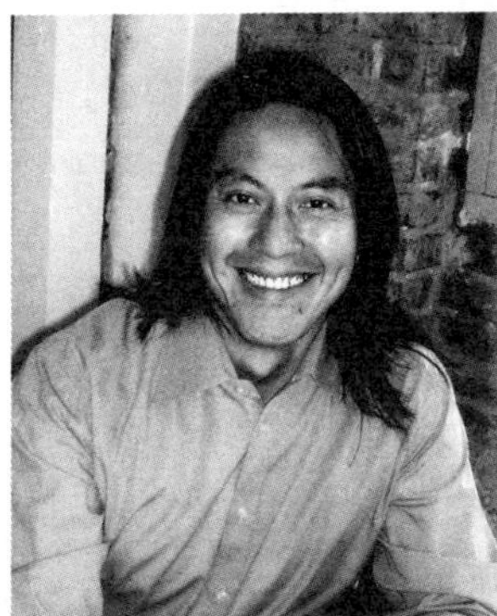

David J. Kuoch, (D.J.) L.Ac.

About the author

David J Kuoch, LAc, (D.J.). began his early training in China. He is a graduate of UCLA as well as a graduate of Emperors College of Traditional Chinese Medicine. David was a student of bodywork at the Massage School of Santa Monica and the Esalen Institute. He was an acupuncture fellow and received tuina training under Dr. Wei Guikang at Guang Xi Traditional Chinese Medical University in Nanning, China in the department of Orthopaedics and Integrative Medicine. Soon after finishing his training, he received advanced hospital training in the Acupuncture and Internal Medicine Departments at Guangzhou Chinese Traditional Medicine in Guangzhou, China. He studied Traditional Thai Massage in Chiang mai Thailand. He is a licensed acupuncturist with a practice in San Francisco, CA specializing in pain management and orthopaedic acupuncture. DJ's work is derived from his passion for the promotion of acupuncture, massage and clinical excellence. When he is not actively involved in clinical practice or writing, he enjoys, yoga, hiking, classic car restoration, riding vintage Ducati's & Moto Guzzi's, NPR, Bruins basketball, running, Chinese food, independent films, and great San Francisco coffee.

To acquire knowledge, one must study;
but to acquire wisdom, one must observe.
~ Marilyn vos Savant

ORDER FORM

MASSAGE DESK REFERENCE

David J Kuoch

Please Print Clearly

Name ....
Address..
City, State, Zip..
Phone...

Books	Quantity	Price	Total
(Massage Desk Reference)		*29.95*	
(Acupuncture Desk Reference V1)		*44.95*	
(Acupuncture Desk Reference V2)		*34.95*	
Subtotal			
California Residents, add 8.25% sales tax			
Shipping & Handling		*5.00*	
Total			$

Make checks or money order or purchase orders payable to **Acumedwest.** We do accept credit cards, however credit cards payments are available through paypal. Visit us at www.massagedeskreference.com to order your copy today.

Please call for wholesale pricing or institutional orders. Massage/bodywork instructor evaluation copies are available upon request for massage course preparation.

Acumedwest Inc.
P.O. Box 14068
San Francisco, CA 94114
(310) 395-9573 Phone
(415) 875-9640 Fax

www.massagedeskreference.com
Email: mdrguide@yahoo.com

Other bestselling books for health-care providers from Acumedwest. Complete clinical guides for herbalist, TCM practitioners and acupuncturist.

Acupuncture Desk Reference
978-0-615-15463-3
by David Kuoch
$44.95 (spiral-bound)

Acupuncture Desk Reference Volume 2
978-0-9815631-1-4
by David Kuoch
$34.95 (spiral-bound)

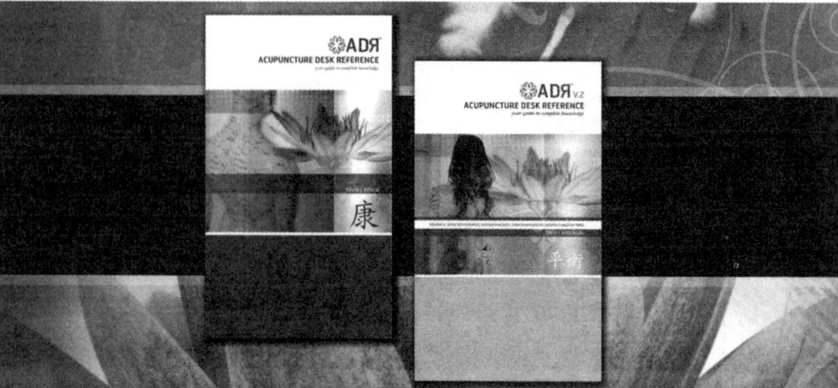

NOTES

NOTES